Hirsch and Brenner's Atlas of EEG in Critical Care

Hirsch and Brenner's Atlas of EEG in Critical Care

Second Edition Edited by

Lawrence J. Hirsch, MD

Professor of Neurology
Chief, Division of Epilepsy and EEG
Co-Director, Comprehensive Epilepsy Center and Continuous EEG Monitoring Program
Yale University School of Medicine
New Haven, CT, USA

Michael W.K. Fong, MBBS

Neurologist and Epileptologist
Westmead Comprehensive Epilepsy Unit, Westmead Hospital
Westmead Clinical School, The University of Sydney
Sydney, NSW, Australia

Richard P. Brenner, MD

Professor of Neurology and Psychiatry (retired)
Director, EEG Laboratories
University of Pittsburgh
Pittsburgh, PA, USA

WILEY Blackwell

This second edition first published 2023
© 2023 John Wiley & Sons Ltd

Edition History
John Wiley & Sons Ltd (1e, 2010)

Registered Office
John Wiley & Sons Ltd, The Atrium, Southern Gate, Chichester, West Sussex, PO19 8SQ, UK

Editorial Office
9600 Garsington Road, Oxford, OX4 2DQ, UK

For details of our global editorial offices, customer services, and more information about Wiley products visit us at www.wiley.com.

Wiley also publishes its books in a variety of electronic formats and by print-on-demand. Some content that appears in standard print versions of this book may not be available in other formats.

Library of Congress Cataloging-in-Publication Data

Names: Hirsch, Lawrence J. author. | Fong, Michael W.K. (Michael Wang
    Keong), 1985- author. | Brenner, Richard P., author.
Title: Hirsch and Brenner's atlas of EEG in critical care / Lawrence J.
    Hirsch, Michael W.K. Fong, Richard P. Brenner.
Other titles: Atlas of EEG in critical care
Description: Second edition. | Hoboken, NJ : Wiley-Blackwell, 2023. |
    Preceded by Atlas of EEG in critical care / Lawrence J. Hirsch, Richard
    P. Brenner. c2010. | Includes bibliographical references and index.
Identifiers: LCCN 2022019908 (print) | LCCN 2022019909 (ebook) | ISBN
    9781118752890 (cloth) | ISBN 9781118752876 (adobe pdf) | ISBN
    9781118752869 (epub)
Subjects: MESH: Electroencephalography – methods | Critical Care | Atlas
Classification: LCC RC386.6.E43 (print) | LCC RC386.6.E43 (ebook) | NLM
    WL 17 | DDC 616.8/047547 – dc23/eng/20220624
LC record available at https://lccn.loc.gov/2022019908
LC ebook record available at https://lccn.loc.gov/2022019909

Cover image: Courtesy of Lawrence J. Hirsch, Michael W.K. Fong and Richard P. Brenner
Cover design by Wiley

Set in 11/14pt TimesLTStd by Straive, Chennai, India
Printed and bound by CPI Group (UK) Ltd, Croydon, CR0 4YY
C9781118752890_061224

Dr. Hirsch dedicates this atlas to his wife Gaetane; his two sons, Calvin and Toby; and Dr. Brenner for teaching him how entertaining EEG reading and teaching could be, and for putting up with his very long delay in completing this edition.

Dr. Fong dedicates this atlas to his loving wife Katherine and his beautiful daughter, Imogen.

Dr. Brenner dedicates this atlas to his wife Elizabeth.

All authors thank their families for putting up with the many hours of work, including at odd hours, required to complete this.

Contents

Preface

The utilization of continuous EEG (cEEG) in critically ill patients has markedly expanded since the first edition of this atlas just over a decade ago. Multicenter collaborative efforts have determined that increases in seizure burden (including nonconvulsive seizures) are independent predictors of worse outcome in many different types of patients, as measured in many ways, including long-term functional outcome, cognition and later epilepsy. These efforts have also shown that even highly epileptiform patterns that do not qualify as seizures are sometimes sufficient to cause progressive neuronal injury, especially in the setting of an acute brain insult. For the vast majority of patients there is little clinical suggestion at the bedside that these patterns or seizures are present (other than impaired alertness), and thus cEEG has a crucial role in patient care. Centers have responded by incorporating new technology and designing highly specialized neuro-intensive care units with the capacity to record EEG at any time of the day, to detect seizures or potentially injurious EEG patterns, and rapidly feed this information back to treating clinicians to best inform management decisions. Continuous EEG has since become a routine part of caring for critically ill patients in many institutions around the world. As a result, neurologists and intensivists need to become familiar with the use of routine brain monitoring with EEG, or 'neurotelemetry', as they have with routine cardiovascular monitoring.

The atlas begins with a section on the basics of EEG interpretation geared towards someone with minimal if any EEG experience (Chapters 1–2). The atlas follows with chapters on: EEG patterns seen in encephalopathy and coma – both nonspecific and specific (Chapter 3); focal abnormalities (Chapter 4); rhythmic and periodic patterns (RPPs), including detailed explanation of the recent American Clinical Neurophysiology Society (ACNS) standardized critical care EEG terminology guideline that was extensively updated in 2021 (Chapter 5); seizures and status epilepticus, including new definitions of electrographic and electroclinical seizures/status epilepticus (Chapter 6), and controversial patterns such as those on the ictal-interictal continuum (now defined); confusing artifacts, including ones that are often misinterpreted or that mimic seizures (Chapter 7); and patterns that are commonly seen post cardiac arrest (Chapter 8).

After the above sections on raw EEG patterns from both a basic and advanced viewpoint, there is an extensive color section on prolonged continuous digital EEG monitoring, including quantitative EEG techniques to assist with interpretation of prolonged recordings (Chapters 9–10). These techniques can aid in efficient recognition of seizures, ischemia and other neurological events, and can help visualize long-term trends. This chapter also contains examples of multimodal brain monitoring in the neurocritical care setting.

Throughout the atlas, EEG findings are highlighted and labeled in detail within the tracings themselves. Each chapter begins with a short section of text and a list of the most important references as suggested reading. In general, the chapters progress from very basic material at the start of the chapter to more advanced. An appendix summarizing the 2021 ACNS terminology is included as well. There is an extensive index as well to help the reader rapidly find what they need.

Who should use this atlas?

This atlas is geared towards all health care professionals involved in critical care medicine, including all clinicians, fellows, residents, EEG technologists and researchers. Although it may be of particular interest to those in neurology, epilepsy and clinical neurophysiology, it is also appropriate for intensivists with an interest in maintaining brain health during critical illness of any etiology. It covers the basics as well as advanced material.

What's new in this edition?

As the volume and variety of patients undergoing cEEG has increased, new patterns of significance have been observed and defined. As a result, the ACNS standardized critical care EEG terminology underwent a major update in 2021. The definition of many of these patterns was established and the definitions of prior patterns refined when necessary. This atlas contains real-world examples of all the terms, past and newly introduced, included in the ACNS terminology. There are extensive new examples of EEGs in all chapters, and the EEGs that were already in the prior version are now re-labeled with the 2021 terminology.

In addition to new electrographic patterns, there have also been new conditions and toxicities since the prior edition. COVID-19-related encephalopathy, anti-checkpoint inhibitor encephalopathy and specific medication effects such as ketamine are all included. New technologies have allowed for rapid-response EEG and examples of using a limited montage as part of a very rapid EEG to triage patients is discussed.

An approach to tackling the cEEG has been introduced, complete with illustrative diagrams to help the reader understand the difference between terms. Quantitative EEG has also progressed drastically since the last edition, and some of these tools are introduced in the QEEG chapter.

Due to the need for expansion of several of the chapters, especially the quantitative EEG ones, and in order to keep the atlas at a reasonable size, we have removed the chapter on evoked potentials.

Lawrence J. Hirsch, MD, Michael W.K. Fong, MBBS
Richard P. Brenner, MD

Acknowledgments

Dr. Hirsch would like to thank those who have helped develop and maintain the continuous EEG monitoring program, both clinical and research aspects, at Yale Comprehensive Epilepsy Center for the past decade, including all the epilepsy/EEG attendings and technologists, with special thanks to Rebecca Khozein and the Yale Epilepsy/EEG/ICU EEG fellows.

Dr. Fong would like to thank all the neurologists, nurses, EEG technologists, epilepsy fellows and neurology advanced trainees involved at the Westmead Health Precinct and the University of Sydney. Special thanks to Andrew F. Bleasel, Chong H. Wong and Melissa Bartley. Their past,

present and future support of this work and many other clinical and research endeavors is greatly valued. Thanks in particular to Markus M. Leitinger for his dedication in generating many of the illustrative diagrams that have helped foster the understanding of critical care EEG across the world.

Dr. Brenner would like to thank those neurologists, EEG technologists, neurophysiology fellows and neurology residents, at the University of Pittsburgh Medical Center, who have helped over many years in this endeavor. Special thanks to Drs. Mark L. Scheuer and Anne C. Van Cott and EEG technologists Susan Burkett and Cheryl Plummer.

1 EEG basics

1.1 Electrode nomenclature, polarity and montages

Electroencephalography is a technique that measures the spatial distribution of voltage fields on the scalp and their variation over time. The origin of this activity is thought to be due to the fluctuating sum of the excitatory postsynaptic potentials and inhibitory postsynaptic potentials. These potentials arise primarily from the apical dendrites of pyramidal cells in the outer (superficial) layer of the cerebral cortex and are modified by input from subcortical structures, particularly the thalamus and ascending projections of the ascending reticular activating system. Structures in the thalamus serve as a 'pacemaker'. This produces widespread synchronization and rhythmicity of cortical activity over the cerebral hemispheres.

When dendritic generators are aligned, they form a dipole. Dipoles are sources of electrical current consisting of two charges of opposite polarity (one positive [current source], and one negative [current sink]), separated by relatively small distances. The easiest way to conceptualize a dipole is by considering the example of a battery; there is one positive end and one negative end that allows current to flow if the ends are connected. In the cortex these dipoles are mostly radially oriented, which means that they are aligned in a way that projects one end of the dipole towards the scalp, and hence can be recorded with EEG. In general, approximately $10\,cm^2$ of cortex needs to be discharging synchronously for the signal to be appreciated on scalp EEG.

The hardware necessary to record the EEG employs differential amplifiers. Each amplifier records the potential difference between two scalp electrodes (the electrode pair is referred to as a derivation or channel). Each amplifier has two inputs connected to scalp electrodes. By convention, when input 1 (historically referred to as grid 1, or G1) is relatively negative compared to input 2 (grid 2, or G2) there is an upward deflection; when input 1 is relatively more positive than input 2 there is a downward deflection. It is the relationship between the two inputs that determines the direction and amplitude, not the absolute values. Simply put, the tracing at each channel (derivation) displays G1 minus G2, with negative values causing upward deflections. Listed below are some examples to help further demonstrate these principles.

TABLE 1.1 **Polarity**

Channel	Input 1	Input 2	Difference	Deflection direction
A	+50	+10	+40	Down
B	+50	+50	0	—
C	+50	+70	−20	Up
D	+50	−50	+100	Down

In the following four examples inputs 1 and 2 have been switched. i.e., channel E is the same as channel A in Table 1.1 with input 1 and input 2 switched and the resultant differences shown.

Hirsch and Brenner's Atlas of EEG in Critical Care, Second Edition. Lawrence J. Hirsch, Michael W.K. Fong, and Richard P. Brenner.
© 2023 John Wiley & Sons Ltd. Published 2023 by John Wiley & Sons Ltd.

TABLE 1.2 **Polarity**

Channel	Input 1	Input 2	Difference	Deflection direction
E	+10	+50	−40	Up
F	+50	+50	0	—
G	+70	+50	+20	Down
H	−50	+50	−100	Up

The EEG is the graphical representation of these differences over time. If taking the timepoint that the above tables were generated, a graphical presentation of this data can be constructed (Figure 1.1).

As can be seen from the above examples, there are no true 'positive' or 'negative' deflections; there are only upward or downward deflections. When there is no deflection, the inputs are equipotential and are either equally active or inactive. For example, taking channel B, if both the inputs were made −50 µV (as opposed to +50 µV) there would still be no resultant deflection as there would remain no difference between input 1 and 2.

When looking at only a single derivation (a one-channel recording of the potential difference between an electrode pair) one can only state the relationship of input 1 to input 2, i.e., it is either more or less negative or positive. However, it is not possible to localize cerebral activity or determine its polarity without further derivations/channels. Understanding polarity, as well as accurately assessing other factors such as the frequency of the activity being evaluated (cycles/second), its morphology, location, voltage, reactivity and symmetry in conjunction with the age and state of the patient, is necessary for proper interpretation of the EEG. In order to adequately represent the topography of the voltage, additional amplifiers and channels are needed for the sequential display of the EEG data, and this display of multiple channels is termed a *montage*. A montage refers to a collection of derivations for multiple channels recorded simultaneously and arranged in a specific order. Montages enable the technologist and electroencephalographer to systematically visualize the field of electrical activity of the brain.

Electrodes are applied to the scalp in accordance with the International 10-20 System. Different regions of the brain are identified as Fp (frontopolar),

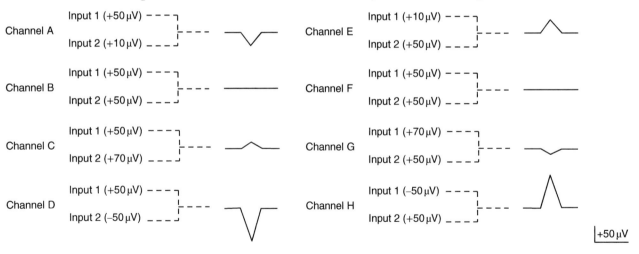

Figure 1.1. Schematic representation of channel inputs. The figure demonstrates how the pen deflections would appear if the voltage inputs from Tables 1.1 and 1.2 were put into an EEG machine. Channels A-D show the resultant inputs from Table 1.1, whereas channels E-H show the deflections if input 1 and input 2 were 'flipped' for each channel, as shown in Table 1.2. The figure exemplifies that if the relative polarity between input 1 and input 2 is flipped from positive to negative, then the resultant waveform is flipped. However, if there is the same relative difference between the two input voltages the height or amplitude of the deflection remains unchanged.

F (frontal), C (central), P (parietal), O (occipital) and T (temporal). Odd numbers refer to the left side, even to the right and z to midline placements. 'A' signifies an ear channel (A1 for left ear, A2 for right). Electrode placement has been standardized with this system, with electrode sites determined by anatomical skull landmarks. Technologists measure the distance from the nasion to the inion and the head circumference, marking precise electrode locations based on 10 or 20% intervals of those distances: hence the name '10-20'. For completeness' sake, a diagram depicting the 10-10 system has been included, this spaces electrodes in 10% intervals from each other (Figure 1.2). The 10-10 system and the 10-20 system use the same electrode labels, just not all electrodes of the 10-10 system are included in the 10-20 system for practical purposes.

Montages may be viewed as software that enhances the use of the EEG machine (hardware) to function as a form of brain imaging. There are two basic types of montages – bipolar and referential. A referential montage compares each individual electrode potential to the potential of a user determined 'referential point'. For this, input 1 (G1) is the electrode position and input 2 (G2) is always the selected referential point. Common referential points include the ear(s), the vertex (Cz) or an average of all electrodes (termed a 'common average reference'). With a bipolar sequential recording, scalp electrodes are linked in straight lines (either anterior-posterior or transverse), and each channel records the difference in potential between electrode pairs.

An analogy that assists with understanding the concept of referential and bipolar montages is to consider a series of buoys floating on waves of the ocean. A bipolar montage is analogous to comparing the relative height of each buoy to that immediately neighboring it. A referential montage is like measuring the absolute height (or altitude) of each buoy in relation to a determined referential point (for example the seabed). This analogy assists with understanding the strengths and weaknesses of the two montage types. A bipolar montage eliminates the signal that is common between two points. This means that when considering a small wave in a deep ocean, the bipolar recording is very sensitive at detecting small differences in height (or potential). The bipolar montage, however, tells you nothing about the depth of the ocean or the actual altitude of the two buoys, merely the height of the small wave. Conversely, a referential montage provides information of the absolute height/altitude (absolute potential) of a waveform.

Consider Figure 1.3, which demonstrates a series of four buoys spaced at equal (predetermined) distances from each other. The height of each buoy measured from a referential point (in this case the seabed) has been provided in units for each buoy. These inputs can be entered into an EEG machine that would generate a series of deflections that cumulatively make up a montage. The resultant deflections for a bipolar and referential montage are shown in Figure 1.4.

There are several points that should be highlighted:

(1) The waveform being measured has not changed in any way when the montage has been changed. The only thing that has changed is how the information from that waveform has been visually displayed.

(2) The reproduction of a wave is limited by the number of sampling points, in this case buoys. The buoys at position 2 and 3 have the same depth (7 units). However, as can be seen by the depiction, neither buoy (despite both having the greatest number of units) sits at the crest of the wave. If two sequential buoys have the same number of units, they could both be positioned at the crest of a very broad wave, but it is possible (as in this case) they both sit an equal difference from the true crest of the wave. It is useful to remember this concept when 'localizing' based on surface EEG. There will always be some spatial limitation. Some of this can be overcome by adding more sampling points. In the case of the buoys, doubling the number buoys would increase the chances that a buoy is positioned at the true crest. In EEG a greater number of electrodes can be applied, for example a 10-10 montage where an electrode is placed every 10% rather than 20% of head measurement, or even a high-density array consisting of 256 or 512 channels. Although this would provide greater spatial resolution it comes at a practical cost.

(3) The vertical scale units of the referential montage are double that of the bipolar; because bipolar montages compare neighboring electrodes, they reject all of the activity that is common between these two points. This means that even very small differences can be more easily

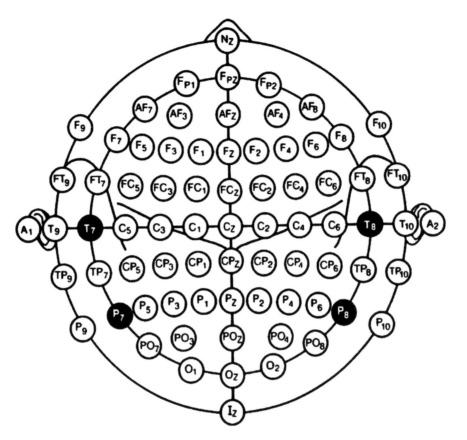

Figure 1.2. International 10-10 system for electrode placement. The figure depicts the standardized international 10-10 system for electrode placement. This system places electrodes at pre-defined positions of the head, relative to the patient's own head measurements (so the positions remain relatively constant between patients, irrespective of head size). In the anterior-posterior (front to back) direction a measurement is taken from the nasion to the inion. This distance forms 100% of a patient's A-P head dimension, and so 10% represents 1/10th of this distance. In the transverse or coronal plane (side to side, or left to right) measurement is taken from the tragus of one ear, across the top of the head, to the tragus of the other ear (tragus to tragus). This distance forms 100% of the head dimensions in the transverse plane. Cz is situated at the approximate vertex (more specifically the intersection between 50% of the nasion-inion distance and 50% of the tragus-tragus distance). Electrodes are then spaced at 10% intervals, so FCz is 10% of the AP distance in front of Cz, and C2 is 10% of the tragus-tragus distance to the right of Cz. All electrodes on the right are assigned even numbers, and all electrodes on the left are assigned odd numbers, with electrodes in the midline allocated a z (for zero). By this nomenclature FC2 is 10% A-P distance in front of Cz, and 10% the tragus-tragus distance to the right. The 10-10 system is presented mostly for reference, with most 'standard' EEG using the modified 10-20 system. This system uses the same electrode naming nomenclature, but mostly only utilizes the electrodes spaced at 20% intervals. Doing so provides a compromise between adequate scalp coverage and the practical application of recording electrodes. The EEG in this book is for the most part recorded using a 10-20 system. The electrodes in bold are those with an historical alternate name (i.e., T7 previously referred to as T3, P7 as T5, T8 as T4 and P8 as T6); these names are still used in some centers.

Reproduced from Acharya JN et al. American Clinical Neurophysiology Society Guideline 2: Guidelines for Standard Electrode Position Nomenclature. J Clin Neurophysiol. 2016;33(4):308–311 with permission.

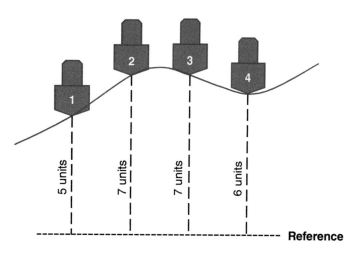

Figure 1.3. Analogy depicting the crest of a wave. In order to conceptually appreciate the difference between bipolar and referential montages, the figure presents an analogy of buoys floating on the surface of an ocean. The waves of an ocean form multiple crests and troughs and this is depicted by the wavy line. Four buoys (numbered 1–4) have been placed at equal distances from each other (similar to how EEG electrodes are placed at predetermined points mostly equidistant from their neighboring electrode). Each buoy has been assigned an arbitrary 'height' or unit (that correlates to amplitude/voltage in EEG). There are two ways of gaining information about the wave.

(1) Compare each buoys height to that of its neighboring buoy (1 compared to 2, 2 compared to 3, etc.). This is equivalent to a bipolar montage.

(2) Compare each buoys height to a set point (reference point) (1 compared to reference, 2 compared to reference, etc.). In this case the reference point has been set as the seabed, but as for the case of any referential montage the set point can be any point determined by the user.

detected, which can be harder to appreciate in a referential montage. The example is the 1-unit difference between buoy 3 and 4. Channel C of the bipolar montage easily shows this difference with a 1-unit deflection, however, to gain this information from the referential montage one would have to compare the height of channel C and D (often done visually).

The above analogy depicts the crest (maximal positivity) of a wave. However, in many cases the activity of interest is oriented so that the resultant radial dipole projects its negative end towards the scalp, therefore in EEG the maximal negativity (trough of a wave) is often the most of interest. This can be conceptualized by flipping the analogy of the waveform on its head

(Figure 1.5). When this information is inputted to a bipolar and referential montage, the result has been shown in Figure 1.6.

These figures highlight the advantages and disadvantages of bipolar vs. referential montages. The bipolar montage is very sensitive for detecting the location of maximal activity, with the deflections of a montage either pointing toward the region of maximal negativity ('negative phase reversal') or away from the region of maximal positivity ('positive phase reversal'). However, the resultant deflections of a referential montage more closely represent the shape (or field) of the waveform being measured, which makes it easier to conceptualize its distribution and potential brain regions involved. Bipolar and referential montages are not used in isolation and should be considered complementary ways of viewing information to (1) detect abnormality,

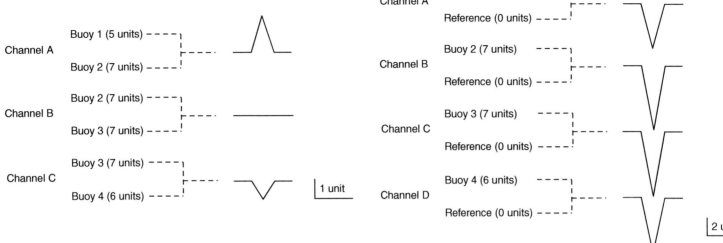

Figure 1.4. Bipolar vs. referential representation of a crest or maximal positivity. The information gained from Figure 1.3 can be represented in bipolar and referential formats/montages. A bipolar montage is shown on the left and referential on the right.

Bipolar montage: each channel of a bipolar montage represents a pair of neighboring buoys. Channel A, input 1 is the height (or altitude) of buoy 1 and input 2 is the height of buoy 2. The resultant deflection for each channel is given by subtracting input 2 from input 1 (5 units − 7 units = −2 units). The resultant deflection is therefore −2 units, which by convention is an upward deflection of 2 units height. Channel B then consists of input 1 (buoy 2 [which was previously input 2 of the prior channel]) and input 2 (buoy 3). In this case buoy 2 (7 units) minus buoy 3 (also 7 units) results in zero, so there is no deflection for that channel; and so on.

Referential montage: each channel of a referential montage represents that buoy compared to a set/referential point. Taking the referential point as zero units: Channel A, input 1 height of buoy 1 (5 units) and input 2 height of the reference point (zero units). Therefore, the deflection of channel A will be positive 5 units (5 units − 0 units = 5 units), which by convention is a downward deflection of 5 units height. Channel B then carries no information about buoy 1, instead channel B is input 1 (buoy 2) compared to input 2 (same referential point), which equates to 7 units minus 0 units, resulting in a positive 7-unit deflection (i.e., a downward deflection of 7 units), and so on.

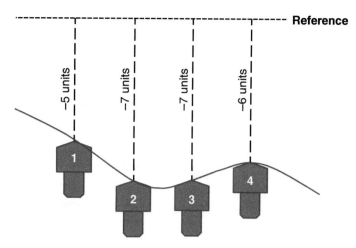

Figure 1.5. Inverse wave analogy. In order to highlight the bipolar and referential depiction of a trough of a wave, the analogy in Figure 1.3 has been inverted (flipped on its head). Here the previous crest of the wave (maximal positivity) now appears as a trough (maximal negativity). Considering these would be theoretically below the seabed the assigned values have become negative.

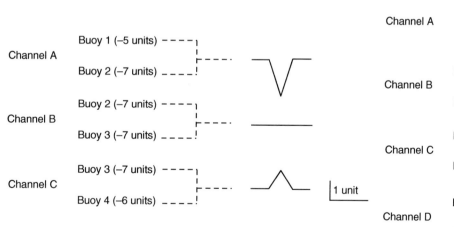

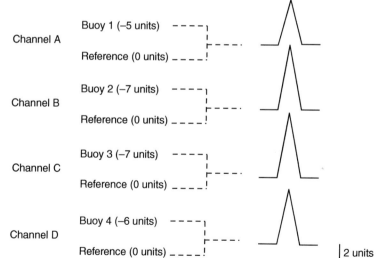

Figure 1.6. Bipolar vs. referential representation of a trough or maximal negativity. The bipolar representation is again shown on the left and referential on the right.

Bipolar montage: considering the reformatted analogy, Channel A, input 1 (buoy 1) is now −5 units and input 2 (buoy 2) is −7 units. Channel A is therefore −5 units − −7 units (with the double negative being equivalent of a +), this results in −5 units + 7 units = +2 units. Hence the 2 unit positive or downward deflection in channel A.

Referential montage: with input 1 of each channel being negative and each compared to input 2, which is zero, the resultant deflections of all channels of the referential montage are negative (upgoing).

(2) identify the region/s most affected, and (3) conceptualize the volume of parenchyma involved.

Listed below are some advantages and disadvantages of each type of recording.

Short distance bipolar recording

Advantages

(1) Value of phase reversal in localization – particularly when this occurs at the same electrode in two montages run at right angles to each other. Phase reversal in a sequential bipolar montage refers to the opposite simultaneous deflection of pens in the channels that contain a common electrode. It is important to realize that a phase reversal does not imply normality or abnormality. This instrumental phase reversal usually, but not always, indicates that the potential field is maximal at or near the common electrode. To be certain that one has accurately defined the site of maximal involvement it is necessary to use an additional bipolar montage at right angles to the first, or a referential recording.

(2) Bipolar montages will usually display local abnormalities well since a phase reversal is often present. The exception occurs when the discharge is maximal at either the beginning or end of the sequential chain and there is no phase reversal.

(3) Can help resolve ambiguous findings on referential montages due to an active reference.

Disadvantages

(1) Amplitudes can be misleading; in any given channel higher amplitude indicates a greater potential difference, not necessarily the most active site, while low amplitude could be due to the two electrodes being equally active and canceling, or to both electrodes being inactive. A flat line in a bipolar pair of electrodes does not mean those channels are not involved, it infers they are equally involved.

(2) Diffuse potentials with relatively flat gradients are not detected well.

(3) Waveforms and frequencies may be distorted.

Referential recording

Advantages

(1) Amplitude can be used to localize site of maximal involvement if the reference is inactive. With referential recordings, when the reference is inactive (or is the least active electrode), the site of maximal involvement is identified as the one having the greatest voltage (i.e., greatest amplitude of deflection).

(2) Little distortion of frequency or waveforms.

(3) Diffuse patterns with flat gradients can be detected. In contrast to focal abnormalities, diffuse discharges are frequently better appreciated on referential montages, particularly when there is a flat gradient.

(4) Can help resolve difficulties in bipolar recordings due to equipotential areas, horizontal dipoles or unevenly sloping gradients.

Disadvantages

(1) The reference electrode may not be inactive or the least active electrode – it may be very active. When the reference electrode is active, because it is located near the peak of the potential being studied, interpretation can be more difficult. A major problem with the use of referential montages is that it is often difficult to use an inactive reference or to realize that the reference is active.

A reference may be active because of artifact, or it may be within the cerebral field under study. With an active reference there often appears to be a 'phase reversal' on a referential montage, i.e., some electrodes are more negative than the reference, while others are more positive. One has to look at relative polarity, as well as amplitude, to decide which is the most active site. For those electrodes that are more active than the reference, the greatest amplitude indicates the site of maximal involvement. In contrast, for sites less active than the reference, the largest amplitude indicates the least active area. The deflection of the maximal and minimal sites will be in opposite directions. When the reference is the most active site the deflections in all channels are in the same direction i.e., there is no phase reversal. Furthermore, the largest amplitudes occur at those sites which are the least active. This type of situation can be confusing since one cannot be sure if the reference is uninvolved or is the most active of all scalp electrodes.

(2) Greater problem with artifact – depending on the reference employed. No single reference electrode is ideal for all situations. The ear electrodes frequently are contaminated by temporal lobe spikes as well as EKG and/or muscle artifact. The Cz electrode, which is often a very good choice in helping to display focal temporal abnormalities, has the least muscle artifact but is very active during sleep. Other midline reference electrodes, such as Fz or Pz, also have limitations: during wakefulness Fz is in the field of vertical eye movements, while Pz may be in the field of the posterior dominant 'alpha' rhythm; thus, these references are often active.

The American Clinical Neurophysiology Society (ACNS) published suggestions for standard montages to be used in clinical electroencephalography. The suggested montages include:

(1) longitudinal bipolar (LB) montages

(2) transverse bipolar (TB) montages

(3) referential (R) montages (such as ipsilateral ear, or Cz reference).

The montages listed are not intended for some purposes, such as neonatal EEG, all-night sleep recordings or for verification of electrocerebral inactivity. Additional guidelines for these specific indications can also be found at www.acns.org/practice/guidelines.

1.2 Normal EEG: awake and asleep

EEGs can be performed on patients of all ages, including neonates. There are marked maturational changes that occur in infancy and early childhood, while in adults, between the ages of 20–60 years, the EEG is relatively stable. Further fairly subtle changes occur in the elderly. Thus, in different age groups different patterns characterize wakefulness, drowsiness and sleep.

The normal adult EEG contains a number of different background rhythms and frequencies. These include alpha, beta, delta, mu, theta and normal sleep activity, such as vertex waves (V waves), spindles, K-complexes and positive occipital sharp transients of sleep (POSTS). EEG activity is conventionally divided into the following frequencies (number of waveforms/second, or hertz [Hz]):

Delta – refers to frequencies under 4 Hz (and ≥0.1 Hz). Delta activity, which is the slowest of the standard waveforms, is normal when present in adults during sleep. In asymptomatic elderly subjects, delta activity is sometimes seen intermittently in the temporal regions during wakefulness, and in a generalized distribution, maximal anteriorly, during drowsiness. It is usually abnormal under other circumstances.

Theta – ranges from 4 Hz to under 8 Hz. It is often present diffusely in young children during wakefulness, whereas in adults it occurs predominantly during drowsiness. Like delta activity, theta activity may occur in the temporal regions in asymptomatic elderly adults during wakefulness.

Alpha – ranges from 8–13 Hz, inclusive.

Beta – ranges from >13 Hz to under 30 Hz. This activity is usually low voltage, most prominent anteriorly, and often increased during drowsiness and in patients receiving sedating medication, particularly barbiturates or benzodiazepines.

In the analysis of the EEG the following need to be evaluated:

(1) frequency

(2) voltage

(3) location

(4) morphology

(5) polarity

(6) state

(7) reactivity

(8) symmetry

(9) artifact.

An important feature of the normal awake EEG is the frequency of the *alpha rhythm*, also known as the *posterior dominant rhythm*. During wakefulness, the alpha rhythm is present over the posterior regions of the head, maximal with the subject relaxed and eyes closed. It attenuates with eye opening. Its frequency ranges from 8.5–13 Hz in normal adults and it is typically sinusoidal. Some normal individuals do not have an alpha rhythm during wakefulness. By itself, this is not abnormal. There is often a mild asymmetry of the alpha rhythm with the right side being of higher voltage. A consistent asymmetry of the alpha rhythm of 50% or more (expressed as a percentage of the higher side) is considered abnormal. Since the right is often somewhat higher in voltage, an asymmetry of 35–50% may be significant and is considered abnormal when the right is the lower amplitude side. Slowing of the alpha rhythm unilaterally is rare and a difference of 1 Hz or greater is significant. An asymmetry of reactivity or frequency is a better indicator of a focal abnormality than is a voltage asymmetry.

Low voltage beta activity is usually present in the normal EEG. Beta activity can show a mild (35%) asymmetry; however, a consistent asymmetry, particularly when associated with other findings, is a sensitive indicator of a cortical abnormality on the lower amplitude side, assuming that there is not an extra-axial collection on that side or a skull defect on the opposite side.

Theta and delta activity are classified as rhythmic (also known as monomorphic) versus arrhythmic (a.k.a. polymorphic or irregular), intermittent versus continuous, and generalized versus lateralized (with lateralized sometimes divided into hemispheric, regional or focal, each involving a smaller volume of brain than the prior term). Lateralized (including regional or focal) slowing (theta or delta), particularly when persistent and of delta frequency, is often associated with a structural lesion. Arrhythmic slowing is classically seen with lesions affecting white matter, whereas rhythmic slowing is more suggestive of subcortical gray matter dysfunction, especially thalamic or upper brainstem, or an epileptic focus (only if lateralized). Attenuation (decreased amplitude) or loss of faster frequencies suggests either cortical dysfunction or a collection between the cortex and the recording electrodes (including extracranial fluid).

The *mu rhythm* (7–11 Hz) is present in some normal individuals in wakefulness and drowsiness; it arises from the Rolandic cortex (primary sensorimotor cortex) at rest. It is often asynchronous and asymmetric and can be unilateral. The mu rhythm attenuates with voluntary movement of the opposite side, such as clenching a fist, or even thinking about moving the opposite side.

Drowsiness could be considered a transition state between wakefulness and sleep. When a patient becomes drowsy there is a decrease in frequency or persistence of the alpha rhythm, appearance of slow lateral eye movements, decrease in myogenic artifact, increased slower frequencies (theta and delta), and often an increase in beta frequencies anteriorly.

As the patient enters sleep there are a number of physiological hallmarks of each stage of sleep. Sleep is split into non-rapid eye movement (REM) and REM sleep. Non-REM sleep includes stages N1, N2 and N3. N3, also known as slow wave sleep, has replaced the prior terms of stage 3 and 4 sleep.

The physiologic hallmarks of sleep include:

POSTS – Positive occipital sharp transients of sleep. These are common in drowsiness and N1 sleep, less common in N2 sleep, and rare in N3 sleep.

Vertex (V) waves – Sharp potential, maximal at the vertex but with a field extending to bilateral fronto-central regions, surface negative, appears at the end of N1 and can persist in deeper stages of sleep.

Sleep spindles – Usually paroxysmal, sinusoidal, low-medium amplitude, 11–15 Hz activity lasting 0.5–2 seconds, and maximal at the vertex and fronto-central regions. Spindles (and K-complexes) mark the beginning of N2 sleep.

K-complexes – High voltage, diphasic slow waves (duration at least 0.5 seconds) frequently associated with a sleep spindle. They are related to the arousal process, usually maximal at the vertex and can occur spontaneously or in response to sudden sensory stimuli.

N3 sleep – Characterized by delta activity ≤2 Hz and >75 μV (peak to peak) occupying at least 20% of the recording.

Stage R, or REM (rapid eye movement) sleep – The EEG is low voltage and there are rapid eye movements. Saw-toothed waves can also be seen in the central regions. Saw-toothed waves are sharply contoured 4–7 Hz theta range activities that resemble the toothed edge of a saw, hence its name.

Figure list

Figure 1.1 Schematic representation of channel inputs.

Figure 1.2 International 10-10 system for electrode placement.

Figure 1.3 Analogy depicting the crest of a wave.

Figure 1.4 Bipolar vs. referential representation of a crest or maximal positivity.

Figure 1.5 Analogy depicting the trough of a wave.

Figure 1.6 Bipolar vs. referential representation of a trough or maximal negativity.

Figure 1.7 Alpha rhythm and blinks.

Figure 1.8 Alpha rhythm reactivity.

Figure 1.9 Mu rhythm and eye movements.

Figure 1.10 Mu rhythm.

Figure 1.11 Lambda waves.

Figure 1.12 Slow lateral eye movements of drowsiness.

Figure 1.13 Positive occipital sharp transients of sleep (POSTS).

Figure 1.14 Vertex waves and sleep spindles.

Figure 1.15 K-complexes and POSTS.

Figure 1.16 N3 sleep.

Figure 1.17 Rapid eye movement (REM) sleep.

EEGs throughout this atlas have been shown with the following standard recording filters unless otherwise specified: LFF 1 Hz, HFF 70 Hz, notch filter off.

Suggested reading

Acharya JN, Hani A, Cheek J, Thirumala P, Tsuchida TN. American Clinical Neurophysiology Society Guideline 2: Guidelines for Standard Electrode Position Nomenclature. *J Clin Neurophysiol.* 2016 Aug;**33**(4):308–311.

Acharya JN, Hani AJ, Thirumala PD, Tsuchida TN. American Clinical Neurophysiology Society Guideline 3: A Proposal for Standard Montages to Be Used in Clinical EEG. *J Clin Neurophysiol.* 2016 Aug;**33**(4):312–6.

Amzica F, Steriade M. The K-complex: its slow (<1-Hz) rhythmicity and relation to delta waves. *Neurology.* 1997;**49**(4):952–959.

Berry RB, Quan SF, Abreu AR, at al. for the American Academy of Sleep Medicine. *The AASM Manual for the Scoring of Sleep and Associated Events: Rules, Terminology and Technical Specifications*, Version 2.6. Darien, IL: American Academy of Sleep Medicine, 2020.

Burgess RC. Localization and field determination in electroencephalography. In: Wyllie E, Gidal B, Goodkin HP, Jehi L, Loddenkemper, T, eds. *Wyllie's Treatment of Epilepsy. Principles and Practice (seventh edition)*. Philadelphia, Wolters Kluwer 2020; 68–90.

Ebersole, JS, Cortical generators and EEG voltage fields. In: Ebersole JS, Husain AM, Nordli DR, eds. *Current Practice of Clinical Electroencephalography (fourth edition)*. Philadelphia, Wolters Kluwer 2014; 72–99.

Gloor, P. Recording principles. Volume conductor theory. *Spike-and-Wave, special issue No. 2*, 1971; 1–48.

Kane N, Acharya J, Benickzy S, et al. A revised glossary of terms most commonly used by clinical electroencephalographers and updated proposal for the report format of the EEG findings. Revision 2017. *Clin Neurophysiol Pract.* 2017;**2**:170–185.

Knott JR. Electrode montages revisited: How to tell up from down. *Am J EEG Technol* 1969;**9**:33–45.

Kozelka JW, Pedley, TA. Beta and mu rhythms. *J Clin Neurophysiol* 1990;**7**: 191–208.

Krishnan V, Chang BS, Schomer DL. Normal EEG in wakefulness and sleep: adults and elderly. In: Schomer, DL, Lopes de Silva F, eds. *Niedermeyer's Electroencephalography: Basic Principles, Clinical Applications and Related Fields.* New York, Oxford University Press 2018; 104–154.

Lesser RP, Luders H, Dinner DS, Morris H. An introduction to the basic concepts of polarity and localization. *J Clin Neurophysiol* 1985;**2**:45–61.

Markand ON. Alpha rhythms. *J Clin Neurophysiol* 1990;**7**:163–189.

Purcell SM, Manoach DS, Demanuele C, et al. Characterizing sleep spindles in 11,630 individuals from the National Sleep Research Resource. *Nat Commun.* 2017;**8**(1):15930.

Radhakrishnan K, Sunku AJ, Donat JF, Klass DW. Pattern-induced negative occipital potentials (PINOP). *J Clin Neurophysiol.* 2007;**24**(3):277–280.

Schomer DL, Epstein CM, Herman ST, Maus D, Gisch BJ. Recording principles: analog and digital principles; polarity and field determinations; multimodal monitoring; polygraphy (EOG, EMG, ECG, SAO). In: Schomer, DL, Lopes de Silva F, eds. *Niedermeyer's Electroencephalography: Basic Principles, Clinical Applications and Related Fields.* New York, Oxford University Press 2018; 104–154.

Tao JX, Baldwin M, Hawes-Ebersole S, Ebersole JS. Cortical substrates of scalp EEG epileptiform discharges. *J Clin Neurophysiol,* 2007;**24**:96–100.

Tatum WO 4th, Husain AM, Benbadis SR, et al. Normal adult EEG and patterns of uncertain significance. *J Clinical Neurophysiol* 2006;**23**:194–207.

Tyner FS, Knott JR, Mayer WB Jr., Artifacts. In: *Fundamentals of EEG Technology*, Volume 1, New York, Raven Press, 1983; 280–311.

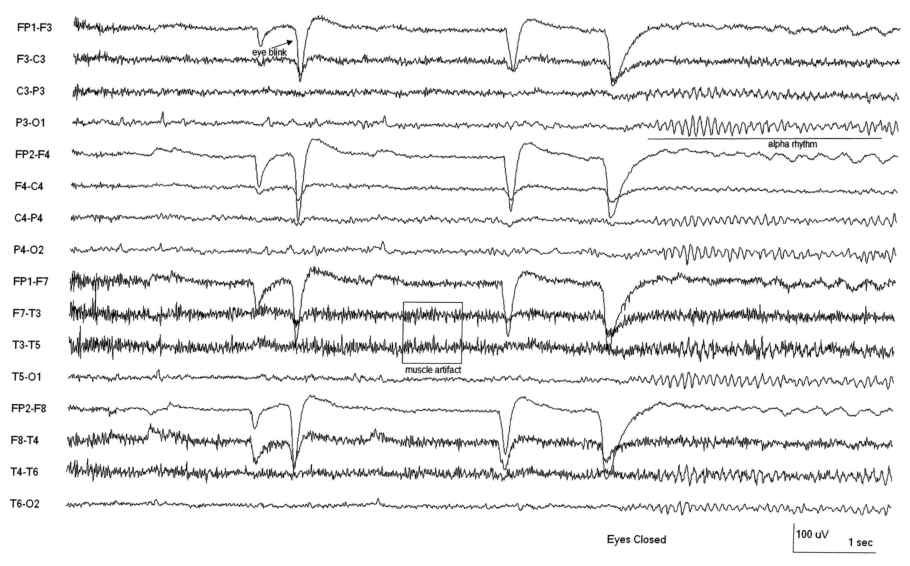

FP1-F3

F3-C3
eye blink

C3-P3

P3-O1
alpha rhythm

FP2-F4

F4-C4

C4-P4

P4-O2

FP1-F7

F7-T3

T3-T5

T5-O1
muscle artifact

FP2-F8

F8-T4

T4-T6

T6-O2

Eyes Closed

100 uV
1 sec

Figure 1.7. Alpha rhythm and blinks. (a) Alpha rhythm, longitudinal bipolar. Following eye closure, rhythmic activity of 10 Hz is present posteriorly. This represents a normal alpha rhythm (sometimes referred to as the posterior dominant rhythm). The activity is maximal in the O1 and O2 electrodes and seen to a lesser extent in the parietal (P3/P4) and posterior temporal (T5/T6) regions. The patient is awake with eye blink artifact (arrow), and muscle artifact more prominent in the temporal regions (box). Additional information on determining eye movement artifact from cerebral activity can be found in Chapter 7: Artifacts. The temporal regions are a common location for muscle artifact given these electrodes overly the temporalis muscle (whereas there is relatively little muscle at the vertex).

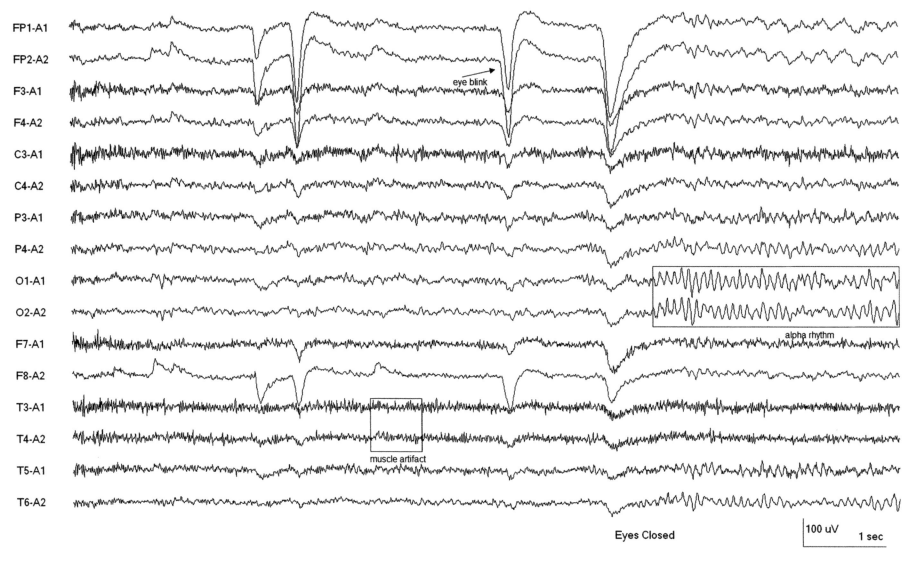

Figure 1.7. (*Continued*) (b) Alpha rhythm, referential. The same epoch in a referential montage, with ipsilateral ear reference. Blinks appear as prominent deflections on the EEG because the eye is a dipole, with the cornea being surface positive and the retina surface negative. During blinks the eyes go upward, due to Bell's phenomenon. This causes the closest electrodes (Fp1 and Fp2) to become relatively positive (as the positive cornea comes into close proximity to these electrodes). As Fp1/Fp2 become grossly positive, a large positive or down-going deflection can be seen in these channels. The opposite occurs if there is a downward movement of the eyes.

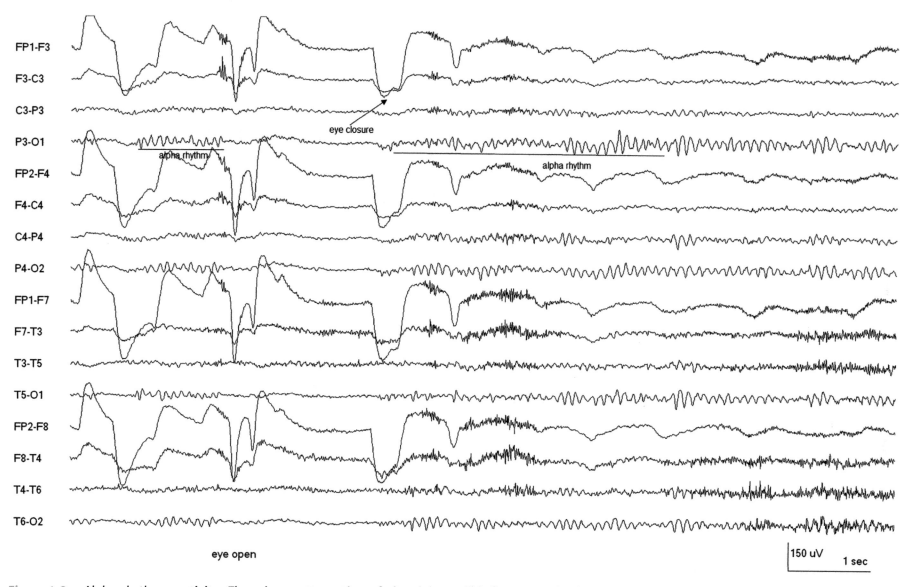

FP1-F3

F3-C3

C3-P3

eye closure

P3-O1

alpha rhythm alpha rhythm

FP2-F4

F4-C4

C4-P4

P4-O2

FP1-F7

F7-T3

T3-T5

T5-O1

FP2-F8

F8-T4

T4-T6

T6-O2

eye open

150 uV
1 sec

Figure 1.8. Alpha rhythm reactivity. There is an attenuation of the alpha rhythm following eye opening in this 72-year-old man. The alpha rhythm then returns following eye closure, best seen in the channels containing O1 and O2.

This feature can be described as 'reactive to eye opening/closure'. Loss of this reactivity can be being an early sign of diffuse dysfunction.

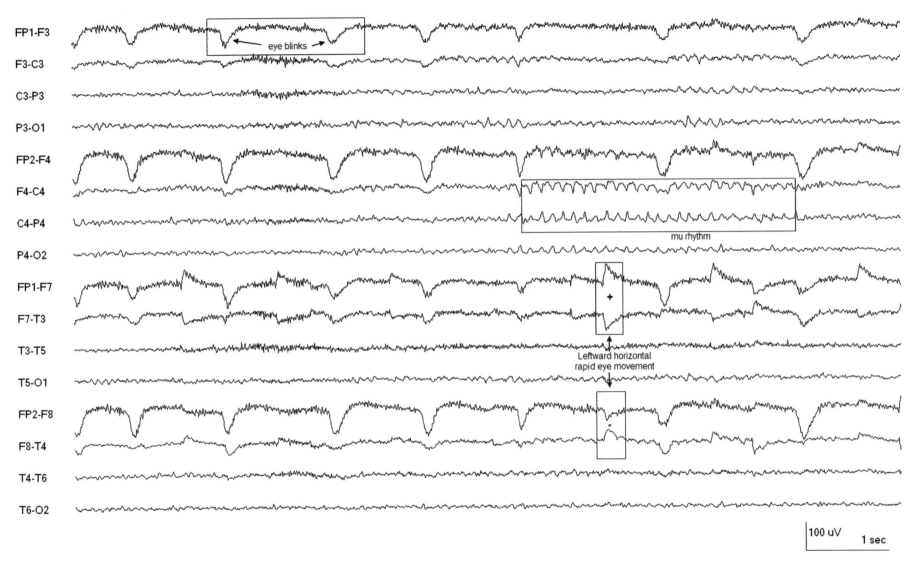

FP1-F3
F3-C3
C3-P3
P3-O1
FP2-F4
F4-C4
C4-P4
P4-O2
FP1-F7
F7-T3
T3-T5
T5-O1
FP2-F8
F8-T4
T4-T6
T6-O2

eye blinks

mu rhythm

Leftward horizontal
rapid eye movement

100 uV
1 sec

Figure 1.9. Mu rhythm and eye movements. (a) Mu rhythm, longitudinal bipolar. A mu rhythm is prominent in the right parasagittal region (box) in this 45-year-old man. The sharp component is surface negative and maximal at electrode C4, as demonstrated by the phase reversal on this bipolar montage. This morphology, containing a sharp negative component alternating with a blunt positive component, as seen in F4-C4 and C4-P4, resembles the Greek letter mu, giving this rhythm its name. There is also a typical leftward horizontal eye movement shown. Again, consider the cornea is positively charged. Eye movement to the left causes the electrode closest to the corner of the left eye (F7) to become positive. Also consider that the electrode closest to the corner of the right eye (F8) would become less positive (more negative) as the right eye moves away from this electrode. Therefore, on the bipolar montage there is a positive phase reversal at F7 with deflections away from each other, whereas at F8 there is a negative phase reversal with the deflections pointing towards each other.

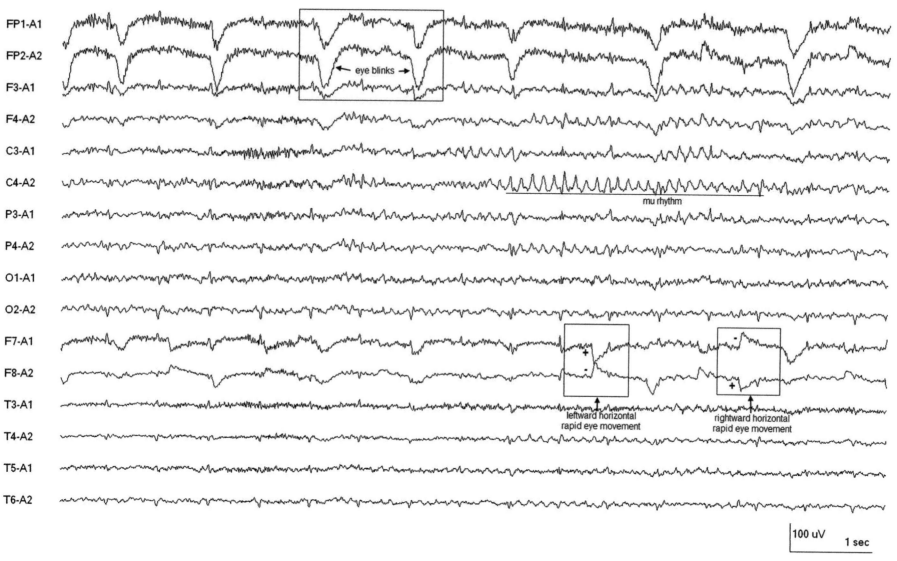

Figure 1.9. *(Continued)* (b) Mu rhythm, referential. In this reformatted referential montage to ipsilateral ears, the same mu rhythm as seen in Figure 1.9a is best seen in the C4-A2 derivation, confirming that the maximum discharge is at C4 (electrode with the greatest amplitude on a referential recording, assuming an inactive reference). The sharp component is upgoing, indicating that C4 (input 1) is more negative than A2. Leftward (positivity at F7) and rightward (positivity at F8) rapid eye movements are shown as well.

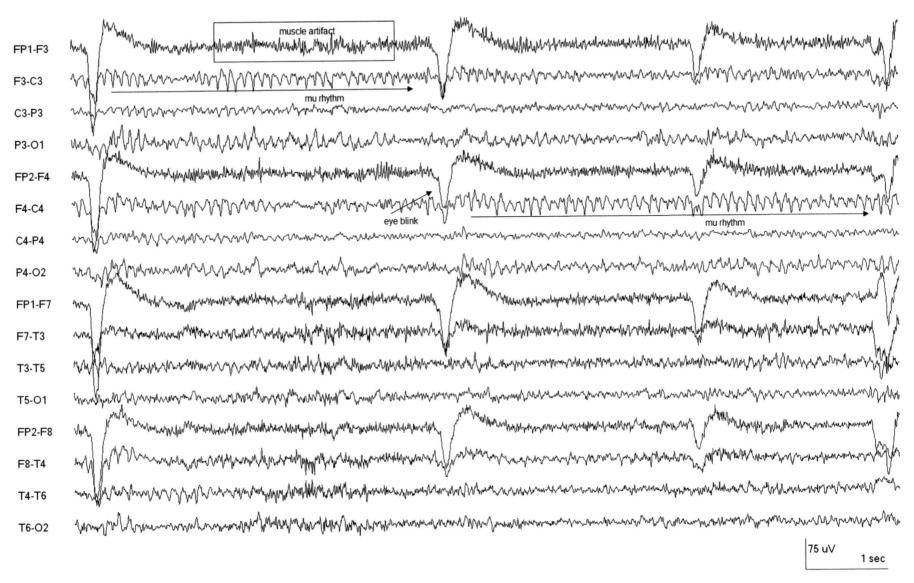

Figure 1.10. Mu rhythm. Rhythmic activity of 9 Hz is present, particularly in the F3-C3 followed by the F4-C4 derivations. This is a normal mu rhythm. Unlike the alpha rhythm, mu can often occur asynchronously, as in this example, and is completely normal. This should be distinguished from asymmetry of the mu, which can be pathological (but can also be normal). Asynchrony refers to a rhythm that sometimes appears on one side of the head, but at other times of the record can appear in the opposite hemisphere. Asynchrony of certain rhythms (such as the mu rhythm, or sleep spindles in infants) can be physiologic, but some (such as infant spindles) should be symmetric over the entire record (seen equally in both hemispheres, though not necessarily at the same time). Thus, rhythms can be asynchronous but symmetric. A rhythm that is only present in one hemisphere over the course of the record or is clearly and consistently more prominent in one hemisphere, is not asynchronous, but rather is asymmetric, and can denote pathology as described in Chapter 4: Focal abnormalities.

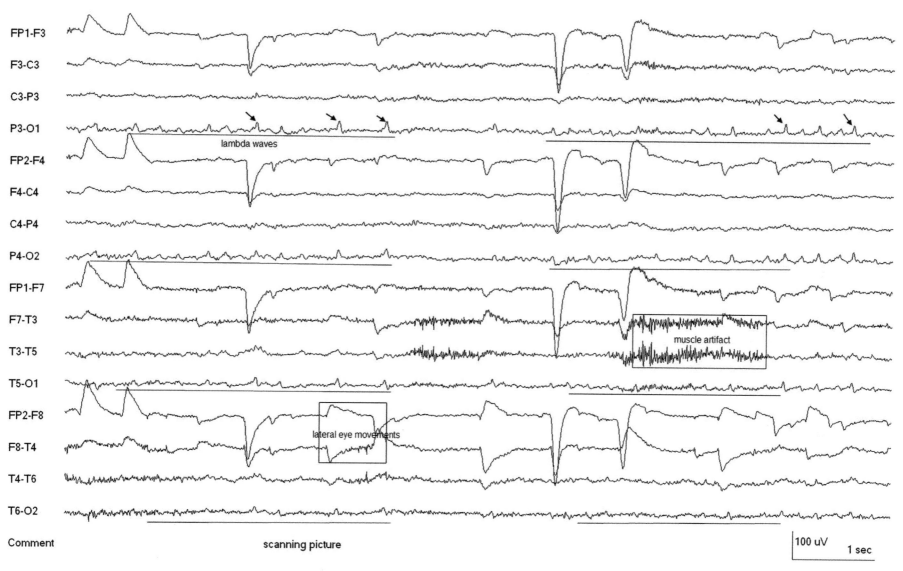

FP1-F3

F3-C3

C3-P3

P3-O1 — lambda waves

FP2-F4

F4-C4

C4-P4

P4-O2

FP1-F7

F7-T3

T3-T5 — muscle artifact

T5-O1

FP2-F8

F8-T4 — lateral eye movements

T4-T6

T6-O2

Comment — scanning picture

100 uV 1 sec

Figure 1.11. Lambda waves. (a) Lambda waves, longitudinal bipolar. Low–voltage sharp waves are present bilaterally in the posterior head regions (derivations P3-O1, P4-O2, T5-O1 and T6-O2; several marked with arrows) in this longitudinal bipolar montage. The sharp component is upgoing. This is because input 1 (electrodes P3, P4, T5 and T6) is relatively negative with respect to input 2 (electrodes O1 and O2). There are two possibilities that could result in this: 1. A negative discharge that is more prominent in input 1, or 2. A positive discharge that is more prominent in input 2 (hence input 1 would be 'relatively negative'). In this case the deflections represent the latter. Lambda waves are surface positive potentials arising in the occipital area; rare negative variants have been described as well. The polarity of lambda waves can be confirmed using a referential montage (Figure 1.11b). Lambda waves are normal and best seen during visual scanning (note: they disappear when the patient stops scanning); they *do not indicate* cortical hyperexcitability.

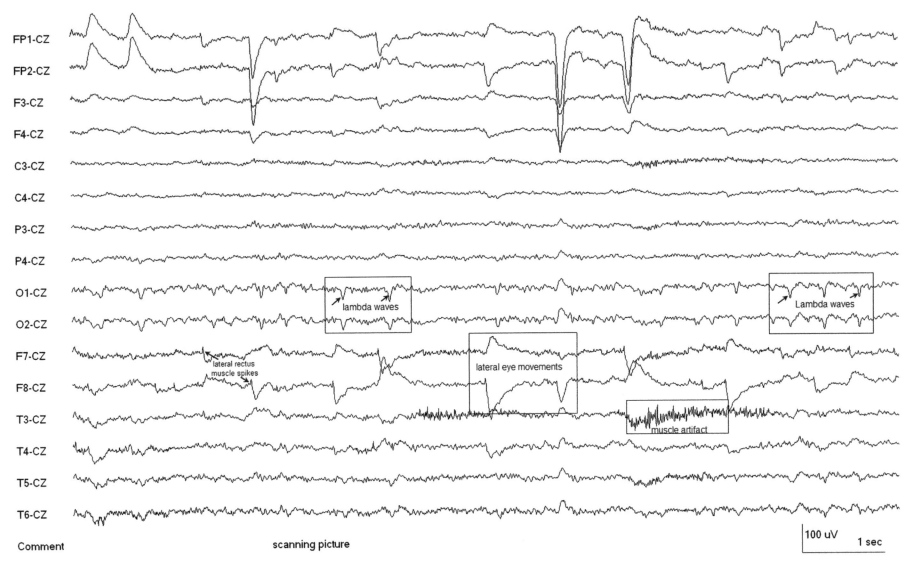

Figure 1.11. (*Continued*) (b) Lambda waves, referential. The polarity of lambda waves can be confirmed with an appropriate referential montage. In a reformatted Cz-referential montage, the same lambda waves are seen as downward (positive) deflections in O1-Cz and O2-Cz derivations. If the alternate explanation for upward deflections in the positive head regions on a bipolar montage were true (i.e., P3, P4, T5 and T6 were surface negative), then upward (negative) deflections would be seen at these derivations in respect to Cz. In this example there is really no additional activity at these channels, and instead it is only the positive deflections at O1 and O2 that are seen. Lateral rectus muscle spikes can be seen at F7 and F8 in association with some of the horizontal eye movements as labeled.

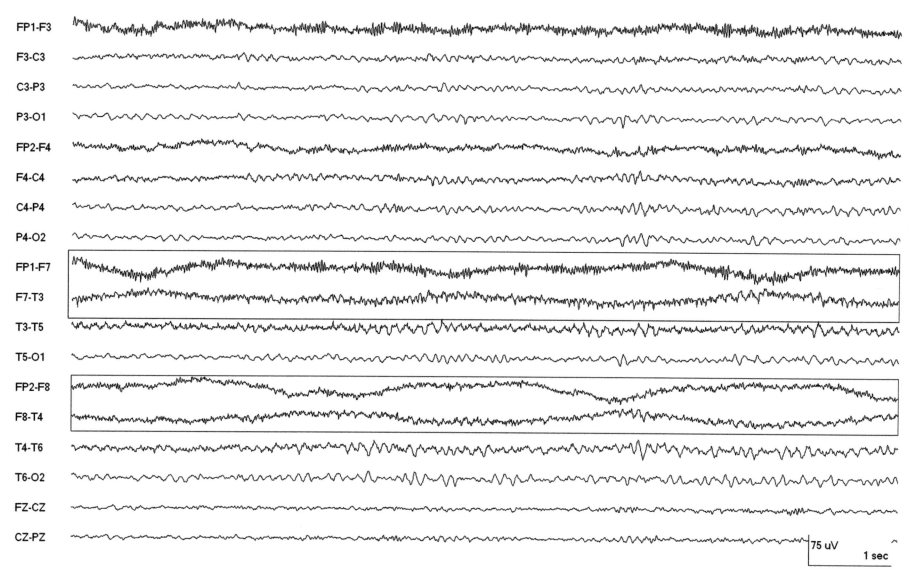

Figure 1.12. Slow lateral eye movements of drowsiness. (a). Slow lateral eye movements of drowsiness, longitudinal bipolar. Slow lateral eye movements are prominent in this 32-year-old man during drowsiness, continuing smoothly in one direction, then the other. This is a normal feature of drowsiness. Note that the F7 and F8 electrodes are out of phase; when one is surface positive (the cornea is moving towards this side), the other is negative (cornea moving away). This is consistent with lateral eye movements. Additional information on determining eye movement artifact can be found in Chapter 7: Artifacts. Slow lateral eye movements are one of the features of drowsiness. Other features include: 1. Loss of eye blinks (note there are no examples of eye blink artifact on this page). 2. Slowing of the posterior dominant rhythm (note on this page the PDR is 7 Hz and there has been some loss of the usual anterior-posterior gradient [where the activity is also seen in C3 and C4]), loss of EMG activity, and the emergence of positive occipital sharp transients of sleep (POSTS) (Figure 1.13).

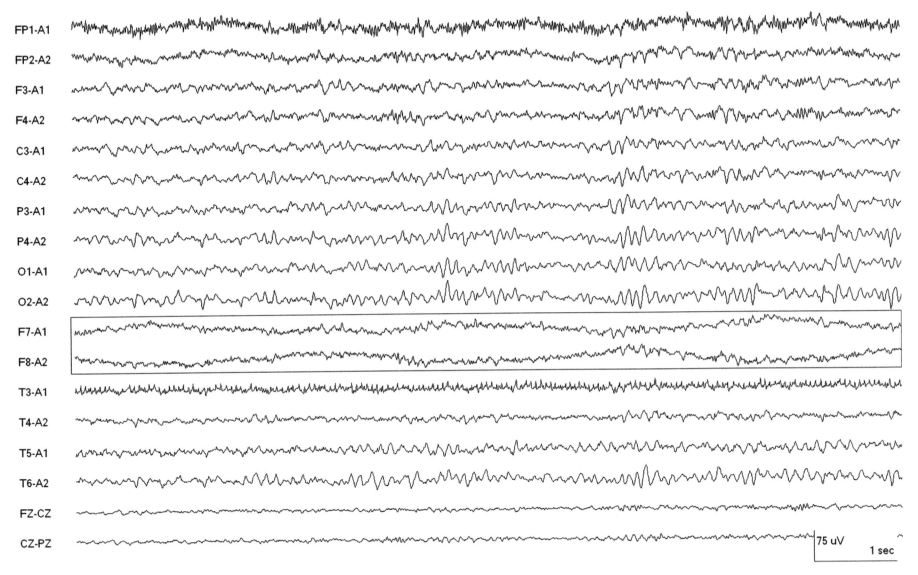

Figure 1.12. (*Continued*) (b) Slow lateral eye movements of drowsiness, referential. A reformatted referential montage to the ipsilateral ear showing the same roving, conjugate horizontal eye movements of drowsiness. Again, the slow deflections in F7 and F8 are out of phase, as one becomes positive, the other becomes negative. This is typical of horizontal eye movements. Vertical eye movements for the most part affect F7 and F8 similarly, therefore vertical eye movements usually generate the same activity in F7 and F8 at the same time [i.e., they remain in phase]).

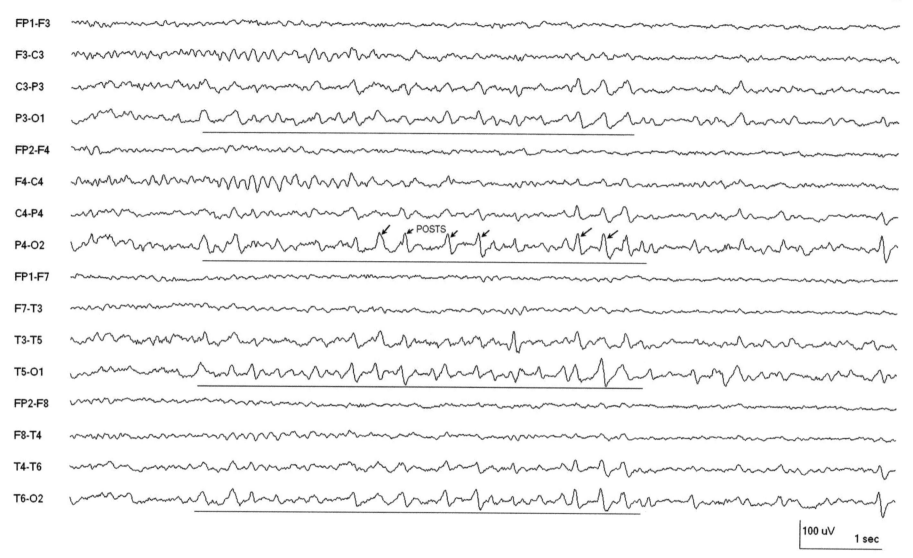

Figure 1.13. Positive occipital sharp transients of sleep (POSTS). (a). POSTS, longitudinal bipolar. Repetitive sharp activity (arrows) is present bilaterally in the posterior head regions in this 31-year-old woman who is drowsy. This activity represents positive occipital sharp transients of sleep (POSTS). POSTS are (by definition) surface positive in O1 and O2, and their polarity can be confirmed with a referential montage (Figure 1.13b). POSTS are normal waveforms of the drowsy state and do not represent cortical hyperexcitability.

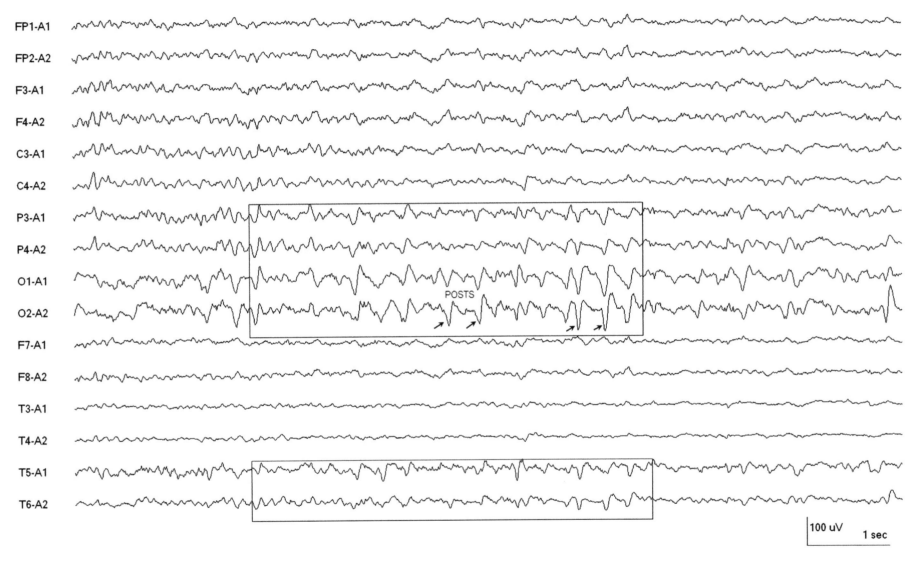

Figure 1.13. *(Continued)* (b) POSTS, referential. In a reformatted montage referenced to ipsilateral ears, the sharp activity is maximal in the O1-A1 and O2-A2 derivations. The sharp activity is down-going since O1 and O2 are relatively positive. The waveforms are also present to a lesser extent in the parietal and posterior temporal areas. It is worth confirming this point as very occasionally surface negative posterior temporal or parietal epileptiform discharges can have a similar appearance. In these cases, the activity would greatly involve T5/T6 or P3/P4 rather than O1/O2, and the deflections would be upgoing on a referential montage (i.e., surface negative).

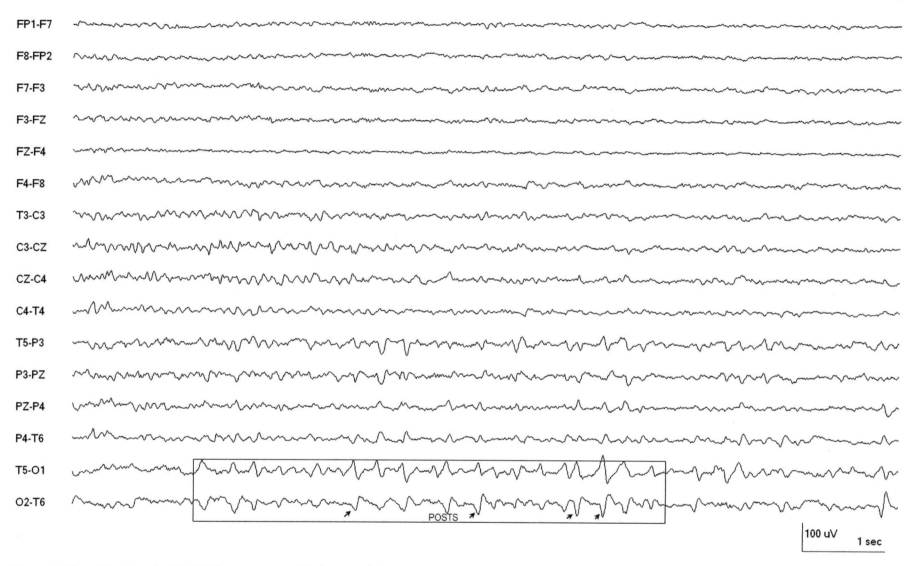

FP1-F7

F8-FP2

F7-F3

F3-FZ

FZ-F4

F4-F8

T3-C3

C3-CZ

CZ-C4

C4-T4

T5-P3

P3-PZ

PZ-P4

P4-T6

T5-O1

O2-T6

POSTS

100 uV

1 sec

Figure 1.13.   (*Continued*) (c) POSTS, transverse bipolar. In this transverse bipolar montage, complexes are seen best in the bottom 2 derivations (T5-O1, O2-T6). The sharp component is upgoing in T5-O1 since T5 is relatively negative when compared to O1 (due to the positivity at O1). In the O2-T6 derivations, since O2 is more positive than T6, there is a down-going deflection. Another way to think of this is that there is a positive phase reversal (i.e., the deflections point away from each other) between O1 and O2, so the region of maximal positivity is between these two electrodes.

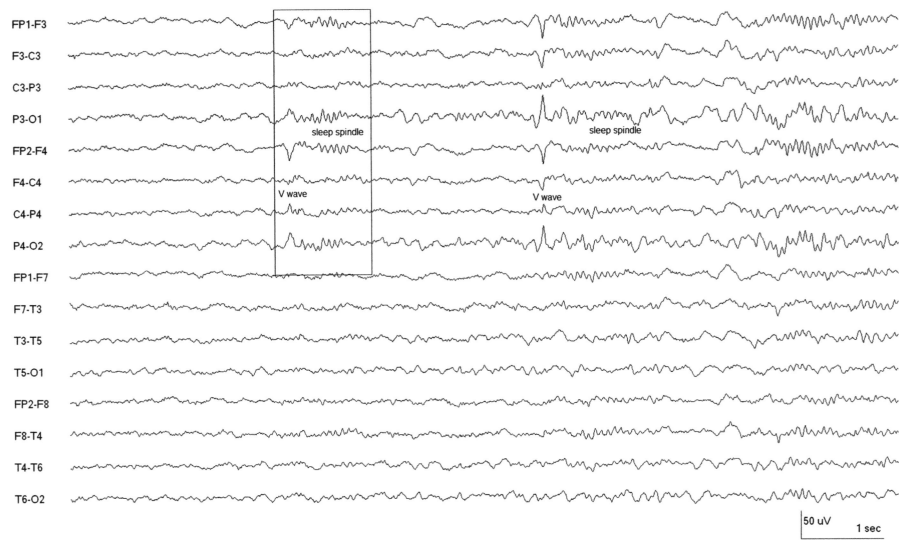

Figure 1.14. Vertex waves and sleep spindles (sleep transients). (a). Vertex waves and sleep spindles, longitudinal bipolar. Vertex waves (V waves) are a feature of N1 sleep but are often present in later stages of sleep (N2, but rarely N3 sleep). This is the case in this 30-year-old woman with both prominent V waves and sleep spindles (the latter being a defining feature of N2 sleep). Regarding the V waves, in the right hemisphere, the activity demonstrates phase reversal at electrode C4, indicating maximal negativity at this site. On the left, the phase reversal is at C3-P3; the C3-P3 derivation does not show this activity since these areas are equipotential and canceling (confirmed in subsequent referential montages). The first labeled V wave is more prominent on the right; this type of asymmetry is not unusual in early sleep and is not abnormal unless it is consistently more prominent in one hemisphere over the course of the record. Sleep spindles (highlighted) are a defining feature of N2 sleep (along with K-complexes). Sleep spindles are usually maximal at the vertex or C3/C4 and consist of a sinusoidal activity usually lasting 0.5–2 seconds, with a frequency of 11–15 Hz (also referred to as the 'sigma band'), typically centered at 13.5 Hz.

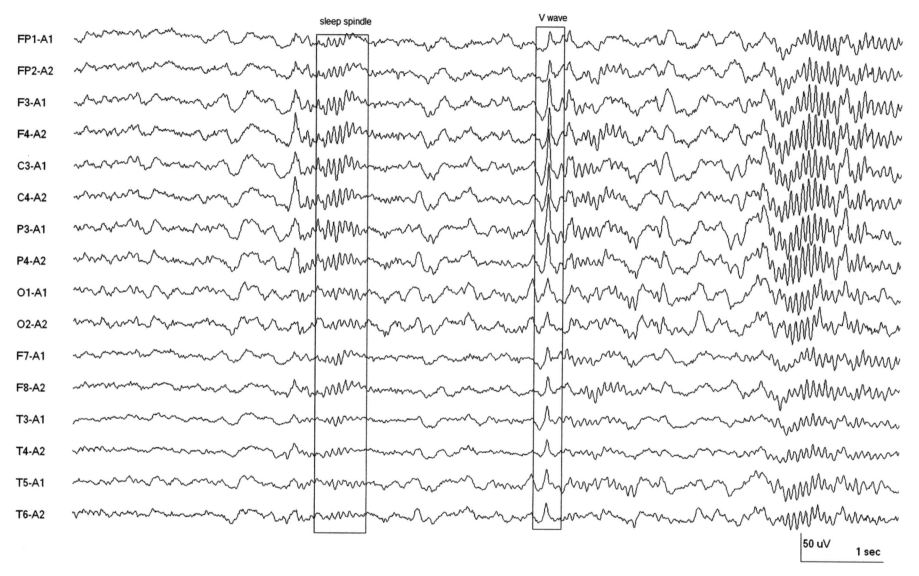

Figure 1.14. (*Continued*) (b) Vertex waves and sleep spindles, referential. A referential montage to ipsilateral ears shows that the V waves and spindles are widespread in distribution in the parasagittal regions, maximal in the fronto-central regions, typical of normal sleep transients.

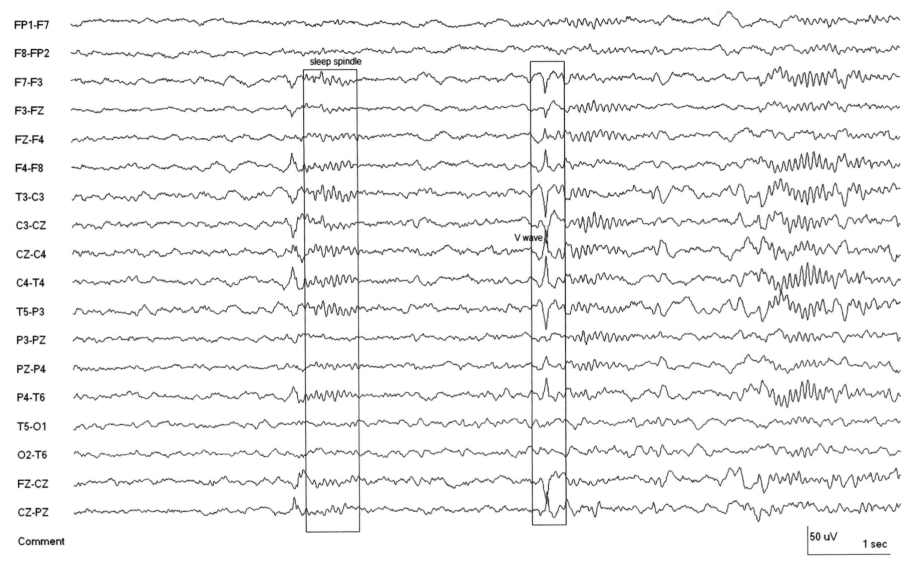

Figure 1.14. *(Continued)* (c) Vertex waves and sleep spindles, transverse bipolar. This montage shows that both the V waves and sleep spindles demonstrate phase reversals at several electrodes (Fz, Cz and Pz) simultaneously. In order to determine where this activity is maximal, one cannot use the amplitude from a bipolar montage, which indicates the difference in potential between two electrodes, to indicate the site of maximal involvement. Fz is being compared to frontal electrodes, Cz to central electrodes and Pz is to parietal electrodes. They need to be compared to each other, or to the same reference. The midline derivations (Fz-Cz and Cz-Pz) are shown in the bottom 2 channels in a longitudinal direction (anterior to posterior). As demonstrated, the Fz-Cz and Cz-Pz derivations display a phase reversal at electrode Cz, with Cz being relatively surface negative compared to Fz or Pz. Thus, Cz is the site of maximal negativity.

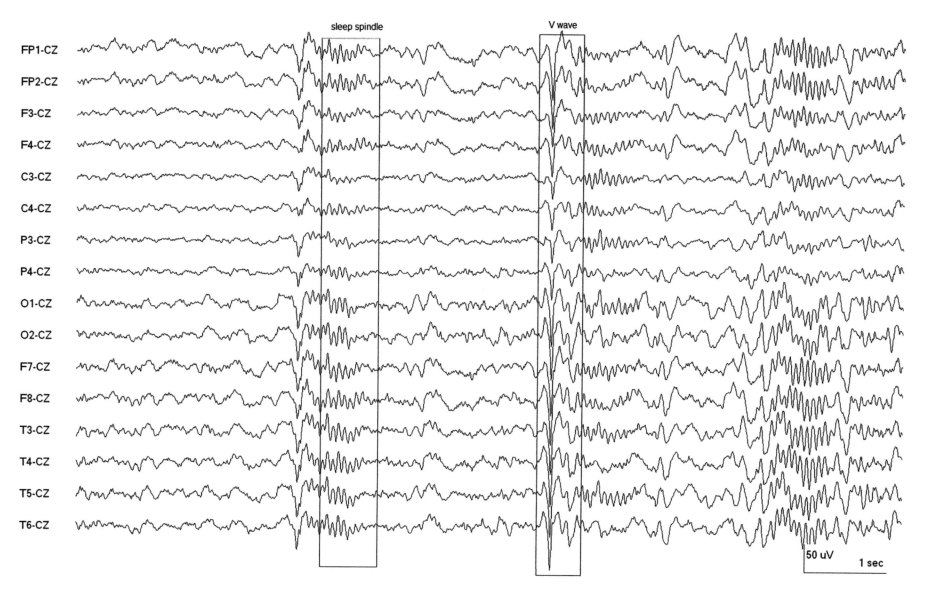

Figure 1.14. (*Continued*) (d) Vertex waves and sleep spindles, referential Cz. In this reformatted referential montage to the Cz, the sharp component of the discharges are down-going in all derivations. This is because electrode Cz is relatively more negative than all other electrodes, which are in input 1. This is an example of an active reference, or 'reference contamination'. If there is no activity at Fp1 (for example), then input 1 (Fp1 = zero) minus input 2 (Cz = strongly negative) = positive/down-going deflection). This is a case where selecting Cz as a reference is sub-optimal, as it includes the activity of greatest interest (i.e., it is an active reference). The result of this is that it falsely leads one to think the V waves at the vertex are generalized and of positive polarity (neither of which is true).

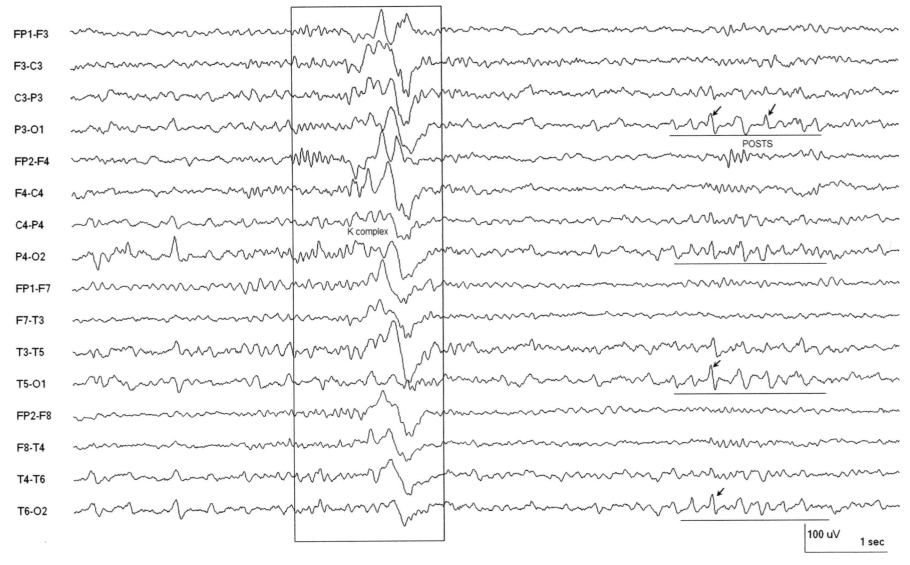

Figure 1.15. K-complex and POSTS. (a). K-complex and POSTS, longitudinal bipolar. A high voltage slow wave (typically diphasic, first phase smaller and negative, second bigger and positive, with a total duration of >0.5 s) preceded by faster activity is prominent in this longitudinal bipolar montage in a 31-year-old woman, who is in N2 sleep. This is typical of a K-complex (a feature of N2 sleep) and the faster activity preceding it is a sleep spindle. Spindle activity preceding or following the high voltage slow wave is common and all form part of the 'complex'. POSTS (positive occipital sharp transients of sleep) are also present, most evident in the last several seconds as labeled.

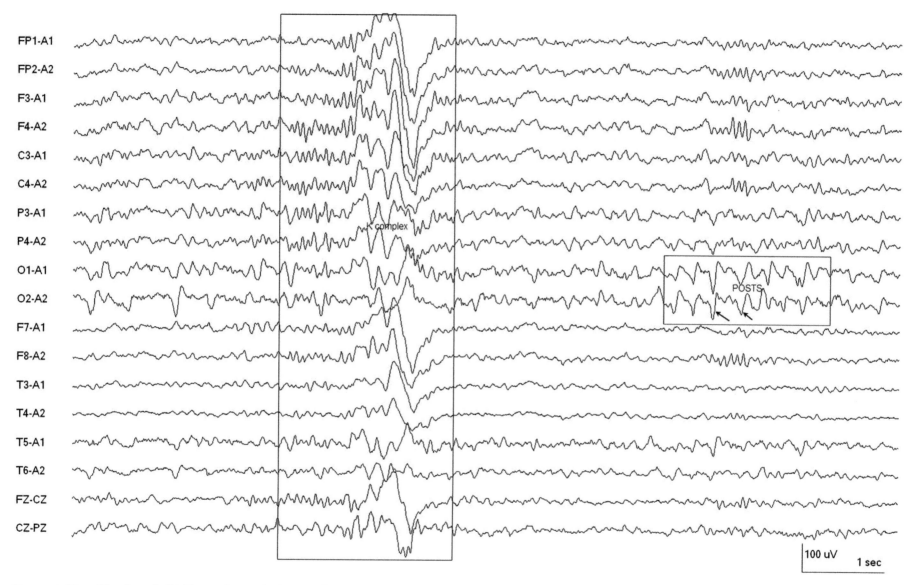

Figure 1.15. *(Continued)* (b) K-complex and POSTS, referential. The referential montage to ipsilateral ears displays this activity, as well as better displaying the preceding sleep spindle. The entire complex is referred to as a K-complex.

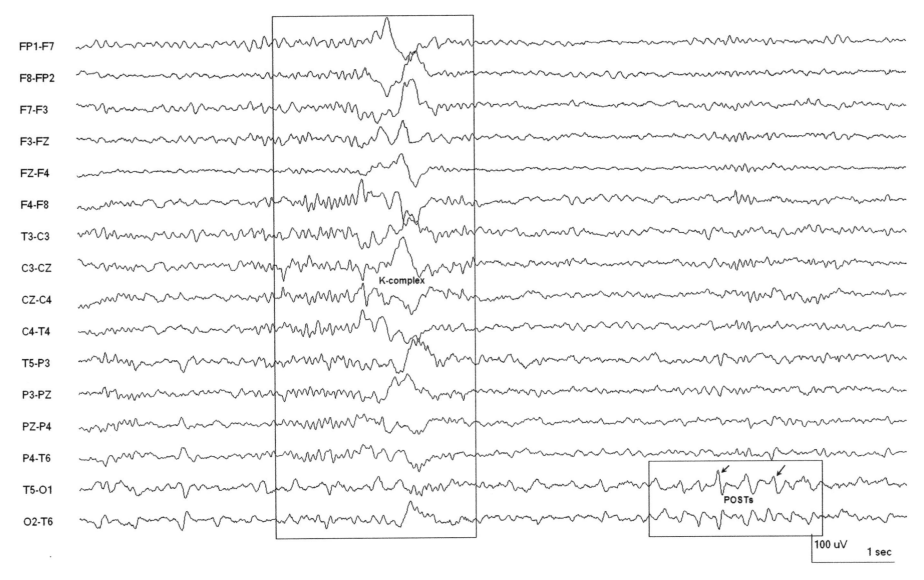

Figure 1.15.   (*Continued*) (c) K-complex and POSTS, transverse bipolar. Here the epoch has been reformatted to a transverse bipolar montage. Here it is easy to appreciate the spindles are centrally maximal, the high voltage slow wave is broadly distributed, and the POSTS are only seen in the occipital regions.

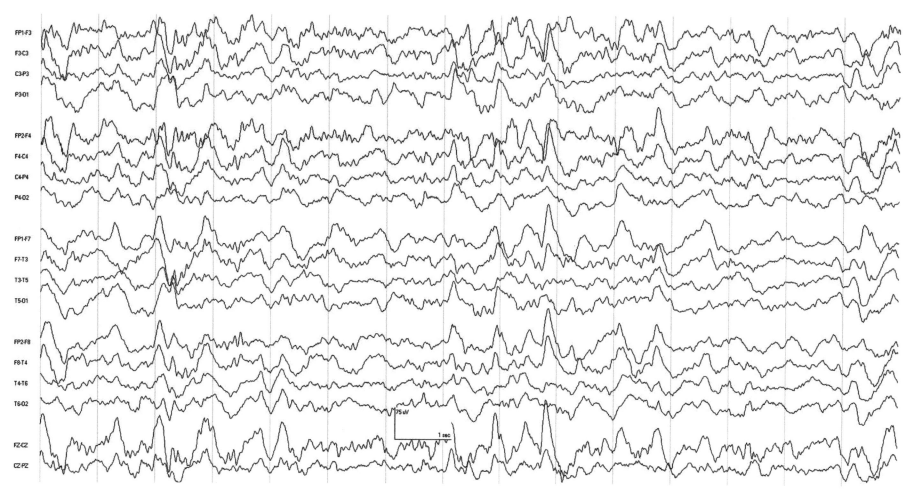

Figure 1.16. N3 sleep. N3 sleep (also known as slow wave sleep) consisting of medium to high voltage polymorphic 1–1.5 Hz delta activity with superimposed 6–7 Hz theta rhythms and some intermittent 13–15 Hz low voltage beta activity. N3 sleep is defined as at least 20% of the epoch consisting of 0.5–2 Hz activity of >75 uV.

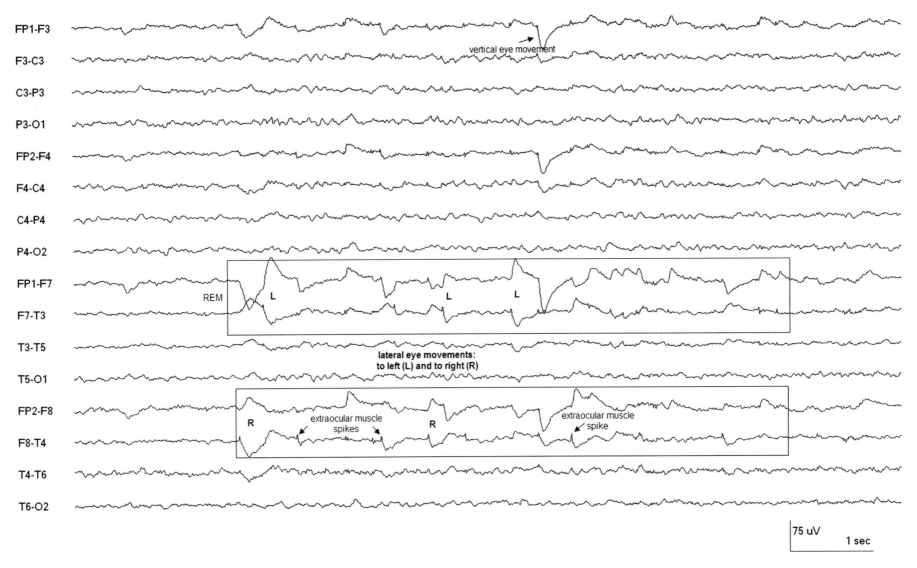

Figure 1.17. Stage R, or REM (rapid eye movement) sleep. (a). REM sleep, longitudinal bipolar. Rapid eye movements are prominent in this 25-year-old man in stage R, or REM (rapid eye movement) sleep. The majority of the movements are lateral, at which time electrodes F7 and F8 are simultaneously out of phase. Leftward and rightward lateral eye movements are labeled, as well as one vertical eye movement. Small, sharp discharges can be seen with some of the rapid eye movements – these represent extraocular muscle spikes (mainly lateral rectus when seen at F7 and F8). Note the actual EEG rhythms in this stage of sleep do not differ greatly from the awake or drowsy states. The characteristic sleep transients of N2 sleep and the striking slowing of N3 sleep are not present. The rapid eye movement artifact is the characteristic EEG finding of REM sleep.

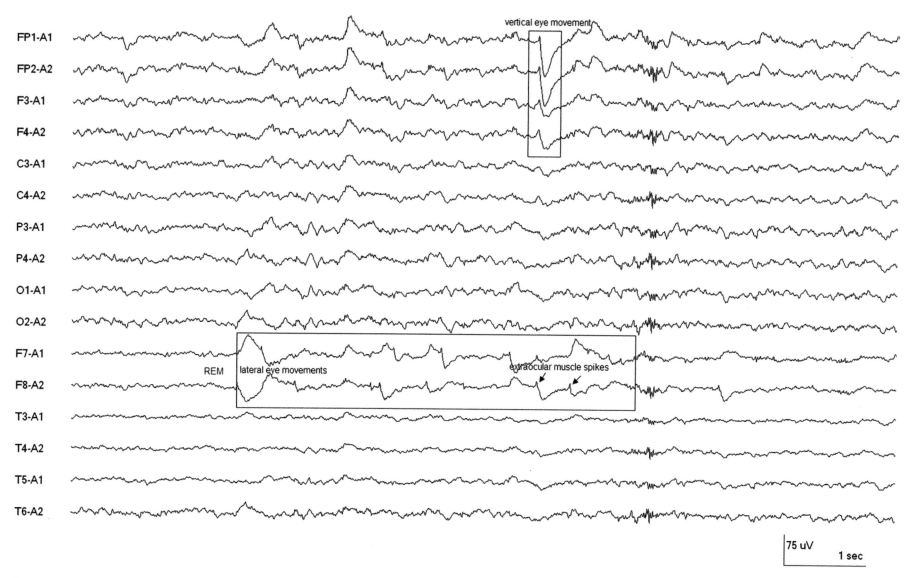

Figure 1.17.   (*Continued*) (b) REM sleep, referential. A reformatted referential montage to ipsilateral ears. The lateral eye movements show up as deflections that are out of phase in F7/F8, contrasted with the blink that is similarly represented in FP1 and FP2.

2 Practical approach to critical care EEG and its classification

The approach to the interpretation of continuous EEG (cEEG) utilizes many of the same principles as any EEG. The major differences are (1) the background features often carry important prognostic implications, (2) the prevalence of rhythmic and periodic patterns (RPPs) is high and features of these patterns determine the probability of subsequent seizures, (3) the distinction between ictal and interictal is much less clear and (4) there are recently defined, complex patterns that only occur in the critical care setting that can be suggestive of certain conditions, be highly associated with seizures, or in themselves may cause clinical signs and/or associated neuronal injury that may warrant treatment. These important differences substantiate the need for tailored critical care EEG terminology and classification.

2.1 Basic approach

Clinical information

An EEG purist will read studies blinded to all clinical information. However, in the ICU there are certain pieces of clinical information that would drastically change the interpretation of the EEG findings. Practically, it is often useful to have some knowledge of the clinical presentation and clinical questions to assist with extracting the greatest amount of information from the EEG. Certain clinical questions are best answered utilizing quantitative EEG, e.g., monitoring for delayed cerebral ischemia after subarachnoid hemorrhage (SAH), and these factors should be considered from the beginning of recording.

A list of clinical information that can be valuable is:

- age

- brief clinical history, especially the primary neurological diagnosis

- sedative medication regimen

- therapeutic temperature management (TTM)

- imaging findings (in particular skull defects)

- clinical spells and phenomena of interest to clinical teams.

Practical approach to EEG interpretation

The physical and in particular neurological examination has a fairly set structure that is taught similarly around the world. When first learning how to examine a patient, a set order helps training clinicians in a thorough assessment as to not miss important clinical signs. With time and experience certain signs are seen more commonly together, and one sign often triggers the search for pertinent associations (including pertinent negatives).

Hirsch and Brenner's Atlas of EEG in Critical Care, Second Edition. Lawrence J. Hirsch, Michael W.K. Fong, and Richard P. Brenner.
© 2023 John Wiley & Sons Ltd. Published 2023 by John Wiley & Sons Ltd.

The interpretation of the EEG uses similar principles. When starting to read an EEG, having a set structure assists greatly with not missing findings. With experience, EEGers start to appreciate findings that often go together, e.g., focal arrhythmic slowing and focal epileptiform discharges. A crucial component, once these findings are documented, is not to get pigeonholed into one diagnosis, but rather to be mindful to continue looking for findings that signify an additional process, e.g., an independent population of epileptiform discharges in another region, or in the opposite hemisphere.

A suggested stepwise approach to the EEG

(1) *Description of the best background* – The description of the awake or most awake (after being stimulated) background usually begins with determination of the alpha rhythm or posterior dominant rhythm (PDR). If a PDR is present, reactivity and symmetry should be specifically assessed in addition to the best awake frequency. Whether or not there is an alpha rhythm, the background still carries a richness of information. The remaining components of the background should be determined and then a severity of dysfunction should be attributed in accordance with a validated encephalopathy scale. The grading of encephalopathy will be addressed in Chapter 3: encephalopathy and coma.

(2) *Focal findings* – In a highly encephalopathic EEG it can be easy to miss focal findings if not specifically looking for them. Focal findings include slowing and attenuation. These hold valuable clues as to where epileptiform patterns may arise in the remainder of the record. Once a focal EEG finding is appreciated it can be useful to integrate the location and extent of the available imaging abnormalities. Focal irregular (synonymous with arrhythmic or polymorphic) slowing concordant with a brain tumor is not surprising. Focal irregular slowing occurring in the face of normal neuroimaging raises the possibility of a purely electrical problem such as epilepsy, and gradually resolving focal slowing is suggestive of a post ictal state; these findings should increase the suspicions of the EEGer that the patient may also have epileptiform patterns. A variety of focal findings can be found in Chapter 4: Focal abnormalities.

(3) *Epileptiform findings* – The remainder of the EEG is then interpreted for epileptiform abnormalities. These include sporadic discharges (SDs, i.e., sharp waves or spikes), rhythmic and periodic patterns (RPPs) and brief potentially ictal rhythmic discharges (BIRDs). Once focal polymorphic/irregular slowing is detected this area should be highlighted as a region where these patterns may arise. For example, lateralized rhythmic delta activity (LRDA) can be missed in the context of medium-amplitude polymorphic slowing in the same region. However, the finding carries a different association with seizures, as rhythmic delta (when not generalized) is associated with seizures, whereas arrhythmic (polymorphic/irregular) is not. These findings are discussed in Chapter 5: Rhythmic and periodic patterns.

(4) *Seizures, status epilepticus and the ictal-interictal continuum* – The EEG interpretation is often sequential. The sensitivity of the EEGer in detecting seizures can be heightened if all the information gathered so far is taken into consideration. Subtle evolution of patterns is often detected more easily when actively looking for the finding in a region of already established cortical hyperexcitability. These topics/patterns are discussed in Chapter 6: Seizures and status epilepticus.

(5) *Long-term trends* – A unique feature of long-term or continuous critical care/ICU EEG is that the brain function (i.e., their neurological state) is often changing over time (and structure is sometimes changing as well) within a single patient's recording session. This provides EEGers the ability to address an additional component of the EEG: changes over time and in particular changes following interventions. A real strength of the long-term EEG is to assess for improvement or deterioration of the patterns and background findings. This can provide clinicians some sense of the trajectory of a patient when the clinical examination is not reliable or when the patient is sleeping. The effects of medication titration, both loading and withdrawal, can be followed. Due to this, it is important to know when certain medications are administered during the EEG recording. Only with this information can responses be conveyed to clinical teams. Many long-term trends are best assessed utilizing quantitative EEG (QEEG) and this will be

covered in the later chapters, especially Chapter 9: QEEG basics and Chapter 10: Special applications and multimodal monitoring.

2.2   Classification using the ACNS Standardized Critical Care EEG Terminology: 2021 version

Careful classification of critical care EEG findings in an objective and quantitative manner has three main strengths:

(1) Allows for the objective comparison of the EEG for any given patient over days to weeks, including across several EEGers. For example, the EEG background continuity changing from discontinuous to near continuous, or the prevalence of periodic discharges (PDs) reducing from abundant to frequent, would be valuable and could signify slow improvement; however, without clear classification standards, it may simply mean there was a different person interpreting the study.

(2) Allows for comparison of findings between patients, to allow clinicians to build an experience base, especially of rare patterns, to determine their clinical associations and help gauge the patterns that may warrant consideration of treatment even when they do not qualify as electrographic seizures.

(3) Allows multicenter research into clinical conditions and electrographic patterns. One of the major limitations with such research in the past, and in EEG teaching in general, is heterogeneity in use of terms. Robust classification minimizes heterogeneity and therefore minimizes the chance of type II error, where the implication of a specific pattern is lost if included in a less stringent (more inclusive) group.

The American Clinical Neurophysiology Society (ACNS) published a guideline that classified mostly RPPs in 2013, with some standards included for reporting background EEG as well. In January 2021, the updated second edition of this guideline was released. The updated guideline is much more comprehensive, with update to previously defined terms and description of many new terms that have emerged since 2013. The content of the terminology has undergone numerous rounds of revisions and validation. The 'reference chart' from the 2021 publication has been reproduced here (Figure 2.1), and many of the diagrams that portray critical concepts have also been reproduced to provide understanding while reading through the remainder of this atlas. All patterns in this book have been described and classified in accordance with this 2021 terminology. The updated terminology now follows a more classical approach to description and classification of all components of the cEEG. This approach is structured in a similar fashion to the approach outlined above (section 2.1). Initially, the background features are described, followed by adding the features of the RPPs, and then seizures. Each term, or descriptor, has been carefully defined in the updated terminology, as a means of forming a strong foundation for cEEG interpretation and reporting, as well as facilitating multicenter research.

Dr. Markus Leitinger MD of the Christian Doppler Medical Centre, Paracelsus Medical University, Salzburg, Austria should be acknowledged for the development of most of the schematic diagrams demonstrating the key features of the ACNS critical care EEG terminology.

The full terminology and related useful tools (reference chart, abbreviated version, EEG examples, training module, access to an online certification test) are available at www.acns.org and are published in the Journal of Clinical Neurophysiology, the official journal of the ACNS.

Figure list

Figure 2.6 State changes and cyclic alternating pattern of encephalopathy (CAPE).

Suggested reading

Gaspard N, Hirsch LJ, LaRoche SM, Hahn CD, Westover MB, for the CCEMRC. Inter-rater agreement for Critical Care EEG Terminology. *Epilepsia.* 2014;**55**(9):1366–1373.

Hirsch LJ, LaRoche SM, Gaspard N, et al. American Clinical Neurophysiology Society's Standardized Critical Care EEG Terminology: 2012 version. *J Clin Neurophysiol.* 2013;**30**(1):1–27.

*Hirsch LJ, Fong MWK, Leitinger M, et al. American Clinical Neurophysiology Society's Standardized Critical Care EEG Terminology: 2021 Version. *J Clin Neurophysiol.* 2021;**38**(1):1–29.

Hofmeijer J, Tjepkema-Cloostermans MC, van Putten MJ. Burst-suppression with identical bursts: a distinct EEG pattern with poor outcome in postanoxic coma. *Clin Neurophysiol.* 2014;**125**(5):947–954.

*Kane N, Acharya J, Benickzy S, et al. A revised glossary of terms most commonly used by clinical electroencephalographers and updated proposal for the report format of the EEG findings. Revision 2017. *Clin Neurophysiol Pract.* 2017;**2**:170–185.

Lee JW, LaRoche S, Choi H, et al. Development and feasibility testing of a critical care EEG monitoring database for standardized clinical reporting and multicenter collaborative research. *J Clin Neurophysiol.* 2016;**33**(2):133–140.

Rodriguez Ruiz A, Vlachy J, Lee JW, et al. Association of periodic and rhythmic electroencephalographic patterns with seizures in critically ill patients. *JAMA Neurol.* 2017;**74**(2):181–188.

Thompson SA, Hantus S. Highly epileptiform bursts are associated with seizure recurrence. *J Clin Neurophysiol.* 2016;**33**(1):66–71.

*Reference defining the terms used in this atlas.

**ACNS Standardized Critical Care EEG Terminology 2021:
Reference Chart**

A. EEG Background									
Symmetry	Background EEG frequency	PDR	Continuity	Reactivity	State Changes	Cyclic Alternating Pattern of Encephalopathy (CAPE)	Voltage	AP Gradient	Breach effect
Symmetric	Beta	Present Specify frequency	Continuous: <1% periods of suppression (<10 µV) or attenuation (≥10 µV but <50% of background voltage)	Reactive	Present with normal stage N2 sleep transients	Present	High ≥150 µV	Present	Present
Mild asymmetry <50% Voltage OR 0.5–1 Hz Frequency	Alpha	Absent		Unreactive	Present but with abnormal stage N2 sleep transients	Absent	Normal ≥20 to <150 µV	Absent	Absent
	Theta	Unclear	Nearly continuous: 1–9% periods of suppression attenuation	SIRPIDs only	Present but without stage N2 sleep transients	Unknown/unclear	Low 10 to <20 µV	Reverse	Unclear
Marked asymmetry ≥50% Voltage OR >1 Hz Frequency	Delta		Discontinuous: 10–49% periods of suppression or attenuation	Unclear	Absent		Suppressed <10 µV		
			Burst-suppression or Burst-attenuation: 50–99% periods of suppression or attenuation	Unknown					
			Suppression: >99% periods of suppression or attenuation						

If Burst-suppression or Burst-attenuation then specify if: ←

Localization of Bursts (G/ L/ Bl/ Ul/ Mf)

Highly Epileptiform Bursts (Present or Absent)

Identical Bursts (Present or Absent)

Figure 2.1. The American Clinical Neurophysiology Society's (ACNS) standardized critical care EEG terminology: 2021 version (reference chart). The reference chart has been reproduced from the ACNS guideline on how to classify findings from prolonged EEG performed in the critically care setting. The various components of the background EEG are first described, followed by rhythmic and periodic patterns (RPPs) and other highly epileptic patterns (i.e., those associated with a high risk of seizures), including seizures themselves, brief potentially ictal rhythmic discharges (BIRDs) and patterns on the ictal-interictal continuum (IIC). Each RPP should be described by combining one of main term 1 (location) and main term 2 (pattern type). In addition, the major modifiers (including Plus modifiers) to RPPs should be documented for each pattern (with the minor modifiers being optional, but helpful). It should then be recorded whether seizures (including the type: electrographic seizure [ESz] and/or electroclinical seizure [ECSz]) and status epilepticus (electrographic status epilepticus [ESE] and/or electroclinical status epilepticus [ECSE]) are present, and/or if there are BIRDs or patterns that are not seizures but fall on the IIC.

Reproduced from Hirsch LJ, Fong MWK, Leitinger M, et al. American Clinical Neurophysiology Society's Standardized Critical Care EEG Terminology: 2021 Version. J Clin Neurophysiol. 2021;38(1):1–29. with permission.

B. Sporadic Epileptiform Discharges	C. Rhythmic and Periodic Patterns (RPPs)	
Prevalence	**Main term 1**	**Main term 2**
Abundant ≥1/10s	**G** *Generalized* - Optional: Specify frontally, occipitally, or midline predominant; or generalized, not otherwise specified.	**PD** *Periodic Discharges*
Frequent ≥1/min but <1/10s	**L** *Lateralized* - Optional: Specify unilateral, bilateral asymmetric, or bilateral asynchronous - Optional: Specify lobe(s) most involved or hemispheric	**RDA** *Rhythmic Delta Activity*
Occasional ≥1/h but <1/min	**BI** *Bilateral Independent* - Optional: Specify symmetric or asymmetric - Optional: Specify lobe(s) most involved or hemispheric	**SW** *Spike and Wave* OR *Polyspike and Wave* OR *Sharp and Wave*
Rare <1/h	**UI** *Unilateral Independent* - Optional: Specify unilateral, bilateral asymmetric, or bilateral asynchronous for each pattern - Optional: Specify lobe(s) most involved	
	Mf *Multifocal* - Optional: Specify symmetric or asymmetric - Optional: Specify lobe(s) most involved or hemispheric	

Figure 2.1. (*Continued*)

Major modifiers								
Prevalence	Duration	Frequency	Phases[1]	Sharpness[2]	Voltage (Absolute)	Voltage (Relative)[3]	Stimulus Induced or Stimulus Terminated	Evolution[4]
Continuous ≥90%	Very long ≥1 h	4 Hz	>3	Spiky <70 ms	High ≥150 μV	>2	SI *Stimulus Induced*	Evolving
		3.5 Hz	3				ST *Stimulus Terminated*	Fluctuating
Abundant 50–89%	Long 10–59 min	3 Hz		Sharp 70–200 ms	Medium 50–149 μV	≤2		
		2.5 Hz	2				Spontaneous only	Static
Frequent 10–49%	Intermediate duration 1–9.9 min	2 Hz	1	Sharply contoured >200 ms	Low 20–49 μV		Unknown	
		1.5 Hz						
Occasional 1–9%		1 Hz			Very low <20 μV			
	Brief 10–59 s	0.5 Hz		Blunt >200 ms				
Rare <1%		<0.5 Hz						
	Very brief <10 s							

Minor modifiers			
Onset	Triphasic[5]	Lag	Polarity[2]
Sudden ≤3 s	Yes	A-P *Anterior-Posterior*	Negative
Gradual >3 s	No		Positive
		P-A *Posterior-Anterior*	Dipole
		No	Unclear

Plus (+) Modifiers
No +
+F *Superimposed fast activity – applies to PD or RDA only* **EDB** (Extreme Delta Brush): A specific subtype of +F
+R *Superimposed rhythmic activity – applies to PD only*
+S *Superimposed sharp waves or spikes, or sharply contoured – applies to RDA only*
+FR *If both subtypes apply – applies to PD only*
+FS *If both subtypes apply – applies to RDA only*

NOTE 1: Phases: Applies to PD and SW only, including the slow wave of the SW complex
NOTE 2: Sharpness and Polarity: Applies to the predominant phase of PD and the spike or sharp component of SW only
NOTE 3: Relative voltage: Applies to PD only
NOTE 4: Evolution: Refers to frequency, location or morphology
NOTE 5: Triphasic: Applies to PD or SW only

Figure 2.1. (*Continued*)

D. Electrographic and Electroclinical Seizures

Electrographic Seizure (ESz)

Either:

A) Epileptiform discharges averaging >2.5 Hz for ≥10 s (>25 discharges in 10 s), OR

B) Any pattern with definite evolution and lasting ≥10 s

Electroclinical Seizure (ECSz)

Any EEG pattern with either:

A) Definite clinical correlate time-locked to the pattern (of any duration), OR

B) EEG _and_ clinical improvement with a parenteral (typically IV) anti-seizure medication

Electrographic Status Epilepticus (ESE)

An electrographic seizure for either:

A) ≥10 continuous minutes, OR

B) A total duration of ≥20% of any 60-minute period of recording.

Electroclinical Status Epilepticus (ECSE)

An electroclinical seizure for either

A) ≥10 continuous minutes, OR

B) A total duration of ≥20% of any 60-minute period of recording, OR

C) ≥5 continuous minutes if the seizure is convulsive (i.e., with bilateral tonic-clonic motor activity).

Possible ECSE: An RPP that qualifies for the IIC (below) that is present for ≥10 continuous minutes or for a total duration of ≥20% of any 60-minute period of recording, which shows EEG improvement with a parenteral anti-seizure medication **BUT** without clinical improvement.

E. Brief Potentially Ictal Rhythmic Discharges (BIRDs)

Focal (including L, BI, UI or Mf) or generalized rhythmic activity >4 Hz (at least 6 waves at a regular rate) lasting ≥0.5 to <10 s, not consistent with a known normal pattern or benign variant, not part of burst-suppression or burst-attenuation, without definite clinical correlate, and that has at least one of A, B or C below:

Definite BIRDs feature either:

A. Evolution ("evolving BIRDs") OR

B. Similar morphology and location as interictal epileptiform discharges or seizures in the same patient

Possible BIRDs are

C. Sharply contoured but without (a) or (b) above

F. Ictal-Interictal Continuum (IIC)

1. Any PD or SW pattern that averages >1.0 Hz but ≤2.5 Hz over 10 s (>10 but ≤25 discharges in 10 s); OR

2. Any PD or SW pattern that averages ≥0.5 Hz and ≤1 Hz over 10 s (≥5 and ≤10 discharges in 10 s), and has a plus modifier or fluctuation; OR

3. Any lateralized RDA averaging >1 Hz for at least 10 s (at least 10 waves in 10 s) with a plus modifier or fluctuation;

AND

4. Does not qualify as an ESz or ESE.

Figure 2.1.   (*Continued*)

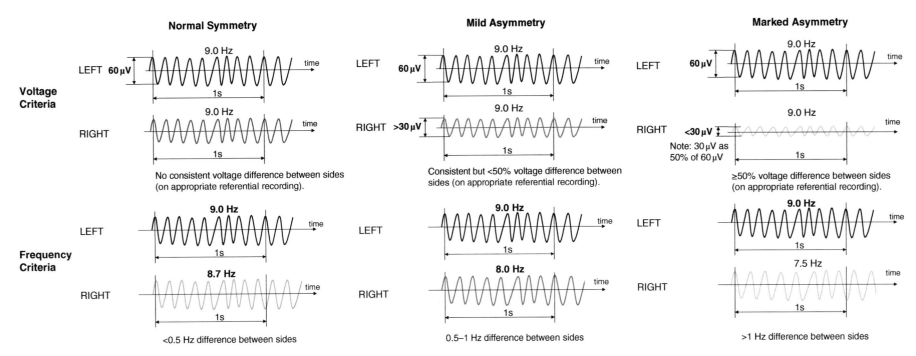

Figure 2.2. Symmetry vs. asymmetry. The background EEG is considered asymmetric if there is a consistent voltage difference between hemispheres or if there is a consistent (≥0.5 Hz) frequency difference between hemispheres. Consistent is defined as being present for ≥80% of the record. Symmetry applies to all background activities (not specifically the posterior dominant rhythm [PDR]). A consistent voltage difference of ≥50% qualifies as a major asymmetry; any visible and consistent asymmetry less than this qualifies as mild asymmetry. Consistent polymorphic slowing in one hemisphere is classified as an asymmetric background; if inconsistent (<80% of the record), it is considered a symmetric background, but with intermittent focal slowing. For example, 7–8-Hz alpha activity in the left hemisphere and 2–3-Hz delta activity on the right throughout a recording is classified as a marked asymmetry in frequency with continuous slowing on the right. If the record was symmetric for >20% of the record and showed this asymmetry for the remainder, this would be considered intermittent slowing on the right with the background being considered symmetric. The prevalence of intermittent slowing is then categorized into abundant, frequent, occasional, etc., as with any other pattern.

Reproduced from Hirsch LJ, Fong MWK, Leitinger M, et al. American Clinical Neurophysiology Society's Standardized Critical Care EEG Terminology: 2021 Version. J Clin Neurophysiol. 2021;38(1):1–29. with permission.

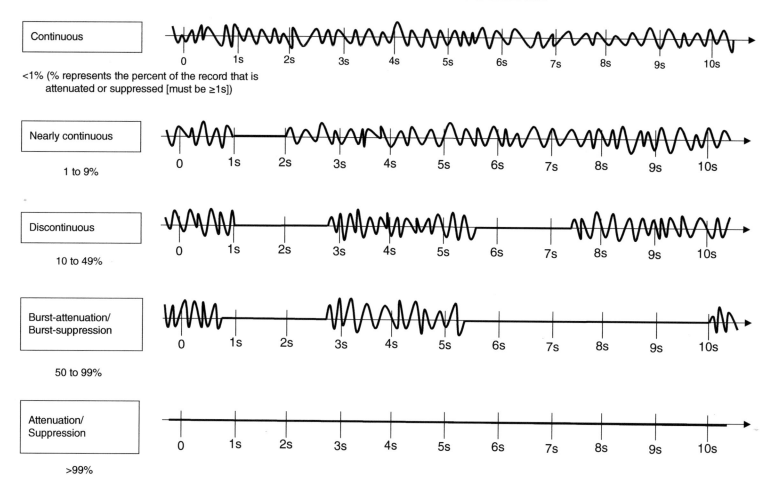

Figure 2.3. Continuity. Continuity refers to the percentage/proportion of the record that is attenuated or suppressed (the exact percentage being referred to as the suppression/attenuation percentage). For example, if for every 10 seconds of the record 2 seconds were attenuated (attenuated is defined as activity ≥10 μV but <50% of the higher voltage background) or suppressed (activity <10 μV), then the suppression/attenuation percentage would be 20% and the record would be 'discontinuous' (because 20% falls between the 10–49% range that defines discontinuity). For an episode of attenuation/suppression to count toward these percentages the episode must last at least one second, i.e., 0.5 s of attenuation/suppression does not count toward the suppression percentage.

Reproduced from Hirsch LJ, Fong MWK, Leitinger M, et al. American Clinical Neurophysiology Society's Standardized Critical Care EEG Terminology: 2021 Version. J Clin Neurophysiol. 2021;38(1):1–29. with permission.

Majority (>50%) of bursts with 2 or more epileptiform
discharges (EDs)

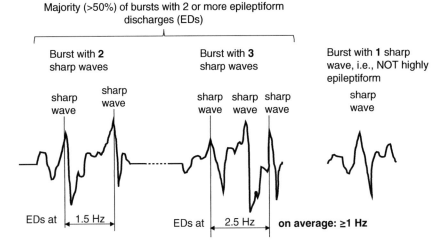

Criterion 1: Two or more
epileptiform discharges (spikes or
sharp waves), within the majority
(>50%) of bursts, and occur at an
average of 1 Hz or faster within a
single burst

Burst with **2**
sharp waves

Burst with **3**
sharp waves

Burst with **1** sharp
wave, i.e., NOT highly
epileptiform

sharp   sharp
wave   wave

sharp   sharp   sharp
wave   wave   wave

sharp
wave

EDs at   1.5 Hz   EDs at   2.5 Hz   **on average: ≥1 Hz**

..... dotted lines represents longer duration of suppression for reasons of presentation

Majority (>50%) of bursts with rhythmic
potentially ictal-appearing pattern

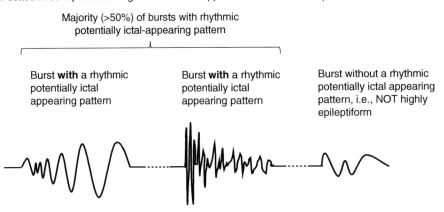

Criteron 2: A rhythmic, potentially
ictal –appearing pattern, within the
majority (>50%) of bursts

Burst **with** a rhythmic
potentially ictal
appearing pattern

Burst **with** a rhythmic
potentially ictal
appearing pattern

Burst without a rhythmic
potentially ictal appearing
pattern, i.e., NOT highly
epileptiform

..... dotted lines represents longer duration of suppression for reasons of presentation

Figure 2.4. Highly epileptiform bursts. The presence of highly epileptiform bursts (HEBs) (as a part of burst suppression/attenuation) influences the probability of status epilepticus recurrence should a highly sedating ASM be weaned. HEBs are defined as present if either of the following two criteria are met:

(1) If 2 or more epileptiform discharges (spikes or sharp waves) are seen within the majority (>50%) of bursts and occur at an average of 1 Hz or faster within a single burst (frequency is calculated as the inverse of the typical interpeak latency of consecutive epileptiform discharges within a single burst). (NOTE: The third burst in the top panel does contain a single epileptiform sharp wave, however, this is not 'highly epileptiform' because it does not contain 2 or more discharges.) OR

(2) If a rhythmic, potentially ictal-appearing pattern occurs within the majority (>50%) of bursts. (NOTE: The first two examples of bursts in the lower panel represent the beginning of ESzs and are therefore 'highly epileptiform' whereas the third burst in the lower panel consists of medium-amplitude polymorphic theta/delta activity, i.e., does not look like the beginning of a seizure, and is therefore not 'highly epileptiform'.)

Reproduced from Hirsch LJ, Fong MWK, Leitinger M, et al. American Clinical Neurophysiology Society's Standardized Critical Care EEG Terminology: 2021 Version. J Clin Neurophysiol. 2021;38(1):1–29. with permission.

Criterion 1: The first 0.5 s or longer of each burst is visually similar in all channels in the vast majority (>90%) of bursts

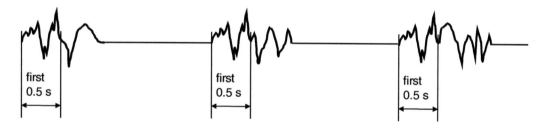

first 0.5 s   first 0.5 s   first 0.5 s

Criterion 2: The first 0.5 s or longer of each of **two or more** bursts in a **stereotyped cluster** are visually similar in all channels in the vast majority (>90%) of bursts

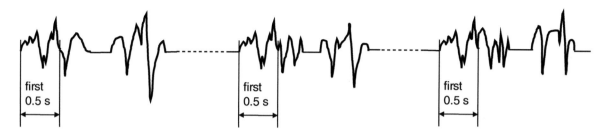

first 0.5 s   first 0.5 s   first 0.5 s

Figure 2.5. Identical bursts. Identical bursts could be conceptually considered as a state of extreme invariance, where all of the bursts are the same, i.e., they lack variability. In this state, the first 0.5 seconds or longer of *each burst*, or the first 0.5 seconds or longer of two or more bursts occurring in a *stereotyped cluster*, are visually similar in all channels in the vast majority (>90%) of bursts or clusters of bursts. A point to make is that only the first 0.5 seconds of each burst or stereotyped cluster needs to be visually similar to be classified as 'identical bursts'. For example, the second half of each burst in the top panel, and the second part of each stereotyped cluster in the bottom panel, are actually different, but the first 0.5 seconds are all identical, so they still qualify.

Reproduced from Hirsch LJ, Fong MWK, Leitinger M, et al. American Clinical Neurophysiology Society's Standardized Critical Care EEG Terminology: 2021 Version. J Clin Neurophysiol. 2021;38(1):1–29. with permission.

State changes

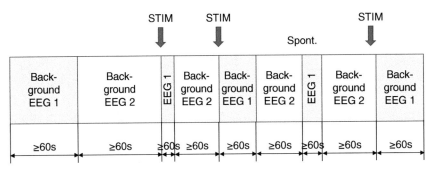

At least 2 sustained types of background EEG:

1. Related to level of alertness or stimulation
2. Each must persist at ≥60 s to qualify as a "state"
3. Stimulation should be able to transition the patient from the less alert to more alert/more stimulated state
4. The more alert/more stimulated state is considered the "reported background" EEG
5. State changes can also occur spontaneously

EEG background 1: stimulated/more awake: used for background feature description ("reported background")
EEG background 2: unstimulated/less awake state; commonly lasts minutes to hours (minimum: 60 s)

STIM = stimulation, Spont. = spontaneous

Cyclic Alternating Pattern of Encephalopathy (CAPE)

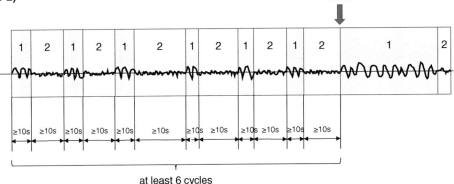

Changes in EEG background patterns 1 and 2:

1. each lasting at least 10 s,
2. **spontanously** alternating between the two patterns in a regular manner,
3. for at least 6 cycles.

at least 6 cycles

Figure 2.6. State changes and cyclic alternating pattern of encephalopathy (CAPE). State changes are present if there are at least 2 sustained types of background EEG related to level of alertness or stimulation; each must persist at least 60 seconds to qualify as a 'state'. Stimulation should be able to transition the patient from the less alert to more alert/more stimulated state. State changes can also occur spontaneously. The more alert/stimulated pattern is considered the primary reported 'background' EEG pattern for the patient. State changes can be characterized as:

a) present with normal stage N2 sleep transients (K-complexes and spindles)

b) present but with abnormal stage N2 sleep transients

c) present but without stage N2 sleep transients

d) absent.

CAPE refers to changes in background patterns, each lasting at least 10 s, and spontaneously alternating between the two patterns in a regular manner for at least 6 cycles (but often lasts minutes to hours). If each pattern of CAPE lasts >60 s this would also qualify as presence of state changes. This is a newly defined pattern, essentially unstudied at this point, but may reflect a better prognosis in the critically ill; it is certainly better than having an unreactive record.

Reproduced from Hirsch LJ, Fong MWK, Leitinger M, et al. American Clinical Neurophysiology Society's Standardized Critical Care EEG Terminology: 2021 Version. J Clin Neurophysiol. 2021;38(1):1–29. with permission.

3 Encephalopathy and coma

3.1 Nonspecific patterns of encephalopathy

There are many nonspecific changes in the EEG that occur during diffuse encephalopathies. Early changes include slowing of the alpha rhythm and excess slowing during wakefulness, first theta and then delta. This is followed by loss of the alpha rhythm, more prominent (mainly delta) slowing, loss of normal faster activity and loss or attenuation of normal sleep transients. Abnormal arousal patterns, such as the cyclic alternating pattern of encephalopathy (CAPE), and generalized rhythmic delta activity (GRDA) may also be seen. GRDA is most commonly seen in diffuse encephalopathy and is nonspecific. Examples of GRDA can be found in Chapter 5: Rhythmic and periodic patterns (RPPs).

As encephalopathy worsens, changes include loss of normal variability and state changes, loss of reactivity to external stimuli including pain, possibly burst suppression, diffuse attenuation and ultimately electrocerebral inactivity (a 'flat' tracing). It is important to recognize that most or all of these patterns can be produced in a normal brain via the use of high dose sedatives such as barbiturates, propofol and benzodiazepines.

3.2 Grading of encephalopathy

Grading the degree of encephalopathy is clinically valuable; and allows for the progress (improvement/deterioration) of a patient to be objectively monitored over time (especially if the clinical examination is unreliable). Although the term 'encephalopathy' is a clinical diagnosis (and therefore does not feature in the ICU EEG terminology), as a patient becomes progressively encephalopathic and enters coma there are a number of sequential (mostly generalized) EEG changes that suggest deeper states of diffuse cerebral dysfunction. Documenting the severity of encephalopathy also provides ancillary information that can assist in patient prognostication.

Two of the most validated encephalopathy grading scales were proposed by Synek, VM in 1988 and Young et al. in 1997. Both scales, which have been replicated in Tables 3.1 and 3.2, mostly described EEG changes that would fall under 'background EEG' in the latest terminology. The inter-rater reliability was good to very good for both scales, and the prognostic implications to the various 'grades and subgrades' of encephalopathy were determined. It should be noted that several specific clinical states, such as 'alpha, theta or spindle coma' do not feature in the ICU EEG terminology. Similar to 'encephalopathy', the terminology provides the descriptive tools to classify the EEG changes and avoids clinical interpretation. For example, the EEG finding of an 'unreactive alpha record without state changes' would infer the clinical state of 'alpha coma', and practically (including at times in this atlas) the EEG and clinical terms are used interchangeably.

Since the publication of the above EEG grading systems there have been several updates in the literature:

(1) The clinical importance of certain features (such as reactivity) has been further studied, and many have become important determinants of prognosis.

Hirsch and Brenner's Atlas of EEG in Critical Care, Second Edition. Lawrence J. Hirsch, Michael W.K. Fong, and Richard P. Brenner.
© 2023 John Wiley & Sons Ltd. Published 2023 by John Wiley & Sons Ltd.

TABLE 3.1 **Synek EEG Coma Scale (1988)**

Grade of encephalopathy	Description	Subgrades or subdivisions
I	Predominantly regular alpha activity with some scattered activity in the theta frequency range (reactive)	
II	Predominantly theta range activity with some alpha and delta waves	a. Normal voltage, reactive b. Low voltage, unreactive
III	Predominantly delta activity (regular or irregular) with little activity in other frequencies. Further divided into 'subgrades' consisting of:	a. High voltage rhythmic delta activity that is maximal frontally (reactive) [Would now be described as GRDA]. b. Spindle coma c. Low voltage irregular delta (non-reactive) d. Medium voltage irregular delta (non-reactive)
IV	a. Burst-suppression	i. With epileptiform activity (epileptiform discharges consisting of polyspikes or clusters of sharp waves) [Now referred to as highly epileptiform bursts] ii. No epileptiform activity
	b. Alpha coma	i. With some reactivity ii. Without reactivity
	c. Theta coma	
	d. Low output EEG, voltages less than 20 μV but not suppressed	
V (Suppression)	Absence of cerebral activity (all activity <2 μV).	

Adapted from Synek VM. *EEG abnormality grades and subdivisions of prognostic importance in traumatic and anoxic coma in adults.* Clin Electroencephalogr. 1988;19(3):160–166. The grading system was originally validated in patients with TBI and post anoxic brain injury, but later tested across a range of disease processes.

(2) Select patterns (e.g., highly epileptiform bursts) have been further characterized, but in order to limit heterogeneity they have been mostly studied in very specific patient cohorts (e.g., in the weaning of highly sedating anti-seizure medications used for treatment of status epilepticus, or in post anoxic brain injury).

(3) The definitions of certain terms have become standardized and some of these differ from historical definitions (such as the definition of burst suppression mentioned above).

(4) New patterns/terms have been identified (such as identical bursts) that were not included in these original classification systems.

(5) Old descriptions (such as triphasic waves) have been further assessed and their specific association with encephalopathy (or any other clinical scenario) placed in question.

The result of the above has meant the above grading systems have been poorly adopted into routine clinical practice and the information included in them possibly outdated. The prior grading systems were not intuitively linear, e.g., in both systems a predominantly theta record (Synek grade II, Young grade I) was classified as either (1) reactive or (2) unreactive. However, if a record is unreactive this has a worse prognosis than GRDA (Synek grade IIIa)

TABLE 3.2 **Young et al.; EEG Classification for Coma (1997)**

Category	Subcategory
I Delta/theta >50% of record (not theta coma)	A) Reactivity
	B) No reactivity
II Triphasic waves	
III Burst-suppression	A) With epileptiform activity
	B) Without epileptiform activity
IV Alpha/theta/spindle coma (unreactive)	
V Epileptiform activity (not in burst-suppression pattern)*	A) Generalized
	B) Focal or multifocal
VI Suppression	A) <20 µV, but >10 µV
	B) ≤10 µV

Reproduced from Young GB, et al., *An Electroencephalographic Classification for Coma.* Canadian Journal of Neurological Sciences. 1997;24(04):320–325.

It should be noted that some of the suggestions differ significantly from the updated definitions of the same term. For example, Young, et al., suggested that burst-suppression pattern should have generalized flattening at standard sensitivity for ≥1 second at least every 20 seconds. Under current terminology 1 second of suppression every 20 seconds equates to a suppression percent of 5% and therefore that record would be classified as 'nearly continuous' rather than burst suppression, which would require a suppression percent between 50–99% of the record. If more than one category applied, then it was suggested that the most 'serious' category should be selected. Therefore the 1997 classification did not account for multiple patterns to be included in the same record.

[a] 'Epileptiform activity' was not specifically defined; however, the example of activity included under this category consisted of a highly epileptiform pattern of fluctuating spiky 1.5–2-Hz GPDs on a suppressed background (i.e., a pattern that would currently be considered on the ictal-interictal continuum).

when this pattern was later studied; or unreactive vs those with epileptiform discharges (Young grade IV). A grading system for encephalopathy should ideally only make comment on the degree of diffuse dysfunction, i.e., should not have implications outside of this discussion. The prior grading systems included terms such as epileptiform discharges, which clearly have implications on the probability of subsequent seizures. One of the main limiting factors of historical studies has been that over the years the definitions of many

of the terms have been debated, refined and standardized. Take the example of 'burst suppression'. As mentioned in the legend of Table 3.2, Young et al.'s definition of burst suppression would have included many patients' EEGs that would now be classified as either 'nearly continuous' or 'discontinuous'. The implication of this is that the 'severity' and clinical prognosis attributed to many of these patterns may no longer be valid.

There is currently no universally accepted scale of encephalopathy. Surveys have shown that most institutions either use no specific scale or utilize center-specific grading systems that are much more basic. These grading systems often use the terms 'mild', 'mild to moderate', 'moderate', 'moderate to severe' and 'severe' to classify severity of diffuse dysfunction. The major benefit of this is that they are much easier to understand and integrate into clinical practice. For example, if the EEG findings for a given patient changed from 'severe' to 'mild', this intuitively suggests improvement. An example of such a grading system is the Yale Adult Background EEG Grading Scale 2021 (Table 3.3). This was generated after a series of multicenter surveys of experts about which features are most important, how many categories to use, etc., and has not yet been validated. These scales specifically only comment on features of the 'background' EEG and allow focal findings, sporadic epileptiform discharges and RPPs to stand independent of this. Additional features of the EEG, such as loss of physiologic sleep transients, are also markers of encephalopathy; however, these were not consistently utilized across centers and therefore were not specifically incorporated into the grading scale.

The grading should begin from severe to normal, i.e., if there is no PDR, no reactivity (with adequate testing), and no state changes the record automatically indicates 'severe dysfunction' irrespective of any other features such as the predominant frequency.

3.3 Findings in specific medical conditions

All metabolic encephalopathies can cause diffuse slowing, generalized periodic discharges (GPDs) including GPDs with triphasic morphology (also known as triphasic waves), and most predispose to seizures as well. Conditions that commonly lead to these findings are hepatic or renal failure, hyponatremia, Hashimoto's encephalopathy and COVID-19-related

TABLE 3.3 **Yale Adult Encephalopathy Scale (2021)**

Required fields highlighted in yellow	Normal	Mild	Mild - Moderate	Moderate	Moderate - Severe	Severe	Complete Suppression of Cerebral Rhythms[c]
Predominant frequency, most awake state	Alpha or LVF[a] with minimal theta, no delta	≥7 Hz or LVF[a] with prominent theta or any delta (whether rhythmic or not)	For patients who do not meet all criteria for either Mild or Moderate but fall somewhere in between	3–6 Hz	For patients who do not meet all criteria for either Moderate or Severe but fall somewhere in between, OR with LVF in a non-interactive patient[a]	Any	NA
Posterior dominant rhythm (PDR)	≥8.5 or LVF[a]	Present (any freq) or LVF[a] background		Absent		Absent	NA
Continuity, most awake state	Continuous	Continuous		Continuous or nearly continuous		NR	NA
Reactivity	NR[b]	NR[b]		Reactive or SIRPIDs-only		Unreactive or SIRPIDs-only	NA
State changes	NR[b]	NR[b]		Present		Absent	NA

[a] LVF = low voltage beta (or faster) activity diffusely: In awake patients with meaningful interaction, LVF can be part of a normal background, mild dysfunction or mild-moderate dysfunction based on other features. In patients without meaningful interaction, LVF should be classified as moderate to severe if EEG is reactive, and severe if unreactive and without state changes.
[b] NR: Not required. These features are not part of the definition of that level of dysfunction, but all records will be reactive and have state changes if a long enough recording is obtained.
[c] Complete suppression: No discernible cerebral rhythms whether or not standards for determination of electrocerebral silence are met. NA: Not Applicable

encephalopathy. Neuroleptic malignant syndrome, serotonin syndrome and some medication toxicities (i.e., cefepime, baclofen, lithium, ifosfamide, CAR-T cell therapy and others) can cause similar patterns. One particular pattern of encephalopathy, the extreme delta brush (EDB) pattern, was initially described in the setting of anti-NMDA receptor mediated encephalitis. Since then, it has been confirmed to have reasonable specificity for the condition (but not 100%) and its features have now been defined in the 2021 ACNS terminology (Figures 3.18, 3.19 and 3.20).

3.4 Medication effects

Many medications exert their effect on the brain and hence can cause changes to the EEG. The number of medications that can alter the EEG is exhaustive. In broad terms these medications can be split into (1) those that cause an

intended effect on the brain or (2) those that have an unintended adverse effect on the brain.

Medications with an intended effect

The most commonly encountered medications with effects on the brain are the highly sedating anti-seizure medications (ASMs), which are often administered intravenously while the cEEG is being recorded in order to control seizures or status epilepticus. Sequentially increasing the dose of any sedative or anesthetic agent will eventually result in diffuse dysfunction of increasing severity (as discussed above). Agents reported to result in marginally more specific EEG changes are:

(1) benzodiazepines and barbiturates, which lead to an excess of fast activity, primarily beta range

(2) dexmedetomidine (selective alpha-2-adrenoreceptor agonist), which is predominantly given for non-opioid sedation in the setting of agitation, induces a state that resembles N2 sleep with prominent spindle-like activity

(3) propofol, which at lower levels causes prominent beta activity, followed by moderate to high amplitude 2–3 Hz delta, and then emergence of 14-Hz spindle-like activity if dosing is maintained and

(4) ketamine, which results in increases in delta activity but with some laboratory evidence of retention of gamma range activity, while attenuating activity in other frequencies.

An important caveat is that most of this information comes from documented use of anesthetic agents in healthy brains. In the critical care setting these medications are being administered to patients with severely altered systemic and cerebral physiology with highly abnormal EEG patterns to start. In this context, administration often leads to an alteration of the EEG pattern, but not necessarily the emergence of the typical EEG response. The second point is that the above descriptions are not absolutely specific. At high enough levels, almost all the agents above can cause burst suppression followed by electrocerebral inactivity.

Medications with an unintended adverse effect

There are also many medications that can cause an unintended adverse effect on the brain and EEG. These medications are administered for an action that is not controlling seizures, but can result in diffuse slowing, epileptiform discharges, GPDs and seizures (similar to the changes described in section 3.3 above that occur in the metabolic encephalopathies). The medications most established to cause such changes are the centrally acting agents of baclofen, lithium and clozapine, as well as the fourth-generation cephalosporin antibiotics, such as cefepime. Medications with a modest association with encephalopathic changes include metronidazole, isoniazid, theophylline, cyclosporine and tacrolimus.

Figure list

Figure 3.1 Mild generalized slowing.

Figure 3.2 Excess beta and an active versus inactive reference.

Figure 3.3 Mild to moderate generalized slowing.

Figure 3.4 Moderate generalized slowing.

Figure 3.5 Continuity (burst suppression, discontinuous, continuous).

Figure 3.6 Frontal intermittent rhythmic delta activity (FIRDA).

Figure 3.7 Moderate to severe generalized slowing.

Figure 3.8 Moderate to severe generalized slowing.

Figure 3.9 Reactivity in coma.

Figure 3.10 Reactivity in coma.

Figure 3.11 Reactivity in coma.

Figure 3.12 Alpha coma.

Figure 3.13 Spindle coma.

Figure 3.14 Diffuse attenuation/suppression.

Figure 3.15 Diffuse suppression.

Figure 3.16 Electrocerebral inactivity.

Figure 3.17 Hepatic failure with 14 Hz positive spikes.

Figure 3.18 Extreme delta brush (EDB).

Figure 3.19 Extreme delta brush (EDB).

Figure 3.20 Extreme delta brush (EDB), periodic variant.

Figure 3.21 COVID-19-related encephalopathy.

Figure 3.22 Phenytoin toxicity.

Figure 3.23 Baclofen toxicity.

Figure 3.24 Cefepime toxicity.

Figure 3.25 Benzodiazepine effect.

Figure 3.26 Mild generalized slowing and dexmedetomidine.

Figure 3.27 Nearly continuous background and propofol effect.

Figure 3.28 Propofol effect on epileptiform pattern in NCSE.

Figure 3.29 Ketamine effect on epileptiform pattern.

Figure 3.30 Barbiturate-induced burst suppression.

Figure 3.31 Electrocerebral inactivity due to barbiturates.

EEGs throughout this atlas have been shown with the following standard recording filters unless otherwise specified: LFF 1 Hz, HFF 70 Hz, notch filter off.

Suggested reading

Akeju O, Song AH, Hamilos AE, et al. Electroencephalogram signatures of ketamine anesthesia-induced unconsciousness. *Clin Neurophysiol.* 2016;**127**(6):2414–2422.

Antony AR, Haneef Z. Systematic review of EEG findings in 617 patients diagnosed with COVID-19. *Seizure.* 2020;**83**:234–241.

Bahamon-Dussan JE, Celesia GG, Grigg-Damberger MM. Prognostic significance of EEG triphasic waves in patients with altered state of consciousness. *J Clin Neurophysiol* 1989;**6**:313–319.

Bickford RG, Butt HR. Hepatic coma: the electroencephalographic pattern. *J Clin Invest* 1955;**34**:790–799.

Blume WT. Drug effects on EEG. *J Clin Neurophysiol* 2006;**23**:306–311.

Capparelli FJ, Diaz MF, Hlavnika A, Wainsztein NA, Leiguarda R, Del Castillo ME. Cefepime- and cefixime-induced encephalopathy in a patient with normal renal function. *Neurology* 2005;**65**:1840

Chatrian GE, White LW, Daly D. Electroencephalographic patterns resembling those of sleep in certain comatose states after injuries to the head. *Electroencephalogr Clin Neurophysiol* 1963;**15**:272–280.

Dhakar MB, Sheikh ZB, Desai M, Desai RA, Sternberg EJ, Popescu C, Baron-Lee J, Rampal N, Hirsch LJ, Gilmore EJ, Maciel CB. Developing a Standardized Approach to Grading the Level of Brain Dysfunction on EEG. *J Clin Neurophysiol.* 2022.

Fisch BJ, Klass DW. The diagnostic specificity of triphasic wave patterns. *Electroencephalogr Clin Neurophysiol* 1988;**70**:1–8.

Foley JM, Watson CW, Adams RD. Significance of the electroencephalographic changes in hepatic coma. *Trans Am Neurol Assoc* 1950;**75**:161–164.

Foreman B, Mahulikar A, Tadi P, et al. Generalized periodic discharges and 'triphasic waves': A blinded evaluation of inter-rater agreement and clinical significance. *Clin Neurophysiol.* 2016;**127**(2):1073–1080.

Fountain NB, Waldman WA. Effects of benzodiazepines on triphasic waves: implications for nonconvulsive status epilepticus. *J Clin Neurophysiol* 2001;**18**:345–352.

Hansotia P, Gottschalk P, Green P, et al. Spindle coma: incidence, clinicopathologic correlates, and prognostic value. *Neurology* 1981;**31**:83–87.

Herkes GK, Wszolek ZK, Westmoreland BF, Klass DW. Effects of midazolam on electroencephalograms of seriously ill patients. *Mayo Clin Proc* 1992;**67**:334–338.

Hockaday JM, Potts F, Epstein E, Bonazzi A, Schwab RS. Electroencephalographic changes in acute cerebral anoxia from cardiac or respiratory arrest. *Electroencephalogr Clin Neurophysiol* 1965;**18**:575–586.

Hormes JT, Benarroch EE, Rodriguez M, Klass DW. Periodic sharp waves in baclofen-induced encephalopathy. *Arch Neurol* 1988;**45**:814–815.

Hughes JR. Correlations between EEG and chemical changes in uremia. *Electroencephalogr Clin Neurophysiol* 1980a;**48**:583–594.

Kaplan PW, Genoud D, Ho TW, et al. Etiology, neurologic correlations, and prognosis in alpha coma. *Clin Neurophysiol* 1999;**110**:205–213.

Kaplan PW, Genoud D, Ho TW, et al. Clinical correlates and prognosis in early spindle coma. *J Clin Neurophysiol* 2000;**111**:584–590.

Kaplan PW, Birbeck G. Lithium-induced confusional states: nonconvulsive status epilepticus or triphasic encephalopathy? *Epilepsia* 2006;**47**:2071–2074.

Karnaze DS, Bickford RG. Triphasic waves: A reassessment of their significance. *Electroencephalogr Clin Neurophysiol* 1984;**57**:193–198.

Lin L, Al-Faraj A, Ayub N, et al. Electroencephalographic abnormalities are common in COVID-19 and are associated with outcomes. *Ann Neurol.* 2021;**89**(5):872–883.

Martinez-Rodriguez JE, Barriga FJ, Santamaria J, Iranzo A, et al. Nonconvulsive status epilepticus associated with cephalosporins in patients with renal failure. *Am J Med* 2001;**111**:115–119.

Mason KP, O'Mahony E, Zurakowski D, Libenson MH. Effects of dexmedetomidine sedation on the EEG in children. *Paediatr Anaesth.* 2009;**19**(12):1175–1183.

Moise AM, Karakis I, Herlopian A, et al. Continuous EEG findings in autoimmune encephalitis. *J Clin Neurophysiol.* 2021;**38**(2):124–129.

Primavera A, Audenino D, Cocito L. Ifosfamide encephalopathy and nonconvulsive status epilepticus. *Can J Neurol Sci* 2002;**29**:180–183.

Rae-Grant AD, Strapple C, Barbour PJ. Episodic low-amplitude events: An under-recognized phenomenon in clinical electroencephalography. *J Clin Neurophysiol* 1991;**8**:203–211.

Rae-Grant A, Blume W, Lau C, Hachinski VC, et al. The electroencephalogram in Alzheimer-type dementia. A sequential study correlating the electroencephalogram with psychometric and quantitative pathologic data. *Arch Neurol* 1987;**44**:50–54

Rubin DB, Danish HH, Ali AB, et al. Neurological toxicities associated with chimeric antigen receptor T-cell therapy. *Brain.* 2019;**142**(5):1334–1348.

San-Juan D, Chiappa KH, Cole AJ. Propofol and the electroencephalogram. *Clin Neurophysiol.* 2010;**121**(7):998–1006.

Schauble B, Castillo PR, Boeve BF, Westmoreland BF. EEG findings in steroid-responsive encephalopathy associated with autoimmune thyroiditis. *Clin Neurophysiol* 2003;**114**:32–37

Schmitt SE, Pargeon K, Frechette ES, Hirsch LJ, Dalmau J, Friedman D. Extreme delta brush: a unique EEG pattern in adults with anti-NMDA receptor encephalitis. *Neurology.* 2012;**79**(11):1094–1100.

Smith SJ, Kocen RS. A Creutzfeldt-Jakob like syndrome due to lithium toxicity. *J Neurol Neurosurg Psychiatry* 1988;**51**:120–123.

Stecker MM, Sabau D, Sullivan L, et al. American Clinical Neurophysiology Society Guideline 6: Minimum Technical Standards for EEG Recording in Suspected Cerebral Death. *J Clin Neurophysiol.* 2016;**33**(4):324–327.

Sundaram MBM, Blume WT. Triphasic waves: clinical correlates and morphology. *Can J Neurol Sci* 1987;**14**:136–140.

Synek VM. Prognostically important EEG coma patterns in diffuse anoxic and traumatic encephalopathies in adults. *J Clin Neurophysiol* 1988;**5**:161–174.

Synek VM. Validity of a revised EEG coma scale for predicting survival in anoxic encephalopathy. *Clin Exp Neurol.* 1989;**26**:119–127.

Westmoreland BF, Klass DW, Sharbrough FW, et al. Alpha-coma: electroencephalographic, clinical, pathologic and etiologic correlations. *Arch Neurol* 1975;**32**:713–718.

Wieser HG, Schindler K, Zumsteg D. EEG in Creutzfeldt-Jakob disease. *Clin Neurophysiol* 2006;**117**:935

Young GB, Blume WT, Campbell VM, et al. Alpha, theta and alpha-theta coma: a clinical outcome study utilizing serial recordings. *Electroencephalogr Clin Neurophysiol* 1994;**91**:93–99

Young GB, McLachlan RS, Kreeft JH, Demelo JD. An electroencephalographic classification for coma. *Can J Neurol Sci* 1997;**24**:320–325.

Zak R, Solomon G, Petito F, Labar D. Baclofen-induced generalized nonconvulsive status epilepticus. *Ann Neurol* 1994;**36**:113–114.

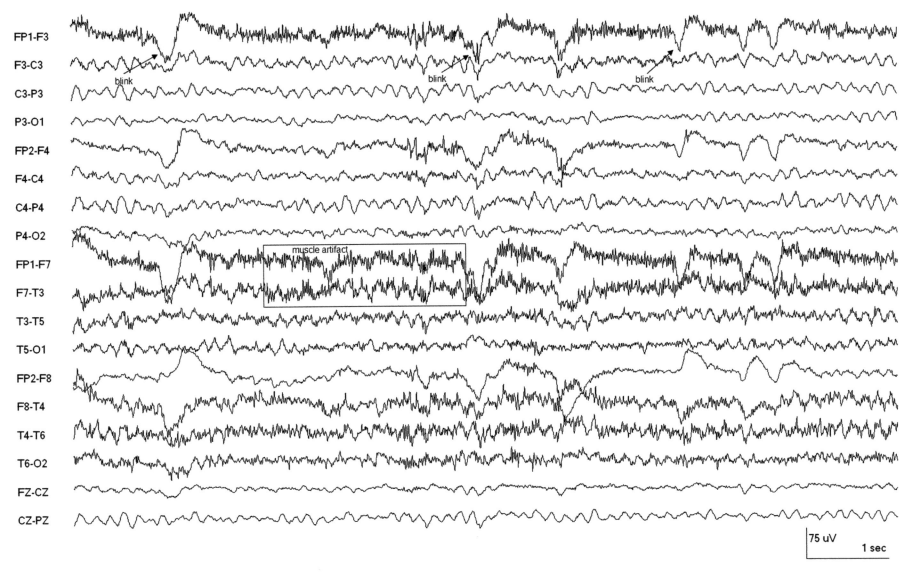

Figure 3.1. Mild generalized slowing. The EEG in this 72-year-old man with renal failure shows mild diffuse slowing of background rhythms (mostly 7 Hz). The patient is awake, as evidenced by muscle artifact (especially at Fp1-F7 and F7-T3) and eye blinks (arrows). There is a probable posterior dominant rhythm of 7 Hz as well., though reactivity is not shown in this sample.

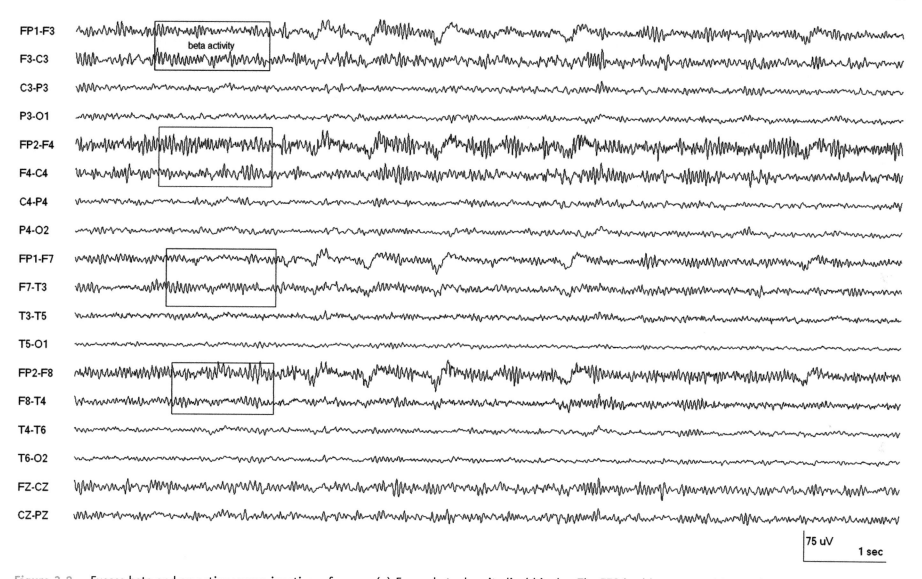

Figure 3.2. Excess beta and an active versus inactive reference. (a) Excess beta, longitudinal bipolar. The EEG in this 18-year-old man shows an excessive amount of beta activity anteriorly (box). The patient was receiving benzodiazepines.

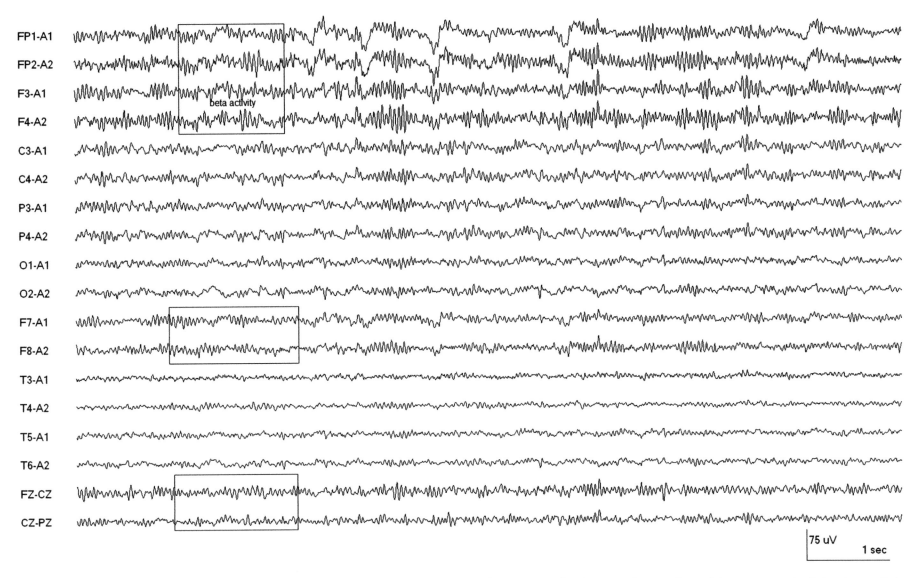

Figure 3.2.   (*Continued*) (b) Excess beta and inactive (good) reference, referential. The same epoch reformatted to a referential montage to ipsilateral ears. Beta activity is most prominent in Fp1-A1, Fp2 -A2, F3 -A1 and F4-A2 (box).

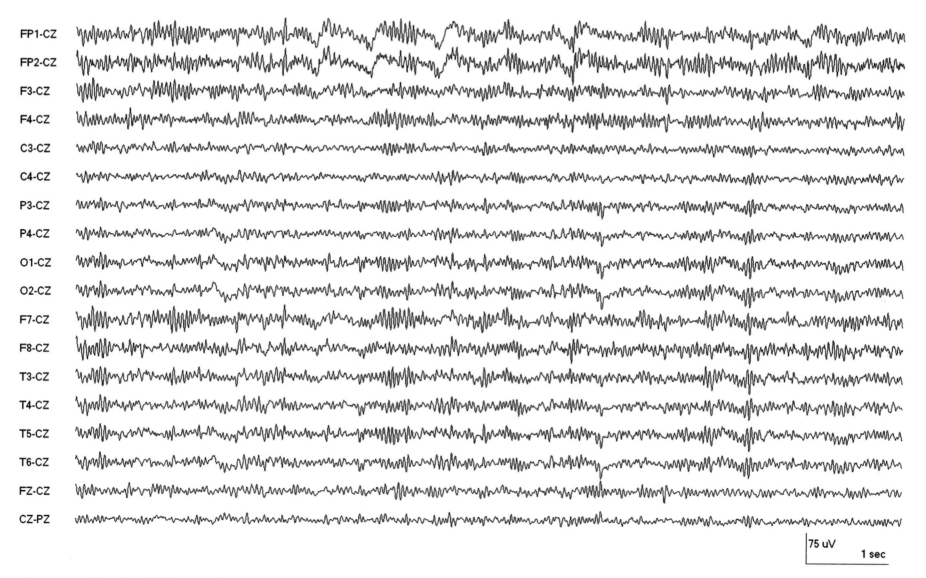

75 uV

1 sec

Figure 3.2. (*Continued*) (c) Excess beta and active (contaminated) reference, referential. The same epoch reformatted to a referential montage to the midline vertex electrode (Cz). Note that in the prior two figures there was relatively little beta activity in the mid and posterior temporal electrodes (T3, T4, T5 and T6). When referenced to Cz however the beta activity appears just as prominent in the temporal electrodes as the frontal electrodes (FP1, F3, FP2 and F4), and relatively reduced centrally (C3, C4). This is an example of selection of a contaminated reference (Cz). In this case the activity of interest is the beta activity, which is maximal fronto-centrally. Selecting Cz as a reference results in the inclusion of that activity in the reference (i.e., Cz includes the activity or interest, or Cz is 'contaminated'). In that case input 1 (region with little activity, e.g., temporal) minus input 2 (Cz that includes the activity) provides a large deflection (not because the temporal region is involved but because the reference is). On the flip side, the activity in neighboring central electrodes (C3, C4) is relatively the same as the activity in Cz, therefore subtracting these electrodes results in little deflection (remember an isoelectric line does not mean that there is no activity present, it means that the activity in both input 1 and input 2 are the same). Thus, selecting an 'active' reference can result in misleading information, suggesting a non-involved region is involved and vice versa.

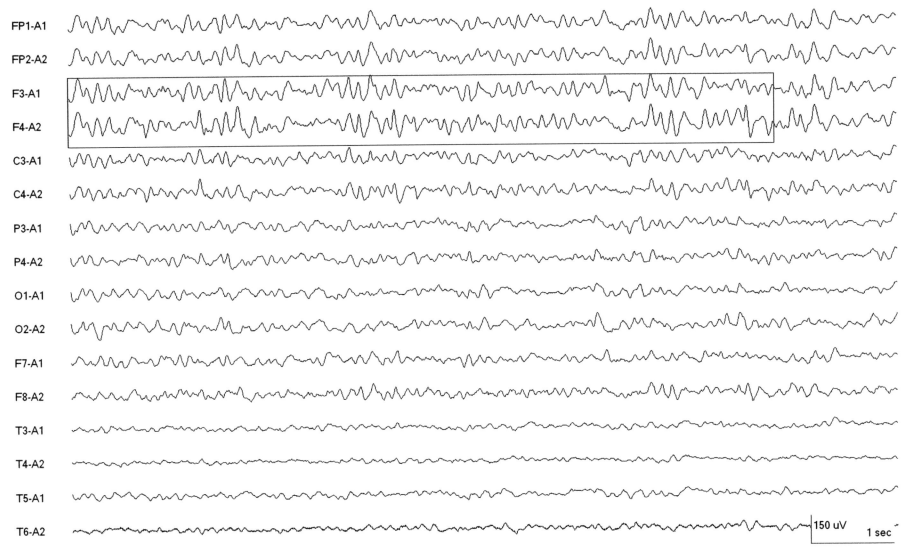

Figure 3.3. Mild to moderate generalized slowing, referential. This is the EEG of a 44-year-old woman with hepatic failure secondary to an acetaminophen overdose. There is again diffuse or generalized slowing of background activity predominantly in the 6–8 Hz range. This demonstrates reversal of the AP gradient utilizing a referential montage to the ipsilateral ear. The activity is higher amplitude and slower in the anterior head regions (box). There is no posterior dominant rhythm; if maximally awake in this segment, this would indicate mild-moderate diffuse dysfunction. A referential montage is useful to confirm reversal of the AP gradient, as apparently low activity (flat tracing) at the back of the head with a bipolar montage could just be due to common mode rejection where there is relatively similar activity at O1/P7 and O2/P8.

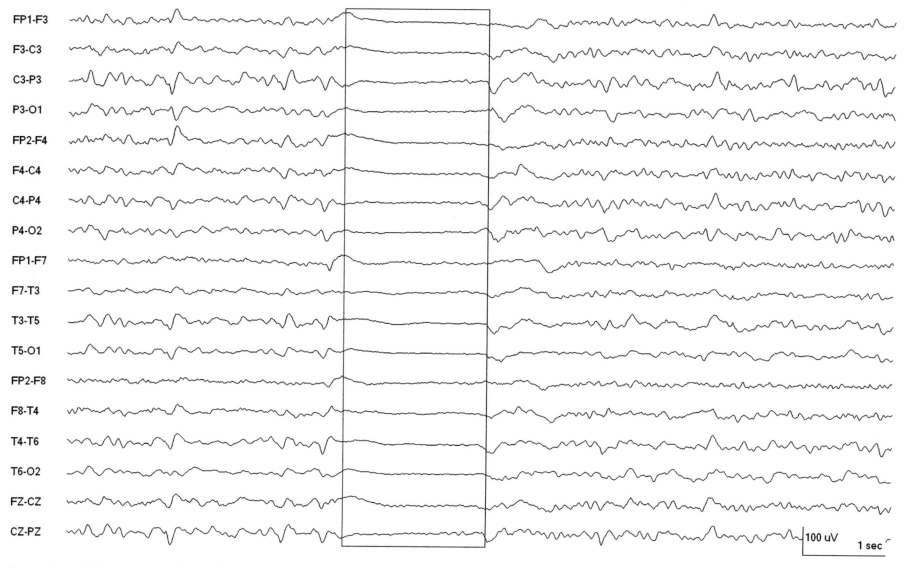

Figure 3.4. Moderate generalized slowing, nearly continuous, longitudinal bipolar. The EEG in this 84-year-old woman shows a sudden 2 second period of suppression, not related to stimulation. She was receiving propofol. Periods of attenuation/suppression are a nonspecific abnormality but usually signifying at least moderate encephalopathy. A background with brief periods of attenuation/suppression occupying 1–9% of the record is classified as nearly continuous. The period of lower voltage activity is considered suppressed if <10 μV peak to peak and attenuated if higher voltage but still <50% of the voltage of the background. If there is a greater degree of dysfunction where the periods of attenuation/suppression constitute 10–49%, then this would be classified as discontinuous; and if 50–99%, it would qualify as burst suppression or burst attenuation. If the periods of attenuation are rare (<1% of the record being attenuated/suppressed), the record is considered continuous; and if they constitute >99% of the record, the whole record is considered attenuated/suppressed.

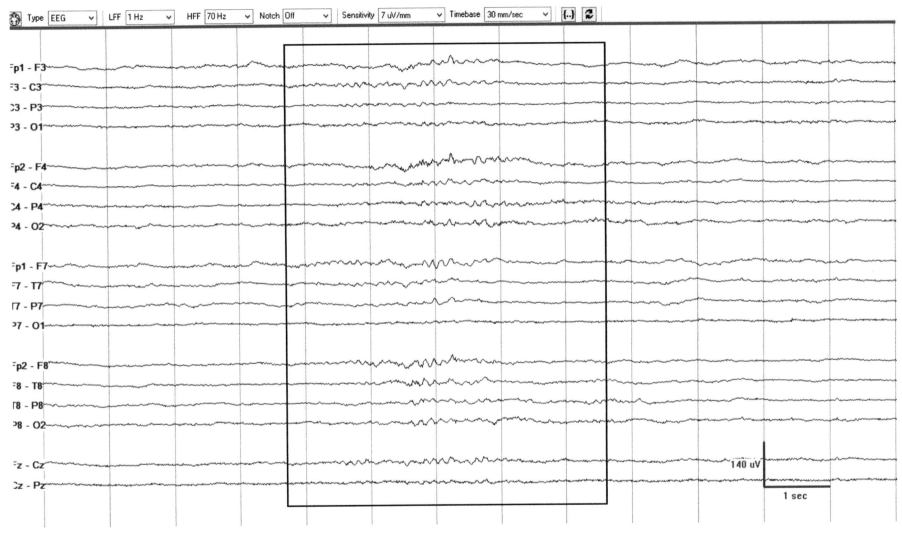

Figure 3.5. Continuity (burst suppression, discontinuous, continuous) (a) Burst suppression, longitudinal bipolar. Similar to Figure 3.4 this EEG was from a 79-year-old woman receiving propofol. The initial EEG was burst suppressed. Here the burst consists of low- to medium-amplitude 7 Hz theta activity with some low-amplitude 1–1.5 Hz delta activity. The activity lasted 4–5 seconds and alternated with periods of 10–15 seconds of attenuation/suppression (only 1 burst shown). Assuming bursts of 5 seconds duration and 15 seconds attenuation, the *suppression percent* would be 15/20, or 75%. 75% falls in the 50–99% range and is therefore considered burst suppression. Note the term 'burst suppression' alone does not provide any information about the content of the bursts, and the further classification of burst suppression will be explored in Chapter 8: Post cardiac arrest EEG.

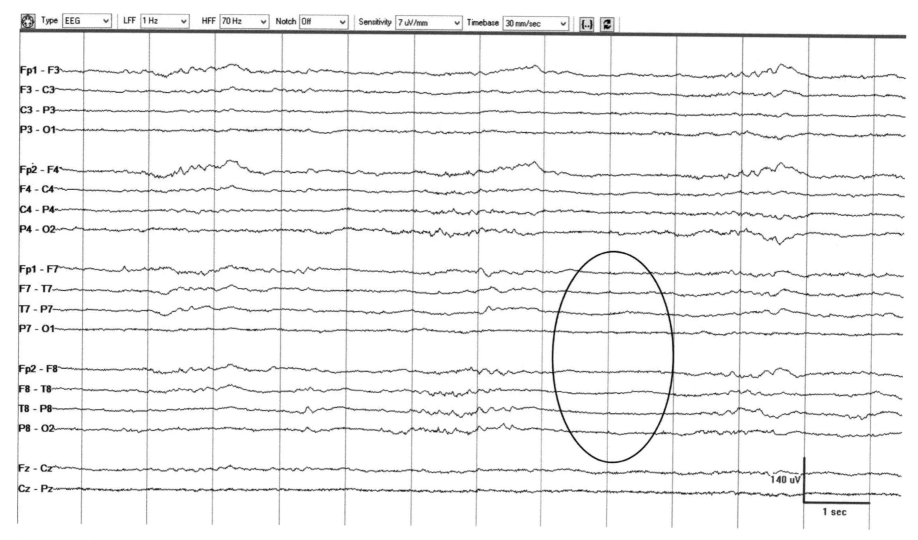

Figure 3.5. (*Continued*) (b) Discontinuous, longitudinal bipolar. The same patient as the prior figure with propofol starting to be weaned. Note: although the activity within the bursts has not changed, the proportion of the record where the activity is present has now improved (increased). Now the periods of attenuation (ellipse) are shorter than the bursts, and thus the suppression percent is <50%, no longer qualifying as burst suppression, but rather as a discontinuous record (with about 25% suppression/attenuation)

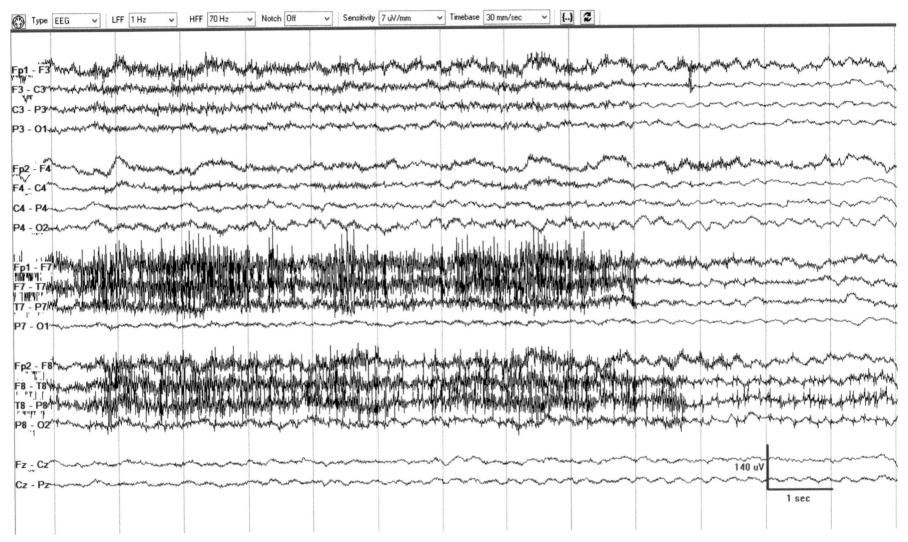

Figure 3.5. (*Continued*) (c) Continuous, longitudinal bipolar. The same patient after cessation of propofol. The patient is starting to wake up, with emergence of EMG artifact, and the record is now continuous (i.e., no further periods of attenuation/suppression) with medium-amplitude 3–3.5 Hz slowing. The sequence of EEG demonstrates the transition from burst suppression, to discontinuous, to a continuous record as sedation was weaned.

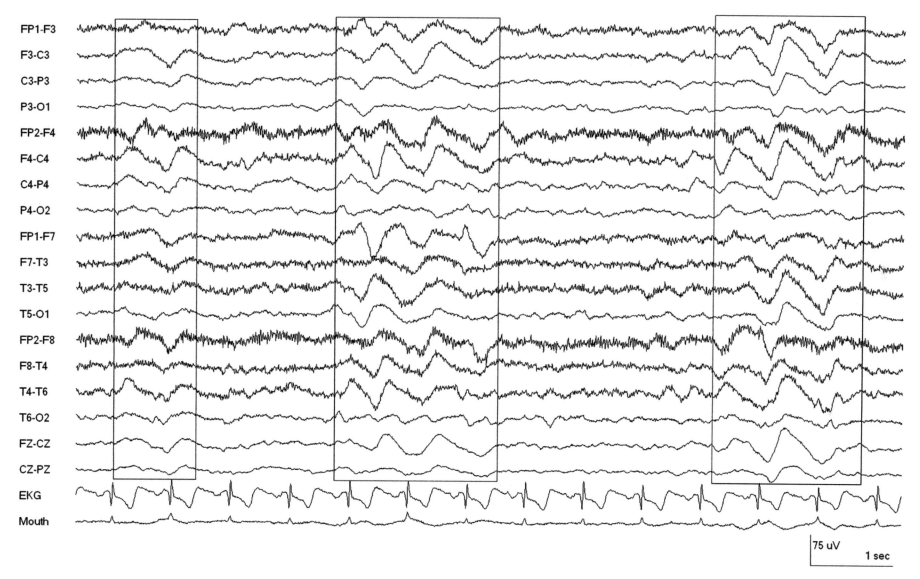

Figure 3.6. Frontal intermittent rhythmic delta activity (FIRDA), longitudinal bipolar. This is the EEG from a comatose 63-year-old woman s/p liver transplant. There is diffuse background slowing and 1–2 second runs of generalized frontally predominant high voltage rhythmic delta activity (boxes) in 2-second bursts (2–4 waves at a time). This activity is FIRDA, a nonspecific marker of diffuse dysfunction. It should be noted that by current terminology this would not classify as generalized rhythmic delta activity (GRDA), mainly because the activity is not sustained for ≥6 cycles. Although this is true, the clinical significance of GRDA is largely synonymous with that of FIRDA (i.e., a marker of diffuse dysfunction with no association with seizures). Patterns that meet definition of GRDA are presented in Chapter 5: Rhythmic and periodic patterns.

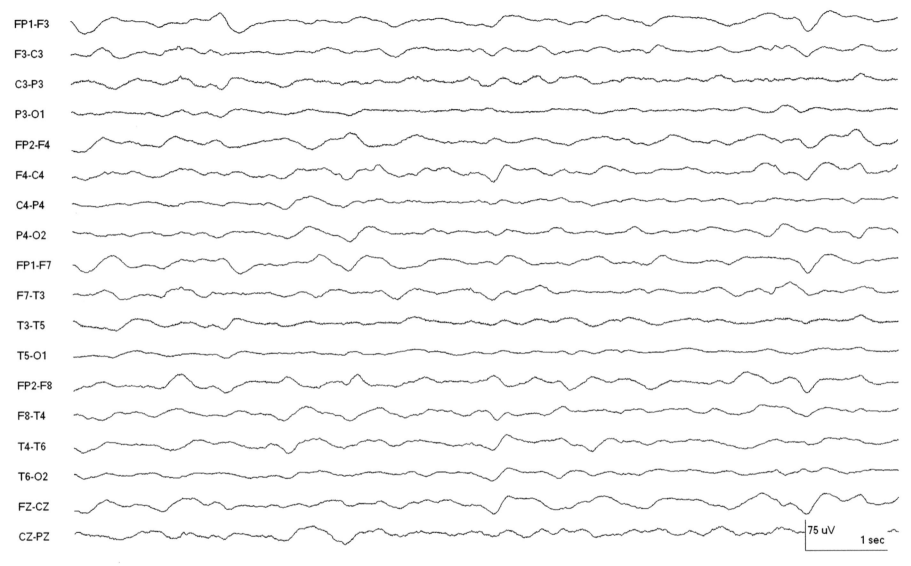

Figure 3.7. Moderate to severe generalized slowing, longitudinal bipolar. The EEG in this 46-year-old man with hepatic encephalopathy shows moderate to severe diffuse symmetrical slowing and attenuation. The activity is predominantly in the slow delta range, with absence of faster frequencies. The lack of activity in the 3–6 Hz range suggests more than moderate dysfunction. There was, however, evidence of reactivity in the record (not shown), therefore not meeting typical criteria for severe dysfunction (such as with the Yale Adult Background EEG Grading Scale, Table 3.3); thus, this would qualify as moderate to severe dysfunction.

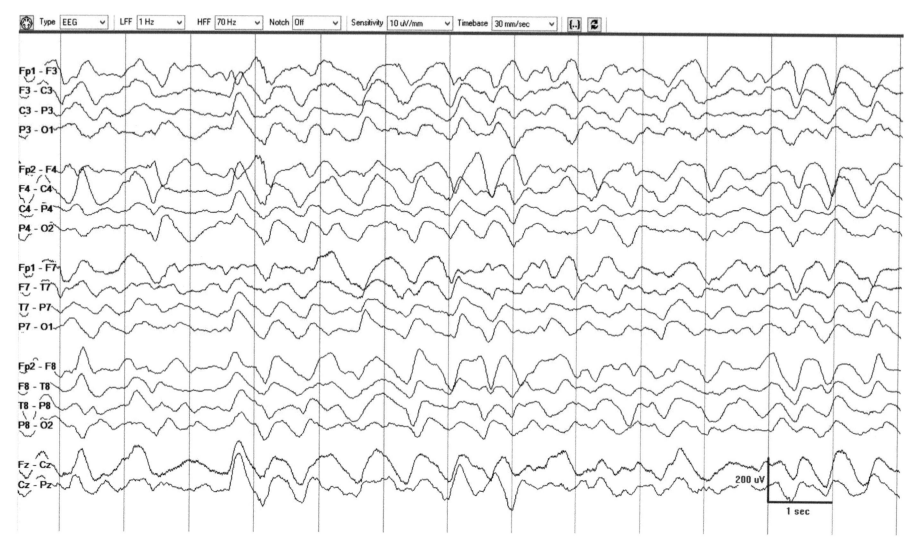

Figure 3.8. Moderate to severe generalized slowing, longitudinal bipolar. The EEG from a 27-year-old woman with cryptogenic NORSE (new onset refractory status epilepticus), after cessation of seizures. The background consists of high amplitude delta activity that is mostly irregular (sometimes rhythmic for a few waves, not sustained enough to be GRDA). This was also reactive to stimulation and therefore suggestive of moderate to severe diffuse dysfunction. The patient was on minimal sedative medication at the time of the EEG, the dysfunction being more reflective of the underlying process, as opposed to medication effect.

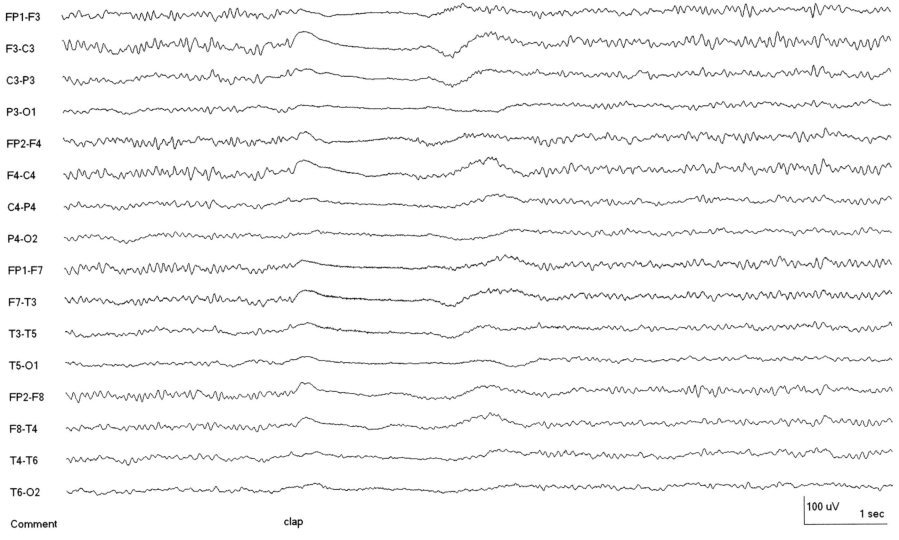

FP1-F3

F3-C3

C3-P3

P3-O1

FP2-F4

F4-C4

C4-P4

P4-O2

FP1-F7

F7-T3

T3-T5

T5-O1

FP2-F8

F8-T4

T4-T6

T6-O2

Comment   clap

100 uV   1 sec

Figure 3.9. Reactivity in coma. A 32-year-old woman with decreased mental status and an elevated ammonia level. Alerting (in this case clapping) resulted in a period of diffuse attenuation, demonstrating a reactive record (albeit an abnormal alerting response). This is an example of stimulus leading to attenuation of activity.

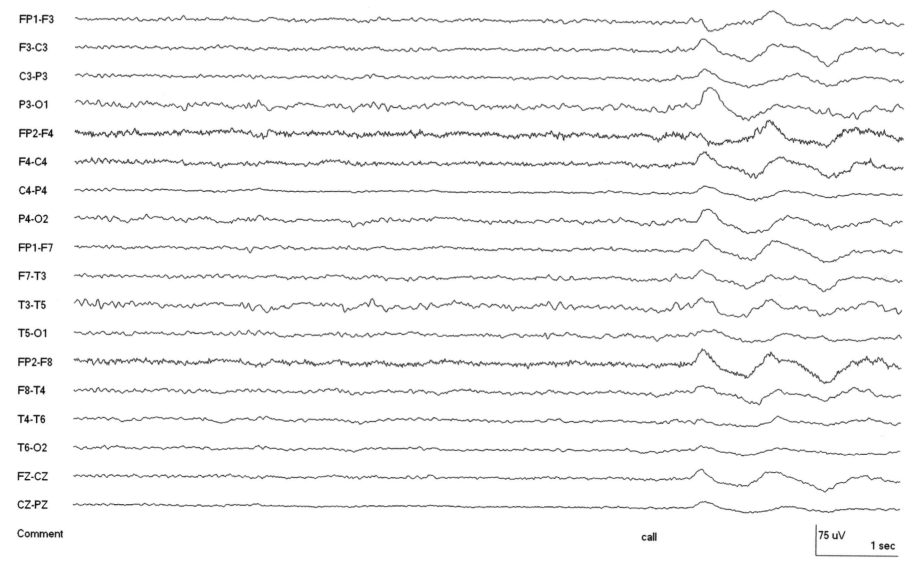

Figure 3.10. Reactivity in coma. The EEG in this 23-year-old comatose woman s/p traumatic brain injury shows the emergence of generalized polymorphic delta activity when called (i.e., due to an auditory stimulus). Although the EEG demonstrates reactivity, clinically the patient was unchanged. Reactivity indicates a lighter level of coma compared to an unreactive record. Reactivity has prognostic significance, with an unreactive record being an independent determinant of poor neurological outcome and mortality in many conditions. Note the stimulation actually brings out a much slower record (slow delta), the opposite of a normal alerting response; this has been referred to as 'paradoxical' arousal.

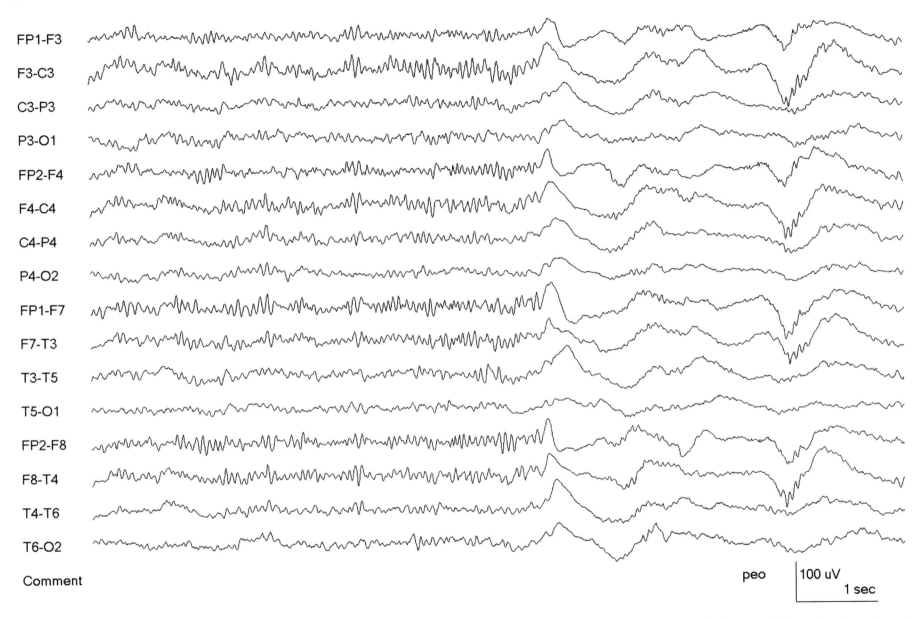

FP1-F3

F3-C3

C3-P3

P3-O1

FP2-F4

F4-C4

C4-P4

P4-O2

FP1-F7

F7-T3

T3-T5

T5-O1

FP2-F8

F8-T4

T4-T6

T6-O2

Comment   peo   100 uV

                                                                                              1 sec

Figure 3.11.   Reactivity in coma. The EEG in this 31-year-old woman receiving propofol shows reactivity when eyes are passively opened. There is attenuation of faster background activity followed by bursts of higher amplitude delta activity.

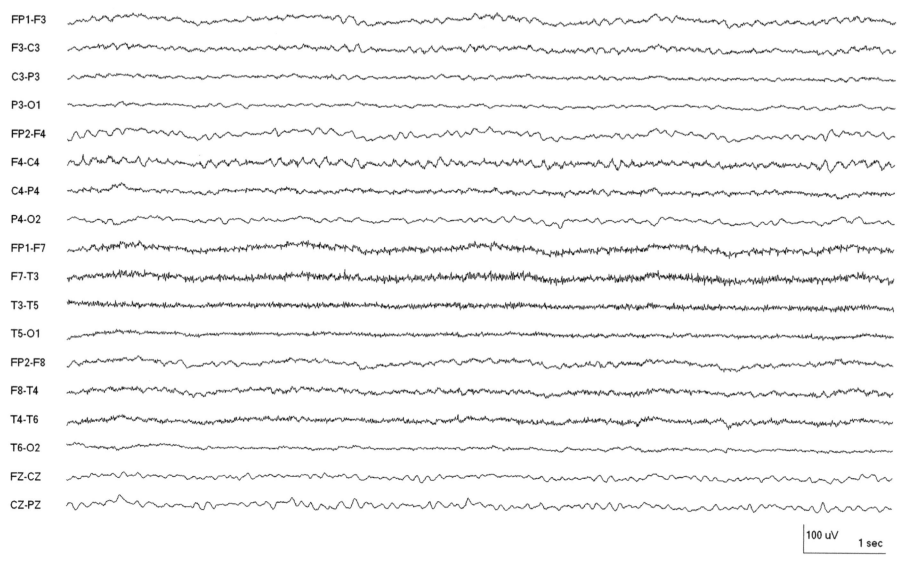

FP1-F3

F3-C3

C3-P3

P3-O1

FP2-F4

F4-C4

C4-P4

P4-O2

FP1-F7

F7-T3

T3-T5

T5-O1

FP2-F8

F8-T4

T4-T6

T6-O2

FZ-CZ

CZ-PZ

100 uV   1 sec

Figure 3.12. Alpha coma. The EEG in this 42-year-old comatose man with a history of cardiac arrest 1 day previously shows an alpha coma pattern, with continuous, frontally predominant, monomorphic 8 Hz activity. The pattern was unreactive. This demonstrates an important point. The absence of reactivity (even though the pattern is in the alpha range) suggests severe diffuse or multifocal dysfunction. Alpha coma can be misinterpreted as mild generalized slowing if the EEGer does not specifically remember to assess for reactivity. The other feature of alpha coma is its invariance (or lack of state change): every page through the record appears like the one before it. Again, if not specifically looking for state changes this feature can be missed.

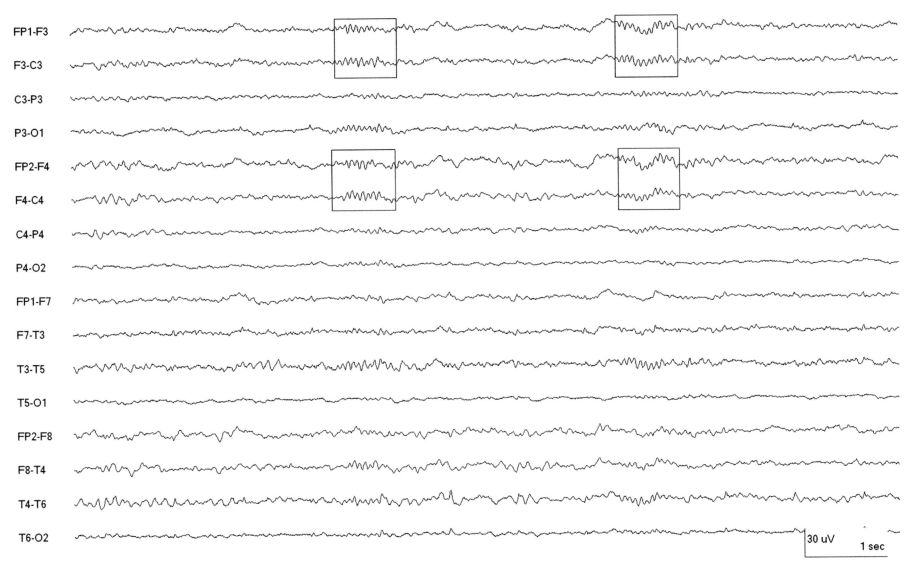

Figure 3.13.   Spindle coma. The EEG in this 61-year-old comatose man with a subarachnoid hemorrhage shows sleep spindles (boxes) consistent with a spindle-coma pattern. This pattern resembles normal sleep, but the patient cannot be awakened. Again, like alpha coma, the pattern is unreactive and without any state changes.

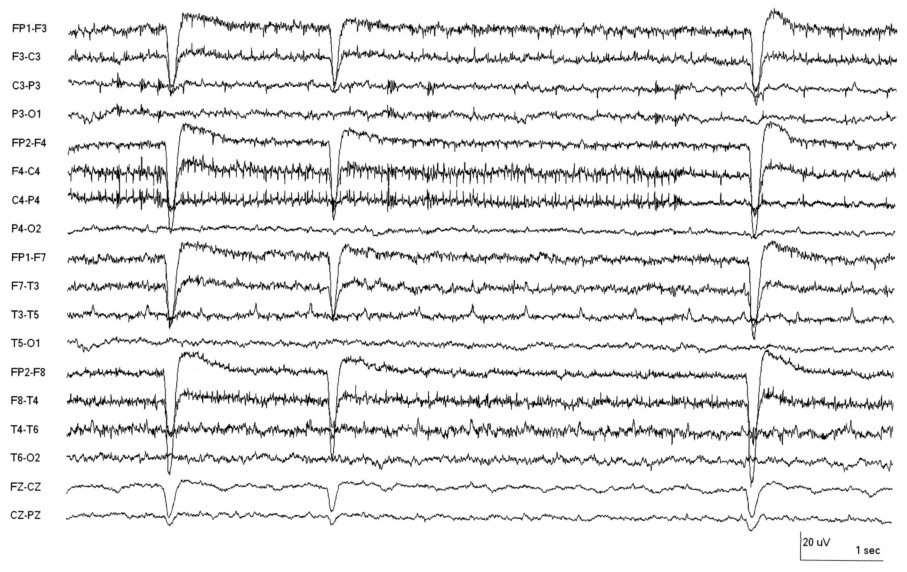

Figure 3.14. Diffuse attenuation/suppression. The EEG in this 48-year-old man in a vegetative state following a cardiac arrest shows marked suppression of background activity even at a high sensitivity (recorded at very high gain, note scale legend). Eye blink artifacts are prominent as well as muscle and EKG (especially at T3-T5); however, there is little if any definite cerebral activity, but with too much artifact to be certain. The finding suggests severe diffuse or multifocal dysfunction.

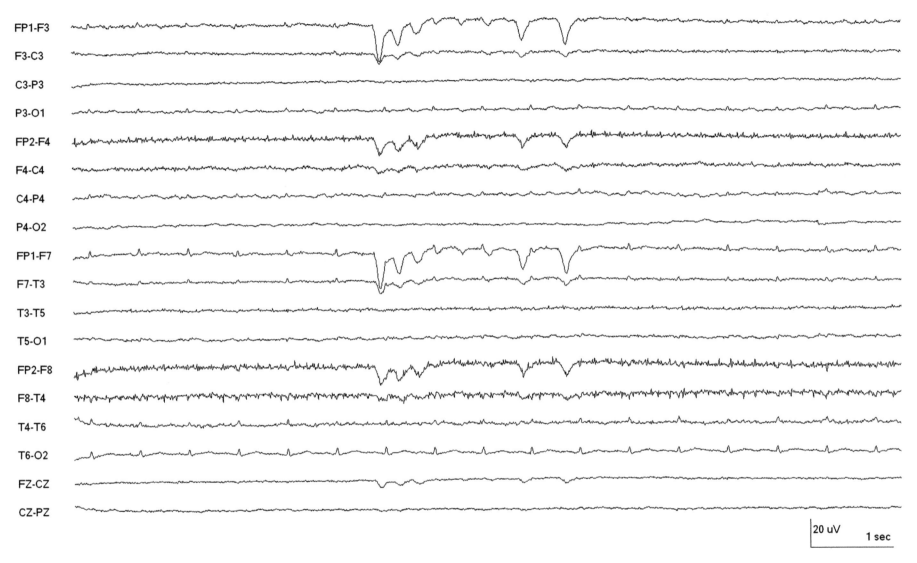

Figure 3.15. Diffuse suppression. Similar to the prior figure, but with less muscle artifact. The EEG in this 44-year-old man in a persistent vegetative state (PVS) shows no evidence of definite cerebral activity (all possible cerebral activity <10 uV) despite very high gain (note scale legend). In the center of the epoch are several eye blinks. EKG artifact is present, especially in T6-O2. Usually, patients in a PVS show more EEG activity than this.

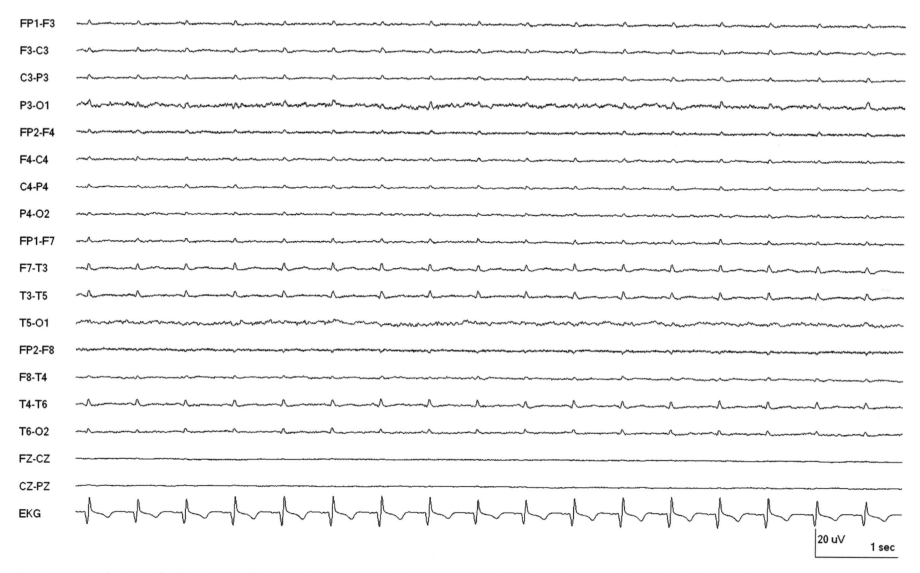

Figure 3.16. Electrocerebral inactivity. The EEG in this 50-year-old woman being evaluated for brain death demonstrates electrocerebral inactivity. There are strict guidelines for performing EEGs for this purpose – see the American Clinical Neurophysiology Society guidelines regarding the technical requirements for using EEG as part of the determination of brain death (in reference list). For example, this montage would not be appropriate for an ECI determination, as inter-electrode distances should be double that of the usual ones. When all of those procedures and criteria are not strictly followed, this should be reported as severe or profound diffuse attenuation, but without mention of electrocerebral inactivity. EEGs are rarely performed as part of the determination of brain death in recent years.

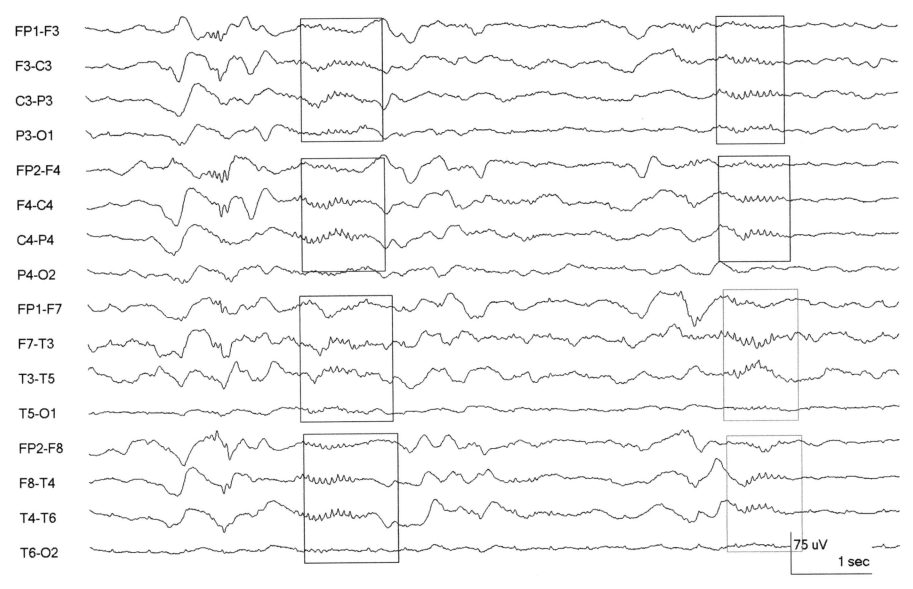

Figure 3.17. Hepatic failure with 14-Hz positive spikes. (a) Hepatic failure with 14-Hz positive spikes, longitudinal bipolar. The EEG in this 38-year-old comatose man with hepatic failure demonstrates 14 Hz positive spikes. Although this is usually a benign variant seen in drowsiness (i.e., 14- & 6-Hz positive spikes), it can also be seen in comatose patients with acute hepatic failure.

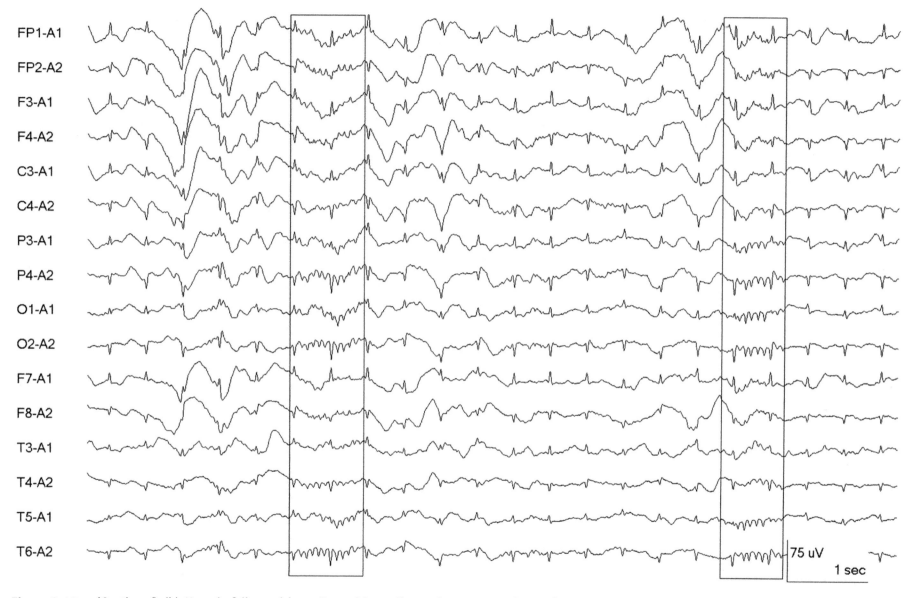

Figure 3.17. (*Continued*) (b) Hepatic failure with 14-Hz positive spikes, referential/ The epoch reformatted utilizing a referential montage to ipsilateral ears. These low-amplitude positive discharges (down-going on this referential montage) are often maximal in the posterior temporal region (e.g., see T6 in this example, within the box; also seen well at O2 in this patient).

Extreme Delta Brushes (EDB)

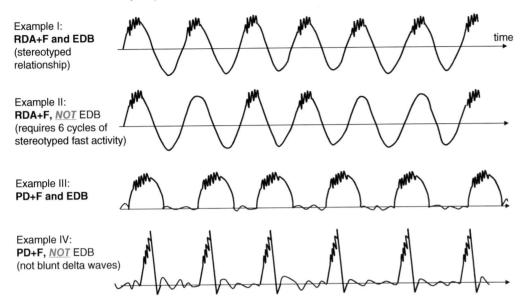

	RDA+F; or PD+F if (and only if) the PDs are blunt delta waves	
	Continuous/ Abundant (≥50% of record/epoch)	*Frequent/Occasional (≥1 to 49% of record/epoch)*
Fast activity WITH stereotyped relationship to delta wave	Definite EDB	Possible EDB
Fast activity WITHOUT stereotyped relationship to delta wave	Possible EDB	RDA+F or PD+F, but NOT EDB

Figure 3.18.   Extreme delta brush (EDB). Extreme delta brushes (EDB) is a plus feature that is classified as a specific subtype of +fast and has been associated with the condition of anti-NMDA receptor-related encephalitis. EDB can either be definite or possible, as demonstrated in the table. The morphological term 'delta brush' is given from the resemblance of the pattern to the delta brush pattern (also known as beta-delta complexes) seen as a part of the normal ontogeny of neonatal EEG. The classical description of EDB was extrapolated from the literature on NMDA encephalitis and consists of continuous or abundant delta brushes, where the delta brushes are either RDA+F where the fast forms a stereotyped relationship with each delta wave (example I); or PD+F where each 'discharge' consists of a blunt delta wave with stereotyped fast activity (i.e., periodic delta brushes) (example III). If there are delta brushes where the pattern (RDA+F or PD+F) is only frequent or occasional, these would count as 'possible EDB', mainly because the pattern is not prevalent enough to qualify as 'extreme'. Similarly, if there is continuous RDA+F or periodic delta brushes where the fast activity does not have a stereotyped relationship to the delta waves (i.e., is present continuously when the pattern is present) then this also qualifies as 'possible EDB'. Examples I and III would qualify as definite EDB if the pattern were continuous or abundant, and possible EDB if less prevalent. Examples II and IV are examples of RPPs that do not qualify as definite or possible EDB.

Reproduced from Hirsch LJ, Fong MWK, Leitinger M, et al. American Clinical Neurophysiology Society's Standardized Critical Care EEG Terminology: 2021 Version. J Clin Neurophysiol. 2021;38(1):1–29. with permission.

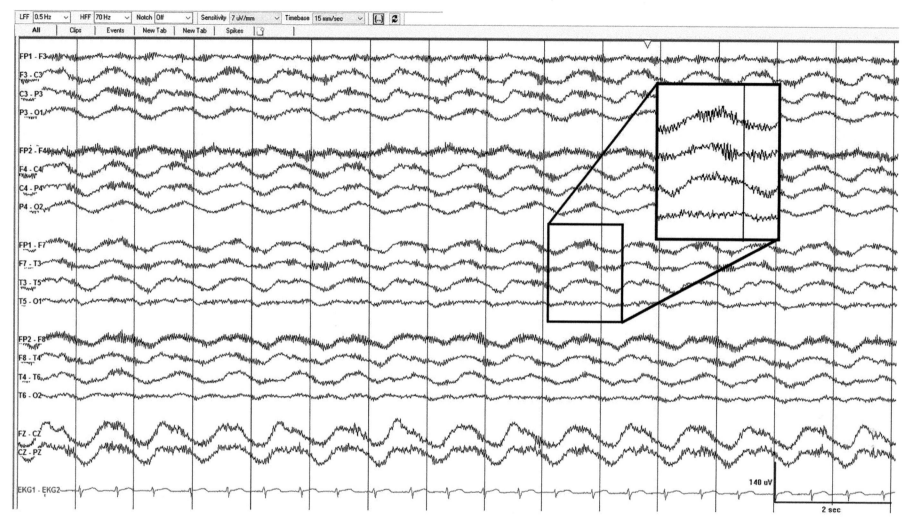

Figure 3.19. Extreme delta brush (EDB). (a) Extreme delta brush (EDB), longitudinal bipolar. EEG from a 27-year-old woman with anti-NMDA receptor encephalitis. The EEG demonstrates continuous medium-amplitude GRDA+F. The fast activity in this case has a stereotyped relationship with each delta wave (maximal at the crest and downslope of each wave) (as highlighted in the expanded box). This meets criteria for 'definite' EDB. NOTE: if the fast activity was present continuously and did not have a stereotyped relationship with the delta waves, or if the observed GRDA+F pattern was only frequent to occasional (as opposed to abundant or continuous), then this would be classified as 'possible' EDB.

Courtesy of Dr. Jennifer Percy, University of British Columbia, Vancouver.

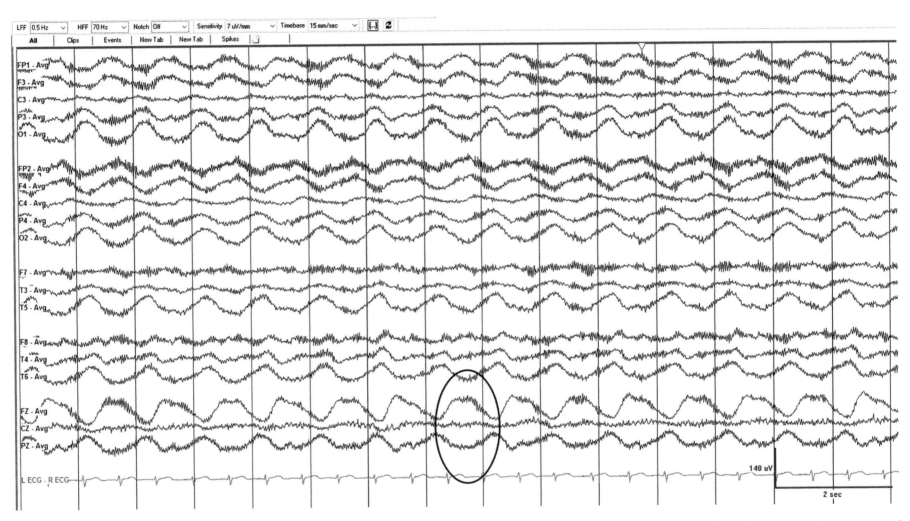

Figure 3.19.   (*Continued*) (b) Extreme delta brush (EDB), reference. The same page as prior reformatted into a common average referential montage. The stereotyped relationship of the fast to each rhythmic delta wave is seen even better in the Fz-Cz channel (ellipse) (occurring at the crest and downslope of each wave).

Courtesy of Dr. Jennifer Percy, University of British Columbia, Vancouver.

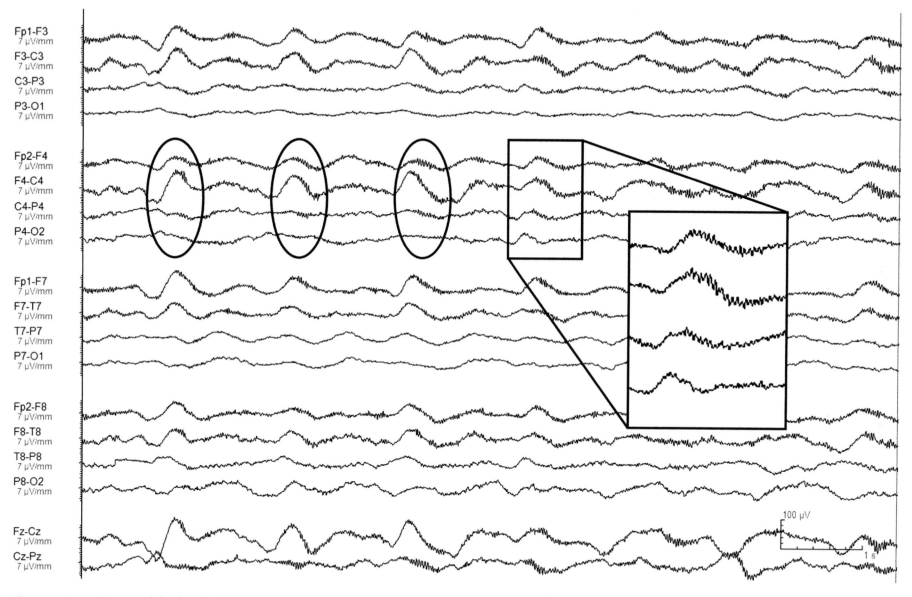

Figure 3.20. Extreme delta brush (EDB), periodic variant, longitudinal bipolar. The EEG demonstrates definite EDB, but in this case the periodic variant. Continuous or abundant PDs+F can also qualify as definite EDB, provided that the PDs are blunt delta waves, and that the fast activity forms a stereotyped relationship to each delta wave (i.e., resembles periodic delta brushes) (ellipses). Note, this pattern is not RDA as there is a clear interval between each consecutive delta brush waveform; thus, it is periodic rather than rhythmic. Again, the fast activity occurs in a stereotyped relation with each delta wave (in this case primarily on the downslope of each delta wave [expanded box]). The same rules apply to the periodic variant of EDB, in that if there was not a stereotyped relationship of the fast to each delta wave, or if the observed pattern were only frequent to occasional, then this could still be classified as 'possible' EDB.

Courtesy of Dr. Nicolas Gaspard, Erasme Hospital, Brussels.

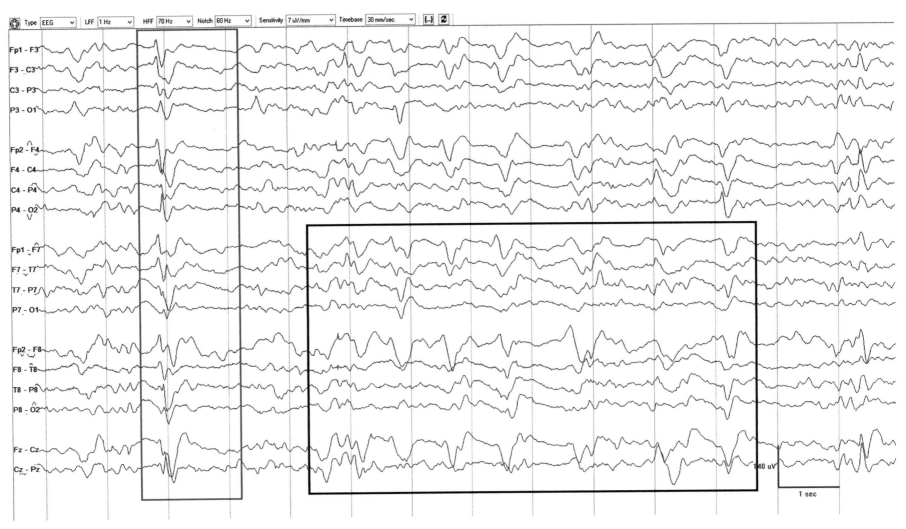

Figure 3.21. COVID-19-related encephalopathy, longitudinal bipolar. The EEG is from a 66-year-old woman with COVID-19 infection who developed encephalopathy, respiratory failure and acute renal failure. The EEG demonstrates mild to moderate diffuse slowing, with frequent generalized sporadic epileptiform discharges (blue box) followed by 1 second of attenuation, and occasional very brief 1-Hz GPDs sometimes with triphasic morphology (black box).

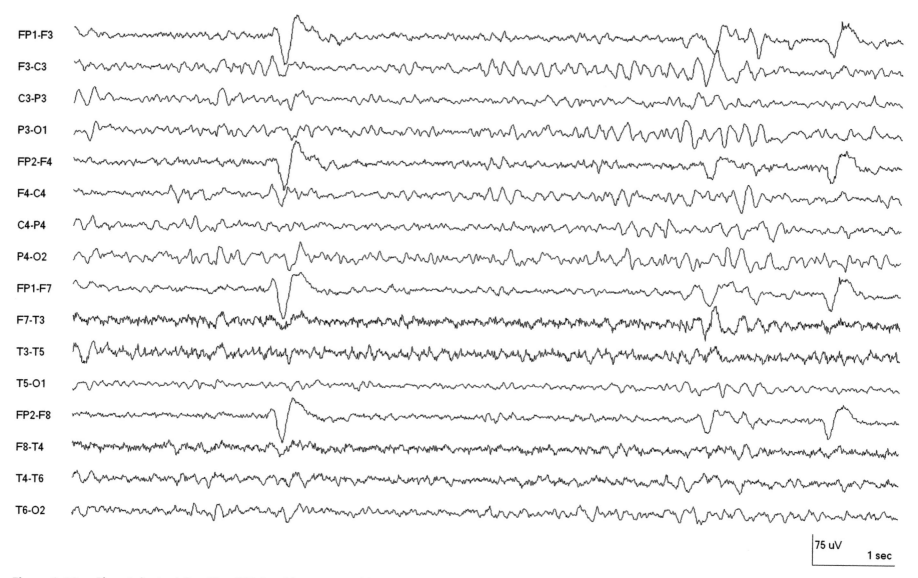

Figure 3.22.   Phenytoin toxicity. The EEG in this 28-year-old woman with phenytoin toxicity shows mild diffuse slowing of background rhythms (mostly 7 Hz or faster) with excess theta activity and occasional bursts of delta slowing. If no PDR is found, we would consider this mild-moderate slowing using the Yale scale.

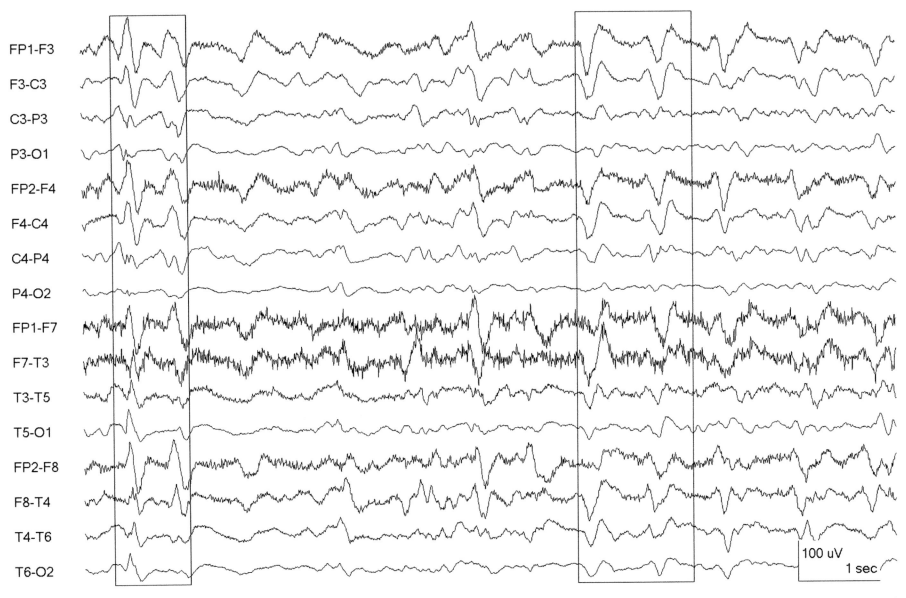

Figure 3.23. Baclofen toxicity. The EEG in this 87-year-old woman being evaluated for a confusional state shows generalized biphasic and triphasic waveforms, sometimes quasiperiodic at ~1 per second for a few waves (see the last few seconds of this sample for example). The patient was being treated with baclofen. Mental status cleared following the discontinuation of this medication and the EEG improved.

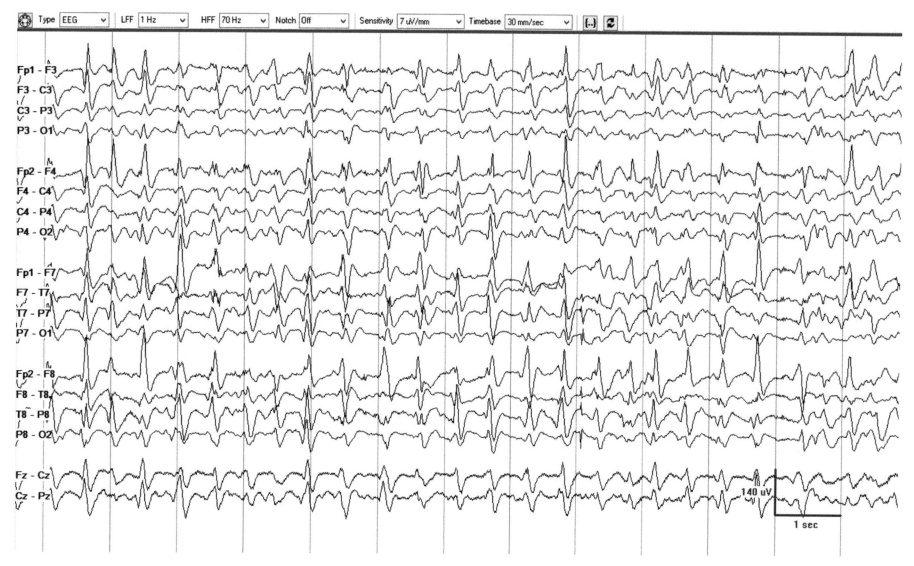

Figure 3.24. Cefepime toxicity. (a) Cefepime toxicity. This 78-year-old man with end-stage renal failure was administered cefepime for a resistant urinary tract infection. On day 3 of treatment, he became progressively obtunded, and an EEG was performed. The EEG demonstrates generalized periodic discharges (GPDs) occurring at 2 Hz. The pattern is highly epileptiform and falls on the ictal end of the ictal-interictal continuum (IIC) (which will be discussed in the later chapter on seizures and status epilepticus); we would consider this probable nonconvulsive status epilepticus (but not definite based on EEG alone).

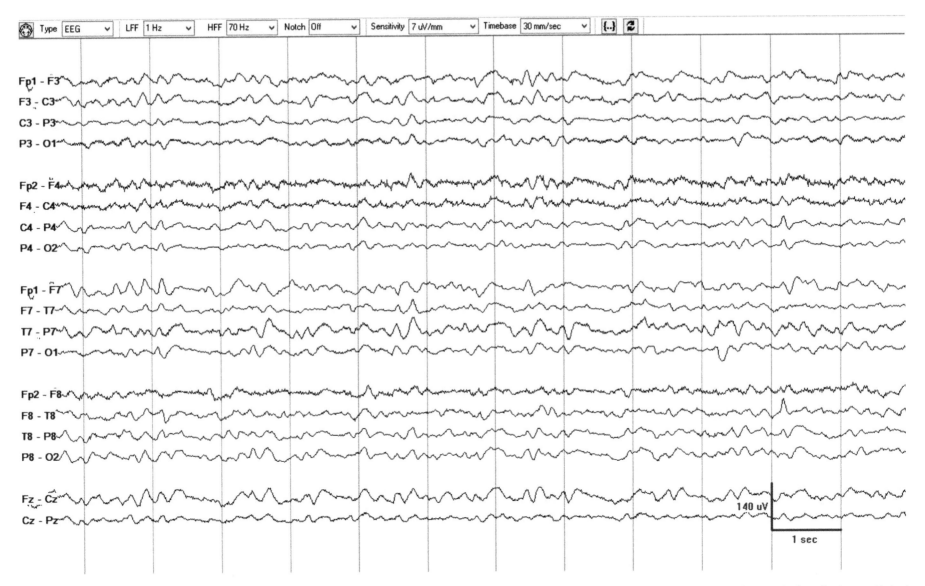

Figure 3.24. *(Continued)* (b) Cefepime toxicity, following treatment. The cefepime-induced highly epileptiform pattern on the prior page was treated with cessation of the cefepime and loading with sodium valproate. 24 hours after these actions, the highly epileptiform pattern resolved, and the EEG demonstrated only mild-moderate generalized slowing (as shown). The patients mental state returned to normal 48 hours after cessation of the epileptiform pattern, inferring the state to be possible cefepime-induced electroclinical status epilepticus (ECSE). However, the slow clinical improvement leaves some doubt as to the relationship between the EEG pattern and the clinical state. If the EEG and patient improved rapidly with IV anti-seizure medication, this would have qualified as electroclinical SE.

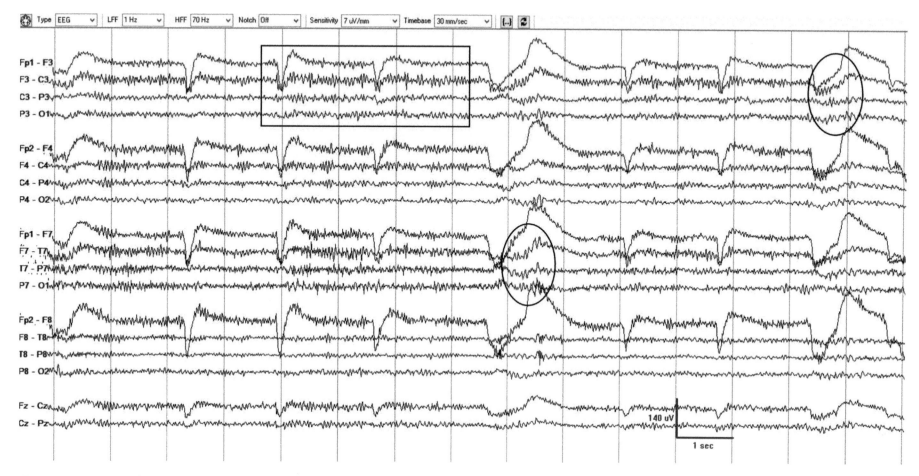

Figure 3.25. Benzodiazepine effect. (a) Normal awake EEG except for excess beta, longitudinal bipolar. This EEG was recorded in the awake state of a 63-year-old man with chronic anxiety who presented with benzodiazepine-related drowsiness. The posterior dominant rhythm has been replaced with medium-amplitude beta activity (in this case 16–20 Hz). Although, 'low voltage fast' can be considered a normal variant of the alpha rhythm, for the finding to be 'physiologic' (rather than pathologic or medication-induced) the low voltage fast activity has to only be in the region where the PDR would normally be (i.e., the posterior head regions). In this patient the beta activity is generalized, and often above 50 µV (i.e., not 'low voltage'). Beta activity can be a feature of the normal drowsy record, but its presence in the awake state is more suggestive of an abnormality. Beta excess (i.e., beta range activity that is generalized [as opposed to only fronto-central], greater than 50 µV, and present in the fully awake state [as opposed to only drowsiness]) can be a marker of benzodiazepine administration, as was the case in this individual. Notably in this example when the patient closes their eyes (ellipses) a very brief PDR is seen (likely a variant of 'alpha squeak', which usually refers to an increase in PDR frequency in the first second after eye closure).

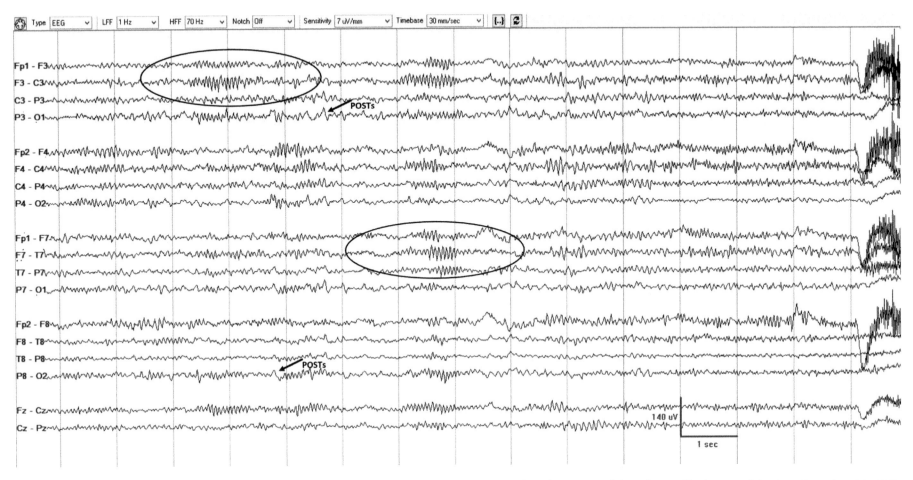

Figure 3.25. (*Continued*) (b) Drowsiness and beta excess, longitudinal bipolar. The same patient in a state of drowsiness. The beta activity has slowed to 14–16 Hz and has become of even greater voltage. Lack of eye blinks and several POSTS (arrows) indicate drowsiness.

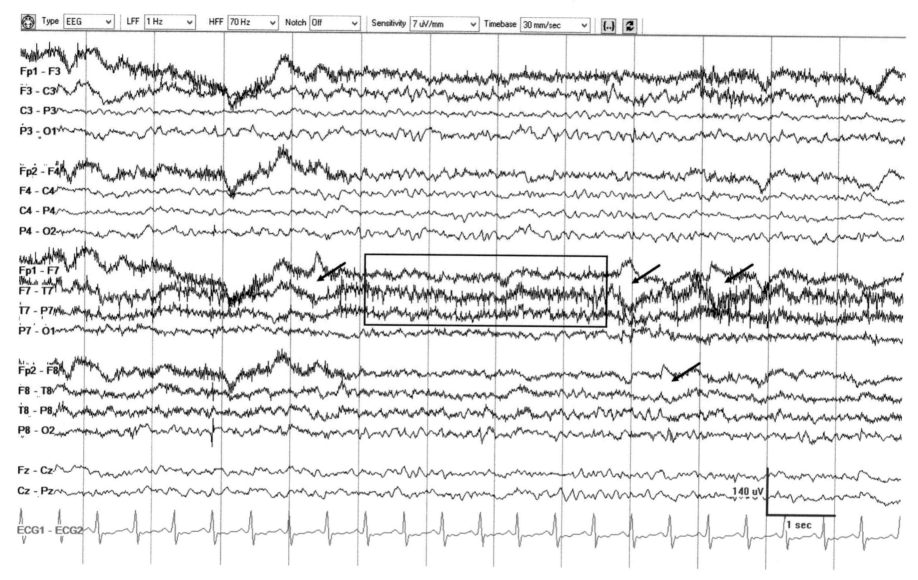

Figure 3.26. Mild generalized slowing and dexmedetomidine. (a) Mild generalized slowing, pre-dexmedetomidine, longitudinal bipolar. This series of EEGs are from a 30-year-old woman with prominent agitation who was subsequently sedated with dexmedetomidine. The initial EEG is with the patient in the awake state with EMG artifact (box) and scanning eye movements (arrows) and shows only mild diffuse slowing with a slow PDR of 7 Hz.

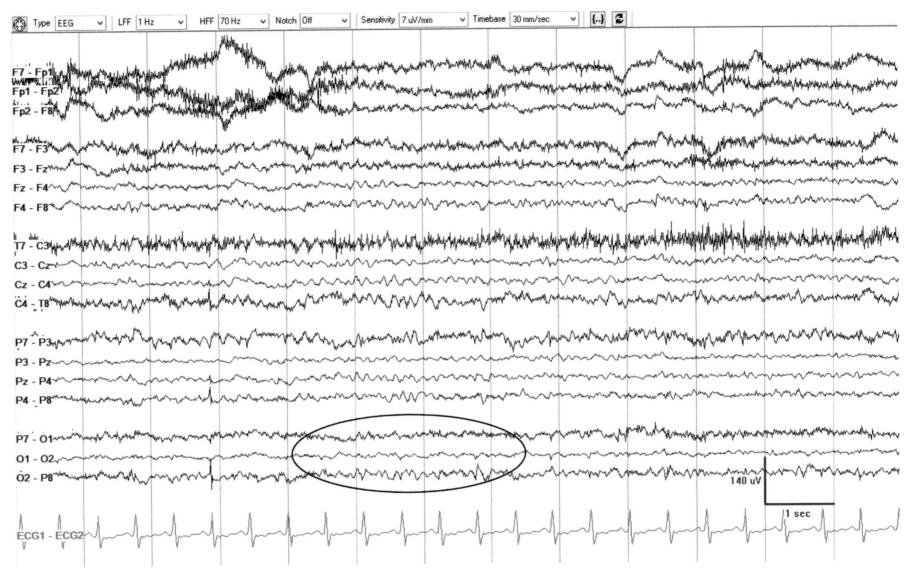

Figure 3.26. (*Continued*) (b) Mild generalized slowing, pre-dexmedetomidine, transverse bipolar. the same page reformatted into a transverse montage. It is easier to appreciate that the AP gradient is still relatively maintained (higher amplitude, slower activity still mostly towards the back of the head with lower voltage, faster frequencies anteriorly), although in the awake state the rhythms are generally slowed and mostly around 7 Hz range (mild generalized slowing).

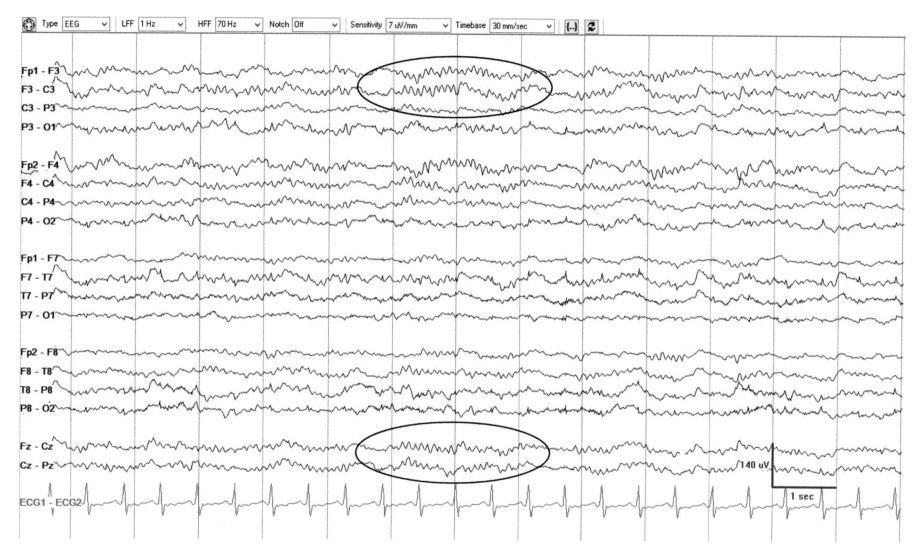

Figure 3.26. (*Continued*) (c) Mild to moderate generalized slowing, post-dexmedetomidine, longitudinal bipolar. Dexmedetomidine was administered for its anti-agitation effect. The patient is now no longer agitated (i.e., no longer blinking, with no EMG activity, although there are few other markers of drowsiness or sleep per se). The new finding is symmetric 10–12 Hz activity that is present in the fronto-central regions (ellipses). There is no longer a PDR (mild-moderate slowing).

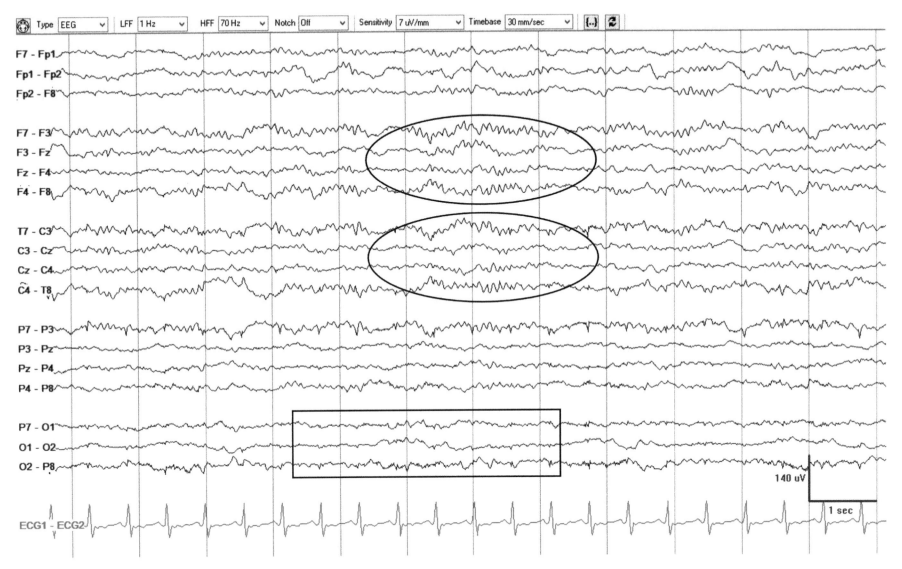

Figure 3.26. (*Continued*) (d) Mild to moderate generalized slowing, post-dexmedetomidine, transverse bipolar: the page prior formatted to a transverse montage. The described activity shares many similarities to sleep spindles. It is symmetric, sinusoidal, of sigma (11–15 Hz) frequency, and fronto-central maximal (ellipses). Note the patient is sedated but is not in N2 sleep (no V waves and no K-complexes). Also, as a result of being mildly sedated there has been loss of the posterior dominant rhythm, despite lack of beta in that region (box highlighting absence). This can be contrasted with prior example of beta excess from benzodiazepine administration (Figure 3.25). In the case of excess beta induced by benzodiazepines, the resultant activity is mostly in the beta range (as previously demonstrated 15–25 Hz); compare this to dexmedetomidine effect, in which there is little activity above 15 Hz, and instead all activity is in the sigma range (11–15 Hz), giving this activity the term 'spindle-like'.

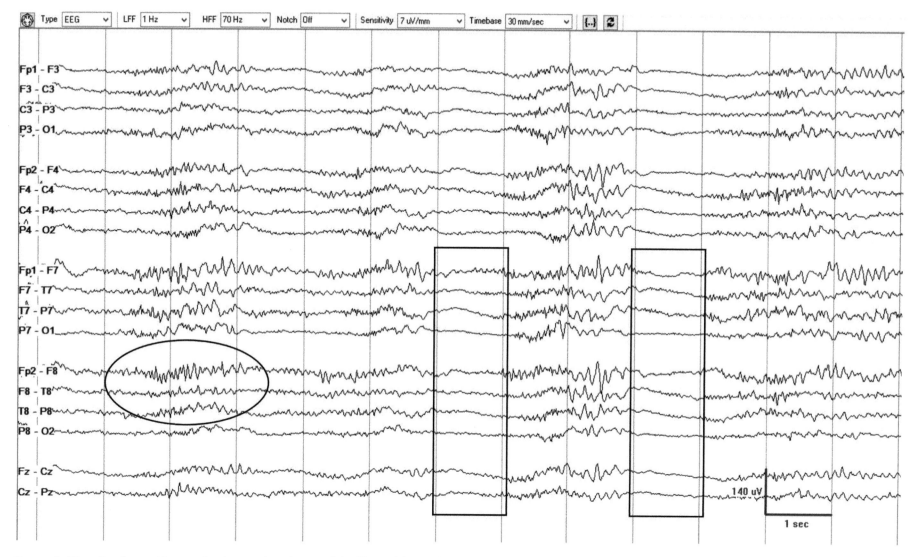

Figure 3.27. Nearly continuous background and propofol effect. (a) Nearly continuous background and propofol effect, longitudinal bipolar. These EEGs are from a 67-year-old woman with end-stage renal disease and opioid abuse. She presented confused and combative requiring sedation and intubation with propofol. The EEG demonstrates 1 second periods of attenuation (boxes) forming 1–9% of the record (i.e., nearly continuous). The activity is a combination of beta and spindle-like activity (almost a combination of the benzodiazepine beta excess and dexmedetomidine spindle-like record) that can sometimes be seen with propofol administration. At higher doses of propofol, this activity can be seen over-riding a discontinuous record with high amplitude delta activity.

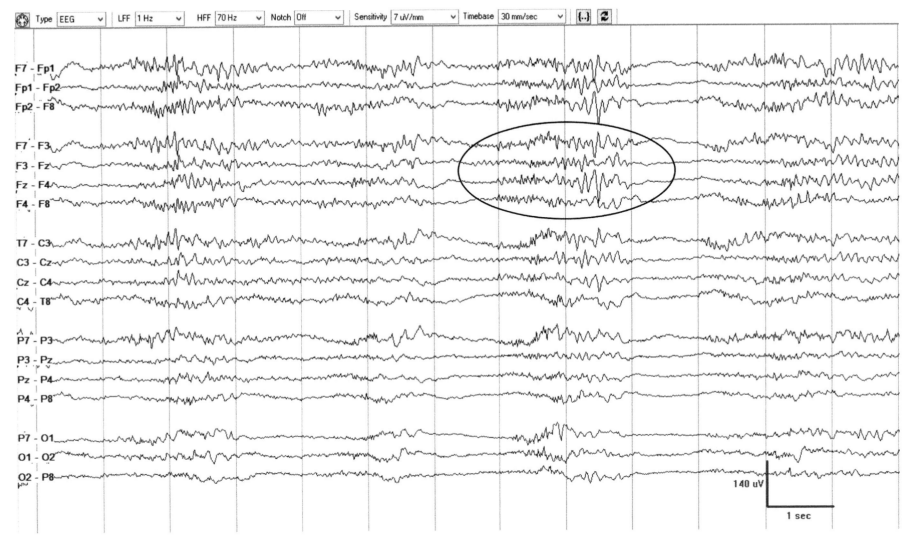

Figure 3.27. (*Continued*) (b) Nearly continuous background and propofol effect, transverse bipolar. The same page as prior reformatted into a transverse montage. Here the generalized low-amplitude beta activity and fronto-central 'envelope' of spindle-like activity is better appreciated (ellipse). This is presented as the combination of rhythms often gives a sharpened appearance (as in this case) that is sometimes misinterpreted as 'epileptiform', and it is valuable appreciating this as a potential effect of propofol (and not epileptiform).

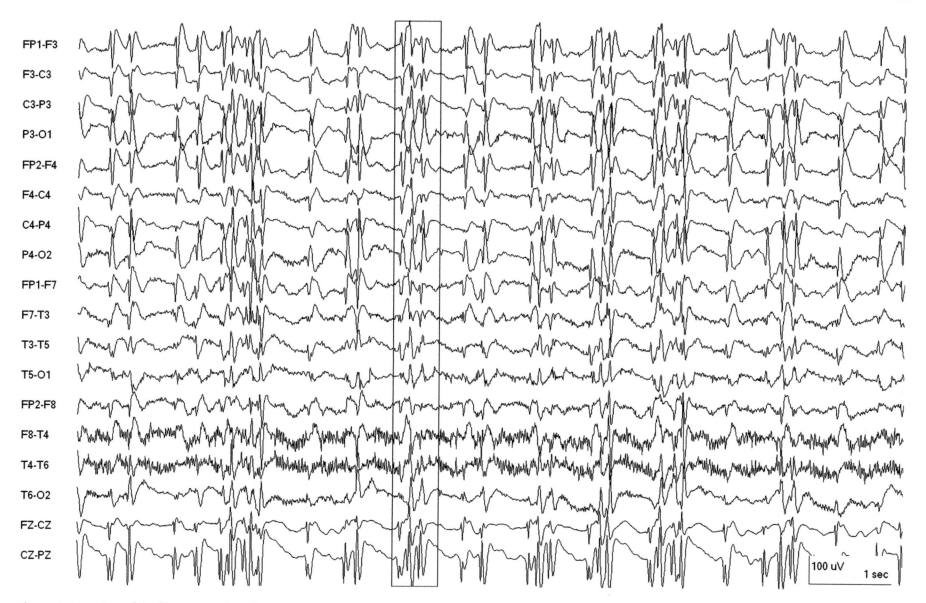

Figure 3.28. Propofol effect on epileptiform pattern in NCSE. (a) Propofol effect on epileptiform pattern in NCSE, pre-treatment. These EEGs are from a 46-year-old man with refractory nonconvulsive status epilepticus (NCSE). There are bursts of generalized spikes and polyspikes (box), only separated by 0.5–1 seconds of attenuation/suppression. Definitions of status epilepticus will be further discussed in the chapter on seizures and status epilepticus, but this qualifies as electrographic SE.

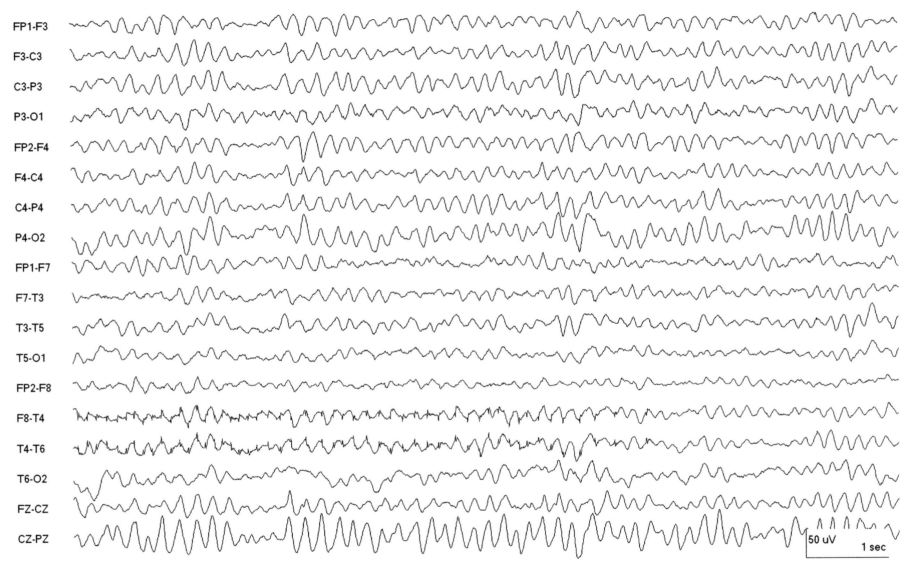

FP1-F3
F3-C3
C3-P3
P3-O1
FP2-F4
F4-C4
C4-P4
P4-O2
FP1-F7
F7-T3
T3-T5
T5-O1
FP2-F8
F8-T4
T4-T6
T6-O2
FZ-CZ
CZ-PZ

50 uV   1 sec

Figure 3.28. *(Continued)* (b) Propofol effect on epileptiform pattern in NCSE, post treatment. The EEG after administration of propofol. Note the epileptiform pattern has been stopped and it has been replaced with generalized theta (6–7 Hz) activity. This is to contrast the propofol effect portrayed in Figure 3.27 with beta and spindle-like activity. These effects can be present when the medication is administered to patients not in NCSE, with most of the descriptions of the effect of propofol on the EEG occurring in normal individuals being administered propofol as a part of anesthesia. In the case of the propofol administered in a patient with a highly epileptiform pattern, the result is hopefully resolution of the pattern, often then resulting in generalized slowing, with the brain being too dysfunctional to generate the 'normal' faster activity in response to medication administration.

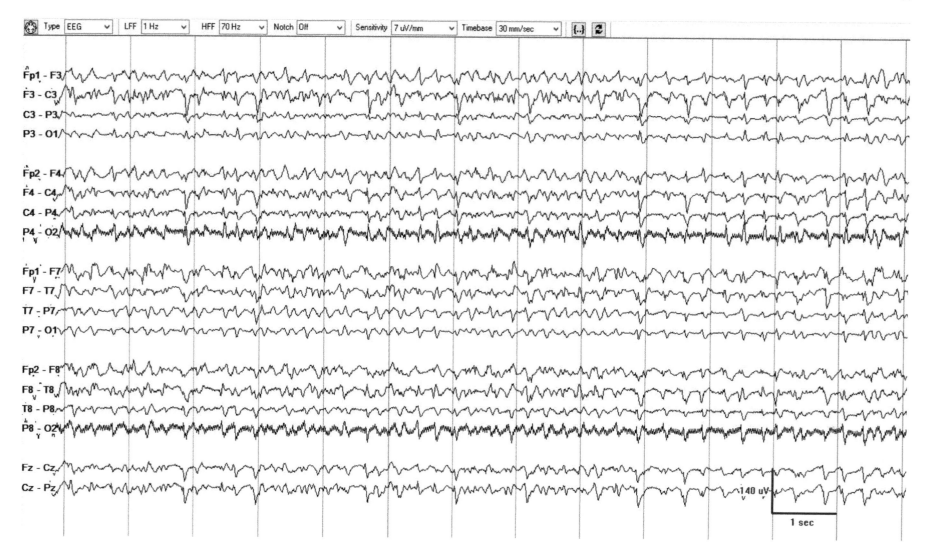

Figure 3.29. Ketamine effect on epileptiform pattern. (a) Ketamine effect on epileptiform pattern, pre-treatment. These EEGs are from a 47-year-old woman s/p prolonged cardiac arrest. The initial EEG demonstrates NCSE with continuous 3–6 Hz low-medium voltage generalized sharp waves. This was refractory to multiple highly sedating anti-seizure medications including benzodiazepine infusion. Significant hemodynamic instability limited the administration of sufficient doses of propofol and barbiturates, therefore ketamine was trialed.

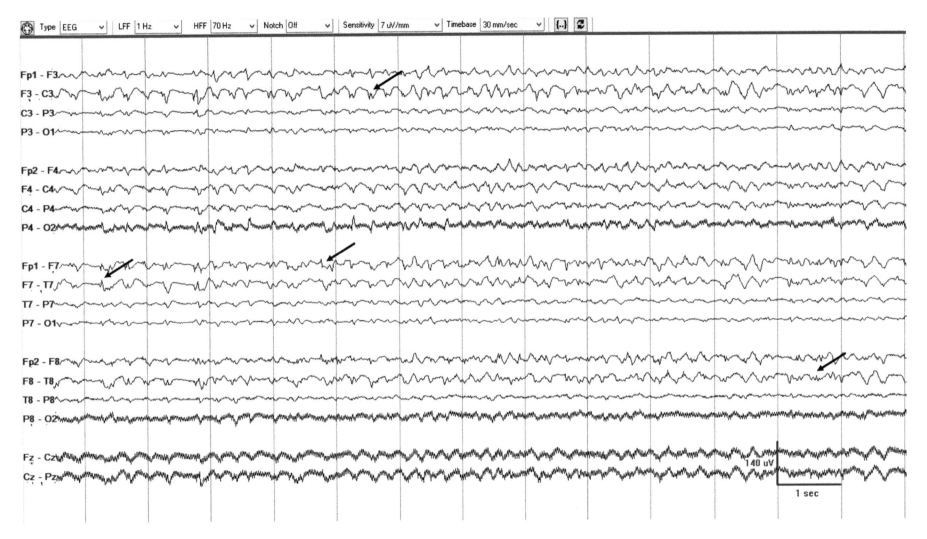

Figure 3.29. (*Continued*) (b) Ketamine effect on epileptiform pattern, post first bolus of ketamine. Ketamine administration led to slowing and mild reduction of the previously seen highly epileptiform pattern. It is however noted that the pattern persists to some degree, lower amplitude and slower, but there is still a reasonable amount of apiculate activity on this EEG page, with several low-amplitude spikes highlighted with arrows. We would interpret this as only partial treatment, with ongoing NCSE.

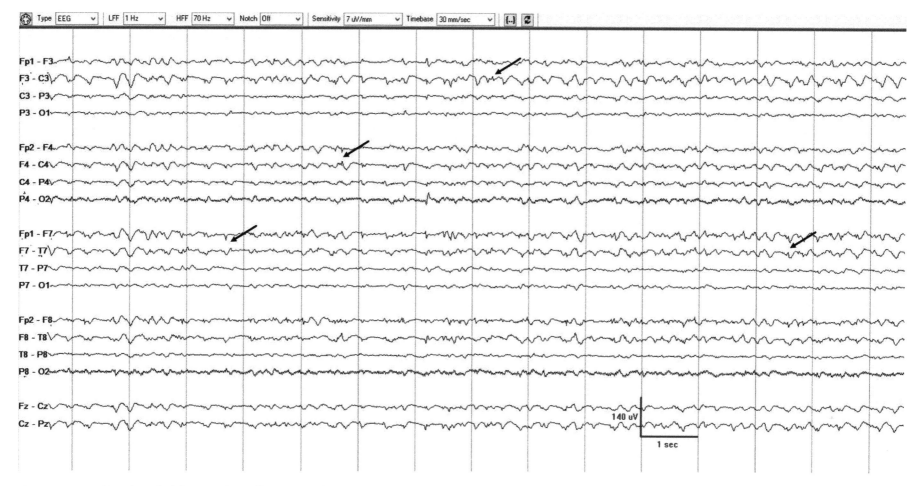

Figure 3.29. (*Continued*) (c) Ketamine effect on epileptiform pattern, post 2nd bolus of ketamine. Additional doses of ketamine have significantly altered the epileptic pattern of Figure 3.29a. Although the electrographic pattern has been significantly attenuated, there are still now very low voltage spikes (arrows), with the same rhythmic activity (again only partially treated). This can occur specifically following ketamine administration. Ketamine administered to normal patients results in a phenomenon known as 'gamma burst', repetitive bursts of gamma range activity with reduction of activities across other frequencies. Theoretically, this may result in persistence of apiculate findings when treating epileptiform patterns, as is seen here. If enough ketamine is administered, the EEG will become suppressed, as was the case with this patient with subsequent boluses.

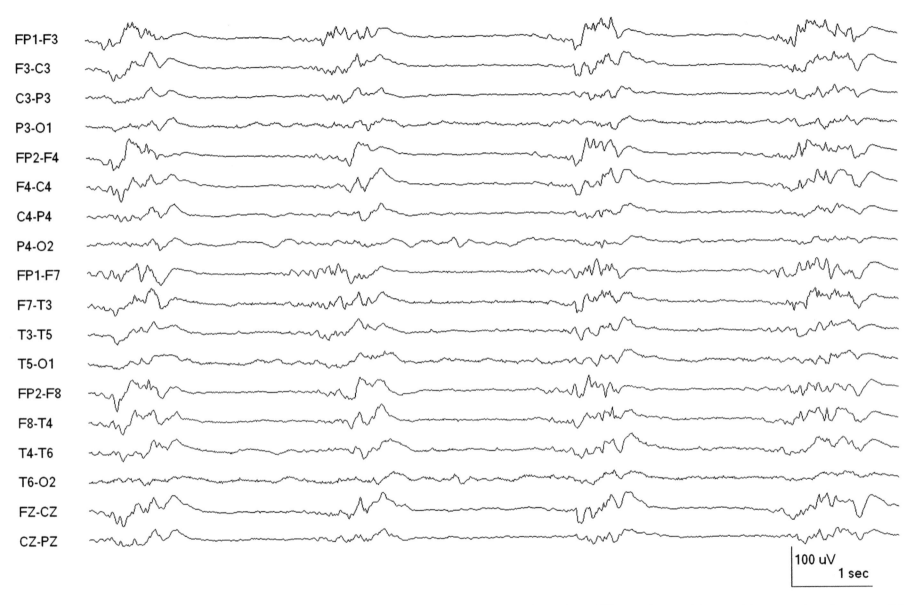

Figure 3.30. Barbiturate-induced burst suppression. (a) Barbiturate-induced burst suppression. These EEGs are from a 65-year-old man undergoing a carotid endarterectomy. The patient had been given pentobarbital prior to intubation, resulting in burst suppression.

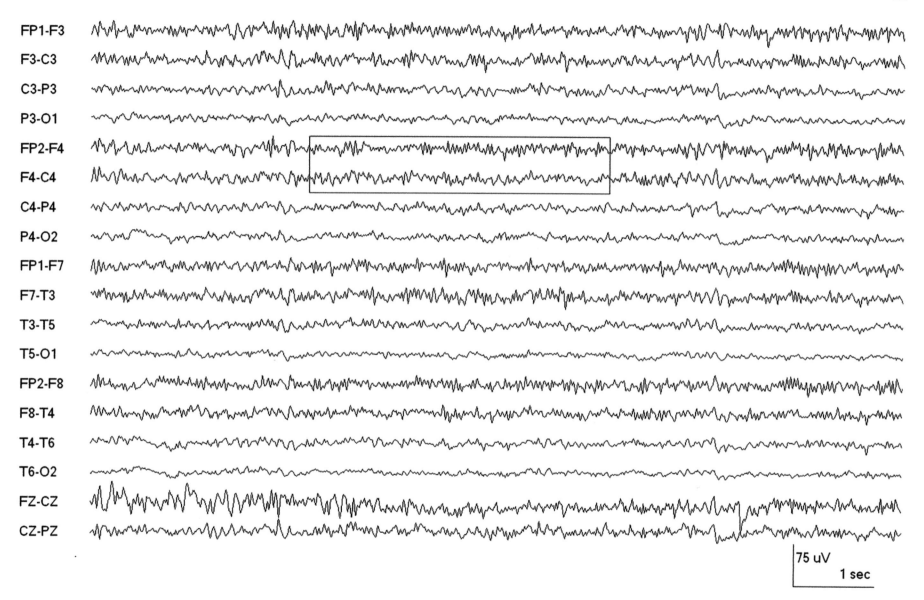

Figure 3.30. (*Continued*) (b) Barbiturate-induced burst suppression, continuous record. Later in the tracing, the EEG shows a lighter level of coma. The background is now continuous with diffuse beta activity (some alpha as well), which is more prominent anteriorly (box), typical of medication-induced beta activity.

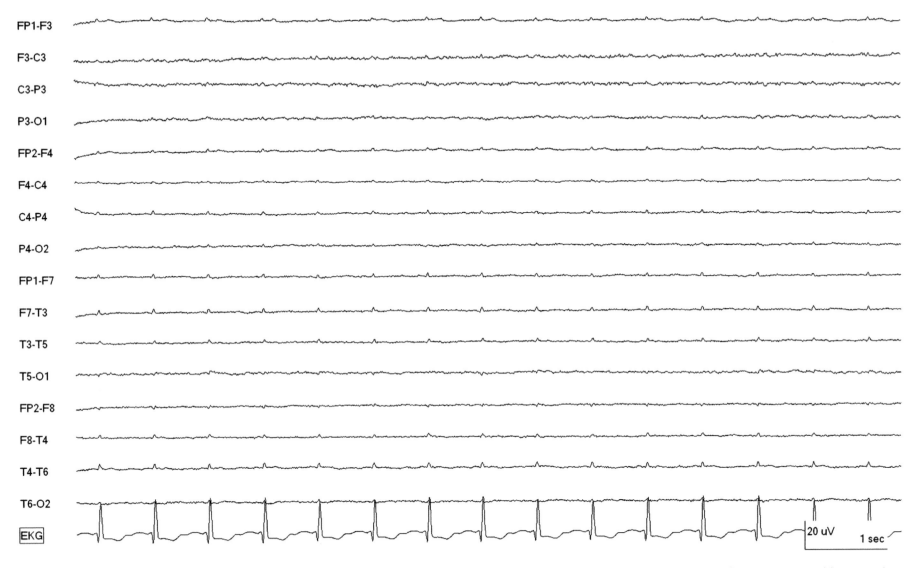

Figure 3.31. Electrocerebral inactivity due to barbiturates. (a) Electrocerebral inactivity due to barbiturates. These EEGs are from a 30-year-old woman in a pentobarbital-induced coma. The EEG shows no evidence of cerebral activity despite the high gain (note the scale legend).

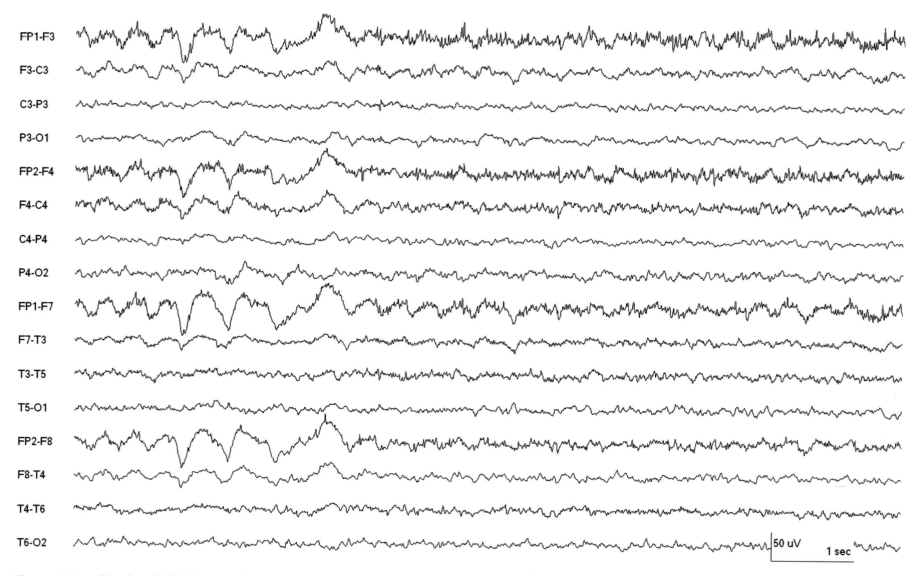

Figure 3.31. (*Continued*) (b) Electrocerebral inactivity due to barbiturates, continuous record. Several days later, following discontinuation of pentobarbital, there is now continuous normal voltage cerebral activity. The EEG is diffusely slow including bursts of higher amplitude frontally predominant delta (first several seconds).

4 Focal EEG abnormalities

Any structural abnormality can cause a focal abnormality on the EEG. There are three EEG findings that suggest a focal abnormality: focal slowing, focal attenuation, and asymmetry of physiologic rhythms (usually reduced on the side of the abnormality). A valuable concept in the localization of focal abnormalities is that a standard 10-20 EEG montage has limited spatial resolution. Abnormalities usually localize to brain regions rather than to a specific gyrus or even lobe. In addition, there are several locations that typically result in EEG abnormalities in neighboring or distant regions. Figure 4.1 helps to understand this concept. The figure demonstrates the position of standard 10-20 electrodes in relation to underlying brain. From this figure it is easy to appreciate how electrodes at F7/8 are more likely to record abnormalities from anterior temporal regions rather than frontal regions, and how electrodes at P7/8 mostly measure activity from posterior temporal structures rather than parietal ones.

4.1 Focal EEG abnormalities

Focal attenuation

Focal attenuation or suppression refers to when the recorded amplitude/voltage in a particular region is reduced (compared to the background amplitude/voltage or that of the homologous region). The terms 'amplitude' and 'voltage' are generally interchangeable, with 'voltage' featuring in the terminology mainly to support consistency.

Focal attenuation can be focal, regional or hemispheric. For example, attenuation can occur in the temporal region, with the voltages relatively preserved in other regions (frontal/parietal/occipital), or hemispheric where the voltages through one side of the head are reduced compared to the other side.

The causes of focal attenuation can be derived from first principles. It can either be caused by:

(1) the dysfunction/destruction of cortical generators of EEG (by any process), or

(2) the obstruction of conduction of that signal to surface recording electrodes (either from an extra-axial collection, most commonly a subdural or epidural collection, but also including extracranial soft tissue swelling [such as a scalp hematoma or subgaleal swelling, common in neonates]).

There are many systemic processes that cause diffuse attenuation of the EEG (i.e., a low voltage record, e.g., Paget's disease of bone, chronic alcoholism, hypothyroidism, Huntington's disease), but these processes rarely result in focal attenuation.

Focal slowing

Although slowing is a common EEG abnormality, its assessment is too often cursory. There are emerging nuances to slowing and the appreciation of these can significantly alter the impression of an EEG.

Hirsch and Brenner's Atlas of EEG in Critical Care, Second Edition. Lawrence J. Hirsch, Michael W.K. Fong, and Richard P. Brenner.
© 2023 John Wiley & Sons Ltd. Published 2023 by John Wiley & Sons Ltd.

Slowing is best classified using the following categories:

(1) continuous (≥90% of the record), or intermittent (<90% of the record; further subdivided into abundant, frequent, occasional or rare, as with all intermittent findings; see ACNS terminology reference chart, Figure 2.1)

(2) polymorphic/irregular/arrhythmic (all synonyms) vs. monomorphic/regular/rhythmic

(3) typical frequency

(4) typical voltage

(5) focal/regional/hemispheric (i.e., lateralized) vs. generalized.

If all of these features are noted, a descriptive summarizing statement can be generated. Examples of summarizing statements are: 'There was continuous polymorphic 2–3-Hz medium-amplitude slowing in the left temporal region'; or 'There was occasional, irregular, sudden-onset, high voltage 1.5–2 Hz right hemisphere slowing, usually lasting 2–5 seconds'.

It is valuable to spend time describing the above features as several form a conceptual dichotomy. Continuous slowing is said to be more associated with structural lesions compared to intermittent slowing; focal slowing is obviously due to vastly different processes compared to generalized slowing; and, importantly, focal rhythmic slowing is highly associated with seizures, whereas focal polymorphic slowing is not. Such is the significance of rhythmic slowing that the terminology includes rhythmic delta activity (RDA) as a main term 2 (examples of which can be found in the chapter on RPPs). Care should be taken when applying these terms as incorrect classification may indirectly result in exposing patients to unnecessary harms. The epitome of this is that focal polymorphic/irregular slowing is often misclassified as rhythmic (LRDA), especially when higher voltage and slower. Several studies have confirmed that LRDA is highly associated with seizures, whereas focal polymorphic slowing is not. Incorrectly concluding that a patient has LRDA potentially results in clinical teams administering ASMs (including highly sedating ones), when this may not have been indicated otherwise.

Speaking of the terminology, all rhythmic delta activity should be classified under RDA (main term 2) as these form specific patterns that have been studied independently and have established associations.

Asymmetry of physiologic rhythms

Most physiologic rhythms are overall symmetric, i.e., they are equally represented in both hemispheres. These rhythms can often have shifting laterality, meaning that they are sometimes seen better formed in one hemisphere, and then at other times of the record better formed in the other hemisphere. However, when taking the record as a whole, most physiologic rhythms should be symmetric.

Persistent asymmetry of these rhythms suggests dysfunction on the side where the rhythm is usually present but instead reduced or absent. Common examples of asymmetries of physiologic rhythms include asymmetry of the PDR and asymmetry of sleep transients (V waves, sleep spindles, K-complexes).

In subtle cases, an asymmetry can be the only finding to suggest regional or hemispheric dysfunction. In even more subtle cases, impaired reactivity of a physiologic rhythm in one hemisphere may be the only finding, i.e., even when voltage and frequency are preserved. The best described (albeit rare) example of this is Bancaud phenomenon: Bancaud described unilateral loss of reactivity of the alpha rhythm (usually to eye opening/closure) in the dysfunctional hemisphere, while preserved in the normal hemisphere. Thus, with eyes open, the alpha rhythm (PDR) ends up higher amplitude and/or better developed in the abnormal hemisphere, since it does not attenuate with eye opening as much as in the healthier hemisphere.

4.2 EEG changes in ischemia

As cerebral blood flow decreases, the EEG changes in the following manner: First, there is subtle loss of faster frequencies (beta and alpha, sometimes including sleep spindles) leading to asymmetry (asymmetry of physiologic rhythms). Then, as flow drops further, slowing appears – first excess theta, then excess delta (focal polymorphic slowing). All of this occurs while ischemia is at a reversible stage and standard anatomical imaging, including MRI with diffusion weighted imaging, can remain normal. As flow continues to decline, there is attenuation/suppression of all frequencies, which, if persistent, corresponds with irreversible neuronal death (infarction), and subsequent focal attenuation. Thus, EEG can detect ischemia before structural neuroimaging can, although perfusion imaging can also detect this. This ability of EEG to detect ischemia early with a procedure that can be done continuously at the bedside, is the basis for continuous EEG monitoring in patients at high risk of developing regional ischemia, such as patients at risk of delayed cerebral ischemia (DCI) in the setting of SAH. These changes are best appreciated with quantitative EEG (QEEG) and continuous monitoring for DCI; these topics will be discussed in Chapter 10: QEEG special considerations.

4.3   Breach effect

Breach effect is a sharply contoured often resembling a mu rhythm (especially when central) that occurs with a skull defect, including a craniotomy, burr hole or skull fracture. A breach effect can even persist after the bone has been replaced. It is often referred to as a *breach rhythm*; however, it is important to realize that the finding itself is not a distinct brain rhythm. Breach effects occur purely as an artifact of surface EEG recording. Removing a piece of the cranium does not lead to the generation of a new cerebral rhythm; it merely alters the way that these rhythms are conducted to the recording electrodes.

A skull defect causes a low-impedance pathway for electrical activity. This results in less attenuation of rhythms before reaching the EEG recording electrode. The result is an accentuation of the underlying EEG, particularly higher frequencies. High-frequency cerebral activity is often low amplitude, even when measured on the cortical surface. This means that these rhythms are often attenuated and often not present on scalp EEG recordings. A skull defect allows all cerebral activity to be enhanced (resulting in higher amplitudes through all frequencies) but the expression of high-frequency activity is the most striking (as it is usually absent). Medium-high amplitude slow activity is minimally affected by a skull defect, but lower amplitude, faster frequencies can be markedly enhanced. This leads to the EEG in the region of breach

appearing sharper (more apiculate) and this can sometimes be misinterpreted as epileptiform. In the presence of a breach effect, there should be a higher threshold for determining that a discharge is 'epileptiform' and features other than how sharp/apiculate it is should be included in this determination (such as the presence of an aftergoing slow wave).

A pure breach effect does not result in focal slowing (mainly because it in itself does not cause disruption of the underlying cerebral rhythms). Although this point is often made, it is in practice fairly uncommon to detect a breach effect without underlying dysfunction. Most often, if a craniotomy is performed, an underlying focal lesion is already present, or a focal lesion is introduced for a neurosurgical indication (e.g., epilepsy surgery). These changes to the brain itself result in underlying focal slowing, but a skull defect alone will not.

Figure list

Figure 4.1 International 10-20 surface electrode positions relative to underlying brain.

Figure 4.2 Unilateral attenuation.

Figure 4.3 Focal slowing.

Figure 4.4 Focal slowing after subarachnoid hemorrhage.

Figure 4.5 Focal slowing and attenuation from stroke.

Figure 4.6 Focal slowing and sharp waves.

Figure 4.7 Hemispheric attenuation.

Figure 4.8 Hemispheric suppression after traumatic brain injury.

Figure 4.9 Unilateral attenuation of physiologic rhythms.

Figure 4.10 Slowing and spindle asymmetry from stroke.

Figure 4.11 Focal attenuation and unilateral visual evoked potential (VEP).

Figure 4.12 Unilateral reactivity.

Figure 4.13 Breach effect.

Figure 4.14 Breach effect.

Figure 4.15 Focal slowing and breach effect after subdural hematoma evacuation.

Figure 4.16 Breach with and without slowing.

Figure 4.17 Breach with and without spikes.

EEGs throughout this atlas have been shown with the following standard recording filters unless otherwise specified: LFF 1 Hz, HFF 70 Hz, notch filter off.

Suggested reading

Alzawahmah M, Fong MWK, Gilmore EJ, Hirsch LJ. Neuroimaging correlates of lateralized rhythmic delta activity, lateralized periodic discharges, and generalized rhythmic delta activity on EEG in critically ill patients. *J Clin Neurophysiol.* 2020.

Cobb WA, Guiloff RJ, Cast J. Breach rhythm: the EEG related to skull defects. *Electroencephalogr Clin Neurophysiol.* 1979;47(3):251–271.

Contreras D, Steriade M. Cellular basis of EEG slow rhythms: a study of dynamic corticothalamic relationships. *J Neurosci.* 1995;15(1 Pt 2):604–622.

Donnelly EM, Blum AS. Focal and generalized slowing, coma, and brain death. In: Blum AS, Rutkove SB, eds. *The Clinical Neurophysiology Primer.* Totowa, NJ: Humana Press; 2007; 127–140.

Faught E. Current role of electroencephalography in cerebral ischemia. *Stroke.* 1993;24(4):609–613.

Gambardella A, Gotman J, Cendes F, Andermann F. Focal intermittent delta activity in patients with mesiotemporal atrophy: a reliable marker of the epileptogenic focus. *Epilepsia.* 1995;36:122–129.

Lundstrom BN, Boly M, Duckrow R, Zaveri HP, Blumenfeld H. Slowing less than 1 Hz is decreased near the seizure onset zone. *Sci Rep.* 2019;9(1):6218.

Noh BH, Berg AT, Nordli DR, Jr., Concordance of MRI lesions and EEG focal slowing in children with nonsyndromic epilepsy. *Epilepsia.* 2013;54(3):455–460.

Panet-Raymond D, Gotman J. Asymmetry in delta activity in patients with focal epilepsy. *Electroencephalogr Clin Neurophysiol.* 1990;75(6):474–481.

Piantoni G, Halgren E, Cash SS. Spatiotemporal characteristics of sleep spindles depend on cortical location. *NeuroImage.* 2017;146:236–245.

Schaul N, Green L, Peyster R, Gotman J. Structural determinants of electroencephalographic findings in acute hemispheric lesions. *Ann Neurol.* 1986;20(6):703–711.

Westmoreland BF, Klass DW. Defective alpha reactivity with mental concentration. *J Clin Neurophysiol.* 1998 Sep;15(5):424–428.

Westmoreland BF, Klass DW. Unusual EEG patterns. *J Clin Neurophysiol.* 1990 Apr;7(2):209–228.

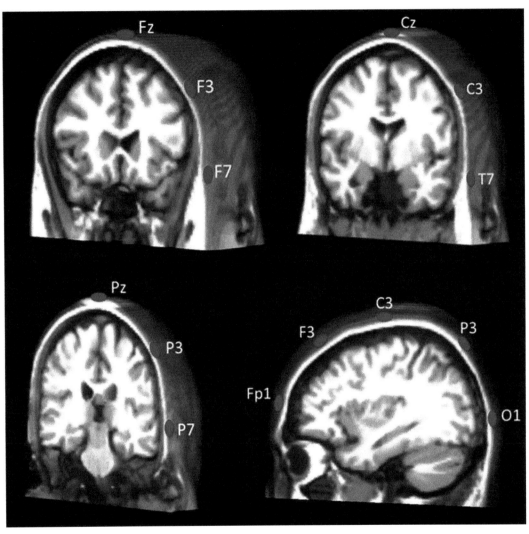

Figure 4.1. International 10-20 surface electrode positions relative to underlying brain. A head reconstructed from an MRI demonstrating the locations of scalp EEG electrodes of a 10-20 montage relative to underlying brain. The notable features are that F7 (and F8 on the right) are fairly low on the head and mostly measure activity projected from the anterior temporal lobe (as opposed to being 'frontal' per se). Most of the frontal activity is recorded by F3 (F4) and Fp1 (Fp2). Similarly, P7 (and P8) are in line with F7/T7 (or F8/T8) and can be seen to largely overly the posterior temporal structures (as opposed to being 'parietal', as suggested by the 'P'). It is important to understand these nuances when attempting to localize abnormalities based on scalp EEG. The International 10-20 System is broadly labeled for standardization and ease of use, and an electrode may not necessarily be named in accordance with the lobe whose activity it is measuring. The 'temporal' electrodes, for example, overlie the Sylvian fissure and superior portions of the temporal lobe. Thus, activity in these channels often includes activity that originates from supra-Sylvian structures, and conversely often does not record well from inferior temporal or basal temporal regions.

Courtesy of Dr Jeremy Moeller, Yale, New Haven, CT.

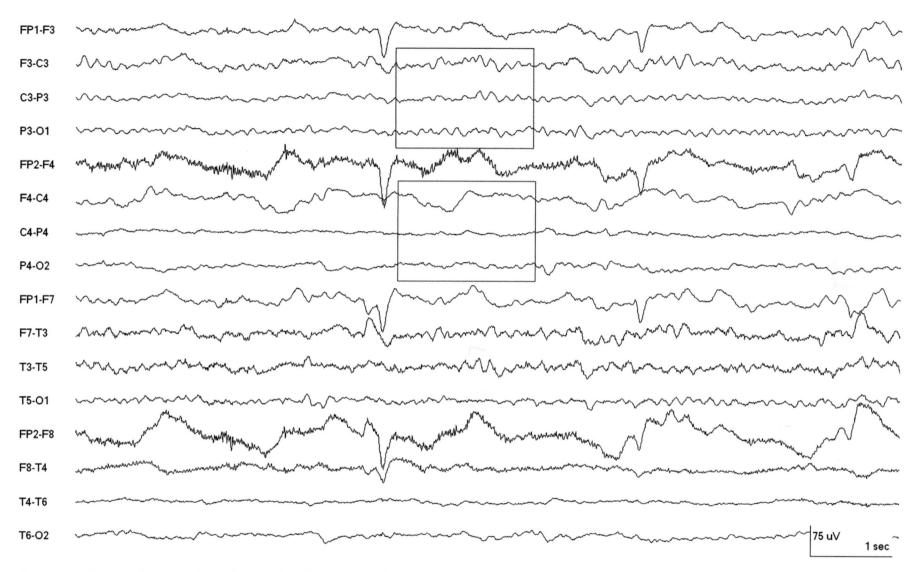

Figure 4.2. Unilateral attenuation. The EEG in this 42-year-old man with a history of a large right MCA/ACA stroke and s/p partial resection of the infarcted tissue shows prominent hemispheric differences. Background activity is markedly suppressed over the right hemisphere. The boxes highlight homologous electrodes, with faster (alpha frequency) activity on the left that is absent on the right. This attenuation of faster activity signifies either cortical dysfunction (such as from an infarct or resection, as in this case) or an extra-axial collection on the right. Note that there is no significant slowing (i.e., no increase in delta activity) in the right centro-parieto-occipital region, just marked attenuation.

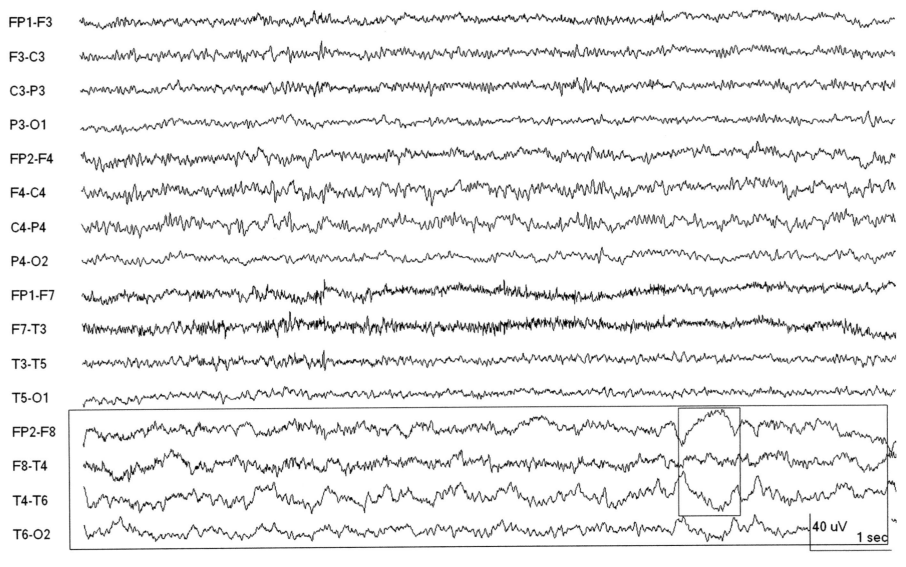

FP1-F3

F3-C3

C3-P3

P3-O1

FP2-F4

F4-C4

C4-P4

P4-O2

FP1-F7

F7-T3

T3-T5

T5-O1

FP2-F8

F8-T4

T4-T6

T6-O2

40 uV
1 sec

Figure 4.3. Focal slowing. (a) Focal slowing, longitudinal bipolar. This EEG demonstrates right temporal slowing consisting of arrhythmic (also known as polymorphic or irregular) delta activity seen in the bottom 4 channels (large box); the small box highlights one particularly prominent slow wave. The slowing is maximal at F8 and T4 equally (best demonstrated by the slow wave in the small box). There is phase reversal of the slow wave across the temporal region, with the F8-T4 channel demonstrating cancellation (i.e., they are equally involved). This can be confirmed in a referential montage.

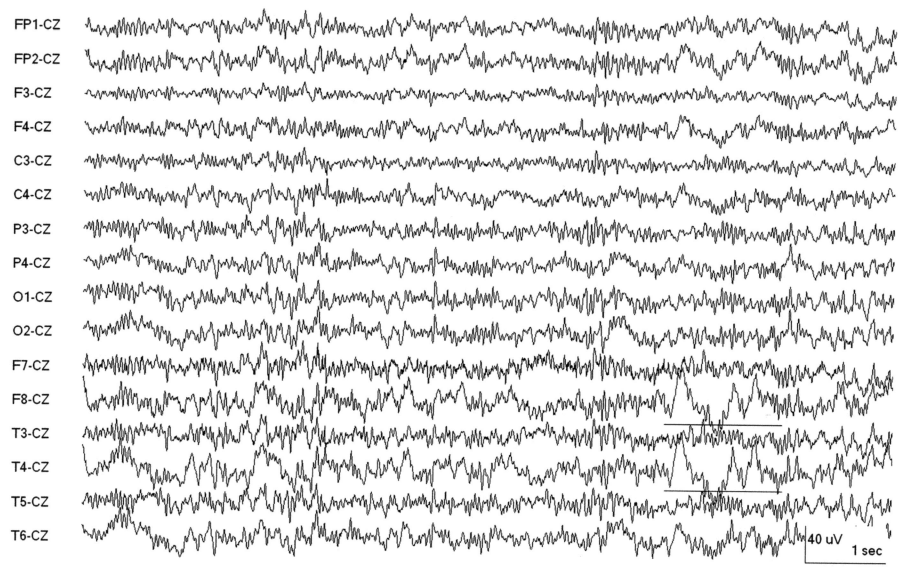

Figure 4.3. (*Continued*) (b) Focal slowing, Cz reference. The midline vertex electrode (Cz) is an excellent choice to display focal slow activity in the temporal region. This is because there is a relatively large physical distance between Cz (vertex) and the temporal electrodes (i.e., they are widely spaced). A large inter-electrode distance increases sensitivity (as the difference between widely spaced electrodes is greater) and allows a good comparison of the two temporal lobes. In addition, abnormalities in the temporal region are usually not present at the vertex (i.e., the Cz reference is unlikely to be active/contaminated). In this case, the intermittent slowing is most marked in the F8 and T4 electrodes (underlined), and they are relatively equally active (as evidenced by the absolute height of the wave being similar on referential montage).

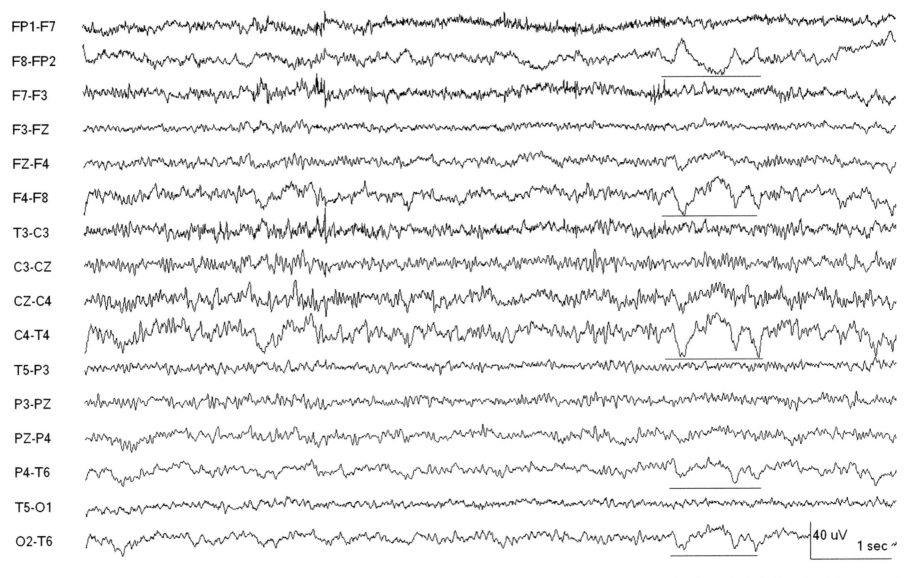

Figure 4.3. (*Continued*) (c) Focal slowing, transverse bipolar. Intermittent delta activity can again be appreciated in the channels including the right temporal electrodes (F8/T4 > T6; underlined).

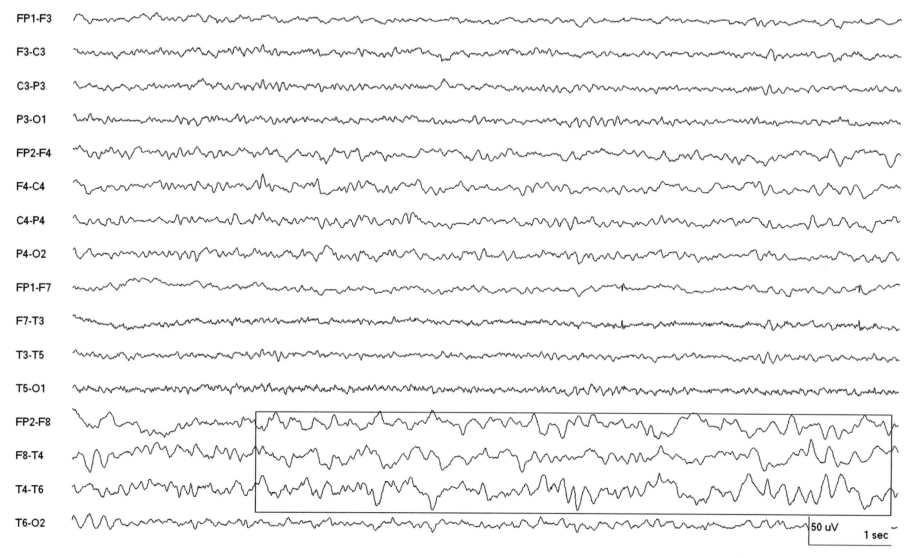

Figure 4.4. Focal slowing after subarachnoid hemorrhage. (a) Focal slowing after subarachnoid hemorrhage, longitudinal bipolar. The EEG in this 40-year-old woman with a history of a subarachnoid hemorrhage, s/p right MCA aneurysm coiling, shows prominent right-sided focal slowing, polymorphic delta, maximal in the temporal region (box).

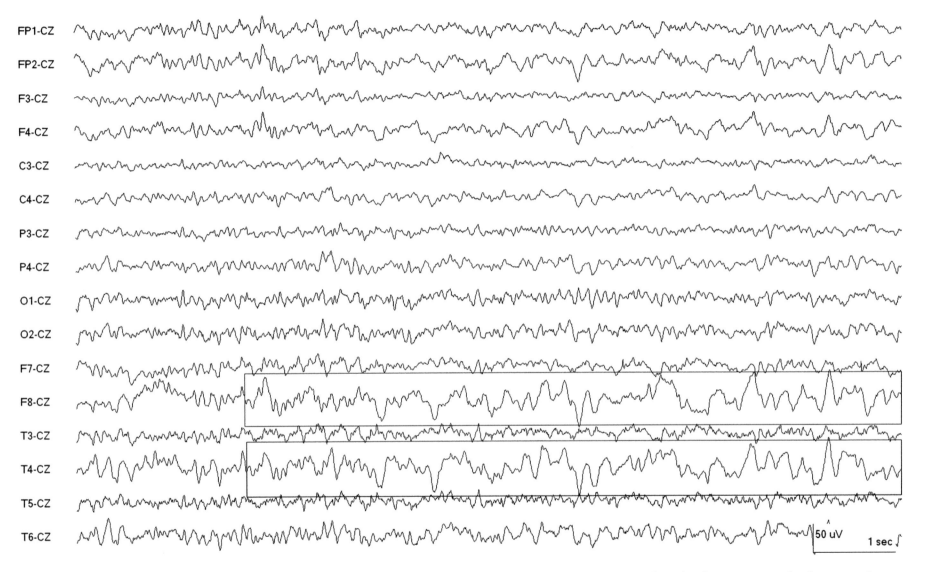

Figure 4.4.   (*Continued*) (b) Focal slowing after subarachnoid hemorrhage, Cz reference: The midline vertex electrode Cz is often a very good reference to demonstrate temporal slowing. The slowing is maximal in the F8 and T4 electrodes (boxes) with lesser involvement of the Fp2 and F4 electrodes.

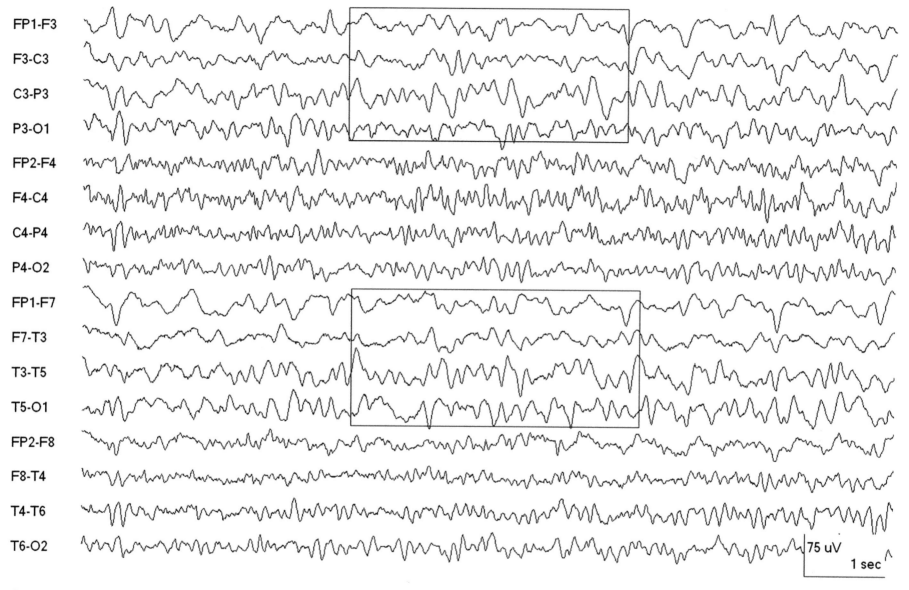

Figure 4.5. Focal slowing and attenuation from stroke. (a) Focal slowing and attenuation from stroke, longitudinal bipolar. The EEG in this 54-year-old woman with a stroke and acute onset of aphasia and right hemiparesis shows prominent slowing (polymorphic delta) and attenuation of faster frequencies over the left hemisphere (box). This suggests both cortical (attenuation) and subcortical (slowing) dysfunction.

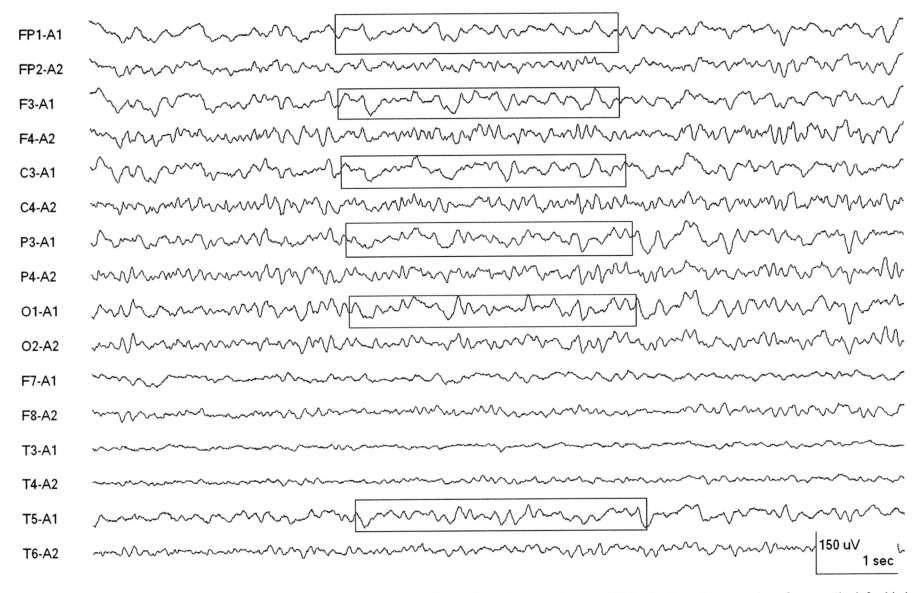

Figure 4.5. *(Continued)* (b) Focal slowing and attenuation from stroke, referential. A reformatted epoch utilizing ipsilateral ears as the reference. The left-sided attenuation (fewer fast frequencies, alpha/beta) and polymorphic slowing (increased delta and theta) are highlighted in the boxes.

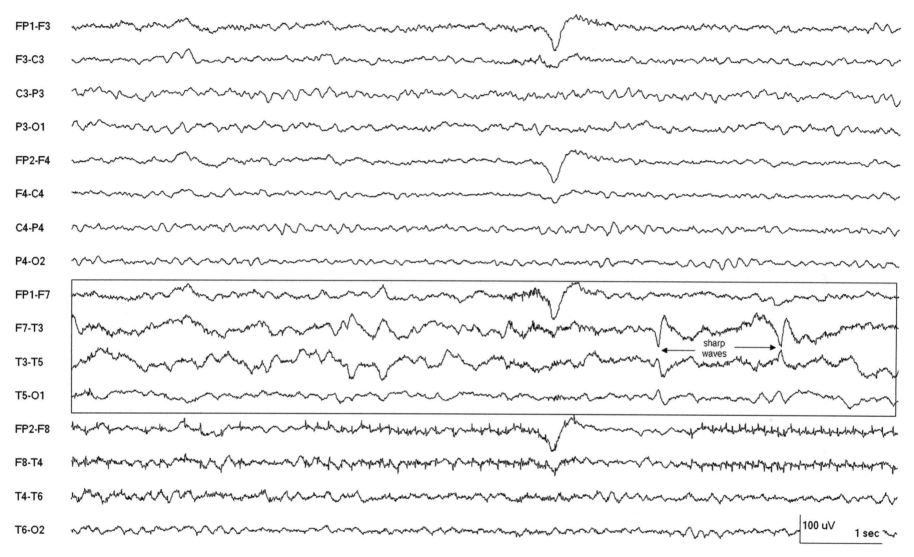

Figure 4.6. Focal slowing and sharp waves. The EEG in this 55-year-old woman with a left-sided cerebral tumor shows prominent focal slowing, polymorphic delta, most marked in the left temporal region (box), as well as sharp waves (arrows) indicating epileptogenic potential, maximal in the mid-temporal area (electrode T3, where it is phase-reversing on this bipolar recording).

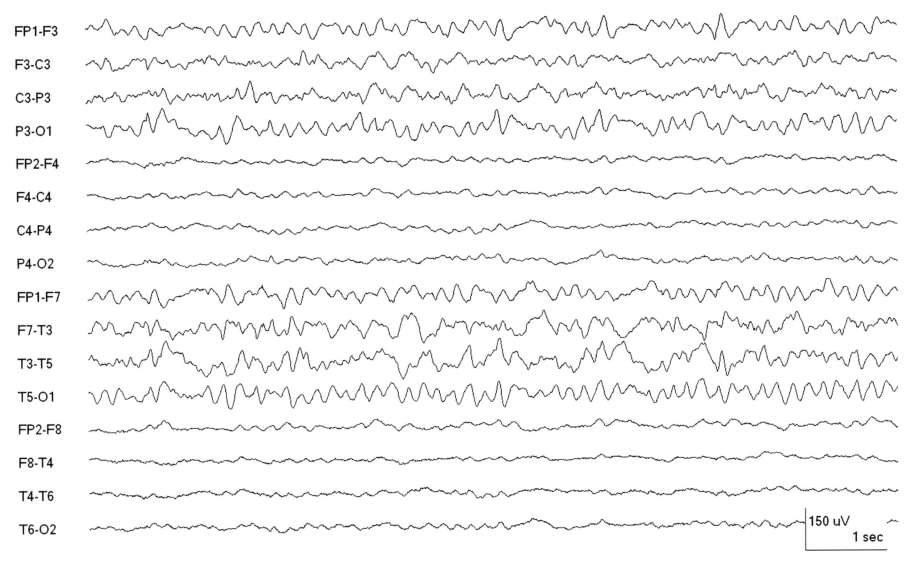

Figure 4.7. Hemispheric attenuation. The EEG in this 48-year-old man shows marked hemispheric differences. Background activity is markedly attenuated on the right. This could also be interpreted as increased voltage on the left and perhaps due to a skull defect (breach effect); however, in this case it was due to a severe right cerebral contusion. If due to breach effect, one can usually see normal activity in the lower voltage hemisphere (just lower voltage than the other side). In this example, there is a marked loss of normal activity on the right, strongly suggesting that the right is the abnormal hemisphere, even if there were a skull defect on the left.

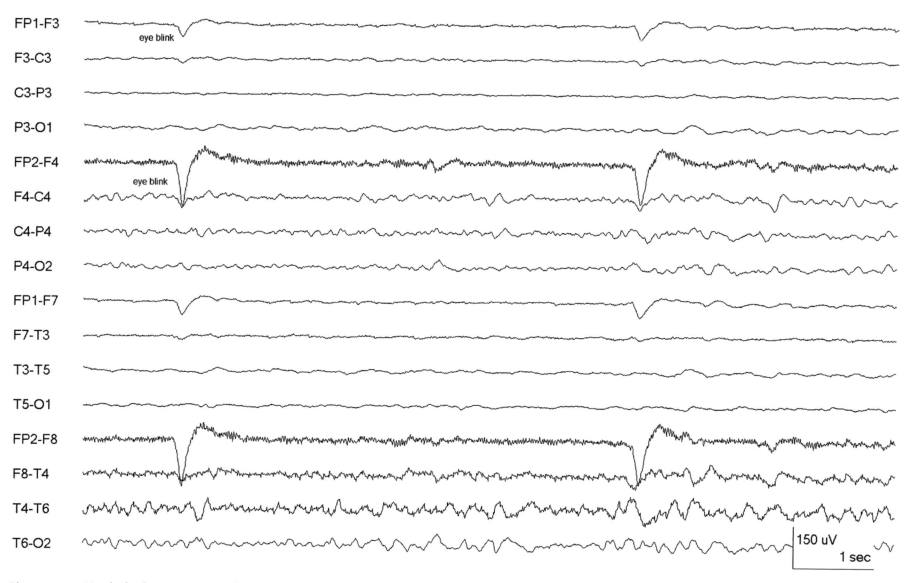

Figure 4.8. Hemispheric suppression after traumatic brain injury. The EEG in this 25-year-old comatose woman involved in a motor vehicle accident shows marked hemispheric differences with activity suppressed over the left side. Faster (more physiologic) frequencies are better developed over the right hemisphere and eye blinks are asymmetric, being decreased on the left. This patient had a left-sided subdural hematoma as well as a left hemispheric infarct. The asymmetric blinks could suggest decreased (but not absent) upgaze on the left (i.e., decreased Bell's phenomenon: upward deviation of the eyes during blinking or eye closure, possibly due to a partial third nerve palsy from trauma, or due to limited eye movement from local swelling), or, alternatively, traumatic injury to the left forehead where Fp1 has been moved away from the eye, or is displaced by scalp hematoma/edema.

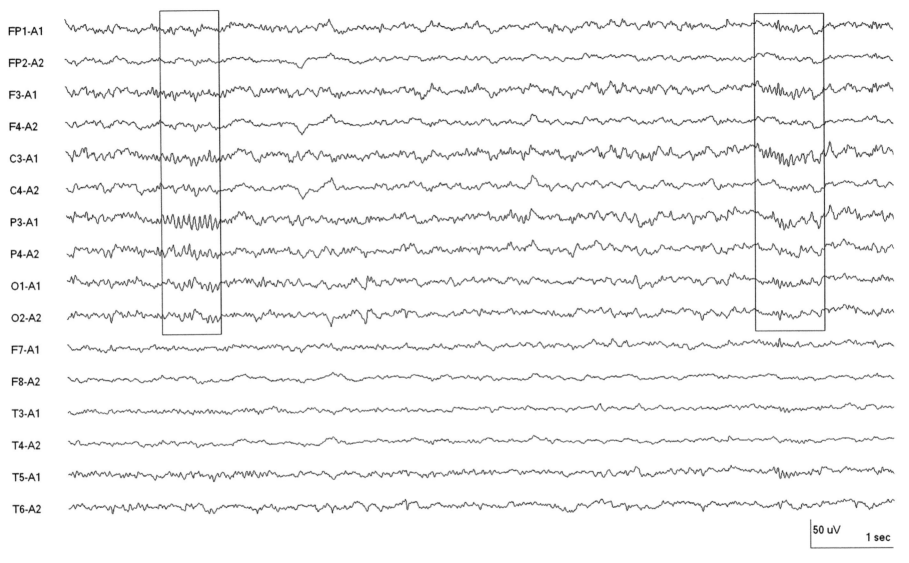

Figure 4.9. Unilateral attenuation of physiologic rhythms. The EEG in this 57-year-old woman s/p large right hemisphere infarct and partial resection shows an asymmetry of beta activity (decreased on the right; shown best in the top 4 channels: compare Fp2-A2 and F4-A2 to Fp1-A1 and F3-A1) and spindles (also decreased on the right, best seen in the 5th–8th channels; compare C4-A2 and P4-A2 to C3-A1 and P3-A1 in the boxes during sleep). The decreased fast activity suggests cortical dysfunction or an extra-axial collection on the right. The decrease in spindles on the right suggests the same, or other involvement of thalamocortical pathways on the right.

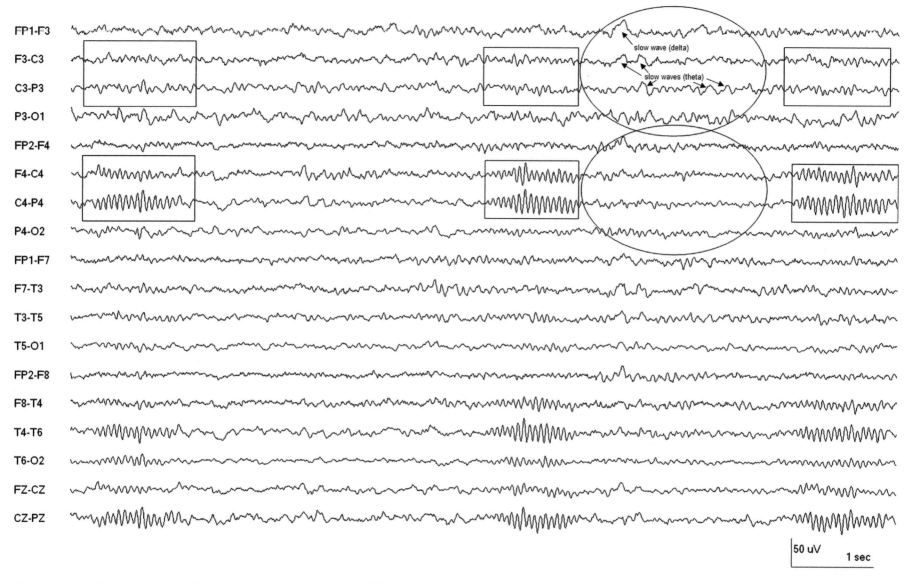

Figure 4.10. Slowing and spindle asymmetry from stroke. An EEG taken during sleep in a 68-year-old woman with an acute left hemispheric stroke shows a prominent asymmetry of sleep spindles, being decreased on the left (compare homologous channels during spindles, in boxes), suggesting dysfunction in the thalamo-cortical pathways involved with spindles. In addition, slower frequencies are present throughout the left hemisphere, maximal in the parasagittal region (compare homologous channels in ellipses), suggesting subcortical white matter dysfunction. Several left-sided slow waves are marked with arrows and labeled.

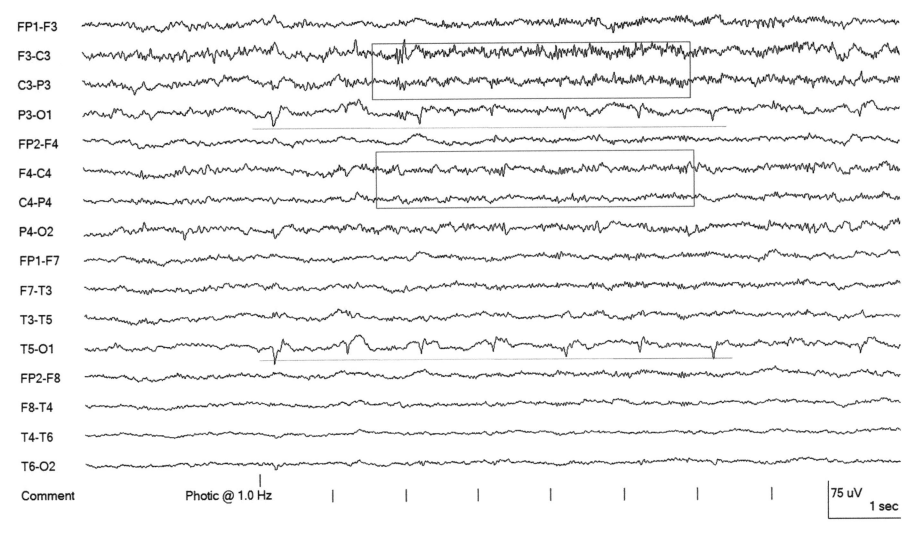

Figure 4.11. Focal attenuation and unilateral visual evoked potential (VEP). The EEG in this 52-year-old man with a history of a prior right-sided hemorrhagic stroke, as well as a recent right occipital ischemic stroke, shows attenuation of fast activity (beta) over the right hemisphere, particularly in the parasagittal area (red), but also apparent in the temporal chains. In addition, visual evoked responses (at the time of 1-Hz photic stimulation, shown at the bottom) are present only on the left (blue underline). Of note, it is unusual to see prominent photic evoked responses on scalp EEG at 1 Hz, and it often suggests either a bad channel (with high impedance in one of the involved channels; O1 in this case) or 'giant' evoked potentials, a sign of cortical hyperexcitability.

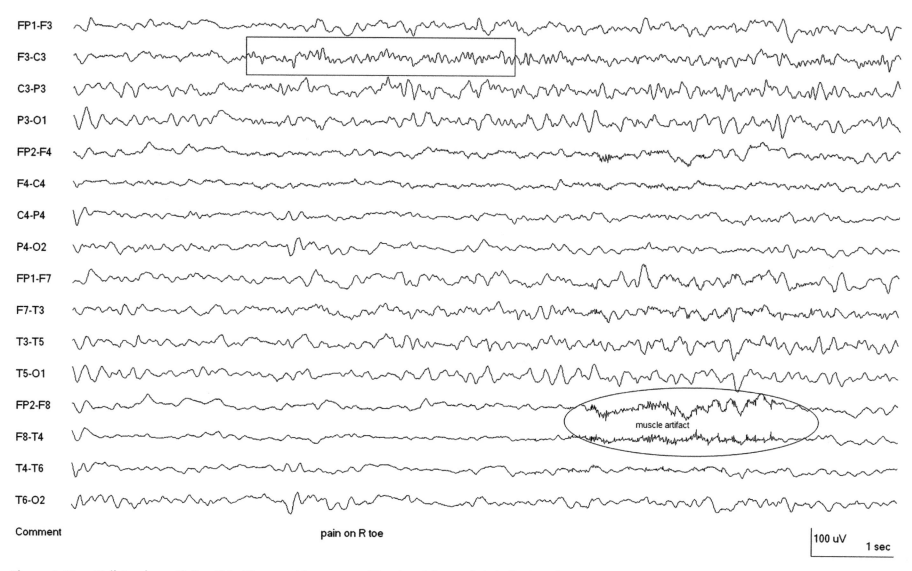

Comment   pain on R toe

100 uV
1 sec

Figure 4.12. Unilateral reactivity. This 80-year-old woman suffered a right hemispheric stroke. The beginning of this EEG shows a mild asymmetry, with attenuation in the right hemisphere. After painful stimulation of the right toe (labeled), there is an increase in faster frequency activity on the left (box), but the right hemisphere remains attenuated.

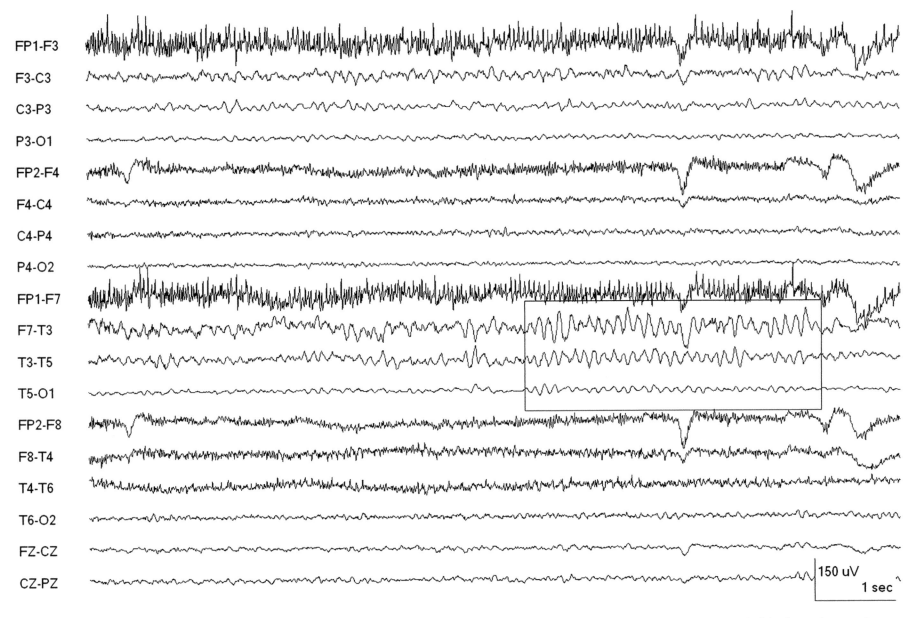

Figure 4.13. Breach effect. This EEG is from a 63-year-old woman s/p left frontal aneurysm clipping. This EEG shows higher amplitudes of faster frequencies on the left compared to the right, most prominent at T3 (left temporal; box). This is due to a skull defect on the left. In the presence of a skull defect (even a small one such as a skull fracture or burr hole), faster frequencies can appear higher amplitude and often sharper, resulting in what is known as a breach rhythm or breach effect.

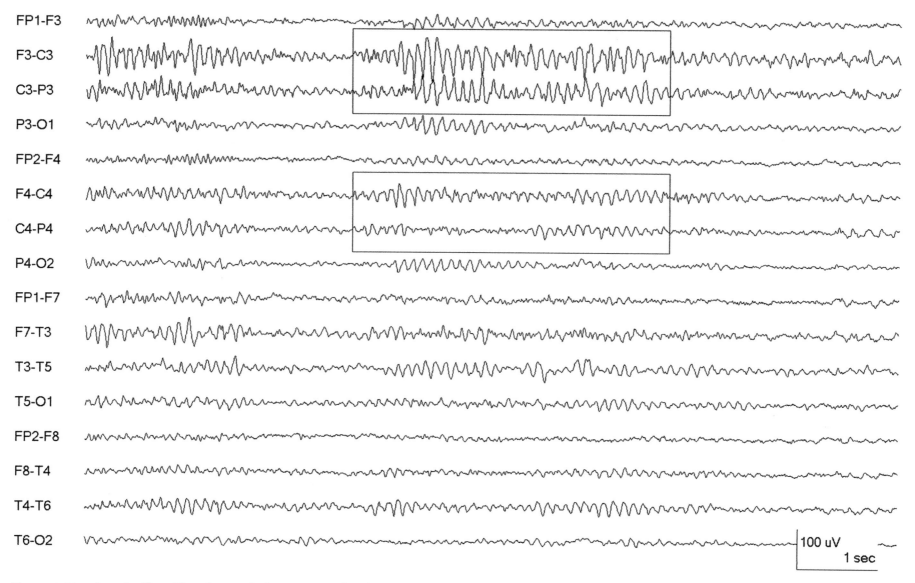

Figure 4.14.   Breach effect. There is a marked asymmetry of background activity in the central areas in this 75-year-old man, with activity being of greater voltage on the left (C3 vs C4, boxes). The patient has had previous surgery in this area, and this represents a breach rhythm due to the skull defect. Although at times this can be spiky/apiculate in appearance, this does not signify epileptic potential.

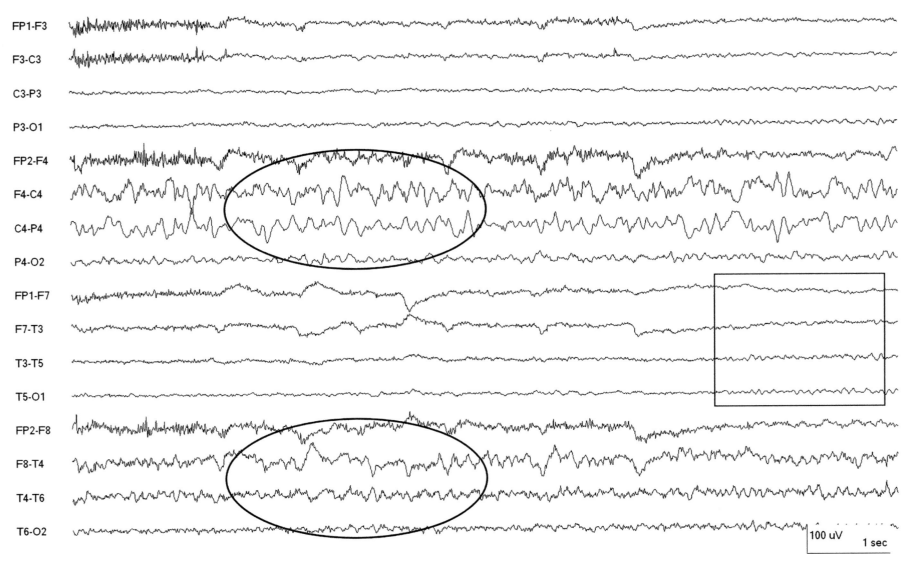

Figure 4.15. Focal slowing and breach effect after subdural hematoma evacuation. The EEG in this 52-year-old man s/p evacuation of a right subdural hematoma shows marked hemispheric differences. The left hemisphere is more 'normal'. At the beginning of the page the activity on the left is largely attenuated, but toward the end there appears what is likely a fragment of the alpha rhythm with preserved A-P gradient (box). The patient had a right craniectomy. This is a prominent example of the effects of a skull defect, where the background activity, including faster frequencies, are of higher voltage over the right side (ellipses). There is also higher voltage slowing on the right that suggests underlying dysfunction in addition to the craniectomy (recalling that a pure breach effect does not generate new rhythms, but rather affects how these rhythms are projected to scalp recording electrodes; thus, slow waves still represent cerebral dysfunction underlying the skull defect).

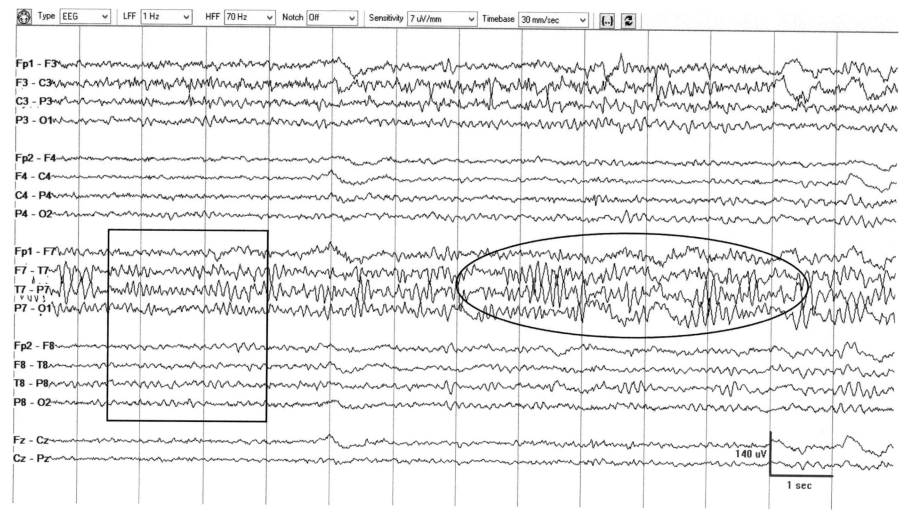

Figure 4.16. Breach with and without slowing. (a) Breach with and without slowing, longitudinal bipolar: These EEGs are from a 78-year-old woman s/p meningioma resection via left temporal craniotomy. The figure contrasts breach effect without slowing (box) and breach effect with underlying focal slowing (ellipse). At the beginning of the page the homologous left temporal region consists of activity that is higher voltage and sharper, with faster frequencies, compared to the right. This is the result of breach effect (skull defect) at a time where there is no concomitant focal slowing. In the later part of the page, intermittent polymorphic 1.5–2-Hz slowing is now present in the left temporal region. The result is that the activity of the breach effect has been overlaid on the delta waves; this indicates cerebral dysfunction in addition to the skull defect.

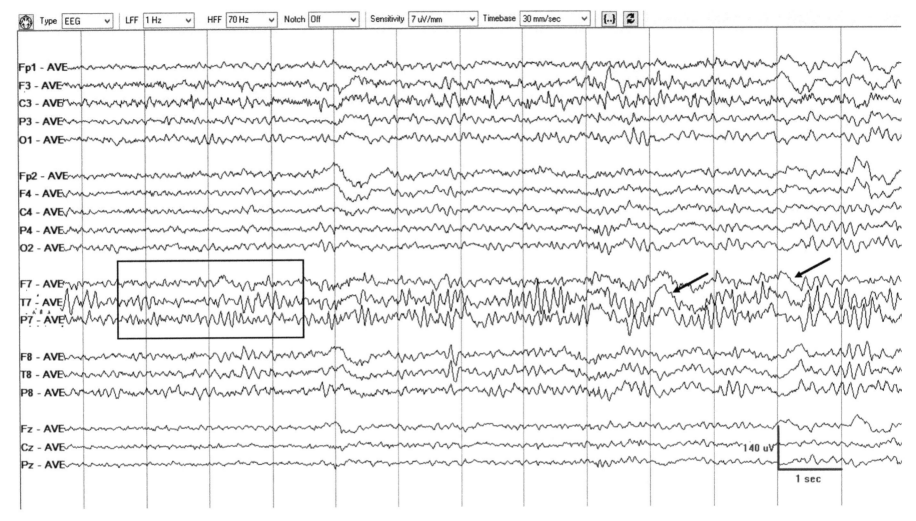

Figure 4.16.   (*Continued*) (b) Breach with and without slowing, referential. The commencement of the focal slowing can be better seen on a referential montage, in this case average reference. Here it is easier to appreciate the emergence of focal delta waves in the left temporal region (arrows). The activity at the beginning of the page (box) is due to breach effect alone, whereas the addition of focal slowing suggests underlying dysfunction.

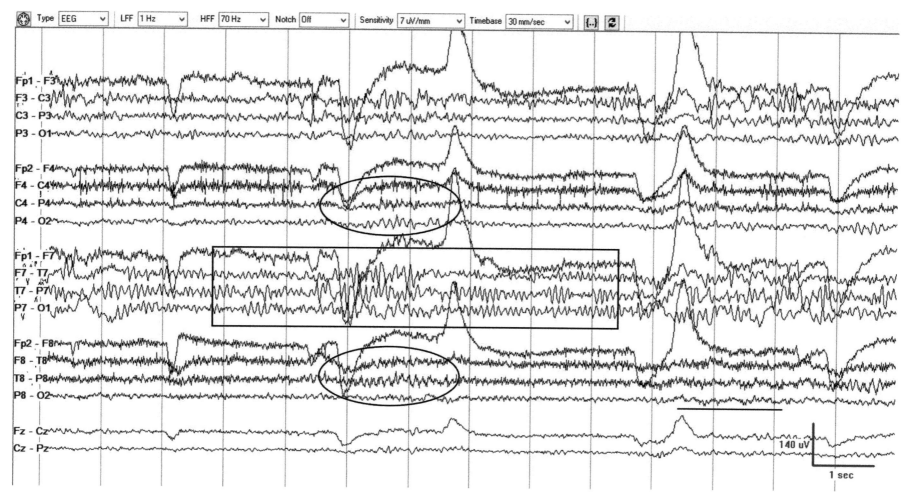

Figure 4.16. (*Continued*) (c) Breach with and without slowing, loss of reactivity, longitudinal bipolar. This EEG is from the same patient at a different stage of the record. In this stage the patient has been asked to blink, and close/open her eyes (as demonstrated by the eye movement artifacts). The EEG demonstrates more physiologic reactivity in the healthy (right) hemisphere. When the patient closes her eyes, the PDR becomes more prominent (ellipses), but predominantly on the right. When she closes her eyes, the activity relatively attenuates (underline), again more clearly on the right. When the patient closes or opens her eyes there is little change to the EEG in the abnormal left hemisphere (box). This phenomenon was initially described by Bancaud, with Bancaud's phenomenon being loss of normal attenuation (reactivity) of the alpha rhythm in the dysfunctional hemisphere (a feature that in this case is accentuated by breach effect); this can cause a paradoxically higher amplitude and more prominent PDR in the abnormal hemisphere, as is seen here.

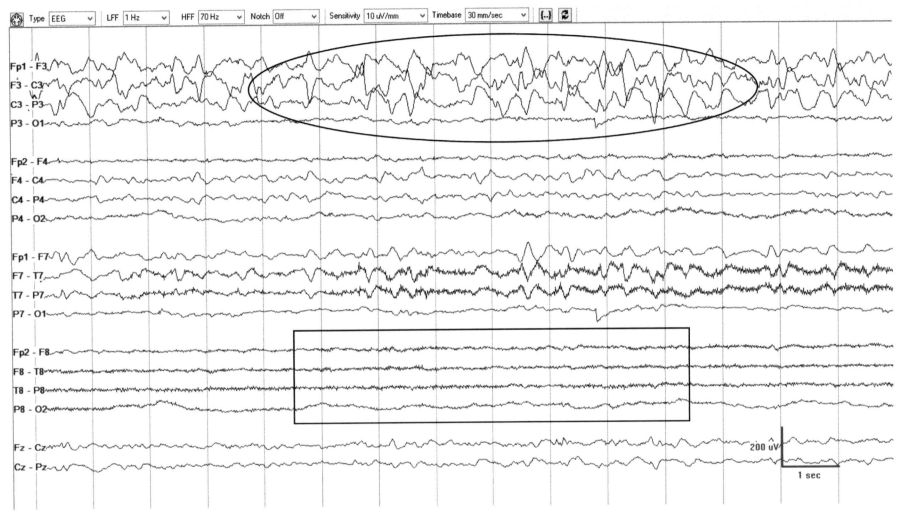

Figure 4.17. Breach with and without spikes. (a) Breach without spikes, longitudinal bipolar. These EEGs are from a 16-year-old boy who suffered from non-accidental trauma in infancy. He has bilateral skull defects and severe encephalomalacia of the right hemisphere. There is suppression of the right temporal region (box). This conveys an important point, which is the EEG is the cumulative result of cortical generators, factors that influence those generators, and factors that influence how that activity is projected to the scalp. A process can impede signals being propagated or accentuate them due to a skull defect. However, even though there is a skull defect over the right hemisphere, the activity in the temporal region is suppressed, and that is because there is simply no cortex underlying this to generate a signal in the first place. This EEG demonstrates a second valuable point; activity within a significant skull defect can be sharply contoured (ellipse) and it can be sometimes difficult to know if this activity is epileptiform. When a skull defect is present, one must have a higher threshold for calling something epileptiform; features such as aftergoing slow waves or other disruption of the ongoing background activity are helpful in this regard.

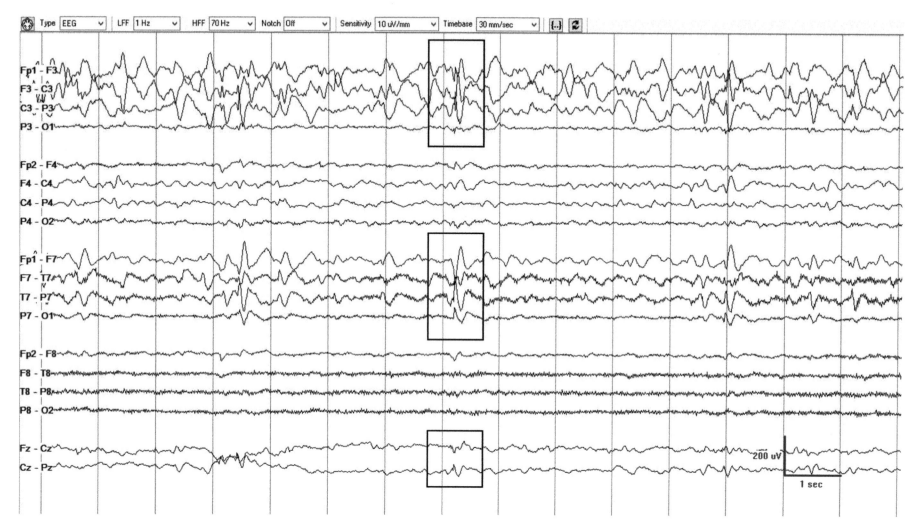

Figure 4.17. (*Continued*) (b) Breach with spikes, longitudinal bipolar. A second page of EEG from the same patient contrasts Figure 4.17a. This page demonstrates definite epileptiform discharges, with one highlighted in the box. Significant caution should be taken to avoid over reporting sharply contoured activity in a breach effect as epileptiform. The same principles apply as to when a discharge should be called epileptiform. Several of these features are highlighted by this example: 1. the discharges should have an asymmetric morphology, usually with rapid upstroke and slow downstroke, though the reverse can also occur; 2. the stereotyped association with an aftergoing slow wave; 3. clearly disrupts and stands out from the background (in this case clearly stands out from the breach rhythm); and 4. has a clear electrographic field (in this case extending into the temporal region with corresponding deflections even seen in the midline).

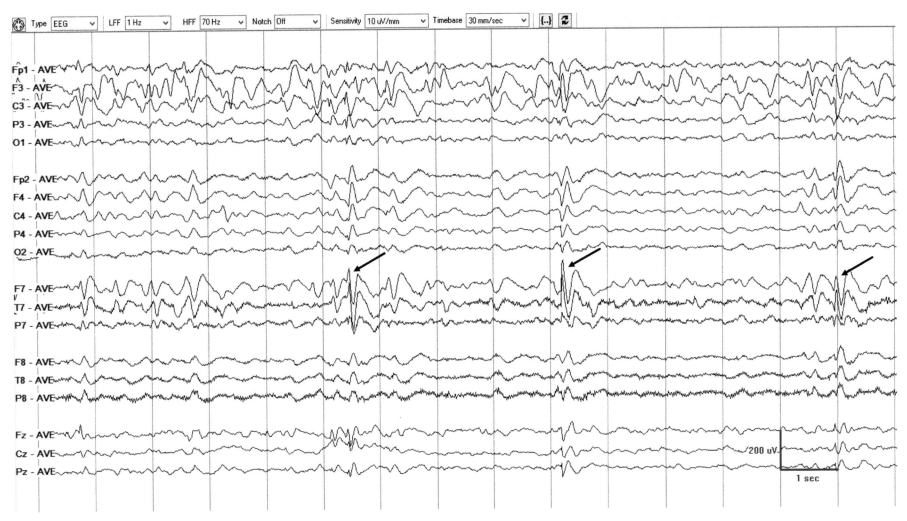

Figure 4.17.   (*Continued*) (c) Breach with spikes, referential. The same page of EEG reformatted into an average referential montage. Note the epileptiform discharges (arrows) that clearly stand out from the underlying breach.

5 Rhythmic and periodic patterns

Much time is spent identifying and classifying rhythmic and periodic patterns (RPPs). Many of these patterns are associated with seizures and can sometimes themselves be considered ictal. They also provide insight into the processes of the brain that may not be apparent with initial imaging. For example, in a patient who sustained a traumatic brain injury (TBI) and the CT head demonstrates a right frontal contusion, an EEG showing bilateral independent periodic discharges (BIPDs) provides information that the injury may in fact be bilateral and that either hemisphere is at risk of generating seizure.

Proper classification/terminology provides the ability to trend the burden of patterns over days to weeks (often across several different EEG readers). A higher pattern burden is one of the factors that is associated with seizures (and outcome) and gradual reduction of this (or changes in other modifiers) can predate clinical improvements. Classification also allows for robust multicenter research collaboration, and the associations and significance of many of these patterns have been determined over the past decade as a result of this.

Rhythmic and periodic patterns are described in accordance with the ACNS critical care EEG terminology 2021 by combining a localization descriptor from 'Main term 1' and a pattern type descriptor from 'Main term 2'. These main terms combined provide a framework for a wide variety of patterns and these can be further refined by applying 'major' and 'minor' modifiers.

5.1 Main term 1 (location)

The first consideration is the location of a pattern (Figure 5.1). The location can be described as either:

- generalized
- lateralized
- bilateral independent
- unilateral independent, or
- multifocal

The most commonly used terms are generalized and lateralized. A generalized pattern is bilaterally synchronous and symmetric, even if it has a restricted field (e.g., bifrontal), and even if it has a shifting predominance. A lateralized pattern is either strictly unilateral, or bilateral but clearly and consistently higher amplitude in one hemisphere (bilateral asymmetric), or bilateral but with a consistent lead-in from one side (bilateral asynchronous). The remainder of the location terms describe several patterns occurring simultaneously, i.e., overlapping in time rather than sequentially,

Hirsch and Brenner's Atlas of EEG in Critical Care, Second Edition. Lawrence J. Hirsch, Michael W.K. Fong, and Richard P. Brenner.
© 2023 John Wiley & Sons Ltd. Published 2023 by John Wiley & Sons Ltd.

with one starting after the other stops. These terms are bilateral independent (BI), during which there are two independent lateralized patterns, one in each hemisphere: unilateral independent (UI), with two independent lateralized patterns both in the same hemisphere; or multifocal (Mf), with at least three independent lateralized patterns, with at least one in each hemisphere (usually meaning two in one hemisphere and one in the other hemisphere).

It is intuitive that a higher number of RPPs signifies a more extensive process, greater association with seizures and worse clinical outcomes. This has been shown in patients with BIPDs that are associated with worse mental status (usually coma), and worse outcome, compared to patients with LPDs. Multifocal RPPs are rare but similarly occur in the setting of significant cerebral insult representing highly epileptic foci through multiple brain regions.

5.2   Main term 2 (pattern type)

Once the location of a RPP is determined, the second descriptor is the pattern type (Figure 5.2). The three descriptors for Main term 2 are rhythmic delta activity (RDA), periodic discharges (PDs), and spike-and-wave or sharp-and-wave (SW).

Rhythmic delta activity (RDA)

Rhythmic delta activity is delta activity (0.5 to ≤ 4 Hz) where the repetition of the waveforms has a relatively uniform morphology and duration, and without an interval between consecutive waveforms. The duration of one cycle (i.e., the period) of the rhythmic pattern should vary by <50% from the duration of the subsequent cycle for the majority (>50%) of cycle pairs to qualify as rhythmic.

The significance of RDA differs if it is generalized (GRDA) vs. lateralized (which includes any lateralized pattern [L, BI, UI and Mf]). GRDA is usually seen in the setting of diffuse dysfunction and encephalopathy, keeping in mind that a subset of the pattern is the previously described FIRDA (frontal intermittent rhythmic delta activity). Even if GRDA is sharply contoured (GRDA+S), it has not been shown to be associated with seizures, a

finding that replicates the associations and teachings historically described of FIRDA. Any lateralized RDA, however, is highly associated with seizures. The best described/recognized historical example is temporal-predominant RDA (known as temporal intermittent rhythmic delta activity [TIRDA] in the epilepsy literature; a subset of LRDA), which is well associated with temporal lobe epilepsy. This association (of any lateralized RDA and seizures) has been robustly confirmed in the critical care setting, with multiple independent publications from numerous centers confirming the finding.

The conceptual dichotomy between generalized and lateralized RDA makes inherent sense. Under normal physiologic conditions, cortical generators of EEG are largely asynchronous and have a relatively small projection to surface recording electrodes. When a sufficient proportion of this cortex becomes 'dysfunctional', then large volumes of the cortex can be synchronized by thalamic mediators, resulting in high-amplitude, symmetric and synchronous rhythmic delta waves (GRDA). Conversely, the pathophysiology of TIRDA has been shown (using intracranial EEG) to be commonly associated with repetitive epileptiform discharges (including bursts of polyspikes) from the temporal lobe on intracranial recordings that are poorly projected to the surface. Limited intracranial EEG in critically ill patients has confirmed the intracranial correlate of LRDA as periodic epileptiform discharges (or even electrographic seizures), hence making sense that the pattern is similarly highly associated with seizures. In fact, the pathophysiology of LRDA does not differ from LPDs (although the surface projections differ), which makes it of no surprise that the clinical, imaging and seizure associations are very similar between the two patterns, if not identical.

Periodic discharges (PDs)

'Discharges' are waveforms that clearly stand out from the background that last <0.5 seconds, or ≥ 0.5 seconds but must have no more than 3 phases (as opposed to 'bursts' that are ≥ 0.5 seconds *and* have at least 4 phases). Periodic discharges (PDs) are the repetition of waveforms with relatively uniform morphology and duration with a clearly discernible inter-discharge interval between consecutive waveforms and recurrence of the waveform at nearly regular intervals. 'Nearly regular intervals' is defined as the cycle length (i.e., period) should vary by <50% from one cycle to the next in most (>50%) cycle pairs.

The dichotomy between generalized and lateralized patterns that exists for RDA does not apply to PDs, i.e., both GPDs and LPDs are highly associated with seizures (though LPDs more so). GPDs (like GRDA) are commonly seen in the context of encephalopathy; however, more than one third of patients will have definite seizures during their acute illness. GPDs can be seen in a variety of settings including in postanoxic coma (when the background is often flat between the discharges), after convulsive status epilepticus, with metabolic disorders, in Creutzfeldt–Jacob disease, during Hashimoto encephalopathy, from medication toxicity (e.g. baclofen, lithium, ifosfamide and cefepime) and in end-stage Alzheimer disease.

Generalized periodic discharges can have triphasic morphology (also known as triphasic waves [TW]). They were initially described in hepatic encephalopathy but as the volume and variety of patients monitored with cEEG has increased, they are commonly seen across a variety of presenting etiologies. One study even demonstrated that patients with TWs were less likely to have a toxic-metabolic encephalopathy compared to a cohort with GPDs without triphasic morphology. When GPDs have a triphasic morphology they tend to recur at 1–2 per second and wax and wane throughout a recording, partly dependent on level of alertness. Nonconvulsive status epilepticus can appear quite similar. Although some have suggested specific features which are more common in patients with metabolic encephalopathy rather than seizures, almost all of these studies suffer from lack of a gold standard for making the final diagnosis, and many have circular logic. It is clear that in a given individual, EEG alone often cannot distinguish between triphasic waves of metabolic encephalopathy (if they exist) and nonconvulsive seizures. Unfortunately, both resolve with benzodiazepines as well. Thus, only EEG *and clinical* improvement with IV anti-seizure medication can prove the presence of nonconvulsive status epilepticus. It is almost impossible to disprove it. Both epileptiform patterns (including seizures) and TWs commonly increase or appear with alerting stimuli in the critically ill; thus, that cannot be used to differentiate them.

Lateralized periodic discharges (LPDs) consist of lateralized complexes usually recurring every 0.5–2 s. The complexes often (but not always) consist of sharp waves or spikes that may be followed by a slow wave. The clinical picture associated with LPDs is usually obtundation, focal seizures, and focal neurological signs. Many patients with LPDs (more than half) will also have seizures during the acute stage of illness. For the majority of cases, LPDs are considered an interictal pattern. There are fewer cases where LPDs are clearly an ictal pattern, mainly when associated with concordant time-locked jerking or focal neurological deficits that resolve when the pattern is treated.

Acute stroke (hemorrhagic and ischemic) is the most common etiology of LPDs, although any acute brain injury that results in focal cortical hyperexcitability can manifest as LPDs. Most patients with herpes simplex encephalitis develop LPDs, maximal in the temporal region(s) and often consisting of prolonged complexes (~0.5 s), often not even sharply contoured, recurring every 1–4 s; however, this pattern is certainly not specific for this diagnosis. Regardless of etiology, LPDs are usually a transient phenomenon. With time (days to weeks), the discharges tend to decrease in amplitude, the repetition rate decreases and ultimately the discharges cease.

'Spike-and-wave' and 'sharp-and-wave' (SW)

SW is defined as a spike, polyspike or sharp wave consistently followed by a slow wave in a regularly repeating and alternating pattern (i.e., spike, then wave, then spike, then wave, etc. for at least six cycles). Technically, this should be called 'spike-and-slow wave', 'sharp wave-and-slow wave' or 'polyspike-and-slow wave', but they are all abbreviated SW for convenience. This specific pattern is much less common than RDA and PDs. The largest difference between SW and PDs, is that in SW there is no inter-discharge interval i.e., the beginning of a subsequent sharp-and-wave complex follows immediately after the end of the sharp-and-wave complex preceding it. The clinical significance, radiographic associations, and association with seizures is probably similar to patients with comparative PDs (i.e., GSW has similar connotations to GPDs, and LSW has similar implications to LPDs), though there are few publications on SW in the critically ill.

5.3   Major and minor modifiers (including *plus* modifiers)

All RPPs can be classified as a combination of main term 1 and 2 above. However, there are multiple features of a pattern that make it more (or less) epileptiform and these are accommodated for in the modifier sections. Major modifiers provide the bulk of description for RPPs, such as how often they occur (prevalence), how long they last (duration), the typical frequency (e.g., 1.5 Hz), or their sharpness.

Plus (+) modifiers describe activity superimposed on RPPs that result in them appearing more 'ictal'. Plus modifiers include admixed sharp waves (+S), added fast activity (+F) or superimposed rhythmic activity (+R) (Figure 5.3). RDA cannot have a +R modifier as the pattern is by definition already rhythmic. PDs cannot have a '+S' since they already have a sharpness modifier that has four categories (spiky, sharp, sharply contoured and blunt). Occasional patterns can have both plus modifiers, for example LPDs+FR. The emergence, or the increase in, plus modifiers can herald the onset of seizures. For example, LPDs changing to LPDs+F can signify that the excitability of underlying cortex has increased, from which transition into an electrographic seizure is probable. Extreme delta brushes (EDB) is an even more specific subset of +, and given its association with NMDA encephalitis has already been presented in Chapter 3 on encephalopathy and coma.

Although there are many descriptors that reside under the modifiers umbrella, it should be noted that their association with seizures is not uniform. Multivariable analysis of nearly 5000 patients revealed that increasing typical frequency (especially ≥2 Hz), and plus modifiers were significantly associated with a higher risk of seizures, whereas modifiers such as voltage, stimulus-induced or not, or triphasic morphology had little independent bearing on the risk of acute seizures.

5.4   Stimulus-induced rhythmic, periodic or ictal discharges (SIRPIDs)

With the advent of continuous video-EEG recordings in the ICU, it became apparent that alerting stimuli (suction, exam, noise, pain) in encephalopathic patients commonly elicit highly epileptiform patterns made up of any of the RPPs described above, or unequivocal evolving electrographic and even electroclinical seizures. These can be focal or generalized. The phenomena of stimulus-induced patterns and seizures is encapsulated within the term SIRPIDs; in the terminology, any pattern can have an 'SI-' prefix, indicating that it can be induced by stimulation (even if it also occurs spontaneously). Note: that the term SIRPIDs no longer features in the terminology except as a specific form of reactivity in which the only change in the EEG is 'SIRPIDs-only'. As patterns and seizures have been further studied, it has become apparent that it is the content of the pattern (i.e., GRDA vs. GPD vs. ESz, etc.) that determines the chance of further seizures, rather than whether or not the pattern is stimulus-induced. The duration and prominence of the pattern often correlate with the duration and degree of stimulation, and the pattern can usually be reproduced with further stimulation (after allowing return to the non-stimulated background). This is usually a purely electrographic finding with no obvious clinical accompaniment, although some patients will have ECSz as well; these are typically focal motor, as other types would be very difficult to detect.

5.5   Brief potentially Ictal Rhythmic Discharges (BIRDs)

Brief potentially Ictal Rhythmic Discharges (BIRDs) represents a group of highly epileptic patterns with a strong association with subsequent seizures. BIRDs are defined as focal or generalized rhythmic activity >4 Hz (at least six waves at a regular rate) lasting ≥0.5 to <10 s, not consistent with a known normal pattern or benign variant, not part of burst suppression or burst attenuation, without definite clinical correlate, and that has at least one of the following features (Figure 5.4):

(1) evolution ('evolving BIRDs,' a form of definite BIRDs)

(2) similar morphology and location to interictal epileptiform discharges or seizures in the same patient (definite BIRDs)

(3) sharply contoured but without (1) or (2) (possible BIRDs).

BIRDs often represent the beginnings of ESzs and their strong association with seizures is not surprising. If a >4 Hz RPP, or a pattern with evolution, lasts for ≥10 s, these would qualify as ESzs. Whether to keep or remove the historical and somewhat arbitrary cut off for ESz to having to be ≥10 s has been discussed at length, but there has not been sufficient consensus by experts to remove this barrier, and currently there is not sufficient evidence in the literature to have discussion of what this cut off should realistically be. Roughly three quarters (75%) of patients with BIRDs will go on to develop definite ESz, and nearly 100% of critically ill patients with evolving BIRDs will have definite seizures during their acute illness. In non-critically ill patients, BIRDs are a sign of poorly controlled epilepsy, and are very useful for localizing the seizure onset zone. In both critically ill and non-critically ill patients, when seizures are fully controlled, BIRDs resolve as well.

Figure list

Figure 5.1 Main term 1 (localization).

Figure 5.2 Main term 2 (pattern type).

Figure 5.3 Plus (+) modifiers.

Figure 5.4 Brief potentially Ictal Rhythmic Discharges (BIRDs).

Figure 5.5 Generalized rhythmic delta activity (GRDA).

Figure 5.6 Generalized rhythmic delta activity (GRDA).

Figure 5.3 Generalized rhythmic delta activity (GRDA).

Figure 5.7 Lateralized rhythmic delta activity (LRDA).

Figure 5.8 Lateralized rhythmic delta activity (LRDA), unilateral.

Figure 5.9 Lateralized rhythmic delta activity (LRDA), unilateral.

Figure 5.10 Lateralized rhythmic delta activity (LRDA), unilateral.

Figure 5.11 Focal irregular (non-rhythmic) slowing.

Figure 5.12 Lateralized rhythmic delta activity (LRDA), bilateral asymmetric.

Figure 5.13 Lateralized rhythmic delta activity (LRDA), bilateral asynchronous.

Figure 5.14 Generalized periodic discharges (GPDs).

Figure 5.15 Generalized periodic discharges (GPDs).

Figure 5.16 Generalized periodic discharges (GPDs).

Figure 5.17 GPDs with triphasic morphology.

Figure 5.18 GPDs with triphasic morphology.

Figure 5.19 Lateralized periodic discharges (LPDs).

Figure 5.20 Lateralized periodic discharges (LPDs).

Figure 5.21 Lateralized periodic discharges (LPDs), bilateral asymmetric.

Figure 5.22 Lateralized periodic discharges (LPDs).

Figure 5.23 Generalized Sharp-and-Wave (GSW).

Figure 5.24 Generalized spike-wave vs. EKG artifact.

Figure 5.25 Lateralized Spike-and-Wave (LSW).

Figure 5.26 Lateralized Sharp-and-Wave (LSW).

Figure 5.27 Unilateral independent rhythmic delta activity (UIRDA).

Figure 5.28 Bilateral independent rhythmic delta activity (BIRDA).

Figure 5.29 Multifocal rhythmic delta activity (MfRDA).

Figure 5.30 Unilateral independent periodic discharges (UIPDs).

Figure 5.31 Unilateral independent periodic discharges (UIPDs).

Figure 5.32 Bilateral independent periodic discharges (BIPDs).

Figure 5.33 Bilateral independent periodic discharges (BIPDs).

Figure 5.34 Bilateral independent periodic discharges with polyspikes.

Figure 5.35 Multifocal periodic discharges (MfPDs).

Figure 5.36 Generalized rhythmic delta activity plus S (GRDA+S).

Figure 5.37 Generalized rhythmic delta activity plus S (GRDA+S).

Figure 5.38 Lateralized rhythmic delta activity plus S (LRDA+S).

Figure 5.39 Lateralized rhythmic delta activity (LRDA) with evolution versus seizure.

Figure 5.40 Symptomatic LPDs mimicking stroke.

Figure 5.41 Stimulus-induced rhythmic, periodic or ictal discharges (SIRPIDs) and SI-GPDs.

Figure 5.42 SIRPIDs: GPDs vs. seizure.

Figure 5.43 SIRPIDs: SI-GSW vs. SI-seizure.

Figure 5.44 Brief potentially Ictal Rhythmic Discharges (BIRDs), with evolution.

Figure 5.45 Brief potentially Ictal Rhythmic Discharges (BIRDs), generalized.

Figure 5.46 Brief potentially Ictal Rhythmic Discharges (BIRDs), evolving BIRDs with similar appearance as the beginning of a seizure.

Figure 5.47 Brief potentially Ictal Rhythmic Discharges (BIRDs), LPDs transitioning into BIRDs.

Figure 5.48 Brief potentially Ictal Rhythmic Discharges (BIRDs), evolving BIRDs, some seizures with similar appearance as BIRDs and others with independent seizure focus.

EEGs throughout this atlas have been shown with the following standard recording filters unless otherwise specified: LFF 1 Hz, HFF 70 Hz, notch filter off.

Additional RPPs can be found in other chapters as follows:

- Additional RPPs in Chapter 6: Seizures, SE and IIC:
  Figure 6.7 LPDs.
  Figure 6.8 LPDs.
  Figure 6.9 Blunt LPDs.
  Figure 6.10 LPDs+F and BIRDs.
  Figure 6.11 LPDs+F.
  Figure 6.16 BIPDs+F, bilateral independent BIRDs.
  Figure 6.17 LPDs+R.
  Figure 6.18 LPDs+F.
  Figure 6.20 GPDs.
  Figure 6.26 GPDs.
  Figure 6.27 GPDs.

- Additional RPPs in Chapter 8: Post cardiac arrest patterns:
  Figure 8.2 GPDs.
  Figure 8.8 GPDs.
  Figure 8.13 GPDs.
  Figure 8.14 GPDs.

- Additional RPPs in Chapter 9: Quantitative EEG: Basics, seizure detection and avoiding pitfalls:
  Figure 9.9 LPDs+F.
  Figure 9.10 BIPDs+F.
  Figure 9.19 GPDs.
  Figure 9.21 LPDs.
  Figure 9.23 BIRDA.
  Figure 9.24 GPDs.
  Figure 9.25 GPDs.
  Figure 9.26 GPDs.
  Figure 9.28 LPDs.
  Figure 9.34 GPDs.
  Figure 9.37 BIPDs+F.

Suggested reading

Alzawahmah M, Fong MWK, Gilmore EJ, Hirsch LJ. Neuroimaging Correlates of Lateralized Rhythmic Delta Activity, Lateralized Periodic Discharges, and Generalized Rhythmic Delta Activity on EEG in Critically Ill Patients. *J Clin Neurophysiol.* 2022;**39**(3):228–234.

Chatrian GE, Shaw CM, Leffman H. The significance of periodic lateralized epileptiform discharges in EEG: an electrographic, clinical, and pathological study. *Electroencephalogr Clin Neurophysiol* 1964;**17**:177–193.

Chong DJ, Hirsch LJ. Which EEG patterns warrant treatment in the critically ill? Reviewing the evidence for treatment of periodic epileptiform discharges and related patterns. *J Clin Neurophysiol* 2005;**22**:79–91.

Cockerell OC, Rothwell J, Thompson PD, Marsden CD, Shorvon SD. Clinical and physiological features of epilepsia partialis continua. Cases ascertained in the UK. *Brain.* 1996;**119**(Pt 2):393–407.

de la Paz D, Brenner RP. Bilateral independent periodic lateralized epileptiform discharges. Clinical significance. *Arch Neurol* 1981;**38**:713–715.

Fong MWK, Jadav R, Alzawahmah M, Hussein OM, Gilmore EJ, Hirsch LJ. The Significance of LRDA With Bilateral Involvement Compared With GRDA on EEG in Critically Ill Patients. *J Clin Neurophysiol.* 2021;Publish Ahead of Print.

Foreman B, Mahulikar A, Tadi P, et al. Generalized periodic discharges and 'triphasic waves': A blinded evaluation of inter-rater agreement and clinical significance. *Clin Neurophysiol.* 2016;**127**(2):1073–1080.

Garcia-Morales I, Garcia MT, Galan-Davila L, Gomez-Escalonilla C, et al. Periodic lateralized epileptiform discharges: etiology, clinical aspects, seizures, and evolution in 130 patients. *J Clin Neurophysiol* 2002;**19**:172–177.

Garzon E, Fernandes RM, Sakamoto AC. Serial EEG during human status epilepticus: evidence for PLED as an ictal pattern. *Neurology* 2001;**57**:1175–1183.

Gaspard N, Manganas L, Rampal N, Petroff OA, Hirsch LJ. Similarity of lateralized rhythmic delta activity to periodic lateralized epileptiform discharges in critically ill patients. *JAMA Neurol.* 2013;**70**(10):1288–1295.

Hirsch LJ, Claassen J, Mayer SA, Emerson RG. Stimulus-induced rhythmic, periodic, or ictal discharges (SIRPIDs): a common EEG phenomenon in the critically ill. *Epilepsia* 2004;**45**:109–123.

Hirsch LJ, Fong MWK, Leitinger M, et al. American Clinical Neurophysiology Society's Standardized Critical Care EEG Terminology: 2021 Version. *J Clin Neurophysiol.* 2021;**38**(1):1–29.

Hirsch LJ, Pang T, Claassen J, Chang C, Abou Khaled K, Wittman J, Emerson RG. Focal motor seizures induced by alerting stimuli in critically ill patients. *Epilepsia* 2008;**49**:968–973.

Kaplan PW, Schlattman DK. Comparison of triphasic waves and epileptic discharges in one patient with genetic epilepsy. *J Clin Neurophysiol.* 2012;**29**(5):458–461.

O'Rourke D, Chen PM, Gaspard N, et al. Response rates to anticonvulsant trials in patients with triphasic-wave EEG patterns of uncertain significance. *Neurocrit Care.* 2016;**24**(2):233–239.

Osman G, Rahangdale R, Britton JW, et al. Bilateral independent periodic discharges are associated with electrographic seizures and poor outcome: A case-control study. *Clin Neurophysiol.* 2018;**129**(11):2284–2289.

Rodriguez Ruiz A, Vlachy J, Lee JW, et al. Association of periodic and rhythmic electroencephalographic patterns with seizures in critically ill patients. *JAMA Neurol.* 2017;**74**(2):181–188.

Yoo JY, Rampal N, Petroff OA, Hirsch LJ, Gaspard N. Brief potentially ictal rhythmic discharges in critically ill adults. *JAMA Neurol.* 2014;**71**(4):454–462.

Yoo JY, Marcuse LV, Fields MC, et al. Brief Potentially Ictal Rhythmic Discharges [B(I)RDs] in noncritically ill adults. *J Clin Neurophysiol.* 2017;**34**(3):222–229.

Yoo JY, Jette N, Kwon CS, et al. Brief potentially ictal rhythmic discharges and paroxysmal fast activity as scalp electroencephalographic biomarkers of seizure activity and seizure onset zone. *Epilepsia.* 2021;**62**(3):742–751.

*Reference defining the terms used in this atlas.

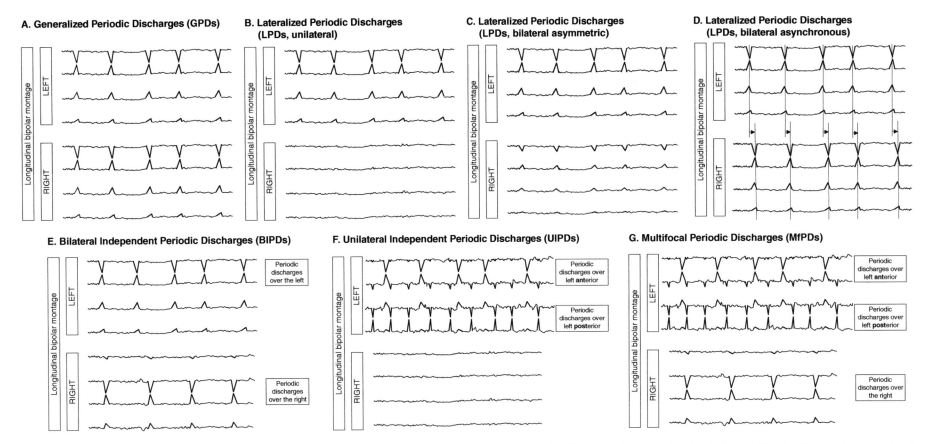

Figure 5.1.   Main term 1 (localization). Main term 1 refers to the localization of a pattern. Most patterns are either 'generalized' (G) (any bilaterally synchronous and symmetric pattern, even if it has a restricted field [e.g., bifrontal]) (panel A); or 'lateralized' (L). 'Lateralized' includes patterns that are purely unilateral (panel B), bilateral but clearly and consistently higher amplitude in one hemisphere (bilateral asymmetric, panel C), or bilateral but with a consistent lead-in from the same side (bilateral asynchronous, panel D). Other less common patterns are: 'bilateral independent' (BI) with two independent lateralized patterns with one in each hemisphere, with both patterns occurring simultaneously (i.e., overlapping in time) (panel E); 'unilateral independent' (UI) with two independent RPPs in the same hemisphere, with both patterns occurring simultaneously (panel F); and 'multifocal'(Mf) with at least three independent lateralized patterns, with at least one in each hemisphere, with all three or more patterns occurring simultaneously (panel G).

Reproduced from Hirsch LJ, Fong MWK, Leitinger M, et al. American Clinical Neurophysiology Society's Standardized Critical Care EEG Terminology: 2021 Version. J Clin Neurophysiol. 2021;38(1):1–29, with permission.

A. Periodic Discharges (PDs)

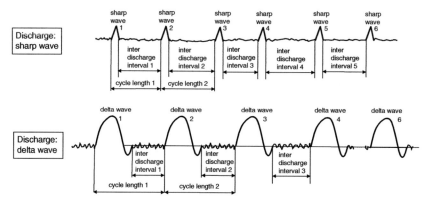

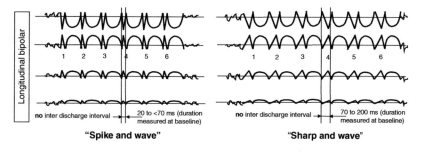

B. Rhythmic Delta Activity (RDA)

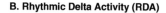

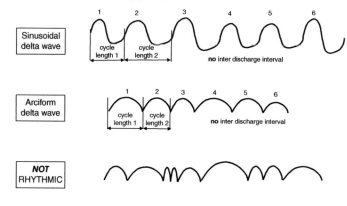

C. "Spike and Wave" or "Sharp and Wave" (SW)

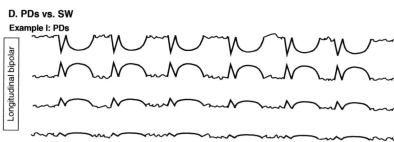

D. PDs vs. SW

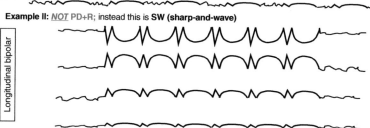

Figure 5.2. Main term 2 (pattern type). Main term 2 refers to the pattern of an RPP, with only 3 possibilities: 'periodic discharges' (PDs) (panel A), 'rhythmic delta activity' (RDA) (panel B), or 'spike-and-wave'/'sharp-and-wave' (SW) (panel C). Periodic discharges consist of repeating waveforms with relatively uniform morphology and duration with a clearly discernable inter-discharge interval (i.e., a break between consecutive waveforms) and recurrence of the waveform at nearly regular intervals (panel A). If there are not breaks between consecutive discharges (i.e., no inter-discharge interval) and the pattern is ≤4 Hz, then it would qualify as either RDA or SW. The more common of these patterns is RDA (i.e., repetition of a waveform with relatively uniform morphology and duration and without an interval between consecutive waveforms, where the activity is in the delta range) (panel B). 'Spike-and-wave' or 'sharp-and-wave' (panel C) is a much less common and more specific pattern defined as a spike, polyspike or sharp wave consistently followed by a slow wave in a regularly repeating and alternating pattern (spike-wave-spike-wave-spike-wave), with a consistent relationship between the spike (or polyspike or sharp wave) component and the slow wave for at least 6 cycles, and with no interval between one spike-wave complex and the next. If spike-wave complexes have an inter-discharge interval (i.e., a break between each complex), these remain PDs (panel D, example I). Only if they are contiguous can they be classified as SW (panel D, example II). If epileptiform discharges are recurring at a faster rate (i.e., >4 Hz), they are either seizures (if lasting 10 seconds or with clinical correlate), BIRDs [if <10 seconds] or highly epileptiform bursts if within burst suppression.

Reproduced from Hirsch LJ, Fong MWK, Leitinger M, et al. American Clinical Neurophysiology Society's Standardized Critical Care EEG Terminology: 2021 Version. J Clin Neurophysiol. 2021;38(1):1–29, with permission.

A. Periodic Discharges PLUS _fast_ activity (PDs+F)

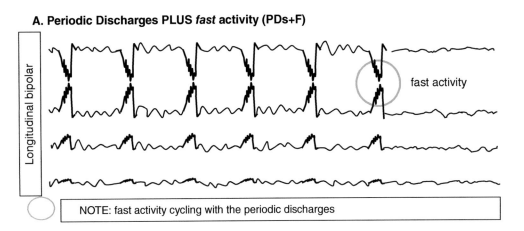

fast activity

NOTE: fast activity cycling with the periodic discharges

B. Periodic Discharges PLUS _fast_ activity (PDs+F)

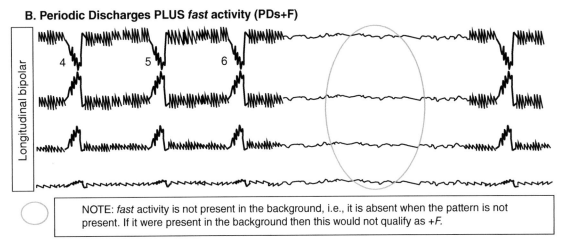

NOTE: _fast_ activity is not present in the background, i.e., it is absent when the pattern is not present. If it were present in the background then this would not qualify as +F.

Figure 5.3. Plus (+) modifiers. Plus (+) modifiers are an additional feature that render a pattern more ictal-appearing (i.e., more closely resembling an EEG pattern seen during seizures) than the usual term without the plus. Plus modifiers include +fast (+F), +rhythmic (+R) or +sharp (+S), as well as combinations of these +FS and +FR. Plus modifiers can only be applied to PDs and RDA, not SW.

Panel A: '+F': with superimposed (some prefer the synonyms of admixed or associated) fast activity, defined as theta or faster, whether rhythmic or not. In this example the fast activity forms a stereotyped relationship with each discharge (i.e., is present on the upstroke and point of each discharge).

Panel B: '+F': fast activity does not have to have a stereotyped relationship with the PDs/RDA to be included. The example qualifies as +F as the fast activity is present when the pattern is present, but then absent when the pattern is absent (i.e., it is associated with the pattern). If, however, the fast activity was present at all times then this would not be considered as +F as it would just be PDs superimposed on a background that already includes fast activity (i.e., not specifically associated with the pattern).

Reproduced from Hirsch LJ, Fong MWK, Leitinger M, et al. American Clinical Neurophysiology Society's Standardized Critical Care EEG Terminology: 2021 Version. J Clin Neurophysiol. 2021;38(1):1–29, with permission.

C. Periodic Discharges PLUS *RDA* (PDs+R)

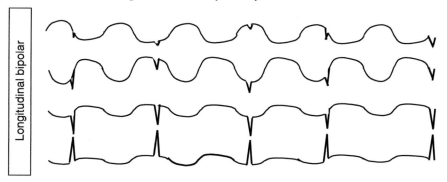

Longitudinal bipolar

NOTE: The delta waves (RDA) are *not* time-locked to spikes, i.e., they are coincident but not related. If the delta waves were time locked with the spikes, with an interdischarge interval, this would remain PDs, where each "discharge" consists of a spike and a wave.

D. Rhythmic Delta Activity PLUS *Spikes* (RDA+S)

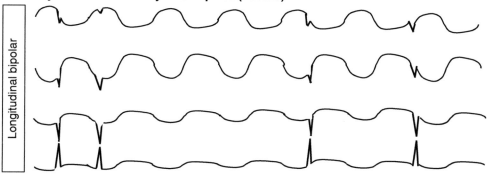

Longitudinal bipolar

NOTE: Rhythmic Delta Activity (RDA) with admixed spikes (RDA+S). Again, the spikes are not time locked to the delta waves, if they were this pattern would be spike-and-wave (SW) as there is no inter-discharge interval.

Figure 5.3. *(Continued)* Panel C: '+R': with superimposed rhythmic or quasi-rhythmic delta activity. This can only be applied to PDs, as RDA is (by definition) already rhythmic. One caveat with +R: If the rhythmic slow waves are time-locked to the PDs, forming a spike-wave complex, then this does not count as PD+R; instead this is either PDs (no +R) or SW (Figure 5.2, panel d): if there is an interval between each sharp-wave complex, it qualifies as PDs; if there is no inter-discharge interval, it would qualify as SW (Example II).
Panel D: '+S': with associated sharp waves or spikes, or sharply contoured morphology. This can only be applied to RDA, as PDs are already have a 'sharpness' modifier. The example demonstrates RDA with admixed spikes. Note the spikes are not time-locked in a regular fashion with each wave (otherwise the pattern would be SW), and the spikes are not periodic (otherwise this is better described as PDs+R, as in panel C). In order to qualify as +S, the spikes, sharp waves or sharply contoured activity need to be present least once every 10 s.
The combinations of the above include +FS (can only be applied to RDA) and +FR (can only be applied to PDs). It is not possible to have +FR for RDA, again because +R cannot be applied to RDA (redundant), and it is not possible to have +FS for PDs, because +S cannot be applied to PDs (instead the sharpness of the PD is described via the major modifier on sharpness: spiky, sharp, sharply contoured or blunt).

Reproduced from Hirsch LJ, Fong MWK, Leitinger M, et al. American Clinical Neurophysiology Society's Standardized Critical Care EEG Terminology: 2021 Version. J Clin Neurophysiol. 2021;38(1):1–29, with permission.

A. Evolving BIRDs (a form of definite BIRDs)

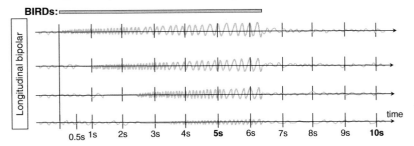

B. BIRDs with similar morphology/location as _interictal epileptiform discharges_ (a form of definite BIRDs)

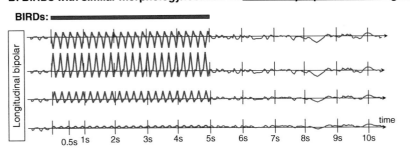

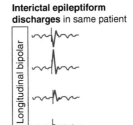

C. BIRDs with similar morphology/location as _seizures_ (a form of definite BIRDs)

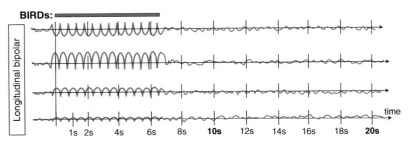

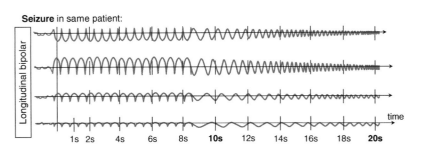

Figure 5.4. Brief potentially Ictal Rhythmic Discharges (BIRDs). BIRDs are defined as focal (including L, BI, UI or Mf) or generalized rhythmic activity >4 Hz (at least 6 waves at a regular rate) lasting ≥0.5 to <10 s, not consistent with a known normal pattern or benign variant, not part of burst suppression or burst attenuation, without definite clinical correlate, and that has at least one of the following features: 1. evolution ('evolving BIRDs', a form of definite BIRDs) (panel A), 2. similar morphology and location to interictal epileptiform discharges (panel B) or seizures (panel C) in the same patient (a form of definite BIRDs), or 3. sharply contoured but without 1 or 2 (e.g., if the highlighted activity in panel B or C was present without recording the interictal discharge or seizure in the same patient) (these are termed 'possible BIRDs'). Definite BIRDs are highly associated with seizures and patients with 'evolving BIRDs' universally had seizures in one study.

Reproduced from Hirsch LJ, Fong MWK, Leitinger M, et al. American Clinical Neurophysiology Society's Standardized Critical Care EEG Terminology: 2021 Version. J Clin Neurophysiol. 2021;38(1):1–29, with permission.

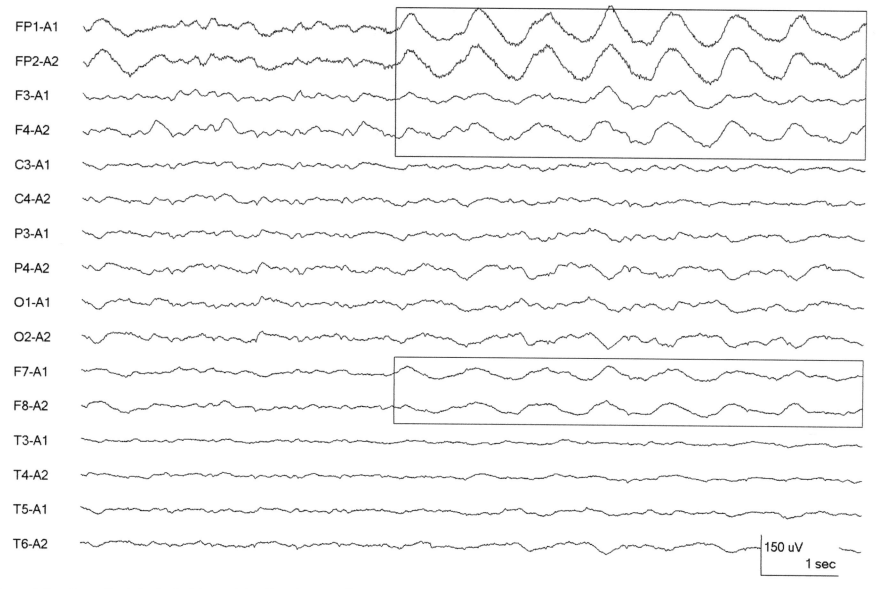

Figure 5.5. Generalized rhythmic delta activity (GRDA). GRDA (boxes) is seen in this 19-year-old woman with an intraventricular hemorrhage. The activity is considered generalized (since bisynchronous and symmetric), frontally predominant (with the greatest voltage in Fp1 and Fp2). In this case the pattern could have also been described by the non-ACNS term of FIRDA (previously described in Chapter 3: Encephalopathy and coma). However, it is valuable appreciating that not all GRDA is synonymous with FIRDA (i.e., not all GRDA is frontally predominant and intermittent), and not all FIRDA equates to GRDA (i.e., not all FIRDA meets the more stringent six consecutive rhythmic waves that is necessary to qualify as GRDA; in fact, FIRDA is commonly only 2–3 s in duration). Although both FIRDA and GRDA are most commonly nonspecific indicators of diffuse dysfunction, typically toxic/metabolic, they can also be seen (much less commonly) with increased intraventricular pressure or with deep midline structures (the setting in which FIRDA was first described).

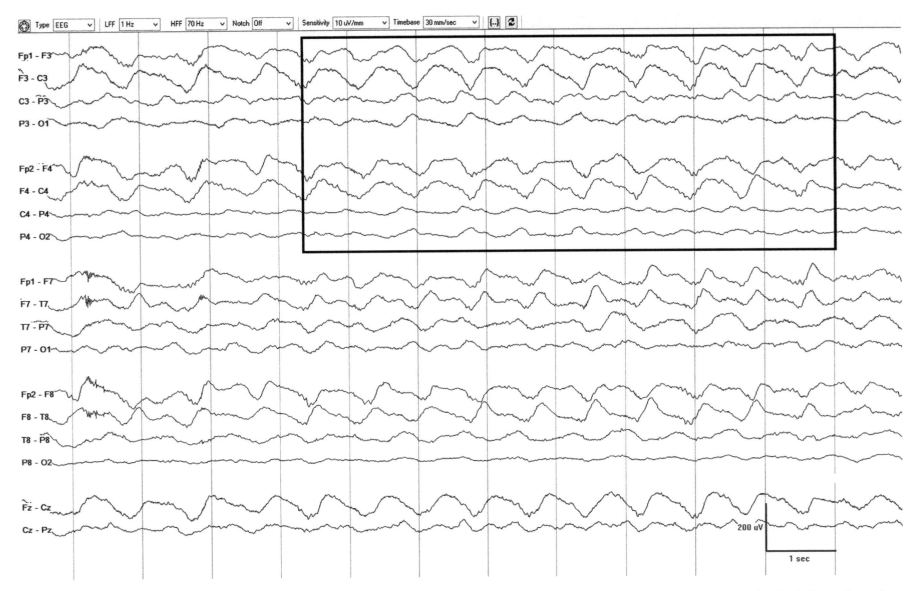

Figure 5.6. Generalized rhythmic delta activity (GRDA). This EEG is from a 36-year-old man with meningo-encephalitis. It demonstrates high voltage (≥150 uV peak to trough) generalized (i.e., symmetric and synchronous) RDA, best appreciated in the parasagittal derivations (box). This is 'frontally predominant', as it is best appreciated in anterior channels.

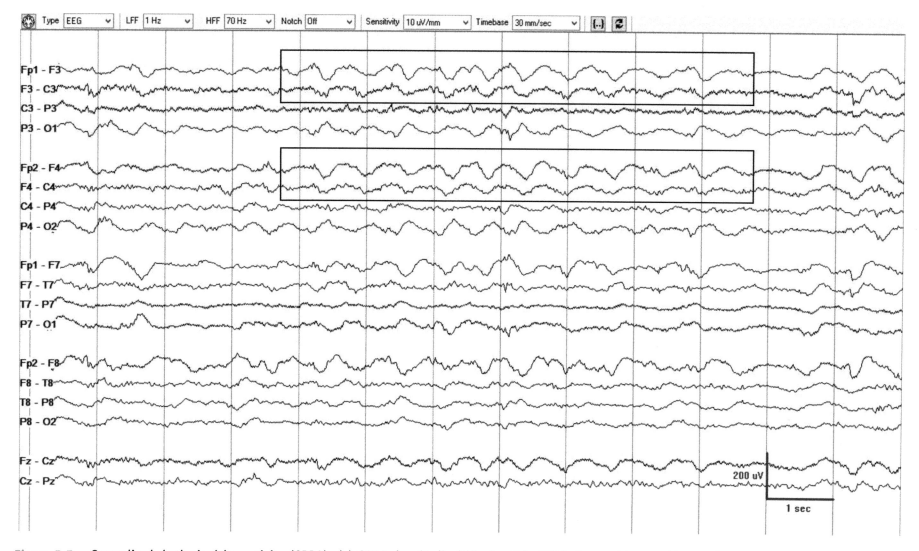

Figure 5.7. Generalized rhythmic delta activity (GRDA). (a) GRDA, longitudinal bipolar. This EEG is from a 35-year-old man that presented following an opioid overdose. The EEG demonstrates GRDA, frontally predominant and very brief (i.e., less than 10 s) (boxes).

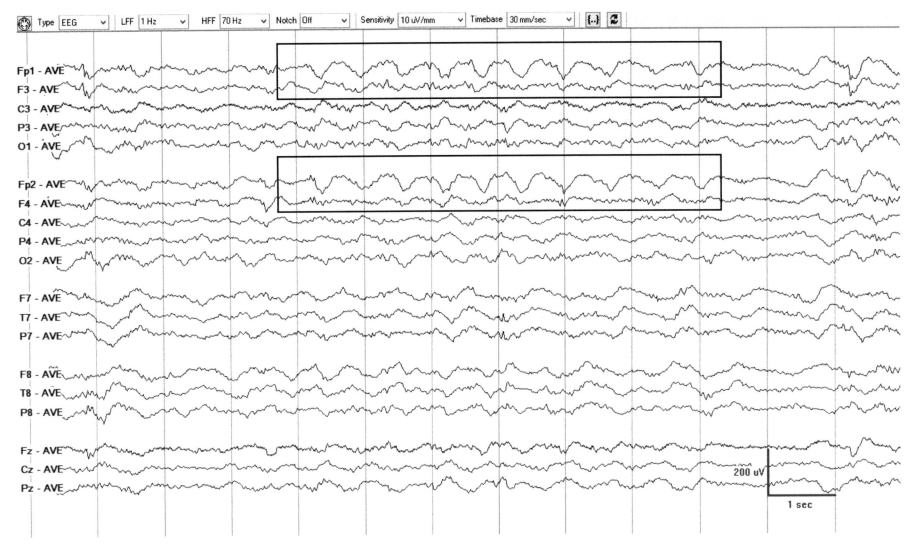

Figure 5.7.   (*Continued*) (b) GRDA, referential. The same page of EEG reformatted into an average referential montage. The rhythmic slowing is largely only seen anteriorly (boxes). There are delta rhythms through the rest of the head; however, these are continuous, low- to medium-amplitude 1–1.5 Hz irregular or polymorphic delta waves as a component of background slowing. The point being made is that GRDA does not always have to be present in all brain regions to be classified as 'generalized', it only has to be symmetric and synchronous.

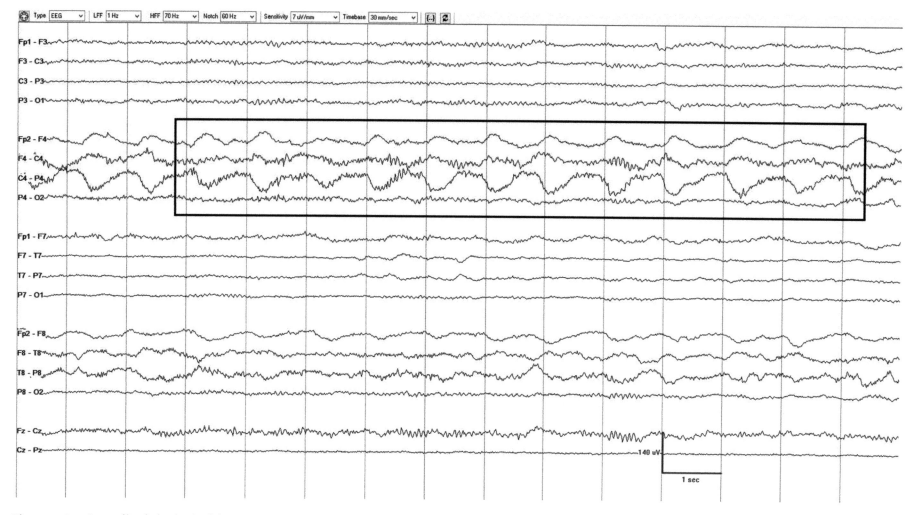

Figure 5.8. Lateralized rhythmic delta activity (LRDA), unilateral. (a) LRDA, longitudinal bipolar. The EEG from this 73-year-old man with a large right frontal subdural hematoma s/p craniotomy demonstrates 1-Hz LRDA in the right fronto-central region (box).

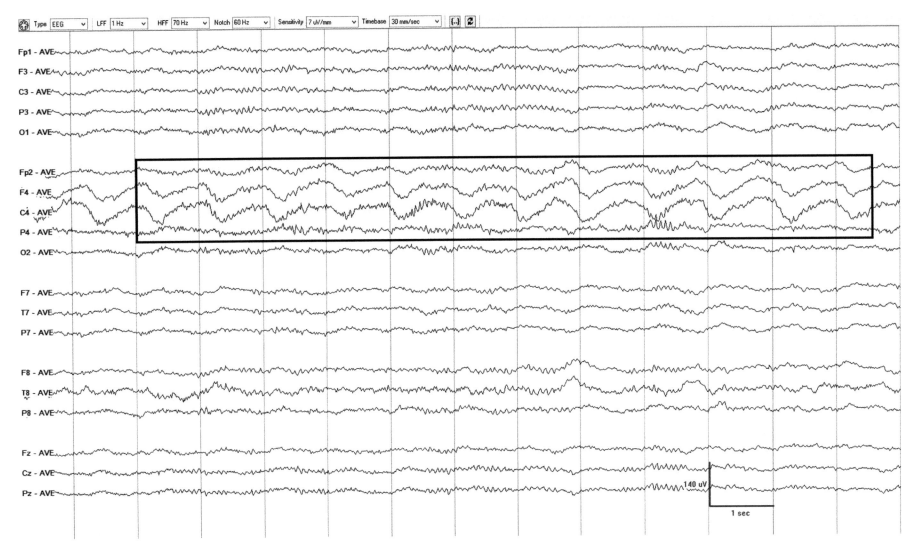

Figure 5.8.   (*Continued*) (b) LRDA, referential. The same page of EEG reformatted to an average referential montage. The monomorphic (also known as rhythmic) delta activity is present at F4/C4. There is the suggestion of additional fast activity in the right parasagittal derivations; however, this was present even when the LRDA was not (i.e., was a part of the background; not shown), so this is not LRDA+F, but is simply a breach effect.

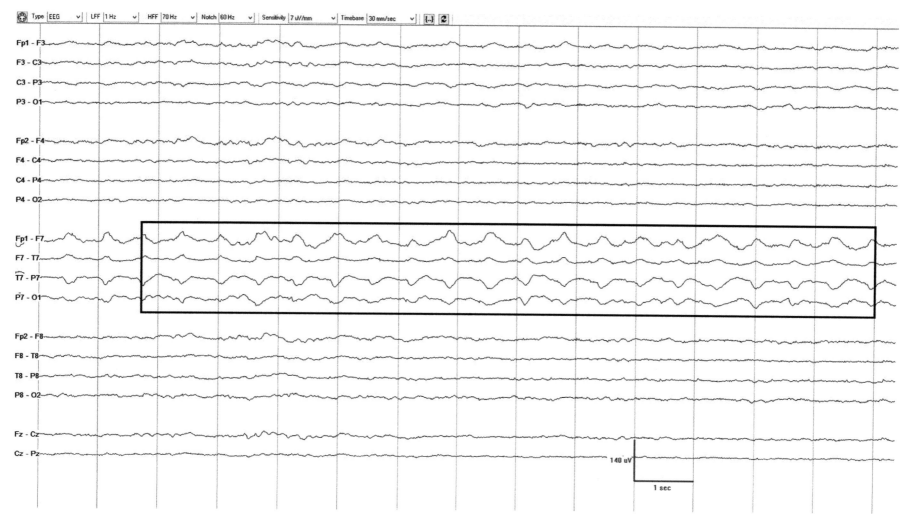

Figure 5.9. Lateralized rhythmic delta activity (LRDA), unilateral. (a) LRDA, longitudinal bipolar. The EEG from this 52-year-old woman s/p resection of large left-sided meningioma demonstrates 1.5-Hz LRDA in the left temporal region (box). The activity is not at all seen in the right hemisphere; therefore, this is LRDA, unilateral.

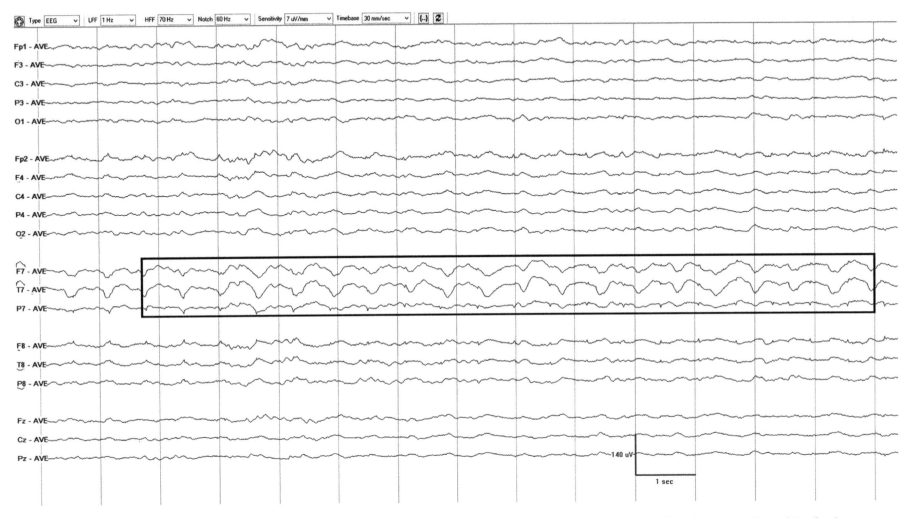

Figure 5.9.   (*Continued*) (b) LRDA, referential. The same page of EEG reformatted to an average referential montage. There is LRDA at F7 and T7 (box).

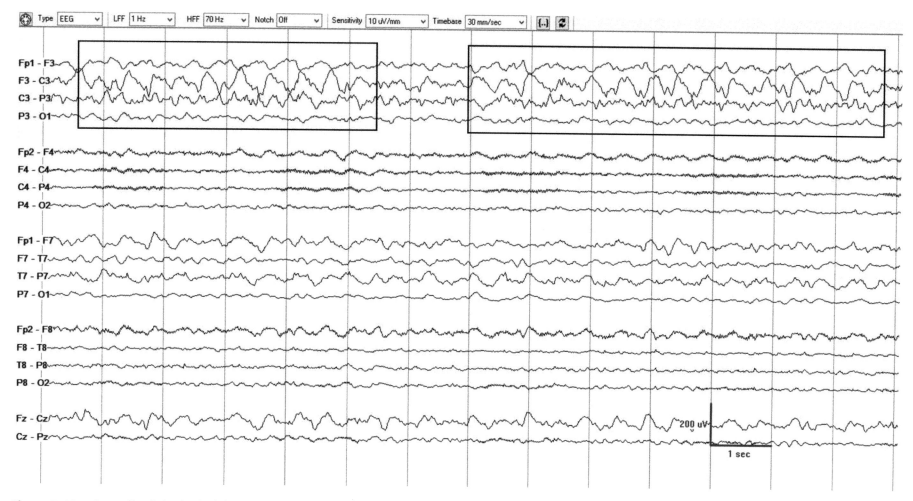

Figure 5.10. Lateralized rhythmic delta activity (LRDA), unilateral. (a) LRDA, longitudinal bipolar. The EEG of this 53-year-old s/p left craniectomy for SDH. There is a breach rhythm through the left hemisphere, best appreciated with the temporal electrodes on the left being of higher amplitude and more sharply contoured compared to the lower amplitude rhythms on the right. In the left central region, there is abundant very brief 2-Hz LRDA (boxes), although the rhythmicity is borderline on this bipolar montage.

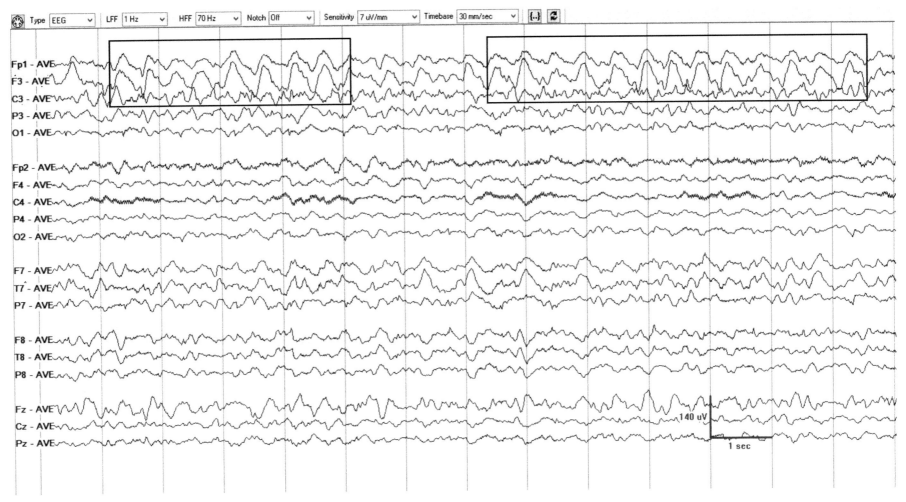

Figure 5.10. (*Continued*) (b) LRDA, referential. The same page of EEG reformatted into referential average montage. The example has been selected as it demonstrates that the morphology of waveforms is often more accurately reproduced when utilizing a referential montage, and the morphology can be distorted by using a bipolar montage. With the referential montage, the LRDA (boxes) appears more monomorphic/rhythmic compared to the bipolar.

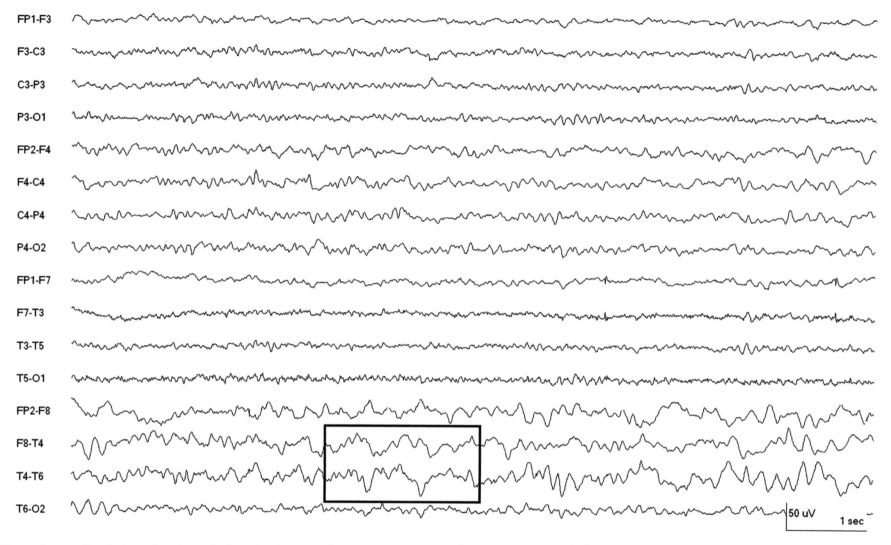

Figure 5.11. Focal irregular (non-rhythmic) slowing. In order to contrast with rhythmic delta (such as LRDA), this figure with focal irregular/polymorphic/non-rhythmic slowing has been duplicated. The figure is from Chapter 4: focal abnormalities, Figure 4.4a. It demonstrates a good example of non-rhythmic slowing in the right temporal region and is valuable to contrast this with Figure 5.9 that demonstrates LRDA in the same region, albeit on the left. In this case there are delta waves in the temporal region; however, the 'period' or 'cycle' of the delta activity and the morphology are not similar for 6 or more cycles. There are at best 2–3 consecutive similar delta waves (box). Within the box and at T4-T6, it could be argued that the second and third waves are similar, but certainly these are different to the first one (i.e., they are not monomorphic, which means they are polymorphic). Delta activity has to be 'monomorphic' for at least 6 cycles to qualify as RDA.

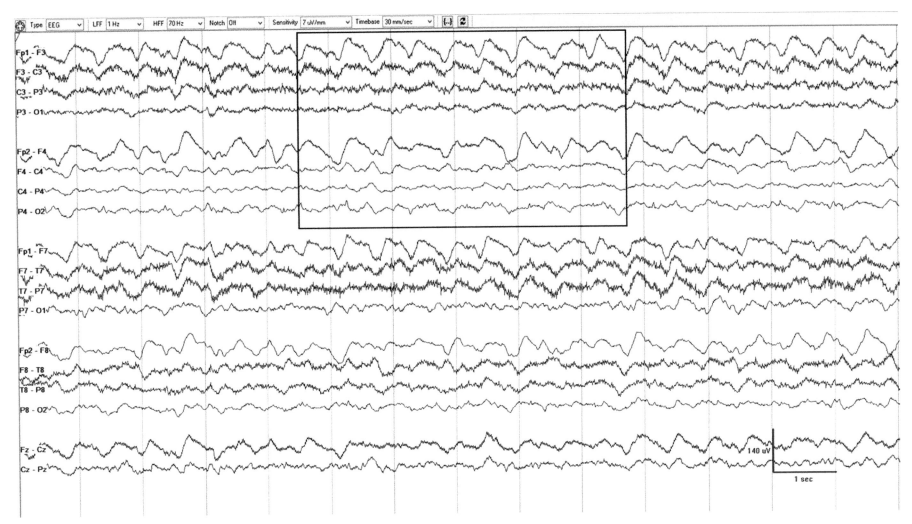

Figure 5.12. Lateralized rhythmic delta activity (LRDA), bilateral asymmetric. (a) LRDA, bilateral asymmetric, longitudinal bipolar. This EEG also demonstrates RDA (box), frontally predominant. In this case, however, the RDA is better formed (i.e., more rhythmic and more apparent) and of higher voltage in the left hemisphere (even more apparent in the referential montage shown next). If a pattern is clearly and consistently of greater voltage in one hemisphere but also seen in the other, this is still considered 'lateralized' (as opposed to 'generalized', which has to be symmetric and synchronous between hemispheres). This is an example of LRDA that is present in both hemispheres so the minor term of bilateral asymmetric can be applied.

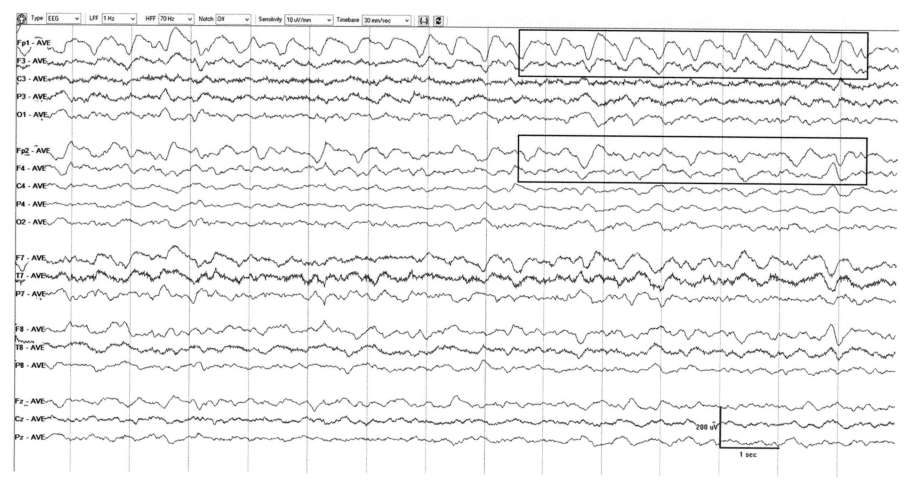

Figure 5.12. (*Continued*) (b) LRDA, bilateral asymmetric, referential. the same page reformatted to a referential average montage. The LRDA is better seen in the left frontal region (Fp1>F3) but there is clearly still reflection of this pattern in the right homologous region (boxes). The pattern is not generalized because it is not symmetric, so it is 'LRDA, bilateral asymmetric'. If the RDA was only present in one hemisphere this would be considered 'LRDA, unilateral'.

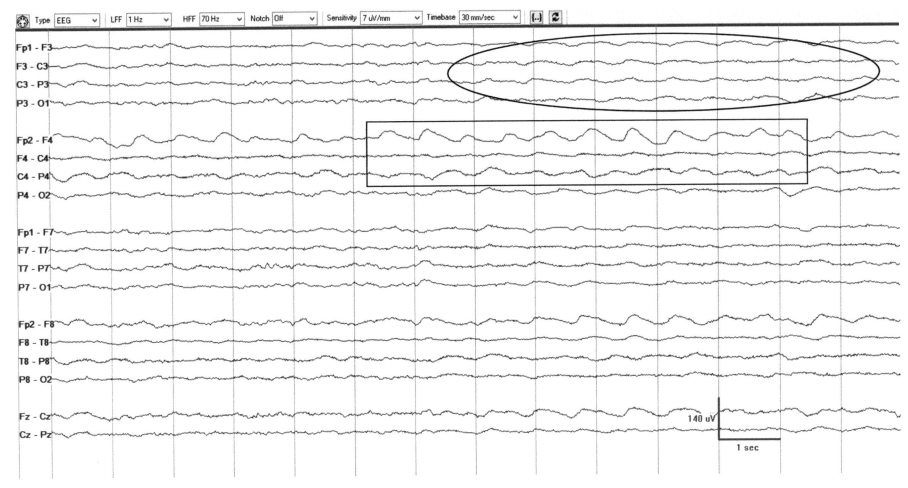

Figure 5.13. Lateralized rhythmic delta activity (LRDA), bilateral asynchronous. (a) LRDA, bilateral asynchronous, longitudinal bipolar. This EEG is from a 73-year-old man s/p right frontal atypical meningioma resection. There is frequent 1.5-Hz LRDA maximal in the right fronto-central region (box). In the second half of the page there is similar rhythmic activity (at the same frequency), lower amplitude in the left fronto-central region (ellipse).

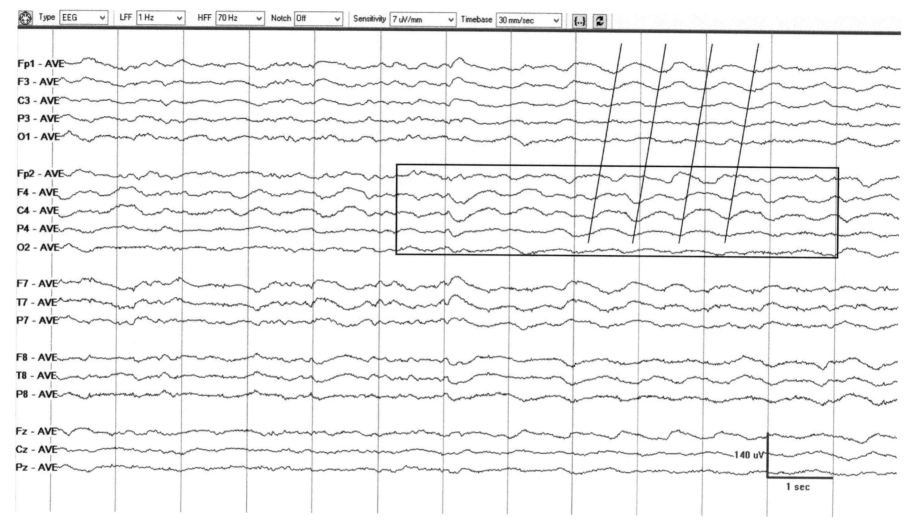

Figure 5.13. (*Continued*) (b) LRDA bilateral asynchronous, referential. The same page of EEG reformatted to a referential average montage. Taking the RDA in the left frontal region, this was subtle with a bipolar montage as it is fairly similar in Fp1 and F3, which means that these activities cancel out in bipolar. With a referential montage it is much easier to appreciate that the RDA is also present in the left frontal region, though still more prominent in the right fronto-central region (F4/C4) (box). What is also appreciated with this montage is that the activity in both hemispheres is the same frequency and time-locked: the pattern on the left is slightly delayed from the pattern on the right. This consistent delay is depicted by parallel diagonal lines that align the troughs of consecutive waveforms at C4 with the troughs of the waveforms at F3. This can be described as 'bilateral asynchronous', the third subtype of lateralized patterns (unilateral, bilateral asymmetric and bilateral asynchronous). In this case the pattern is both bilateral asymmetric (consistently of greater voltage in the right hemisphere) and bilateral asynchronous (consistently starting earlier in the right hemisphere). Note the pattern is *not* bilateral independent (BIRDA), as the patterns in each hemisphere are not independent since they are time-locked (and therefore dependent).

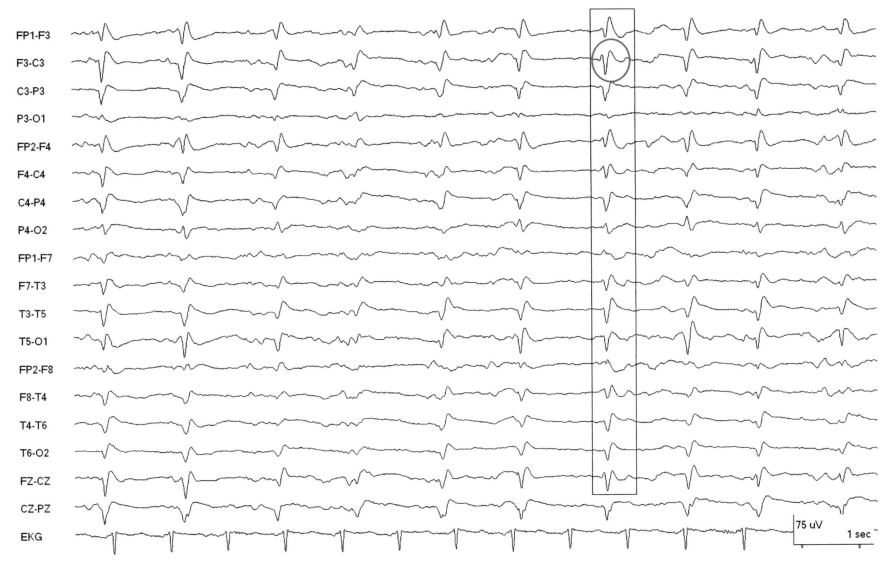

Figure 5.14.   Generalized periodic discharges (GPDs). The EEG in this 45-year-old man shows GPDs. The patient was receiving propofol and had been in status epilepticus. Note the triphasic morphology (one example in box, especially at F3-C3 [red circle]), which is not rare in seizure-related GPDs despite the traditional teaching that they suggest metabolic encephalopathy and are unrelated to seizures, mostly proven inaccurate in blinded, controlled studies. Those studies have shown that in patients with GPDs, regardless of the morphology, metabolic disorders (seen in more than half the patients) and seizures (about 25%) are both very common.

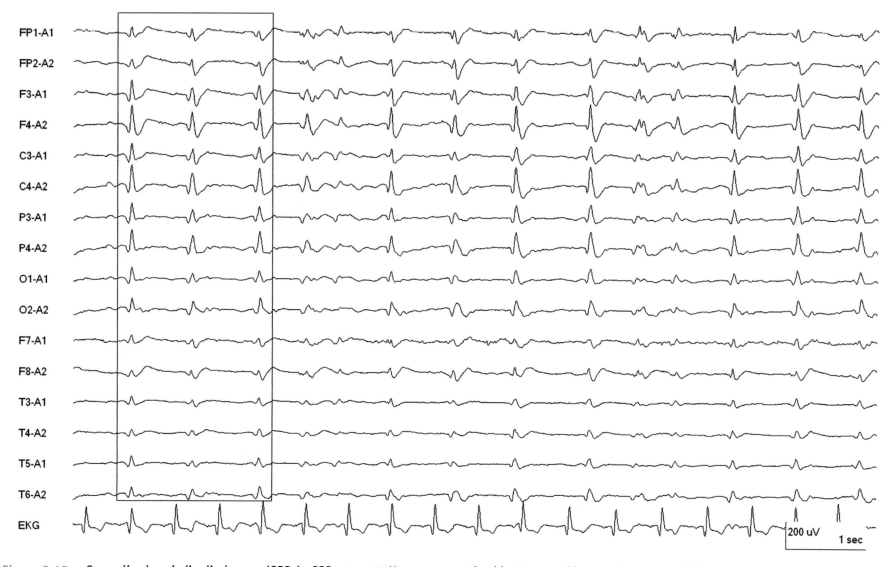

Figure 5.15. Generalized periodic discharges (GPDs). GPDs at ~1.5 Hz are present in this 33-year-old man s/p motor vehicle accident and anoxia. The first 3 discharges are included in the box.

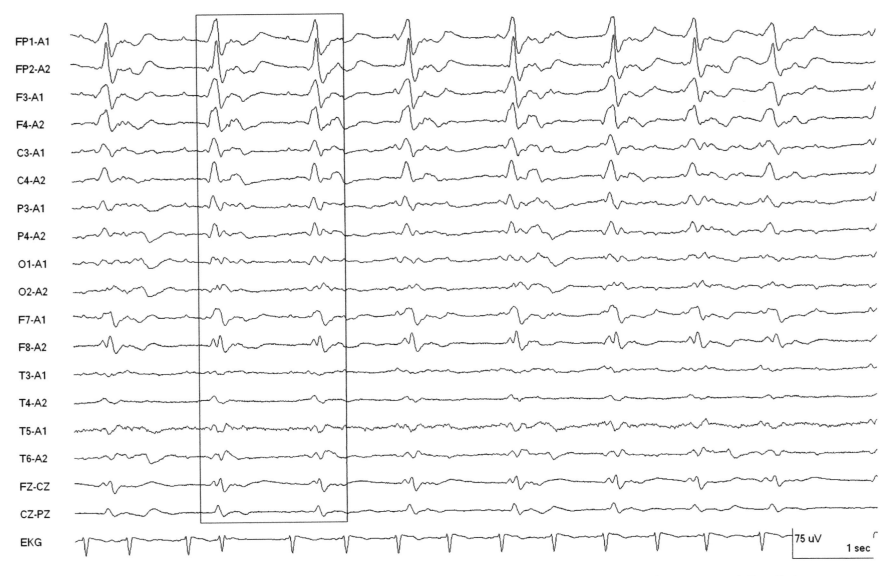

Figure 5.16. Generalized periodic discharges (GPDs). GPDs are present in this 75-year-old comatose woman at just under 1 per second. Two discharges are present in the box. As is typical, they are frontally predominant.

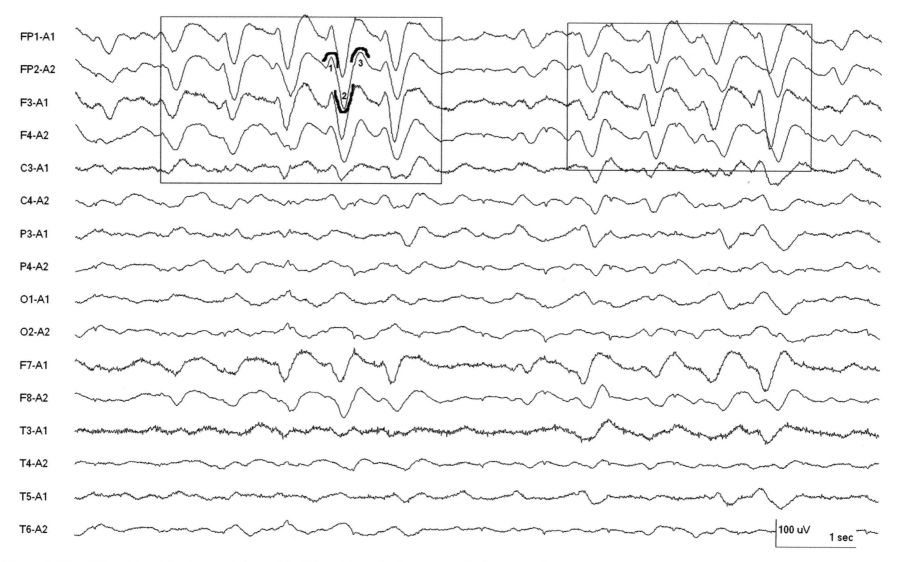

Figure 5.17. GPDs with triphasic morphology. (a) GPDs with triphasic morphology, referential. The EEG in this 66-year-old woman awaiting a liver transplant shows clusters of triphasic waves at 1.5 per second. Note the typical frontal predominance, waxing and waning quality, and the three phases of each discharge: small negativity (upgoing on this referential montage), then larger positivity (main component), then long slow negativity (see sample wave with all three phases labeled).

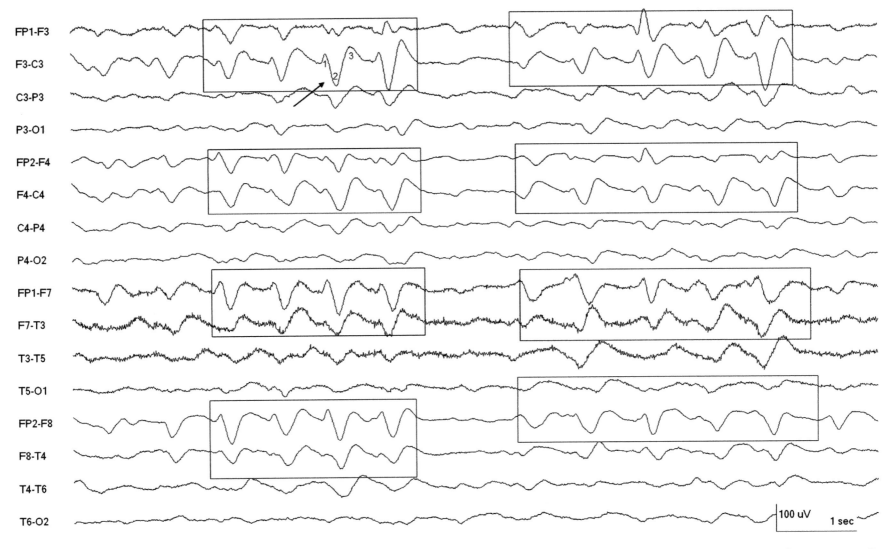

Figure 5.17. *(Continued)* (b) GPDs with triphasic morphology, longitudinal bipolar. The boxes highlight the triphasic morphology. The arrow points out a waveform with the three phases labeled.

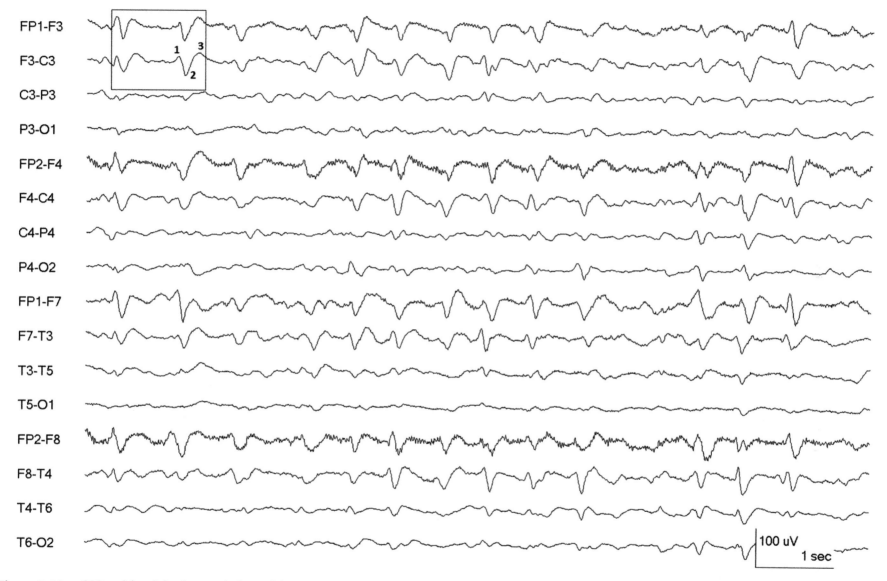

Figure 5.18. GPDs with triphasic morphology. (a) GPDs with triphasic morphology, longitudinal bipolar. Waxing and waning generalized periodic discharges at 1–2 Hz with a triphasic morphology are present, maximal anteriorly, in this 72-year-old man s/p cardiac arrest. The three phases are labeled with numbers in the box.

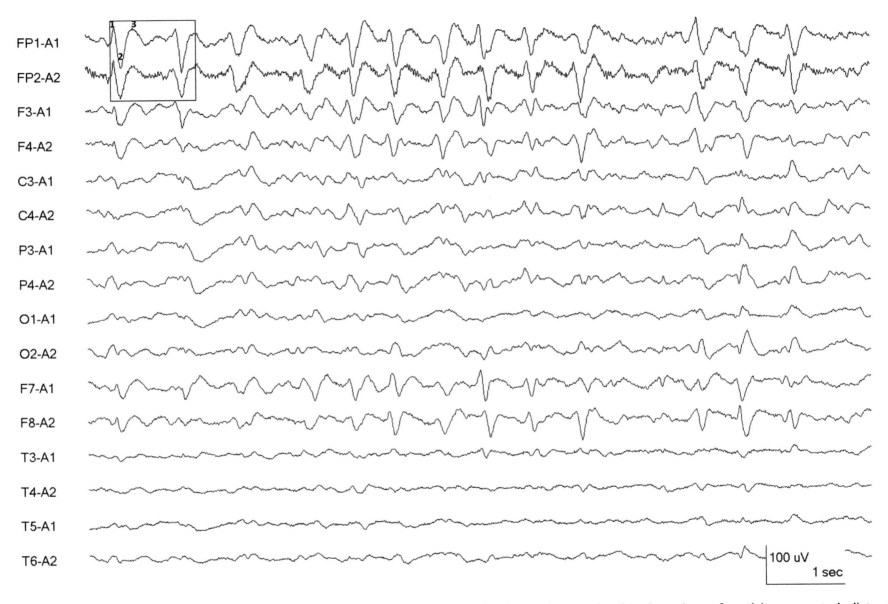

Figure 5.18. (*Continued*) (b) GPDs with triphasic morphology, referential. The epoch has been reformatted and is shown in a referential montage to ipsilateral ears. The three phases of a triphasic wave have again been labeled within the box.

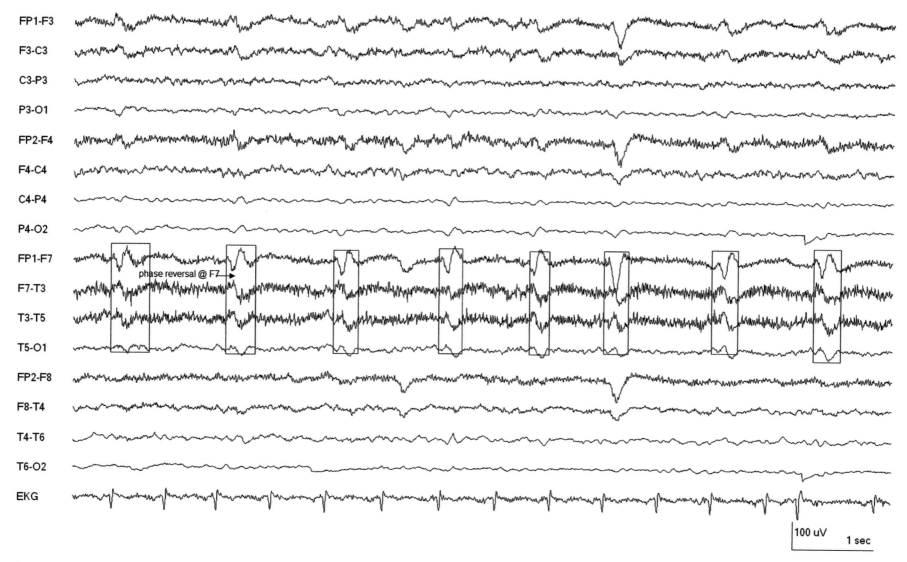

Figure 5.19. Lateralized periodic discharges (LPDs). Left-sided LPDs, maximal at electrode F7, are present in this 54-year-old woman. The discharges have been highlighted with boxes, demonstrating a frequency of about 0.75 Hz.

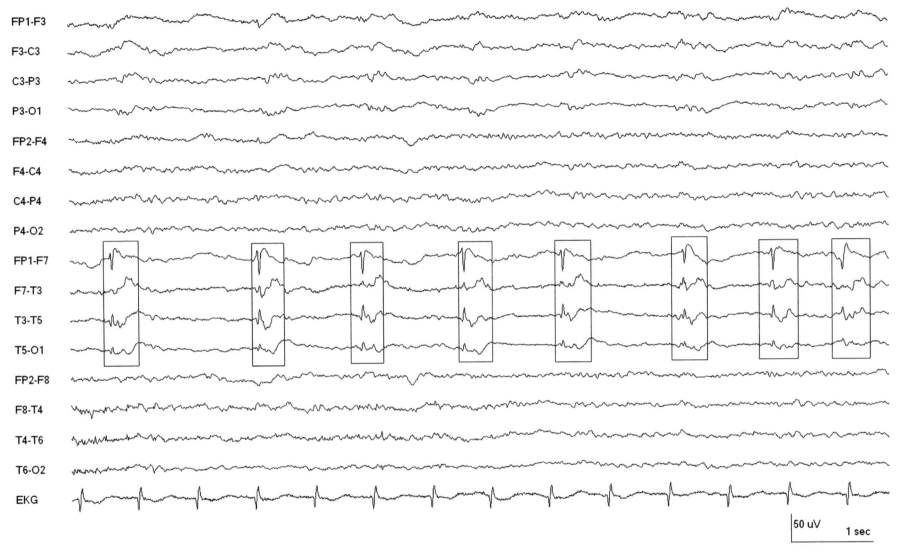

Figure 5.20. Lateralized periodic discharges (LPDs). The EEG in this 64-year-old man demonstrates LPDs (boxes), maximal in the left temporal region, usually phase-reversing (and therefore maximal) at F7-T3. The patient had new onset seizures and a stroke 6 months before. The frequency is about 1 Hz, and the sharpness is 'spiky'.

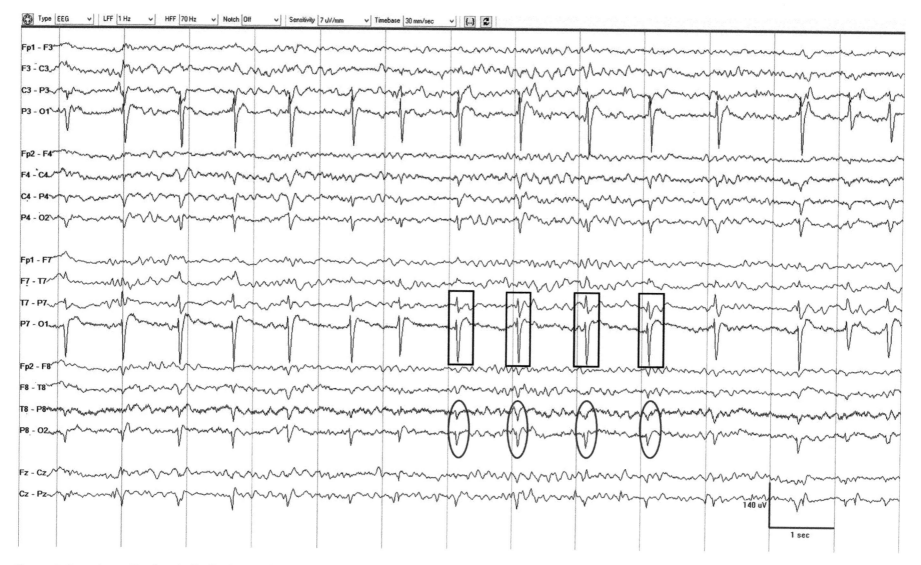

Figure 5.21. Lateralized periodic discharges (LPDs), bilateral asymmetric. This EEG is from a 68-year-old woman with malignancy who developed encephalopathy after being given a check-point inhibitor. The EEG demonstrates LPDs maximal at O1 (boxes). There is also a consistent time-locked component in the right hemisphere (ellipses) that did not have any relationship with the EKG (not shown). The PDs are present in both hemispheres but clearly and consistently of greater voltage on the left. This is therefore *lateralized* (LPDs), but bilateral asymmetric (rather than unilateral).

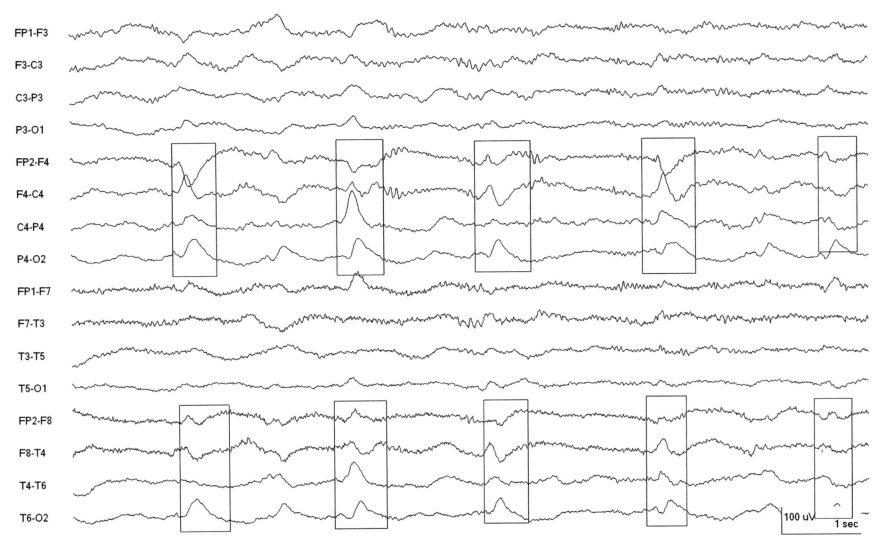

Figure 5.22. LPDs. The EEG in this 26-year-old man shows LPDs consisting of broad periodic slow waves over the right hemisphere. The patient had two bilateral tonic-clonic seizures the evening before the EEG. This EEG demonstrates that not all LPDs have to be sharp or spiky; even blunt complexes still qualify as LPDs and are still highly associated with seizures. In this example, the frequency is 0.5–0.75 Hz, and the sharpness is 'sharply contoured' (some of them might be 'blunt').

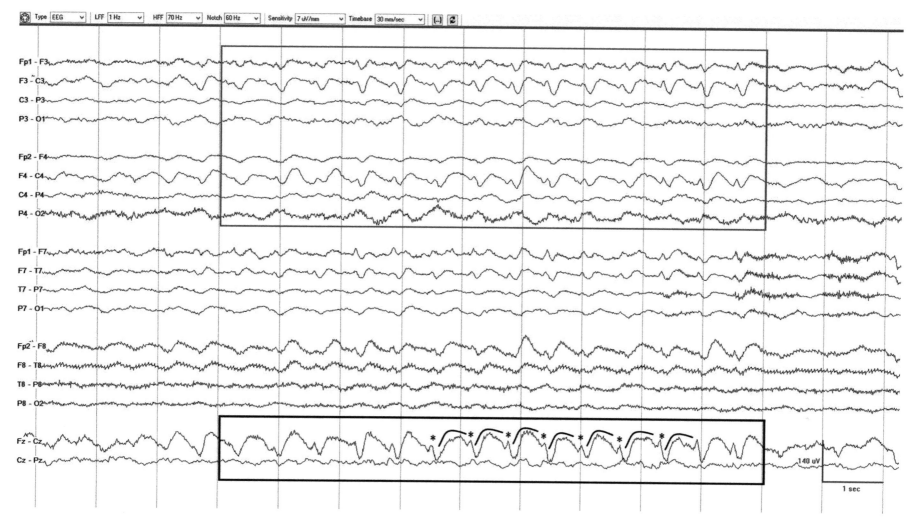

Figure 5.23. Generalized sharp-and-wave (GSW). The EEG from this 55-year-old man with meningo-encephalitis demonstrates 1.75 Hz GSW. The pattern consists of a sharp wave followed by a rhythmic delta wave with no break or inter-discharge interval between one complex and the next, and with a consistent relationship between the sharp wave and the slow wave. Six consecutive sharp waves are marked with asterisks in the Fz-Cz channel, with an arc over the crest of each of the corresponding slow waves. The pattern is 'midline predominant' as it is most prominent at Fz (black box); however, the pattern is symmetric and synchronous (i.e., it looks the same in both hemispheres) (blue box showing it to be the same in the parasagittal derivations). Midline predominant patterns are considered a subtype of generalized patterns.

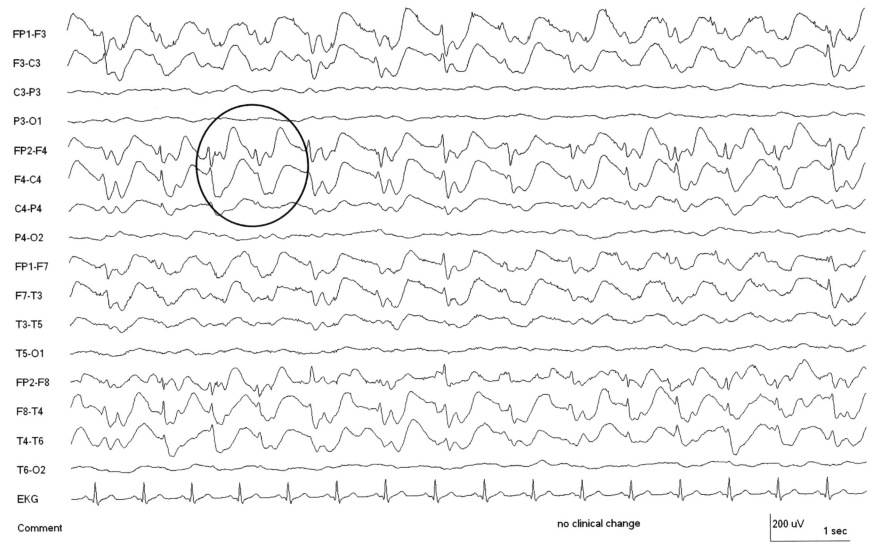

Figure 5.24. Generalized spike-wave (GSW) vs. EKG artifact. Rhythmic polyspike-and-wave activity (a type of GSW) is present in a widespread distribution, maximal anteriorly, fluctuating around 1.5 Hz, in this 21-year-old woman. Two examples of the polyspike-and-wave complexes are circled. Although this rhythmic activity is regular and has a rate of approximately that of the EKG, it does not represent EKG artifact (monitored in the bottom channel). This pattern is on the ictal-interictal continuum (IIC) but does not qualify as definite electrographic seizure on its own (though it would if it were faster than 2.5 Hz). See Chapter 6: Seizures and status epilepticus for more on the IIC. The patient was later shown to be in generalized nonconvulsive status epilepticus, as she improved clinically (and on EEG) with IV anti-seizure medication.

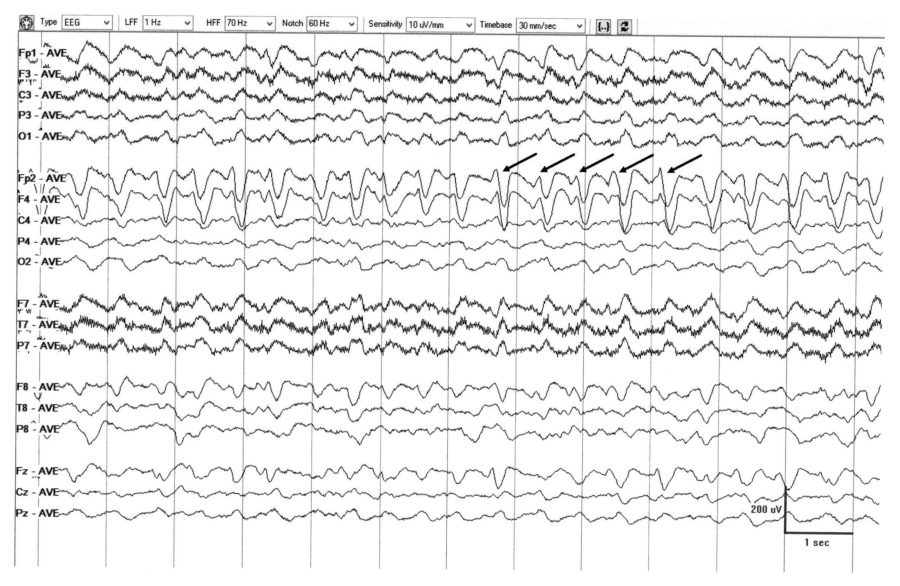

Figure 5.25.   Lateralized spike-and-wave (LSW). This EEG is from a 63-year-old man s/p hemicraniectomy for right frontal intraparenchymal hemorrhage (IPH). It has been shown in a referential montage to retain the morphology of the pattern. There is a repeating pattern characterized by a sharp wave maximal at Fp2/F4 (arrows) followed by a slow wave. There is no break to 'background' between the sharp-and-wave complexes (i.e., no inter-discharge interval), and thus this is not LPDs (not periodic). This pattern is therefore LSW. Note the pattern is not considered LRDA+S. Although there is RDA in the pattern, each rhythmic delta wave occurs as a stereotyped part of a sharp-and-wave complex. The use of the term LRDA+S would be more appropriate if there was no stereotyped association between the sharp waves and the slow waves.

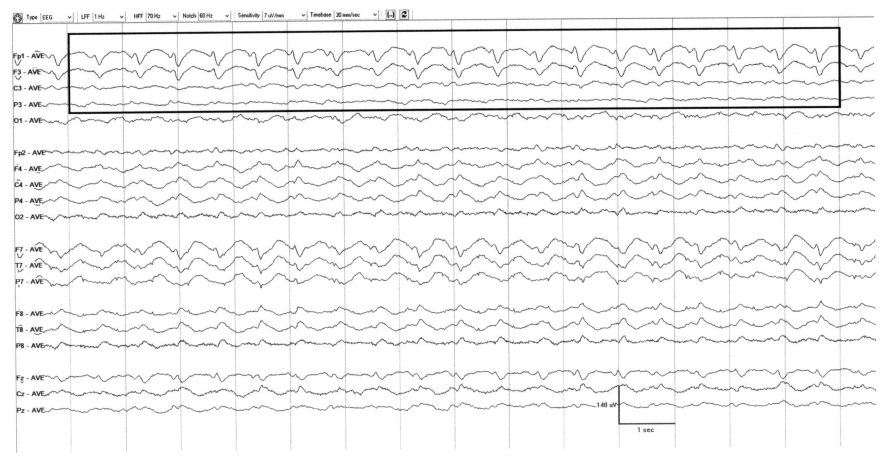

Figure 5.26. Lateralized sharp-and-wave (LSW). This EEG from a 55-year-old man with a left SDH demonstrates left frontal LSW (Fp1 maximal) at 1.5 Hz (box). Each sharp is followed by a delta wave with no break or inter-discharge interval from one complex to the next, and with a stereotyped relationship between the sharp wave and the slow wave.

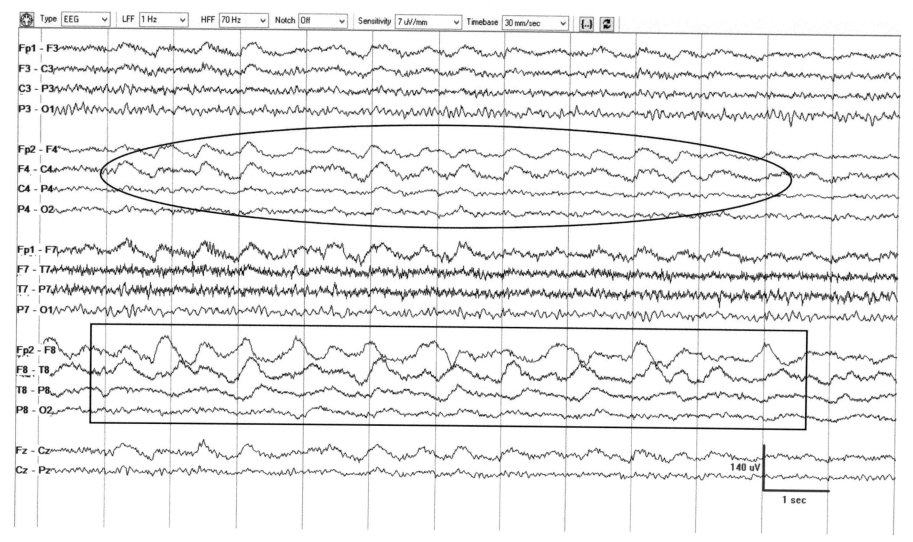

Figure 5.27. Unilateral independent rhythmic delta activity (UIRDA). (a) Unilateral independent rhythmic delta activity (UIRDA), longitudinal bipolar. This EEG is from a 57-year-old man that presented with seizures with a PMHx of a high-grade glioma in his right temporal lobe. There is LRDA in the right anterior temporal region (box). At the same time there is faster LRDA maximal in the right fronto-central region (ellipse). The patterns have different typical frequencies (clearer in the referential montage following this), so one cannot be a propagated or reflected pattern of the other (i.e., they are independent). The occurrence of two simultaneous populations of LRDA in the same hemisphere qualifies as UIRDA.

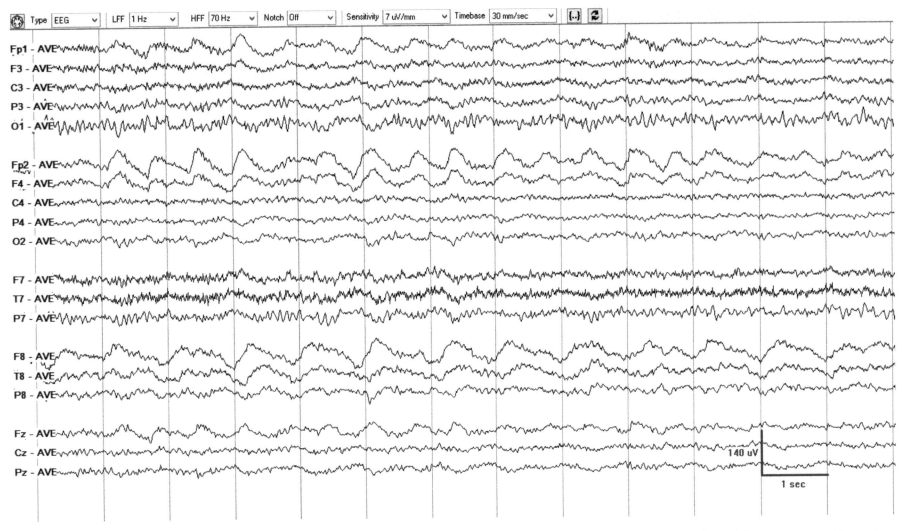

Figure 5.27.   (*Continued*) (b) Unilateral independent rhythmic delta activity (UIRDA), referential. When the EEG is reformatted to a referential montage it is again easier to appreciate the two clearly independent populations of LRDA at Fp2/F4 (≥1.5 Hz) and F8/T8 (slower, close to 1 Hz). The activity also appears more rhythmic in this montage as the referential montage provides a truer depiction of the morphology of waveforms (i.e., there is less distortion from cancellation compared to a bipolar montage).

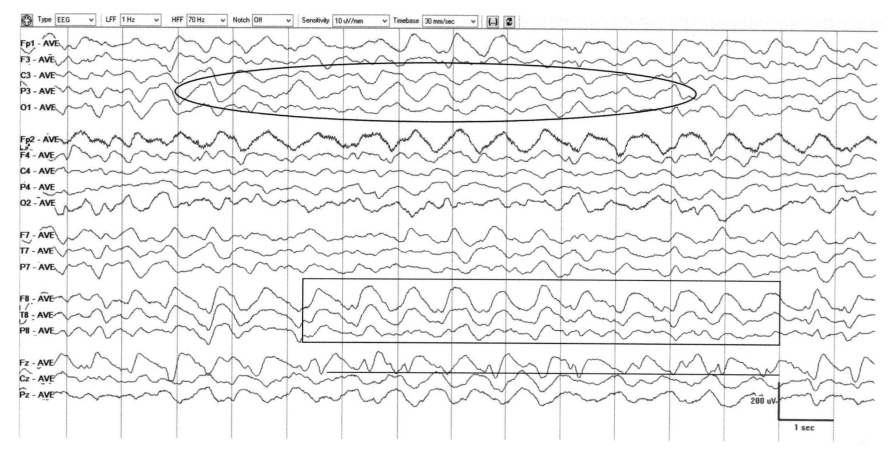

Figure 5.28. Bilateral independent rhythmic delta activity (BIRDA). This EEG is from a 29-year-old woman following TBI. This referential average montage demonstrates two independent foci of LRDA occurring at the same time (BIRDA). There is medium-amplitude 1.5-Hz LRDA maximal in the left centro-parietal region (C3/P3) (ellipse). There is also high amplitude 1–1.5-Hz LRDA in the right fronto-temporal region (F8>T8>Fp2). Although the two patterns have similar frequencies, they were seen independently over the course of the record, including on this page. The independent nature is perhaps best appreciated in the midline derivations at the bottom of the page. Fz (above the line) contains the activity maximal in the right fronto-temporal region, whereas Cz and Pz (below the line) contains the activity of the left centro-parietal region. Each wave at Fz does not have a time-locked relationship with a wave at Pz. Two independent populations of LRDA occurring at the same time (i.e., overlapping in time), with one in each hemisphere, is classified as BIRDA.

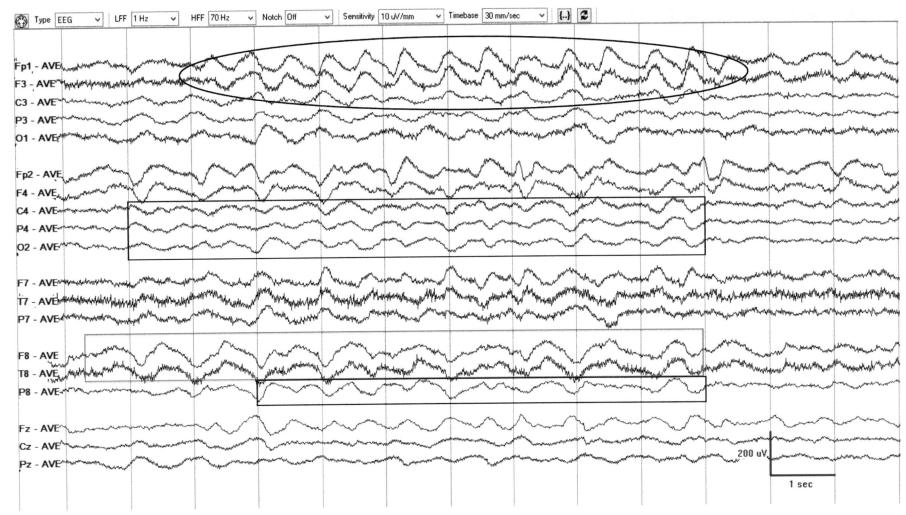

Figure 5.29. Multifocal rhythmic delta activity (MfRDA). This EEG presented in referential average demonstrates MfRDA. There are three independent populations of RDA occurring at the same time, with at least one in each hemisphere (i.e., occurring on both sides of the head). The three populations are 1. 1.75-Hz RDA in the left frontal region (Fp1/F3) (ellipse), 2. Similar frequency but non-time-locked subtle RDA in the right posterior quadrant (P8/O2) (black boxes; admittedly only equivocally qualifying as rhythmic), and 3. 1-Hz RDA in the right temporal region (F8/T8) (red box).

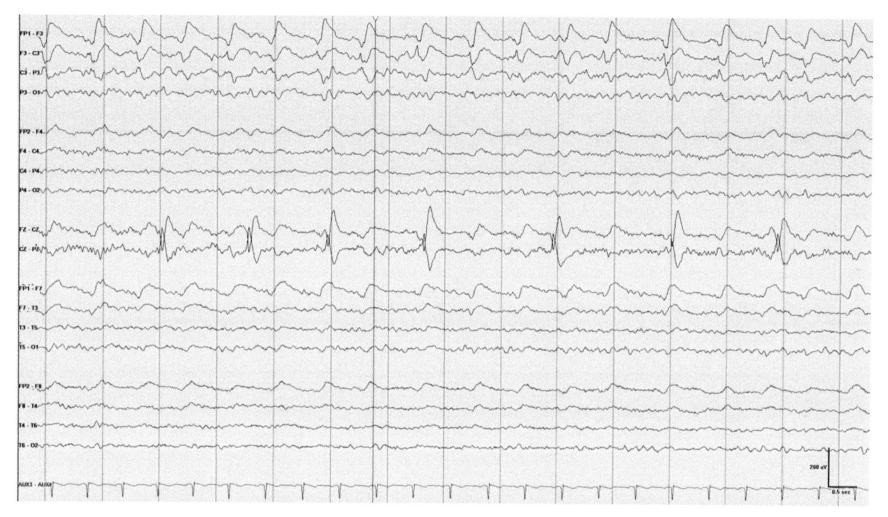

Figure 5.30. Unilateral independent periodic discharges (UIPDs). This EEG is presented in a longitudinal bipolar montage with the midline derivations in the center of the page. The EEG demonstrates UIPDs, two independent populations of PDs occurring simultaneously within the same hemisphere. In this example, there are 1–1.5-Hz PDs occurring in the left fronto-central region (mostly phase-reversing at F3), and a separate population of ~0.5-Hz PDs occurring at Cz. Note, a focal midline pattern may still be classified in the same hemisphere (unilateral) as an independent pattern in either the right or left hemisphere, so this pattern is UIPDs. If there were two independent PD populations with one in each hemisphere, then this would instead be classified as bilateral independent periodic discharges (BIPDs).

Courtesy of Dr. Jong Woo Lee, Brigham and Women's Hospital, Boston, MA.

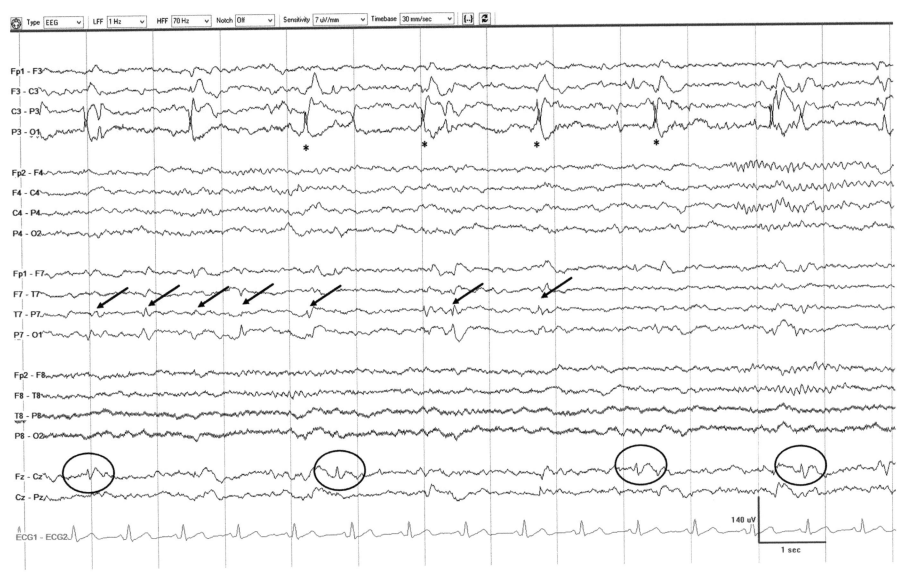

Figure 5.31. Unilateral independent periodic discharges (UIPDs). This EEG is from a 65-year-old man with a left SDH s/p hemicraniectomy. Following resolution of focal electrographic status epilepticus (ESE), there were two definite and one possible independent populations of periodic discharges all within the same hemisphere (assuming midline to be classified in the same hemisphere as the other populations). 1. 0.5–0.75-Hz PDs at P3 (asterisks), 2. 1–1.5-Hz PDs at T7/P7 (arrows), and 3. Almost periodic 0.25-Hz discharges at Fz (ellipses). Two or more independent populations of PDs within the same hemisphere qualify as UIPDs. There are no discharges in the right hemisphere, so this would not qualify as multifocal PDs (MfPDs).

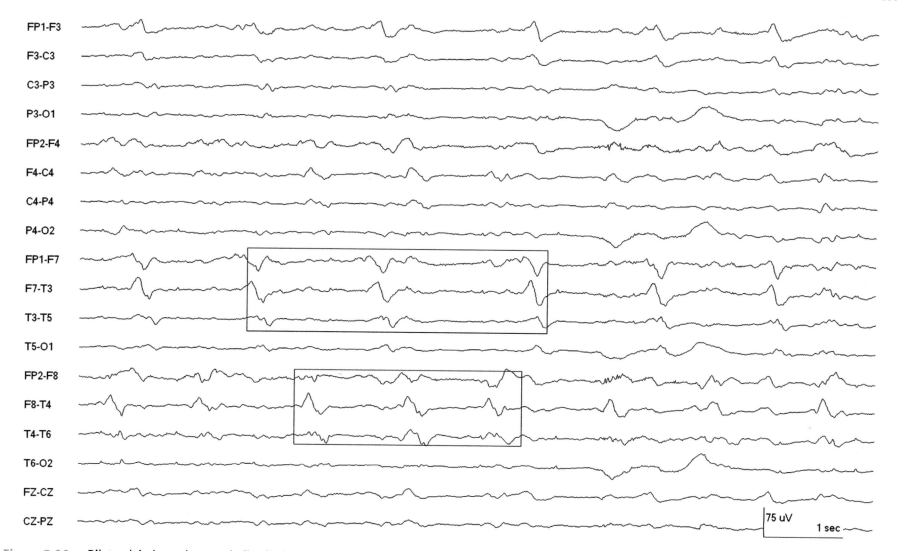

Figure 5.32. Bilateral independent periodic discharges (BIPDs). The EEG in this 75-year-old comatose woman shows BIPDs (3 discharges on each side are boxed). There are LPDs in the left fronto-temporal region (F7 maximal) but clearly an independent population of LPDs in the right fronto-temporal region (F8 maximal) that have no association with the pattern in the other hemisphere.

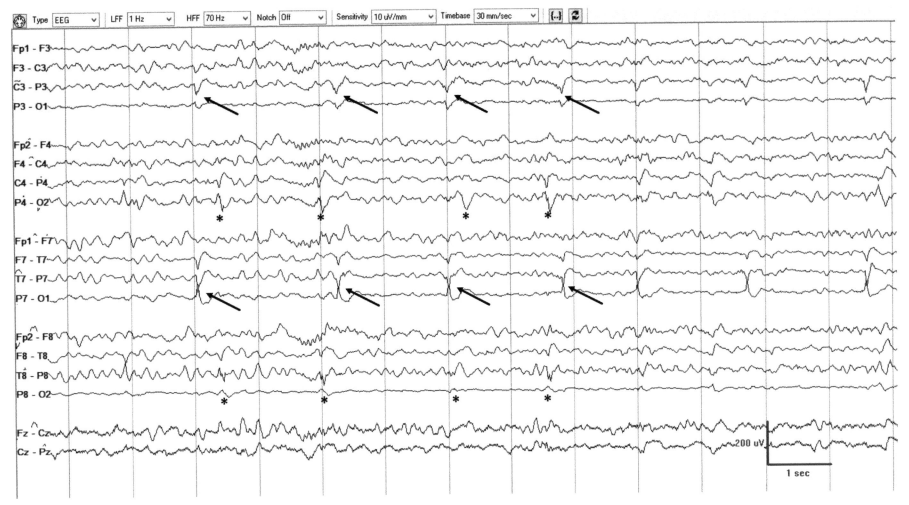

Figure 5.33.   Bilateral independent periodic discharges (BIPDs). This EEG is from a 69-year-old woman with Posterior Reversible Encephalopathy Syndrome (PRES) that was complicated by bilateral occipital strokes. She has one population of LPDs in the left posterior quadrant (P7/P3) (arrows) and another independent population of LPDs in the right posterior quadrant (P4/T8/P8) (asterisks). This is another example of BIPDs.

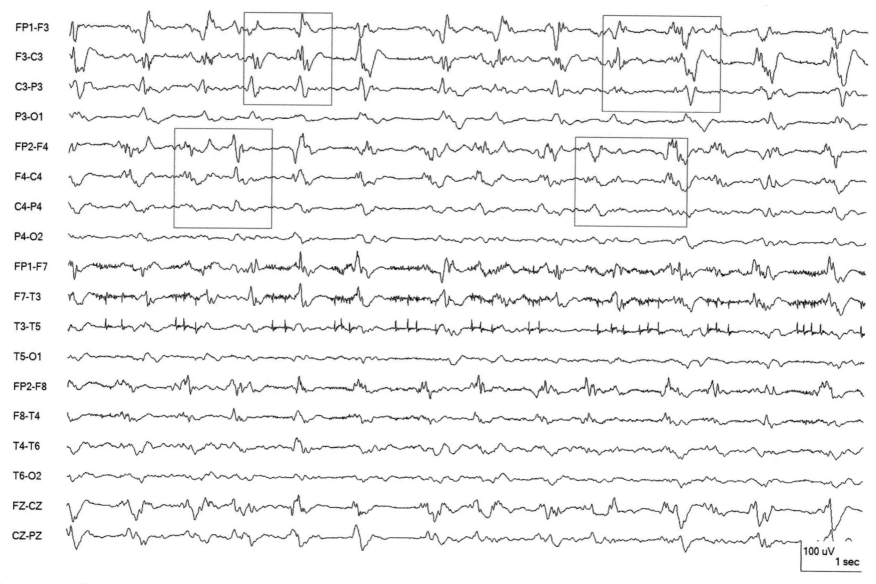

Figure 5.34. Bilateral independent periodic discharges with polyspikes. The EEG shows BIPDs in this 77-year-old woman with an encephalopathy due to sepsis. Both the left and right hemispheric populations are polyspikes (boxes).

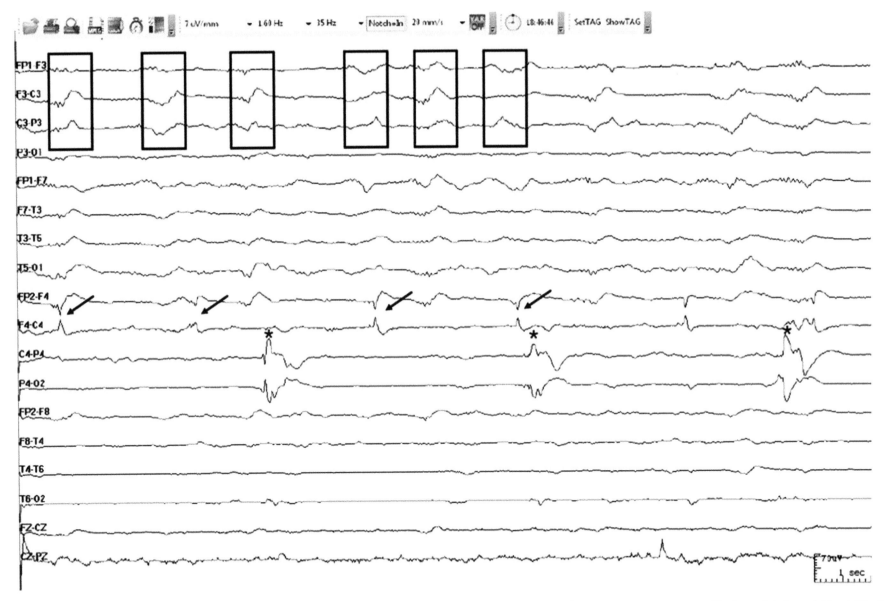

Figure 5.35. Multifocal periodic discharges (MfPDs). This EEG is presented in bipolar longitudinal montage left over right (left central, left temporal, right central, right temporal, then midline). The EEG demonstrates three independent populations of LPDs occurring at the same time with at least one in each hemisphere (two on the right and one on the left). There are sharp PDs at F4 at 0.33 Hz (arrows), spiky PDs at P4 at 0.2–0.25 Hz (asterisks), and blunt PDs in the left fronto-central region at 0.75 Hz (boxes).

Courtesy of Dr. Luis Octavio Caboclo, Albert Einstein hospital, Sao Paulo, Brazil.

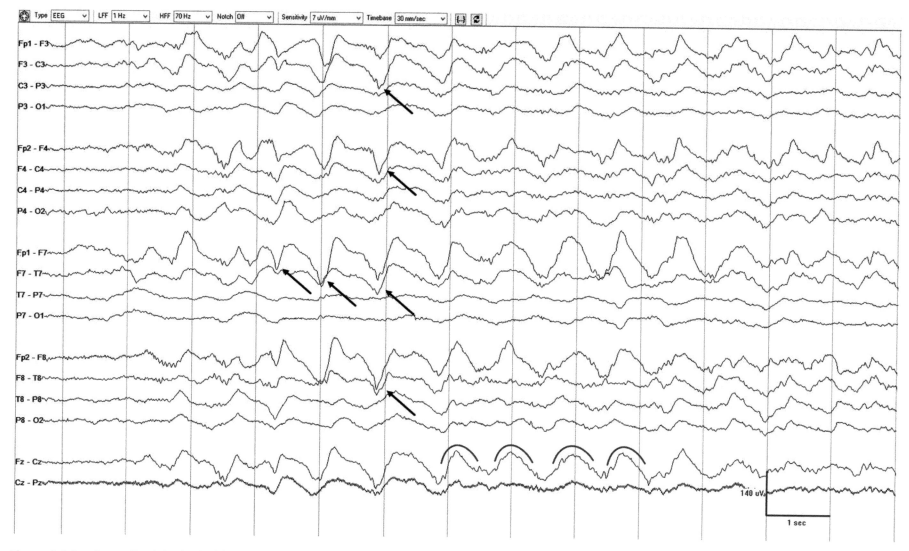

Figure 5.36. Generalized rhythmic delta activity plus S (GRDA+S). The EEG from this 43-year-old woman with altered mental status s/p left temporal encephalocele repair demonstrates GRDA (highlighted with the blue arcs in the midline derivation) that is sharply contoured at times (arrows), qualifying as GRDA+S.

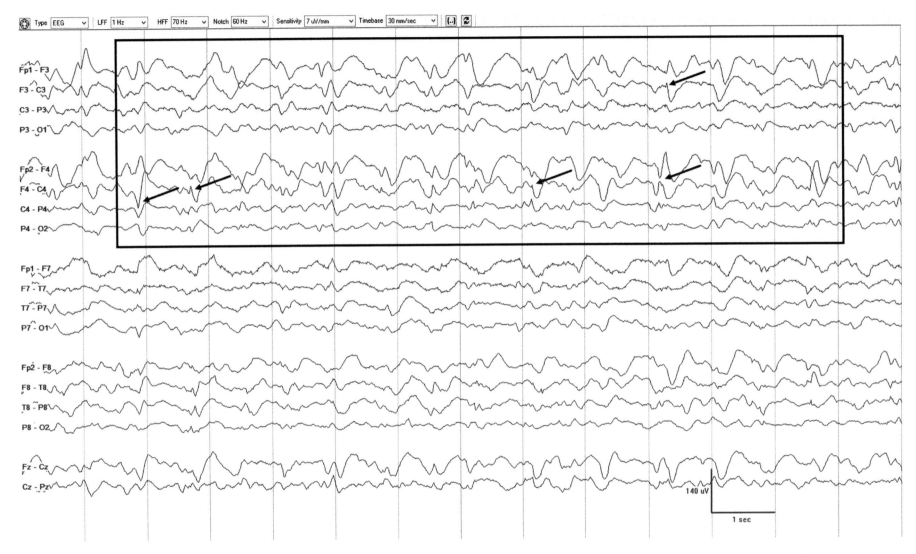

Figure 5.37.　Generalized rhythmic delta activity plus S (GRDA+S). The EEG from this 74-year-old woman s/p rupture of basilar tip aneurysm demonstrates GRDA (box) with admixed sharp waves (arrows), qualifying as GRDA+S. Contrast this to Figure 5.36 where the GRDA is sharply contoured, another form of GRDA+S.

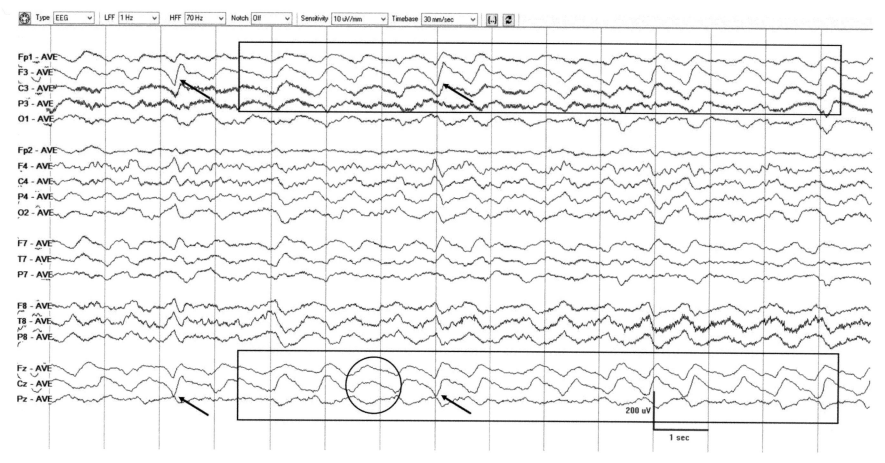

Figure 5.38.   Lateralized rhythmic delta activity plus S (LRDA+S). This EEG is from a 65-year-old man with a large left-sided SDH. There is 1.5-Hz LRDA in the left fronto-central region (F3, C3, Cz) (boxes). The pattern is sometimes sharply contoured (arrows), qualifying as LRDA+S.

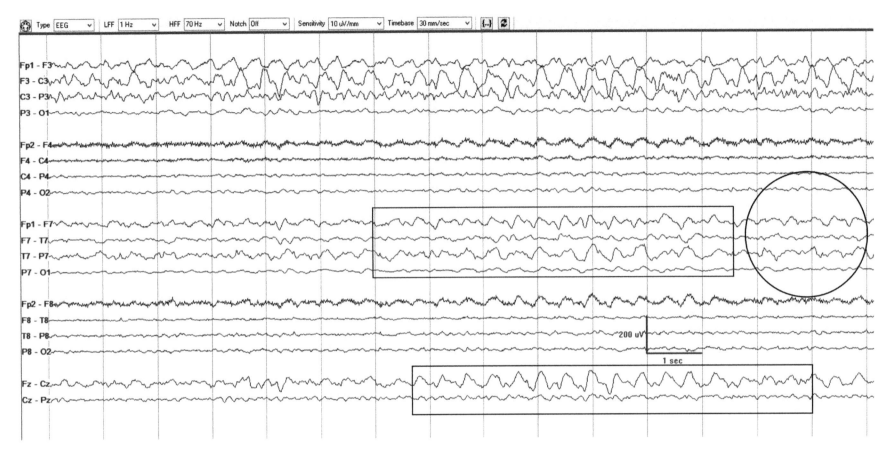

Figure 5.39. Lateralized rhythmic delta activity (LRDA) with evolution versus seizure. (a) Lateralized rhythmic delta activity with evolution, longitudinal bipolar. This EEG demonstrates LRDA with evolution. Note in the first 2–3 seconds of the page there is polymorphic mixed frequency slowing with breach effect in the left fronto-central region. After the third second, the activity becomes rhythmic (LRDA) at ~2 Hz. In the bipolar montage there is clearly evolution of location, spreading first to the left temporal region, and then a few seconds later the midline derivations (boxes). The ellipse highlights the activity waning again and not persisting. However, as there is definite evolution, and the pattern overall lasts >10 s (still ongoing at end of page), this qualifies as an electrographic seizure (ESz). If the pattern ended after <10 s, this would be referred to as LRDA with evolution, but not seizure. (It is not a BIRD since BIRDs have to be >4 Hz.)

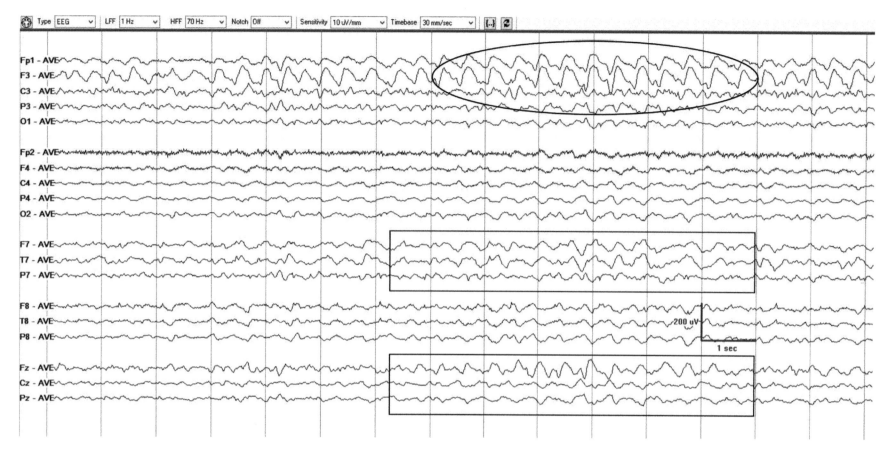

Figure 5.39. (*Continued*) (b) Lateralized rhythmic delta activity with evolution, referential. When reformatted into a referential average montage it is easier to appreciate evolution in morphology (ellipse), becoming higher voltage and sharply contoured (qualifying as LRDA+S). The evolution in location is also confirmed (boxes). Initially the LRDA is only present at F3/Fp1, then spreads to F7/T7, and then a second additional region becomes involved at Fz. Two sequential additional regions involved on a standard 10-20 montage qualifies as evolution in location. The pattern remains 2–2.5-Hz throughout, so there is not evolution in frequency. Evolution in frequency requires two sequential increases/decreases in frequency by 0.5-Hz, i.e., 2 Hz, increasing to 2.5 Hz, and then increasing again to 3 Hz.

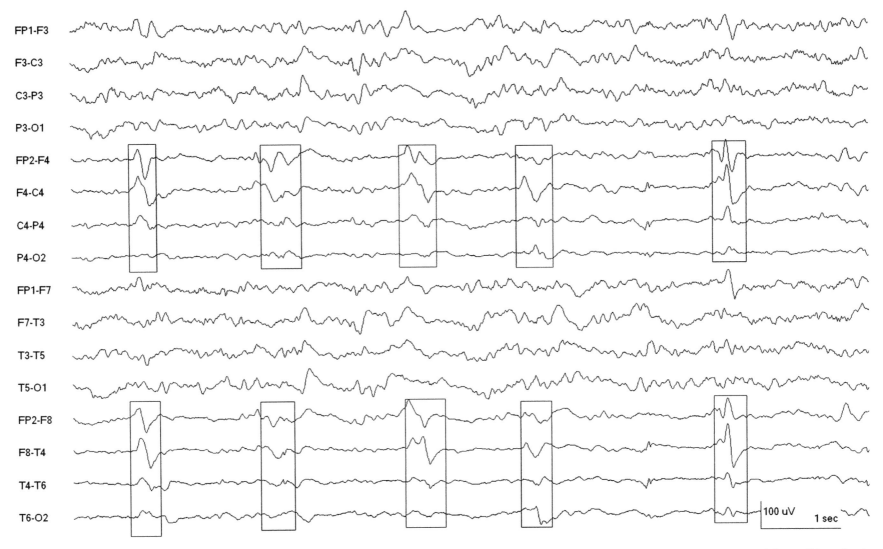

Figure 5.40. Symptomatic LPDs mimicking stroke. This 56-year-old woman with a history of epilepsy since childhood was found unresponsive and not moving her left side. She was felt to have a probable stroke, but imaging was negative. EEG shows right-sided LPDs, about 0.5 Hz and sharply contoured, with attenuation of background activity on the right between the periodic discharges. This is an example of a focal either ictal or postictal state (ictal could be proven via intracranial recordings or via rapid improvement with an IV anti-seizure medication) mimicking an infarct, not an unusual occurrence. The patient's neurological deficit resolved with time and additional anti-seizure medication, leaving it unclear whether this was an ictal or postictal process. Even if not definitively ictal, the PDs likely delayed the recovery of function in that region of the brain.

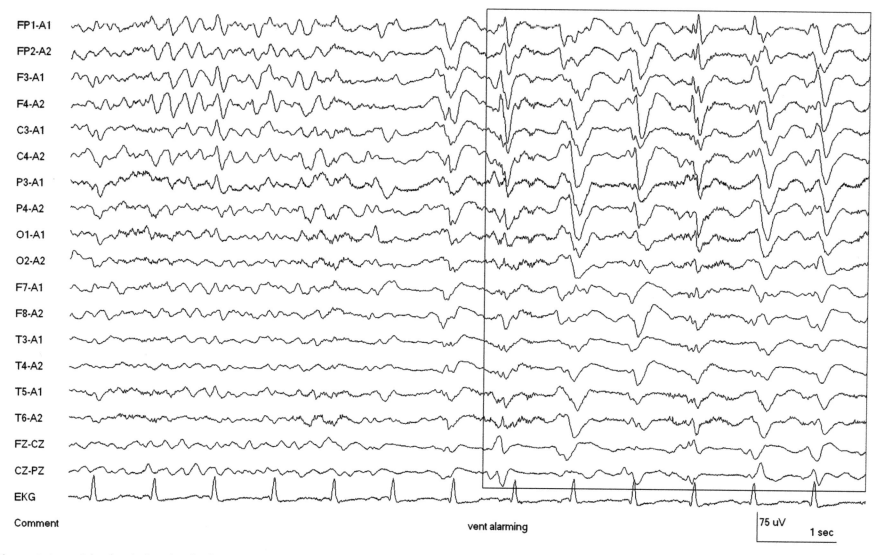

FP1-A1

FP2-A2

F3-A1

F4-A2

C3-A1

C4-A2

P3-A1

P4-A2

O1-A1

O2-A2

F7-A1

F8-A2

T3-A1

T4-A2

T5-A1

T6-A2

FZ-CZ

CZ-PZ

EKG

Comment

vent alarming

75 uV

1 sec

Figure 5.41. Stimulus-induced rhythmic, periodic or ictal discharges (SIRPIDs) and SI-GPDs. SIRPIDs are present in this 62-year-old comatose man. The patient had become unresponsive following abdominal surgery. There is a change in the EEG following alerting stimulation, with the appearance of GPDs. This is best described as SI-GPDs, a more specific term than the broader 'SIRPIDs'.

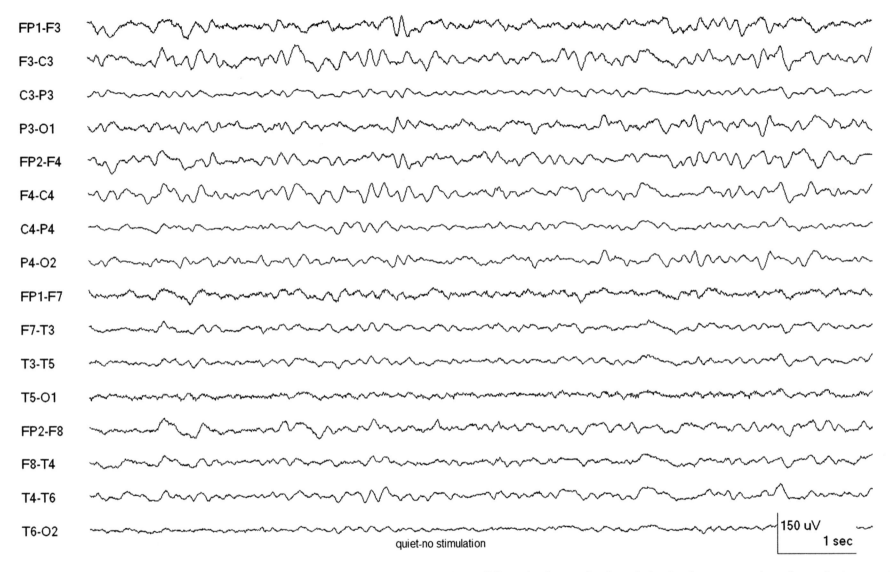

quiet-no stimulation

150 uV

1 sec

Figure 5.42.   SIRPIDs: GPDs vs. seizure. (a) The EEG in this 52-year-old woman shows diffuse slowing predominantly in the theta range when the patient was not stimulated.

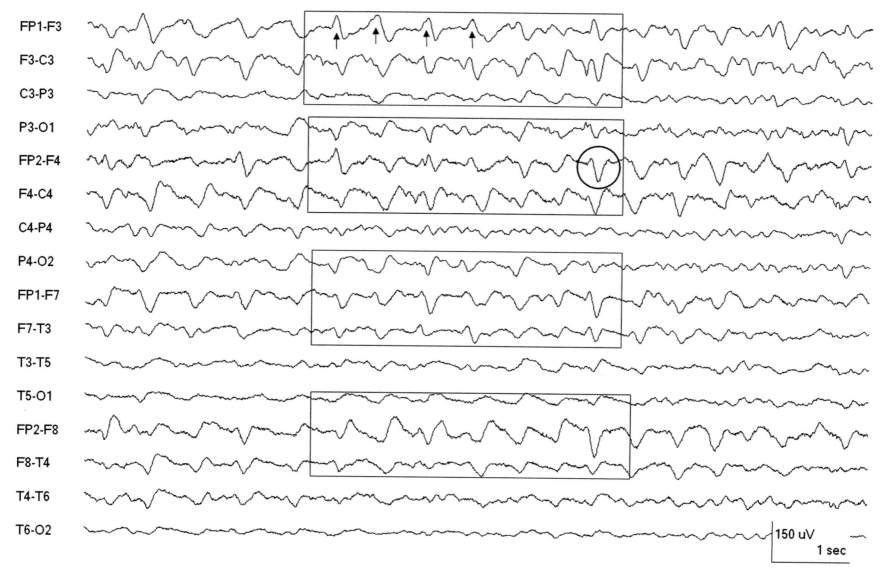

Figure 5.42. (*Continued*) (b) Following stimulation, GPDs at ~2 per second are seen (boxes, with four discharges in a row marked with arrows), sometimes with triphasic morphology (example circled), maximal anteriorly, with a quasi-rhythmic slow background, qualifying as SI-GPD+R. This pattern is potentially ictal and is on the ictal-interictal continuum (discussed in Chapter 6: Seizures and status epilepticus).

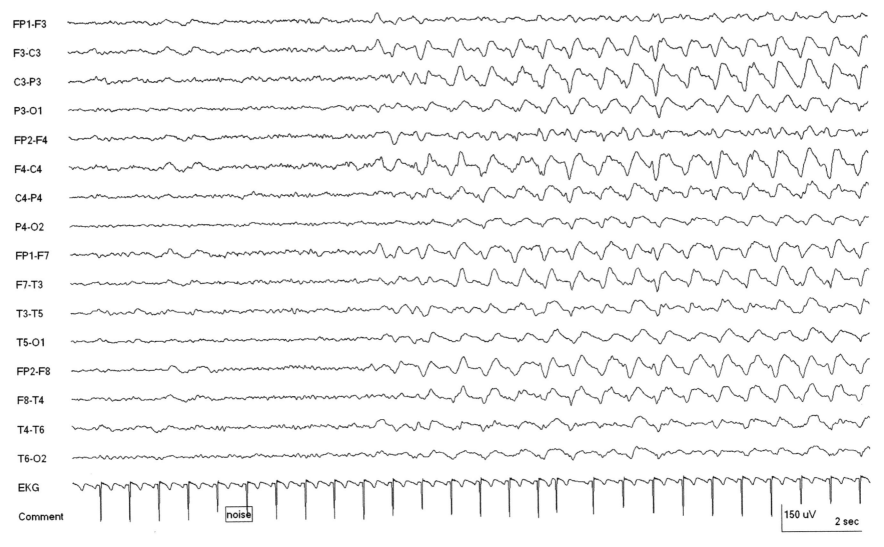

Figure 5.43. SIRPIDs: SI-GSW vs. SI-seizure. (a) This EEG is from a 65-year-old woman with recent bilateral convulsive seizures being evaluated for decreased mental status. When the patient is stimulated by noise, there is the emergence of a generalized spike wave (GSW) pattern at 1.5 Hz; this is GSW as opposed to GPDs as there is no consistent break in between discharges. If the sharp waves/spikes did not have a regular relationship to the slow waves, this would be considered either GRDA+S (if the RDA was more prominent than the PDs) or GPD+R (if PDs more prominent or both equal). This EEG almost qualifies for all three of these patterns (GSW, GRDA+S and GPD+R), though GSW is the best fit. Note this is a compressed EEG at slower 'paper speed' (see scale in lower right).

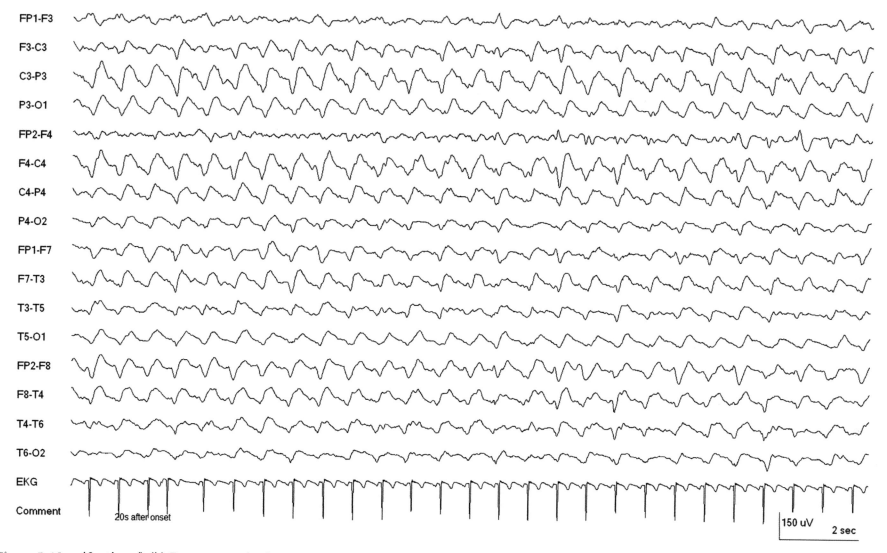

Figure 5.43. (*Continued*) (b) Twenty seconds after onset, the pattern is similar but slightly slower and slightly different in morphology.

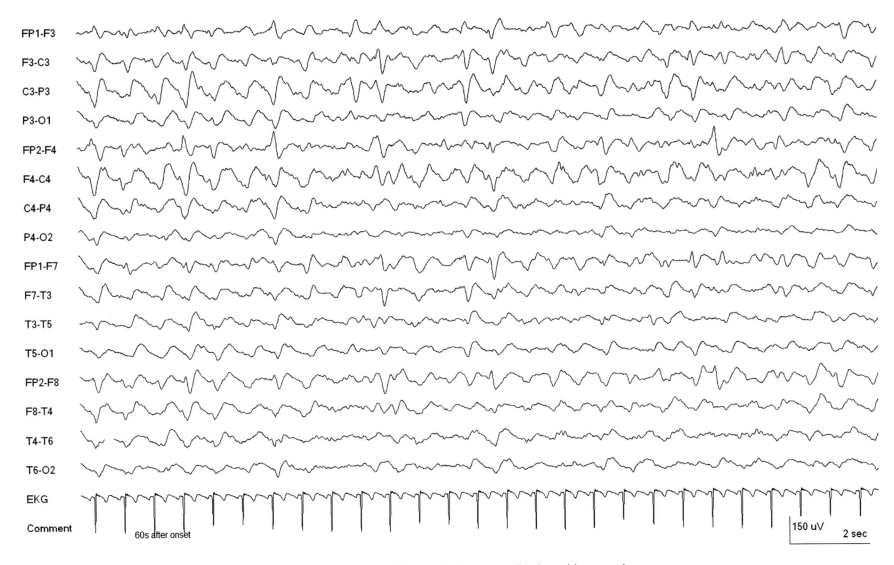

Figure 5.43. (*Continued*) (c) Sixty seconds after onset, the pattern is becoming lower amplitude and less regular.

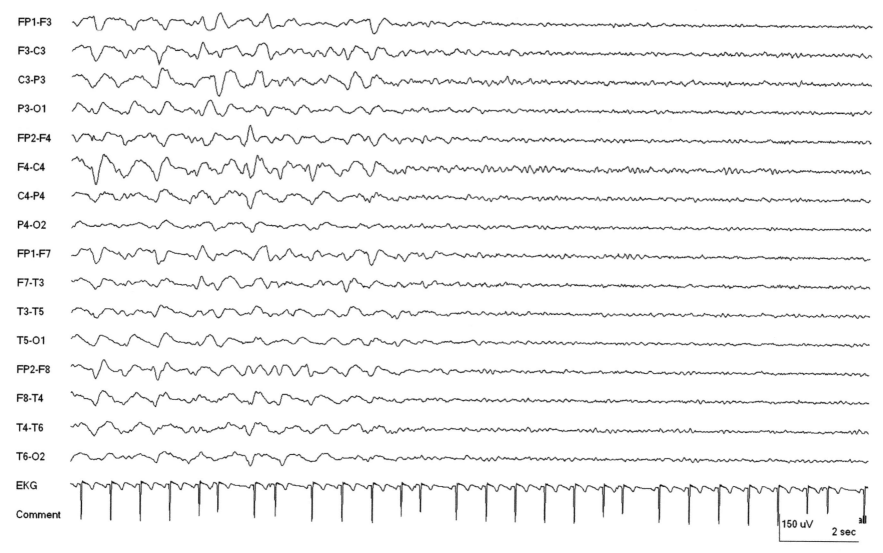

Figure 5.43. (*Continued*) (d) Eighty-three seconds after onset the discharge ceases. There was no clinical accompaniment. This is another example of SIR-PIDs. It is unclear if this represents stimulus-induced seizure activity or not but given the probable subtle evolution in morphology and frequency, and with a history of recent clinical seizures, it probably represents seizure activity. In that case, this would be considered SI-seizures, not an unusual phenomenon in the critically ill; see Chapter 6: Seizures and status epilepticus as well.

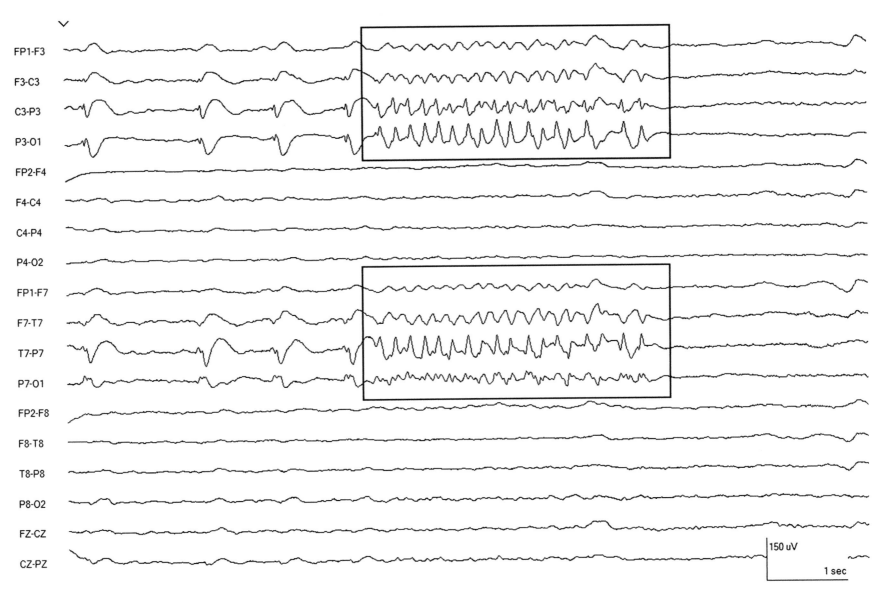

Figure 5.44.   Brief potentially Ictal Rhythmic Discharges (BIRDs), with evolution.

The EEG shows LPDs in the left centro-parietal region. In the middle of the page there is then a 3-second run of 5–6-Hz rhythmic discharges (box). There is some subtle evolution toward the end of the box with a change in morphology and the frequency slows. The finding looks like the beginning of a seizure; however, it is only 3 s, with seizures being defined as lasting at least 10 s; instead, this is referred to as BIRDs (>4 Hz and <10 seconds). Note that even though it cannot be classified as an electrographic seizure, it holds several seizure characteristics. It replaces the pattern of LPDs in the same region preceding it and there is post 'ictal' attenuation after the BIRDs. BIRDs with evolution, or 'evolving BIRDs' are a form of definite BIRDs and are highly associated with definite seizures.

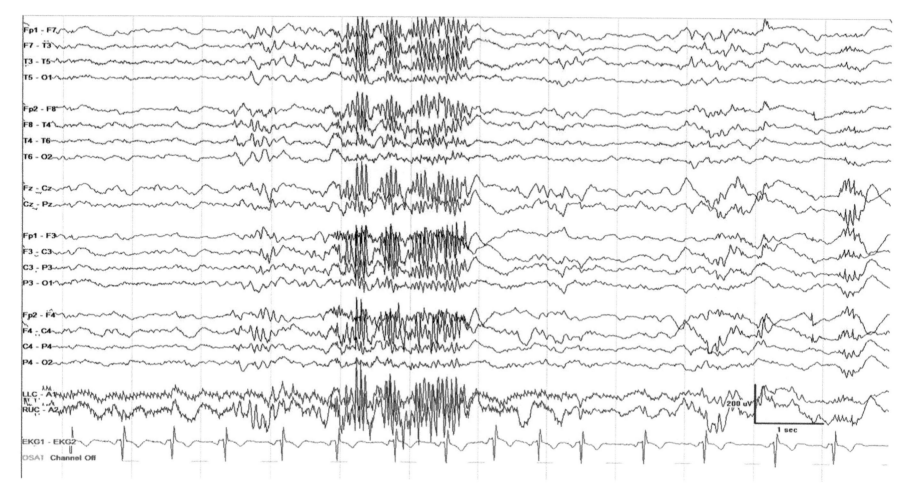

Figure 5.45. Brief potentially Ictal Rhythmic Discharges (BIRDs), generalized. (a) Brief potentially Ictal Rhythmic Discharges (BIRDs), generalized. This EEG is from a 40-year-old woman with medically refractory genetic generalized epilepsy. The montage is longitudinal bipolar (left temporal, right temporal, midline, left parasagittal, right parasagittal). The activity in the center of the page consists of 2 s of generalized high voltage polyspikes, which meet criteria for BIRDs; in the non-critically ill, this is also referred to as generalized paroxysmal fast activity (GPFA). Its presence suggests poorly controlled seizures.

Courtesy of Dr Ji Yeoun Yoo, Mt. Sinai Hospital, New York, NY.

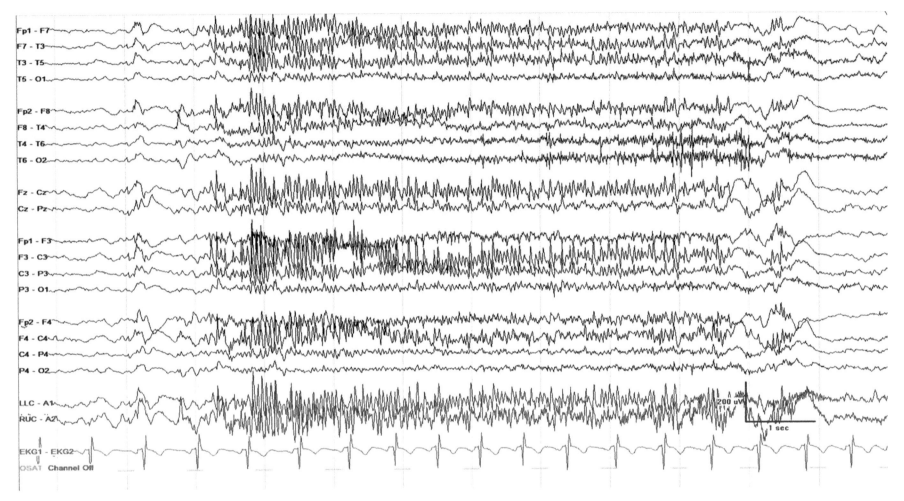

Figure 5.45. (*Continued*) (b) Brief potentially Ictal Rhythmic Discharges (BIRDs), generalized. At other times of the record the activity would reach up to 9 s and demonstrate evolution (as shown in this example). The activity never reached 10 s and so did not qualify as an electrographic seizure. The patient was tested through this activity and there was no suggestion of impaired awareness or recall; thus, with no clinical correlate this could not be classified as an electroclinical seizure. Even though it does not meet strict criteria for an ESz or ECSz, the finding is clearly highly epileptic and highly associated with definite seizures.

Courtesy of Dr Ji Yeoun Yoo, Mt. Sinai Hospital, New York, NY.

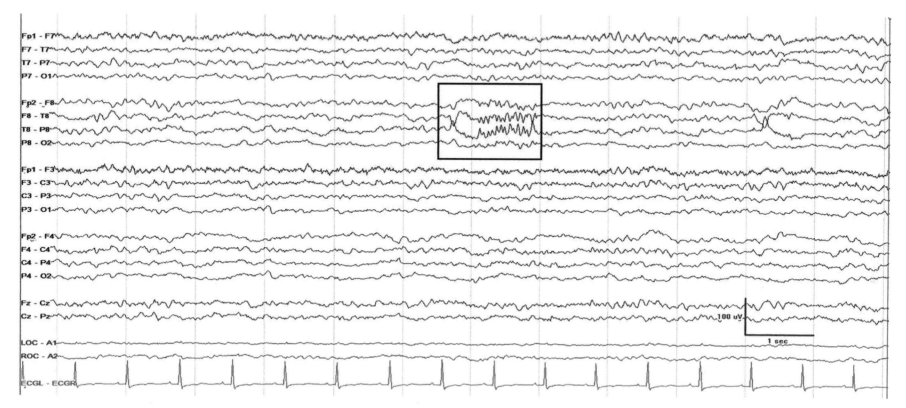

Figure 5.46. Brief potentially Ictal Rhythmic Discharges (BIRDs), evolving BIRDs with similar appearance as the beginning of a seizure. (a) Brief potentially Ictal Rhythmic Discharges (BIRDs), possible BIRDs. This EEG demonstrates a run of BIRDs, beginning with a medium-amplitude sharp wave, associated with low-amplitude fast activity, which changes into spiky 14–16 Hz activity (box), lasting 1.5 s. For these discharges to be classified as definite BIRDs they would have to either show evolution or share the same morphology/location as interictal discharges or electrographic seizures in the same patient.

Courtesy of Dr Ji Yeoun Yoo, Mt. Sinai Hospital, New York, NY.

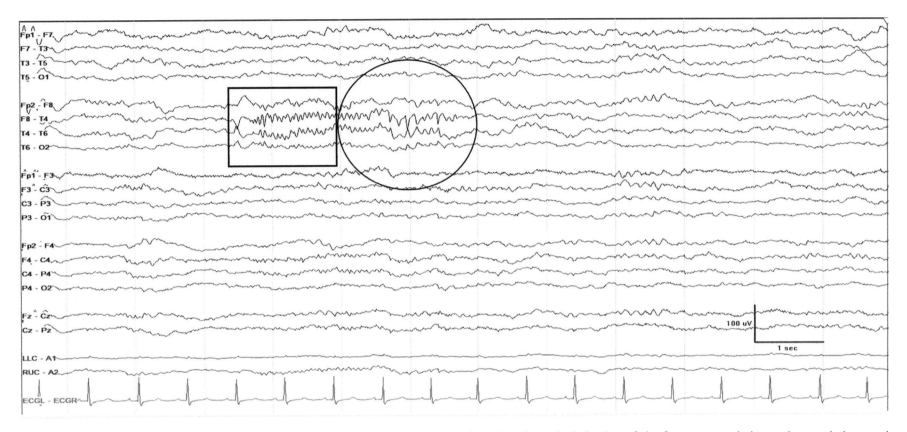

Figure 5.46. (*Continued*) (b) Brief potentially Ictal Rhythmic Discharges (BIRDs), evolving BIRDs. The same patient had evolving BIRDs. The box in the figure is the same size as in Figure 5.46a. This demonstrates that when the BIRDs lasted 1–1.5 s, they did not demonstrate evolution; however, if they were longer than this, they did. The ellipse highlights the second half of the BIRDs, showing that there is gradual slowing of the frequency and change in morphology to be less spiky (i.e., evolving). Evolving BIRDs are a form of definite BIRDs.

Courtesy of Dr Ji Yeoun Yoo, Mt. Sinai Hospital, New York, NY.

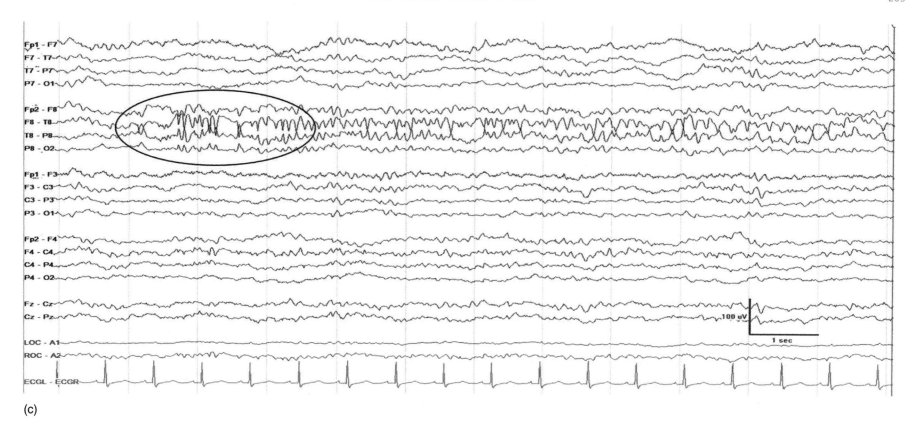

(c)

Figure 5.46. (*Continued*) (c-d) Seizure, with onset identical to the Brief potentially Ictal Rhythmic Discharges (BIRDs). A further way to qualify as definite BIRDs would be to demonstrate that the pattern was similar to the morphology/location of the beginning of a seizure in the same patient. These figures demonstrate a seizure in the same patient. The ellipse highlights that the beginning of the seizure appears very similar to the BIRDs, allowing all BIRDs resembling this pattern in this patient to be classified as definite (including those demonstrated in Figure 5.46a, now definite rather than possible).

Courtesy of Dr Ji Yeoun Yoo, Mt. Sinai Hospital, New York, NY.

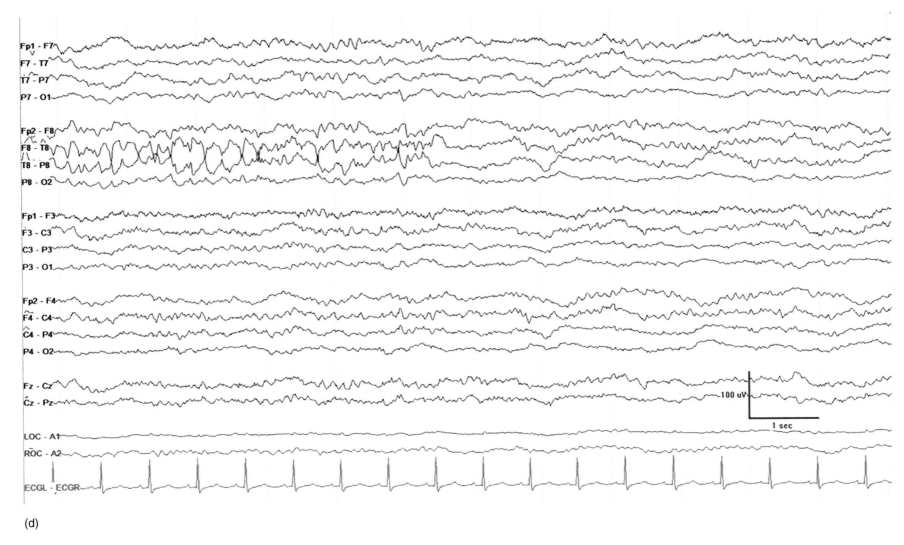

(d)

Figure 5.46.   (*Continued*)

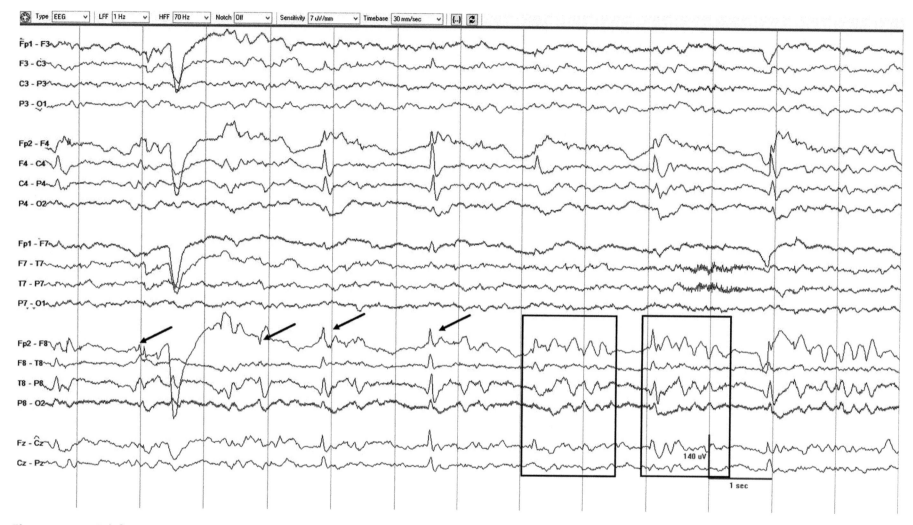

Figure 5.47. Brief potentially Ictal Rhythmic Discharges (BIRDs), LPDs transitioning into BIRDs. (a) Brief potentially Ictal Rhythmic Discharges (BIRDs), LPDs transitioning into BIRDs: This EEG is from a 65-year-old man following TBI and seizures. The EEG demonstrates the transition from LPDs (arrows) to BIRDs (boxes).

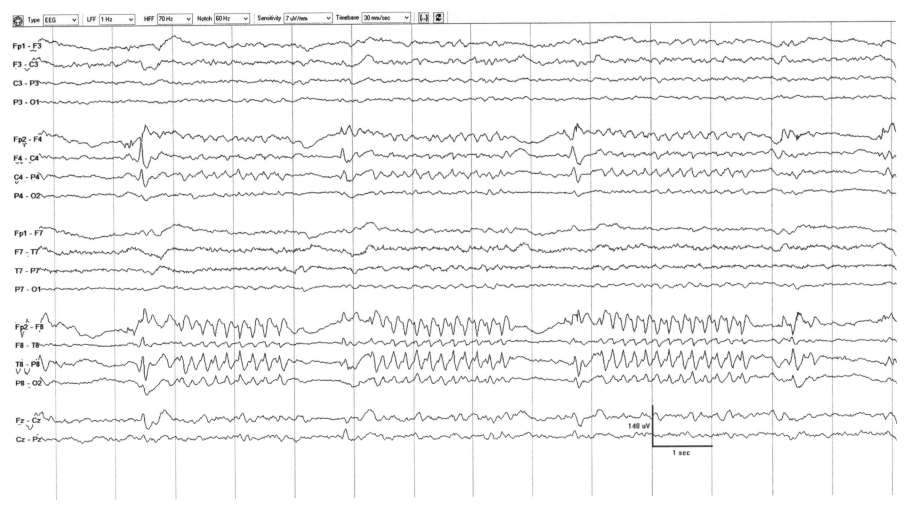

Figure 5.47. (*Continued*) (b) Brief potentially Ictal Rhythmic Discharges (BIRDs), LPDs transitioning into BIRDs: Later in the record, BIRDs became more prolonged and abundant, lasting up to 3–4 s as shown here. Additional anti-seizure medication was administered and the pattern returned to LPDs.

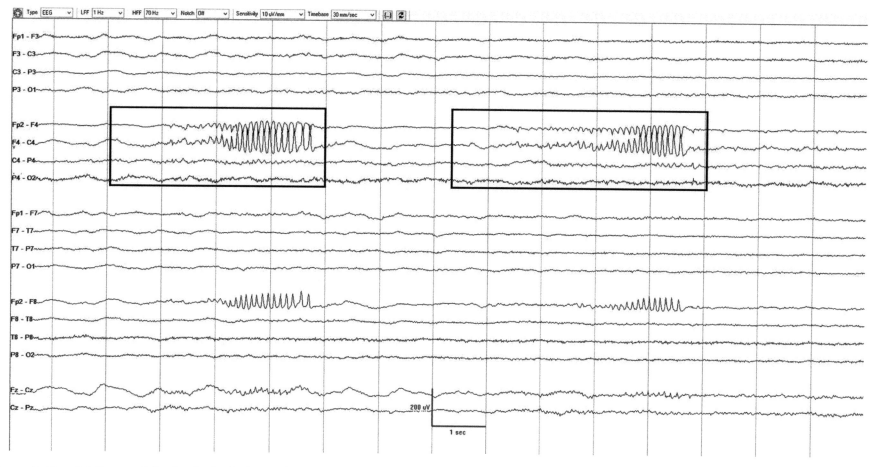

Figure 5.48. Brief potentially Ictal Rhythmic Discharges (BIRDs), evolving BIRDs, some seizures with similar appearance as BIRDs and others with independent seizure focus. This series of EEGs is from a 55-year-old man with a right subdural hematoma. (a) Brief potentially Ictal Rhythmic Discharges (BIRDs), evolving BIRDs. There were frequent evolving BIRDs (boxes).

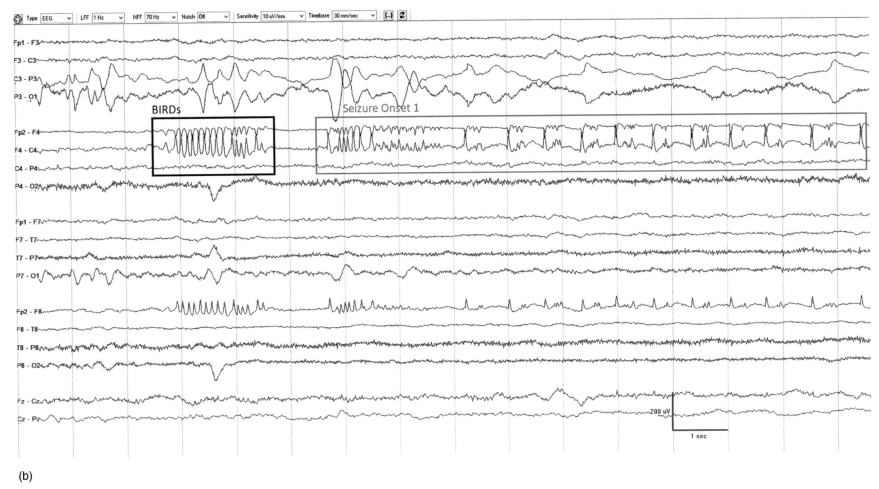

(b)

Figure 5.48.   (*Continued*) (b)–(e) Brief potentially Ictal Rhythmic Discharges (BIRDs), evolving BIRDs with same appearance at beginning of seizures in the same patient. Figure 5.48b demonstrates the seizure onset (red box) with the same location and morphology as BIRDs (black box). Figures 5.48c-e demonstrate evolution of the ESz over the right hemisphere. Note that at the time of this seizure the BIRDs disappear.

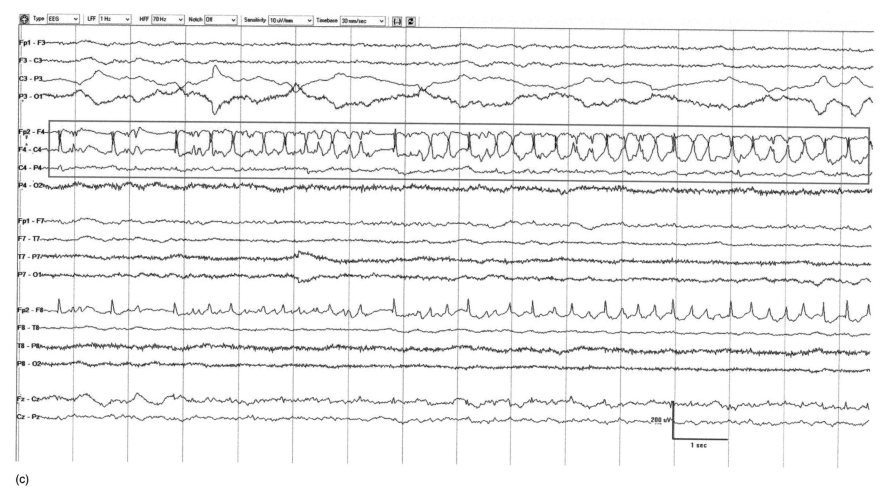

(c)

Figure 5.48. (Continued)

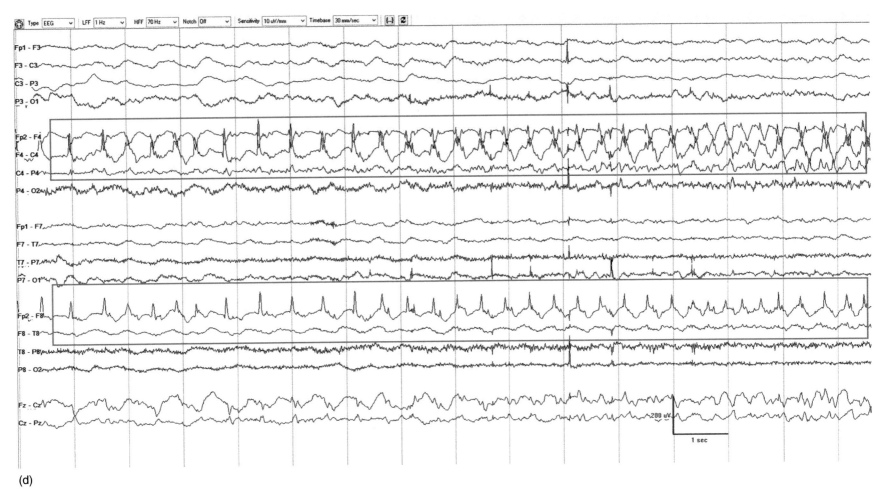

(d)

Figure 5.48.   (Continued)

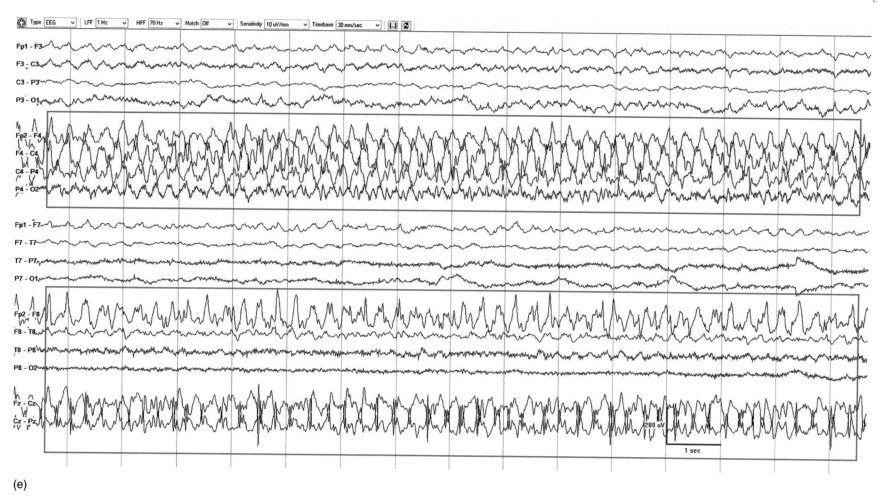

(e)

Figure 5.48. (*Continued*)

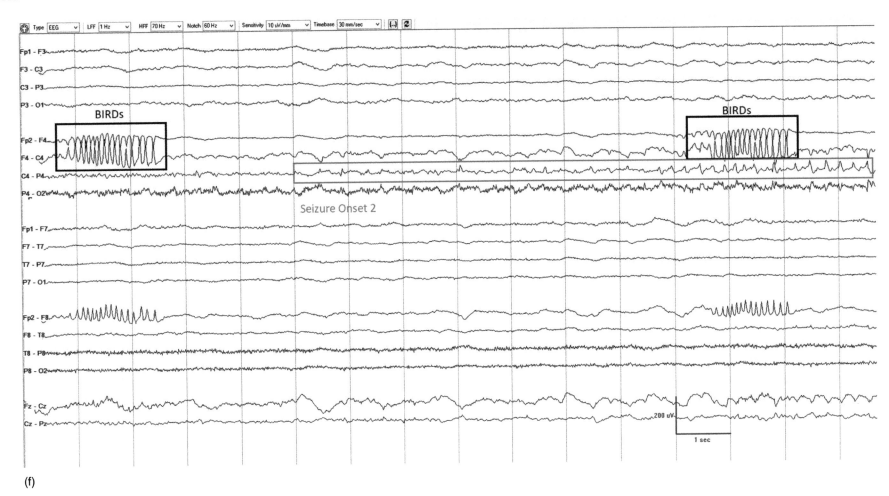

(f)

Figure 5.48. (*Continued*) (f)–(h) Brief potentially Ictal Rhythmic Discharges (BIRDs), evolving BIRDs, independent to a seizure focus in the same hemisphere. Figure 5.48f demonstrates evolving BIRDs (black boxes). In this case the seizure begins in a region (red box) that is posterior to the population of BIRDs. Figures 5.48g and 5.48f demonstrate the seizure propagating to C4/O2/Pz, but still not involving F4 where the BIRDs are located (black boxes). Here the BIRDs and electrographic seizure are independent (i.e., have no relationship to each other), an unusual occurrence. In general, BIRDs are a highly reliable indicator of the seizure onset zone in both critically ill and people with chronic epilepsy.

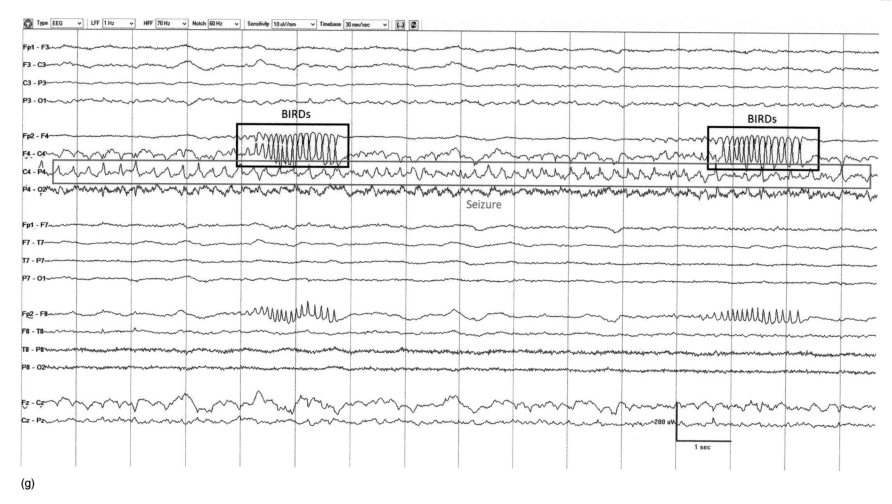

(g)

Figure 5.48. (*Continued*)

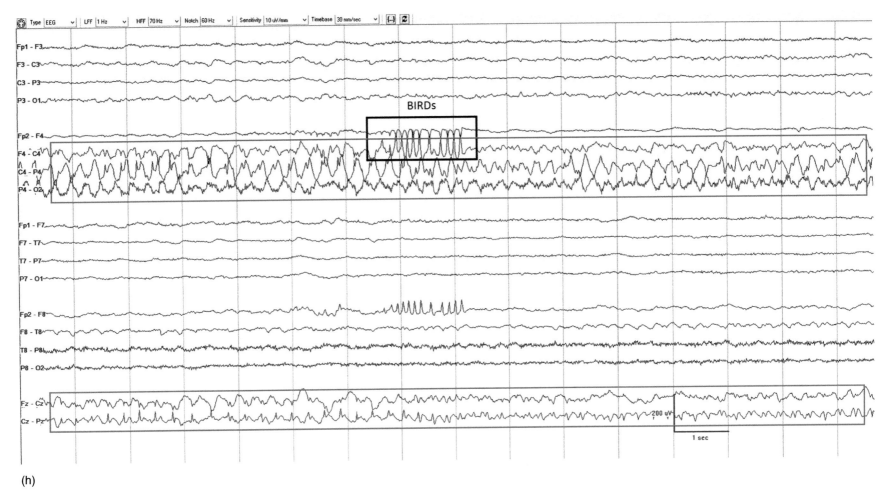

(h)

Figure 5.48.   (Continued)

6 Seizures, status epilepticus and the ictal-interictal continuum

6.1 Electrographic and Electroclinical seizures

Seizures are very common in the ICU, particularly in patients with acute or chronic brain injuries. The prevalence of seizures in those undergoing continuous EEG monitoring (generally for 24 hours or more) ranges from 8% in those without prior seizures and with no subtle signs of seizures to 48% after convulsive status epilepticus. Most studies of acute brain injury (including traumatic brain injury, intraparenchymal hemorrhage and subarachnoid hemorrhage) show a prevalence of seizures of 15–40%. It is clear from many studies now that the majority of seizures in the critically ill are nonconvulsive and can therefore only be diagnosed via EEG. Seizures appear to be an independent predictor of worse outcome in multiple populations, including worse long-term functional outcomes, cognition, hippocampal atrophy and later epilepsy.

Electrographic seizures (ESz) are defined by the ACNS critical care EEG terminology 2021, as either (Figure 6.1):

(1) epileptiform discharges[1] averaging >2.5 Hz for ≥10 seconds (>25 discharges in 10 seconds), or

(2) any pattern with definite evolution (in either frequency, morphology, or location) and lasting ≥10 seconds.

Electroclinical seizures (ECSz) are defined as any EEG pattern with either (Figure 6.1):

(1) definite clinical correlate[2] time-locked to the pattern (of any duration), or

(2) EEG *and* clinical improvement with a parenteral (typically IV) anti-seizure medication.

Seizures in the critically ill with encephalopathy tend to be of slower frequencies, last longer and have less clearly defined onset, evolution and offset than seizures in awake patients. Thus, they can be more difficult to recognize, both visually and via computer-based detection. In general, there must be clear evolution in frequency, morphology or location of an ongoing EEG pattern to be sure it represents seizure activity. However, in prolonged nonconvulsive seizures, the evolution can be subtle or even absent.

---

[1] Electrographic seizures can consist of sharply contoured discharges that are not technically 'epileptiform.' For example, >25 sharply contoured discharges in 10 seconds is still a seizure, although each discharge can be >200 ms duration (and therefore technically not 'epileptiform').

[2] A 'definite clinical correlate' can be subtle, including face twitching, eye deviation or nystagmus. Provided that the clinical sign is clearly time-locked to the EEG pattern (and absent when the pattern is absent), then it should be considered an electroclinical seizure.

Hirsch and Brenner's Atlas of EEG in Critical Care, Second Edition. Lawrence J. Hirsch, Michael W.K. Fong, and Richard P. Brenner.
© 2023 John Wiley & Sons Ltd. Published 2023 by John Wiley & Sons Ltd.

6.2   Status epilepticus

Status epilepticus in concept basically refers to ongoing and prolonged seizure activity. A strong misconception among clinicians is that all status epilepticus is the same. It must be stressed that just as seizures can be highly variable (e.g., absence vs. focal seizure with impaired awareness vs. generalized tonic-clonic), the states and patterns that meet criteria for status epilepticus are also highly variable. These varied presentations have significantly different associations with neuronal injury and therefore can vary greatly with regard to how aggressively/urgently they need to be treated. This diversity was reflected in the ILAE position statement on the definitions and classification of status epilepticus.

Electrographic status epilepticus (ESE) is defined by the ACNS as an ESz for ≥ 10 continuous minutes, or for a total duration of $\geq 20\%$ of any 60-minute period of recording. Previously, it was common to require ESzs to occupy ≥ 30 minutes (or $\geq 50\%$) total duration of any 60-minute period of recording to qualify as ESE. The reduction to $\geq 20\%$ is largely based on one large study that demonstrated that a seizure burden of $>20\%$ was associated with significantly increased chance of neurological decline in a cohort of critically ill children. A similar cutoff was identified in neonates with hypoxic ischemic encephalopathy. Multiple other studies in a variety of ages and conditions have shown a 'dose-response' effect, with greater seizure burden (either measured as peak burden in 1 hour or in 12 hours, or cumulative number of hours) resulting in worse outcomes, both short-term and long-term.

Electroclinical status epilepticus (ECSE) is defined as an ECSz for ≥ 10 continuous minutes, or for a total duration of $\geq 20\%$ of any 60-minute period of recording. An ongoing seizure with prominent bilateral motor activity (and impaired awareness) only needs to be present for ≥ 5 continuous minutes to qualify as ECSE. This can also be referred to as 'convulsive SE', a subset of 'SE with prominent motor activity'. In any other clinical situation, the minimum duration to qualify as SE is 10 minutes.

Some of the more common types of status epilepticus include:

(1) Convulsive (synonymous with 'tonic-clonic', a form of 'SE with prominent motor activity'): with 'episodes of excessive abnormal muscle contractions, usually bilateral, which may be sustained, or interrupted'. It is well established that convulsive SE represents a medical emergency, can cause irreparable neurological damage, and should be treated urgently. This is why convulsive activity only needs to be present for ≥ 5 minutes before meeting criteria for convulsive SE (as opposed to ≥ 10 minutes for any other type of SE).

(2) Nonconvulsive (NCSE, a form of 'SE without prominent motor activity'): can equally represent a prolonged focal seizure in a patient that has a brain tumor, a continuous generalized pattern in a patient with primary generalized epilepsy that is mildly interactive but slightly confused, or a >2.5 Hz pattern of GPDs in a medically ill severely obtunded or comatose patient.

(3) Myoclonic SE: often seen in hypoxic ischemic encephalopathy and discussed further in Chapter 8: Post cardiac arrest EEG.

(4) Focal motor SE (a subtype of which is epilepsia partialis continua [EPC]): A patient in EPC represents a specific class of focal motor status where there is periodic jerking of one particular part of the body and fully retained awareness (focal aware motor status epilepticus). This can be associated with periodic discharges or no scalp EEG correlate (as with any focal aware seizure, lack of scalp EEG correlate is common). EPC can be present for weeks to months, even years on rare occasion, without progressing to any other type of seizure. The finding is often associated with a discrete structural abnormality/lesion resulting in a very limited circuit of re-entrant seizure activity.

In the ICU there are many patients where it is uncertain if the ongoing electrographic pattern is contributing to their clinical signs. These patients are classified in the category of 'possible ECSE'. It should be noted that if it is certain that the electrographic pattern is causing clinical signs (irrespective of the pattern), this would qualify as ECSE. 'Possible ECSE' is defined as a RPP that qualifies for the ictal-interictal continuum (IIC) (i.e., it does not qualify as a ESz/ESE: further discussed and defined below) that is present for ≥ 10 continuous minutes, or for a total duration of $\geq 20\%$ of any 60-minute period of recording, which shows EEG improvement with a parenteral anti-seizure medication BUT without clinical improvement. This remains largely in line with 'possible NCSE' as defined by the Salzburg criteria, commonly accepted criteria for electrographic SE that were largely incorporated into the ACNS terminology.

A specific population that can pose diagnostic challenge are patients with a known prior epileptic encephalopathy. In these patients the baseline EEG is often severely abnormal (at times meeting criteria for ESE). For these patients to qualify as having ECSE, the EEG pattern needs to represent either:

(1) an increase in prominence or frequency of epileptiform discharges compared with baseline with an observable decline in clinical state, or

(2) EEG and clinical improvement with a parenteral (typically IV) anti-seizure medication.

6.3 Ictal-interictal continuum (IIC)

The definitions of what constitutes seizures are mostly based on historical consensus. For example, there is little evidence that a 2.3-Hz pattern causes less neuronal injury than a 2.7-Hz pattern. Yet one is classified as an ESz (or ESE if persistent) and the other is not. There are many patterns (that do not qualify as ESz/ESE) that appear clinically worrisome, can cause subtle clinical signs, are associated with ictal physiology (e.g., increased blood flow and metabolism), and could contribute to additional neuronal injury, especially in the setting of acute brain injury. Thus, they are potentially ictal in some sense. These patterns fall on the 'ictal-interictal continuum', a synonym for 'possible status epilepticus'. When patients with chronic epilepsy are monitored in the epilepsy monitoring unit (EMU) there is a clear distinction between ictal and interictal states (i.e., what is seizure, and what is not). There is also, for the most part, a crisp and immediate transition between these two states, with a clearly identifiable seizure onset, and offset. In critically ill patients the mechanisms of seizure generation, and perhaps more importantly the maintenance of seizure cessation, is often severely impaired. In these patients there is commonly a gradual waxing and waning between patterns, ranging from those that are fairly benign and those that are more epileptic, and at times ESz/ESE.

This phenomenon resulted in the term ictal-interictal continuum (IIC). The definition of the IIC is broad and deliberately inclusive, mostly to stimulate further studies into differentiating between patterns that are potentially injurious vs. those that are not. Patterns currently thought to qualify as the IIC, based on the ACNS definition in 2021, include (Figure 6.2):

(1) any PD or SW pattern that averages >1.0 Hz and ≤ 2.5 Hz over 10 s (>10 and ≤ 25 discharges in 10 s); or

(2) any PD or SW pattern that averages ≥ 0.5 Hz and ≤ 1.0 Hz over 10 s (≥ 5 and ≤ 10 discharges in 10 s), and has a plus modifier or fluctuation; or

(3) any lateralized RDA averaging >1 Hz for at least 10 s (at least 10 waves in 10 s) with a plus modifier or fluctuation

and

(4) does not qualify as an ESz or ESE.

6.4 Rapid EEG

For the most part, the primary goal of cEEG is to detect seizures as quickly as possible, and have this information fed back to clinicians to allow prompt treatment in order to improve outcomes. Although many centers have a dedicated service in order to do this, there are often delays in setting up the EEG, which requires technical training, and reviewer feedback to clinicians. To avoid these delays, there have been systems/devices (caps, belts, headbands, etc.) developed that allow for the rapid application (within a few minutes) of EEG with minimal training that allows instant review by clinicians and/or has automated interpretation. There is even the feature to 'sonify' the EEG (i.e., convert the EEG waves into sound waves) so clinicians can learn to distinguish the constant hum of a non-epileptiform record, versus a louder, more irregular and sometimes crescendo pattern of seizures or status epilepticus, which requires little to no knowledge of the EEG to interpret. Through these means detection of seizures and feedback to clinicians can often occur markedly faster (minutes rather than hours or longer) compared to conventional cEEG. The limited montages of several of these devices do have a mildly reduced sensitivity and specificity compared to traditional full montage; however, rapid EEG is becoming an important supplement to conventional cEEG in many centers for the benefits described, and an important new option for centers without capability for rapid EEGs (especially off-hours) or continuous EEG monitoring.

Figure list

EEGs throughout this atlas have been shown with the following standard recording filters unless otherwise specified: LFF 1 Hz, HFF 70 Hz, notch filter off.

Suggested reading

Beniczky S, Hirsch LJ, Kaplan PW, et al. Unified EEG terminology and criteria for nonconvulsive status epilepticus. *Epilepsia.* 2013;**54** Suppl 6:28–29.

Chong DJ, Hirsch LJ. Which EEG patterns warrant treatment in the critically ill? Reviewing the evidence for treatment of periodic epileptiform discharges and related patterns. *J Clin Neurophysiol.* 2005 Apr;**22**(2):79–91.

Claassen J, Mayer SA, Kowalski RG, Emerson RG, Hirsch LJ: Detection of electrographic seizures with continuous EEG monitoring in critically ill patients. *Neurology* 2004; **62**(10):1743–1748.

Claassen J, Mayer SA, Kowalski RG, Emerson RG, Hirsch LJ. Detection of electrographic seizures with continuous EEG monitoring in critically ill patients. *Neurology.* 2004;**62**(10):1743–1748.

DeLorenzo RJ, Waterhouse EJ, Towne AR, et al: Persistent nonconvulsive status epilepticus after the control of convulsive status epilepticus. *Epilepsia* 1998;**39**(8):833–840.

De Marchis GM, Pugin D, Meyers E, et al. Seizure burden in subarachnoid hemorrhage associated with functional and cognitive outcome. *Neurology.* 2016;**86**(3):253–260.

Drislane FW, Blum AS, Schomer DL. Focal status epilepticus: clinical features and significance of different EEG patterns. *Epilepsia.* 1999 Sep;**40**(9):1254–1260.

Granner MA, Lee SI. Nonconvulsive status epilepticus: EEG analysis in a large series. *Epilepsia.* 1994 Jan-Feb;**35**(1):42–47.

Hirsch LJ, Fong MWK, Leitinger M, et al. American Clinical Neurophysiology Society's Standardized Critical Care EEG Terminology: 2021 Version. *J Clin Neurophysiol.* 2021;**38**(1):1–29.

Jette N, Claassen J, Emerson RG, Hirsch LJ. Frequency and predictors of nonconvulsive seizures during continuous electroencephalographic monitoring in critically ill children. *Arch Neurol.* 2006;**63**(12):1750–1755.

Kamousi B, Grant AM, Bachelder B, Yi J, Hajinoroozi M, Woo R. Comparing the quality of signals recorded with a rapid response EEG and conventional clinical EEG systems. *Clin Neurophysiol Pract.* 2019;**4**:69–75.

Leitinger M, Trinka E, Gardella E, et al. Diagnostic accuracy of the Salzburg EEG criteria for non-convulsive status epilepticus: a retrospective study. *Lancet Neurol.* 2016;**15**(10):1054–1062.

McKay JH, Feyissa AM, Sener U, et al. Time Is Brain: The use of EEG electrode caps to rapidly diagnose nonconvulsive status epilepticus. *J Clin Neurophysiol.* 2019;**36**(6):460–466.

Nei M, Lee J-M, Shanker VL, Sperling MR. The EEG and prognosis in status epilepticus. *Epilepsia.* 1999;**40**(2):157–163.

Payne ET, Zhao XY, Frndova H, et al. Seizure burden is independently associated with short term outcome in critically ill children. *Brain.* 2014;**137**(Pt 5):1429–1438.

Privitera M, Hoffman M, Moore JL, Jester D: EEG detection of nontonic-clonic status epilepticus in patients with altered consciousness. *Epilepsy Res* 1994;**18**(2):155–166.

Sivaraju A, Gilmore EJ. Understanding and managing the ictal-interictal continuum in neurocritical care. *Current Treatment Options in Neurology.* 2016;**18**(2)8.

Struck AF, Westover MB, Hall LT, Deck GM, Cole AJ, Rosenthal ES. Metabolic correlates of the ictal-interictal continuum: FDG-PET during continuous EEG. *Neurocrit Care.* 2016;**24**(3):324–331.

Swingle N, Vuppala A, Datta P, et al. Limited-montage EEG as a tool for the detection of nonconvulsive seizures. *J Clin Neurophysiol.* 2020.

Towne AR, Waterhouse EJ, Boggs JG, et al: Prevalence of nonconvulsive status epilepticus in comatose patients. *Neurology* 2000;**54**(2):340–345.

Treiman DM, Walton NY, Kendrick C. A progressive sequence of electroencephalographic changes during generalized convulsive status epilepticus. *Epilepsy Res.* 1990;**5**(1):49–60.

Trinka E, Cock H, Hesdorffer D, et al. A definition and classification of status epilepticus – Report of the ILAE Task Force on Classification of Status Epilepticus. *Epilepsia.* 2015;**56**(10):1515–1523.

Vespa PM, Nuwer MR, Nenov V, et al: Increased incidence and impact of nonconvulsive and convulsive seizures after traumatic brain injury as detected by continuous electroencephalographic monitoring. *J Neurosurg* 1999;**91**(5):750–760.

Vespa PM, O'Phelan K, Shah M, et al: Acute seizures after intracerebral hemorrhage: a factor in progressive midline shift and outcome. *Neurology* 2003;**60**(9):1441–1446.

Vespa PM, McArthur DL, Xu Y, et al. Nonconvulsive seizures after traumatic brain injury are associated with hippocampal atrophy. *Neurology.* 2010;**75**(9):792–798.

Vespa P, Tubi M, Claassen J, et al. Metabolic crisis occurs with seizures and periodic discharges after brain trauma. *Ann Neurol.* 2016;**79**(4):579–590.

Vespa PM, Olson DM, John S, et al. Evaluating the clinical impact of rapid response electroencephalography: The DECIDE multicenter prospective observational clinical study. *Crit Care Med.* 2020;**48**(9):1249–1257.

Westover MB, Gururangan K, Markert MS, et al. Diagnostic value of electroencephalography with ten electrodes in critically ill patients. *Neurocrit Care.* 2020;**33**(2):479–490.

Witsch J, Frey HP, Schmidt JM, et al. Electroencephalographic periodic discharges and frequency-dependent brain tissue hypoxia in acute brain injury. *JAMA Neurol.* 2017;**74**(3):301–309.

Young GB, Jordan KG, Doig GS: An assessment of nonconvulsive seizures in the intensive care unit using continuous EEG monitoring: an investigation of variables associated with mortality. *Neurology* 1996;**47**(1):83–89.

Zafar SF, Subramaniam T, Osman G, Herlopian A, Struck AF. Electrographic seizures and ictal–interictal continuum (IIC) patterns in critically ill patients. *Epilepsy & Behavior.* 2020;**106**:107037.

Zafar SF, Rosenthal ES, Jing J, et al. Automated annotation of epileptiform burden and its association with outcomes. *Ann Neurol.* 2021;**90**(2):300–311.

*Reference defining the terms used in this atlas.

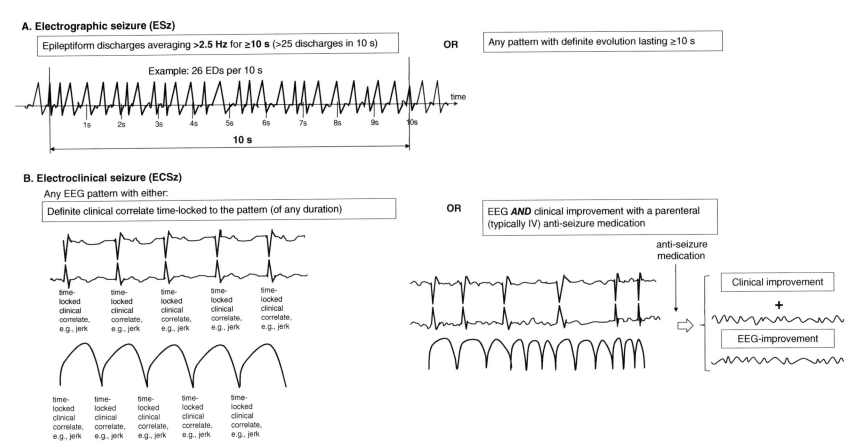

A. Electrographic seizure (ESz)

Epileptiform discharges averaging **>2.5 Hz** for **≥10 s** (>25 discharges in 10 s)   **OR**   Any pattern with definite evolution lasting ≥10 s

Example: 26 EDs per 10 s

time

1s   2s   3s   4s   5s   6s   7s   8s   9s   10s

10 s

B. Electroclinical seizure (ECSz)

Any EEG pattern with either:

Definite clinical correlate time-locked to the pattern (of any duration)   **OR**   EEG **AND** clinical improvement with a parenteral (typically IV) anti-seizure medication

anti-seizure medication

Clinical improvement

+

EEG-improvement

time-locked clinical correlate, e.g., jerk   time-locked clinical correlate, e.g., jerk   time-locked clinical correlate, e.g., jerk   time-locked clinical correlate, e.g., jerk   time-locked clinical correlate, e.g., jerk

time-locked clinical correlate, e.g., jerk   time-locked clinical correlate, e.g., jerk   time-locked clinical correlate, e.g., jerk   time-locked clinical correlate, e.g., jerk   time-locked clinical correlate, e.g., jerk

Figure 6.1.   Electrographic and electroclinical seizures. Electrographic seizures (ESz) are defined as either: 1. epileptiform discharges averaging >2.5 Hz for ≥10 s (>25 discharges in 10 s) (panel A), or 2. any pattern with definite evolution and lasting ≥10 s. Electrographic status epilepticus (ESE) is defined as an electrographic seizure for >10 continuous minutes or for a total duration of >20% of any 60-minute period of recording.

Electroclinical seizure (ECSz) is defined as any EEG pattern with either: 1. definite clinical correlate time-locked to the pattern (of any duration, including subtle clinical correlate as long as it is time-locked to the pattern) (panel B), or 2. EEG *and* clinical improvement with a parenteral (typically IV) anti-seizure medication. The EEG pattern during an 'electroclinical seizure' does not necessarily need to qualify as an 'electrographic seizure'. For example, if static 1-Hz PDs have a clinical correlate, this would not qualify as an electrographic seizure, but would qualify as an electroclinical seizure (as shown in panel B). Many seizures would however qualify for both 'electrographic' and 'electroclinical' seizures, and these should be reported under both terms. Electroclinical status epilepticus (ECSE) is defined as an electroclinical seizure for >10 continuous minutes or for a total duration of >20% of any 60-minute period of recording. An ongoing seizure with bilateral tonic-clonic (BTC) motor activity only needs to be present for >5 continuous minutes to qualify as ECSE. This is also referred to as 'convulsive SE', a subset of 'SE with prominent motor activity'. In any other clinical situation, the minimum duration to qualify as SE is >10 minutes. 'Possible ECSE' is an RPP that qualifies for the IIC that is present for ≥10 continuous minutes or for a total duration of >20% of any 60-minute period of recording, which shows EEG improvement with a parenteral anti-seizure medication BUT without clinical improvement. This remains largely in line with 'possible NCSE' as defined by the Salzburg criteria.

Reproduced from Hirsch LJ, Fong MWK, Leitinger M, et al. American Clinical Neurophysiology Society's Standardized Critical Care EEG Terminology: 2021 Version. J Clin Neurophysiol. 2021;38(1):1–29, with permission.

The Ictal-Interictal Continuum (IIC):

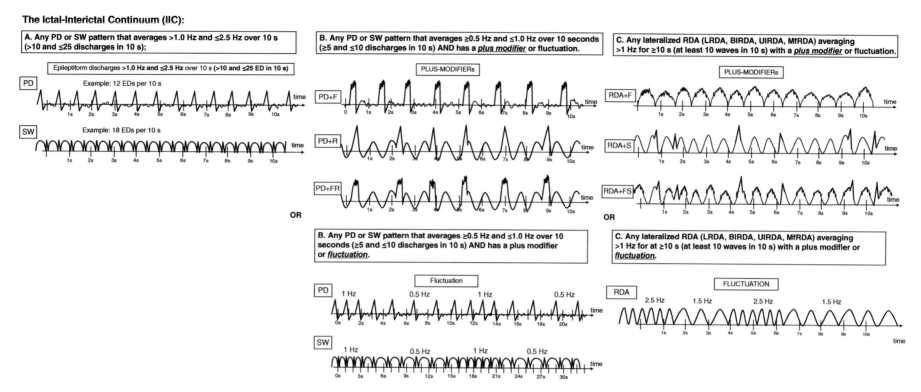

Figure 6.2. Ictal-interictal continuum (IIC).

As an increasing number of patients in the critical care setting are monitored with prolonged EEG it is becoming evident that there are many patterns that behave as seizures, may affect level of alertness, or may be associated with neuronal injury if prolonged, but do not qualify as definite electrographic seizures. Thus, these patterns are 'possibly ictal' in at least some manner. This gray zone has stemmed the term ictal-interictal continuum (IIC). The IIC consists of a group of patterns that 'might' be ictal. The term is largely inclusive, which is deliberate given our lack of certainty and in order to permit research into further defining what makes a seizure and which patterns require treatment (or more aggressive treatment). These efforts hope to further refine the particulars of the term, and by doing so determine the exact components of a pattern that denote the potential for ongoing neuronal injury. At this stage the IIC is defined as: 1. any PD or SW pattern that averages >1.0 Hz and ≤2.5 Hz over 10 s (>10 and ≤ 25 discharges in 10 s) (panel A), or 2. any PD or SW pattern that averages ≥0.5 Hz and ≤1.0 Hz over 10 s (≥5 and ≤10 discharges in 10 s), and has a plus modifier or fluctuation (panel B), or 3. any lateralized RDA averaging >1 Hz for at least 10 s (at least 10 waves in 10 s) with a plus modifier or fluctuation (panel C). This includes any LRDA, BIRDA, UIRDA and MfRDA, but not GRDA. These patterns must not qualify as ESzs or ESEs; otherwise, they should be referred to as such.

Reproduced from Hirsch LJ, Fong MWK, Leitinger M, et al. American Clinical Neurophysiology Society's Standardized Critical Care EEG Terminology: 2021 Version. J Clin Neurophysiol. 2021;38(1):1–29, with permission.

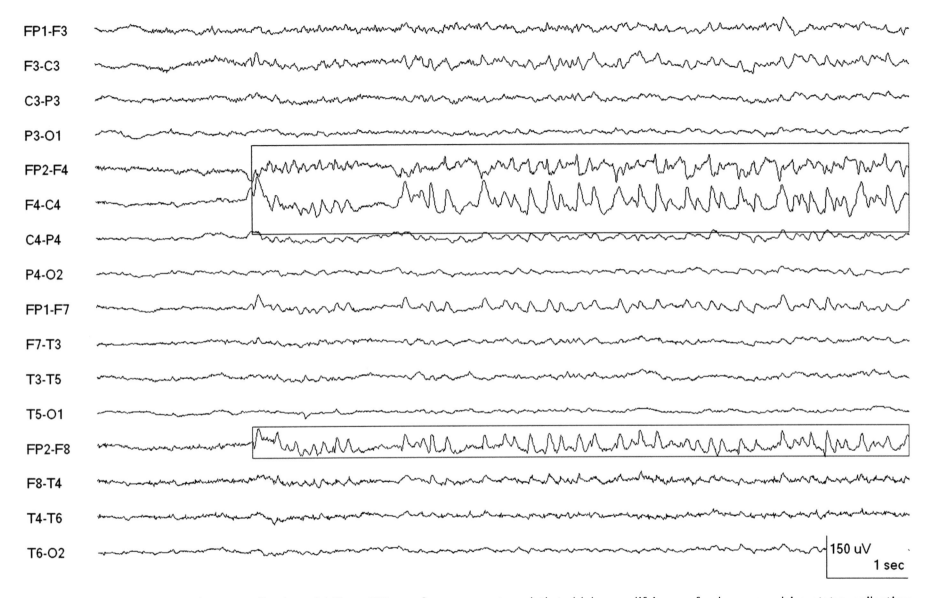

Figure 6.3. Focal seizures and status epilepticus. (a) These EEGs are from a 49-year-old woman with a history of head trauma, seizures and strokes was being evaluated for decreased mental status. During this recording, she had repetitive right-sided electrographic seizures occupying more than half the recording beginning in the right frontal region (highlighted) with rhythmic, sharply contoured theta/alpha, qualifying as focal nonconvulsive status epilepticus (NCSE). Of note, this would qualify as electrographic SE if the prevalence was >20% of any hour (which it was in this case), or if any individual seizure lasted 10 minutes or longer.

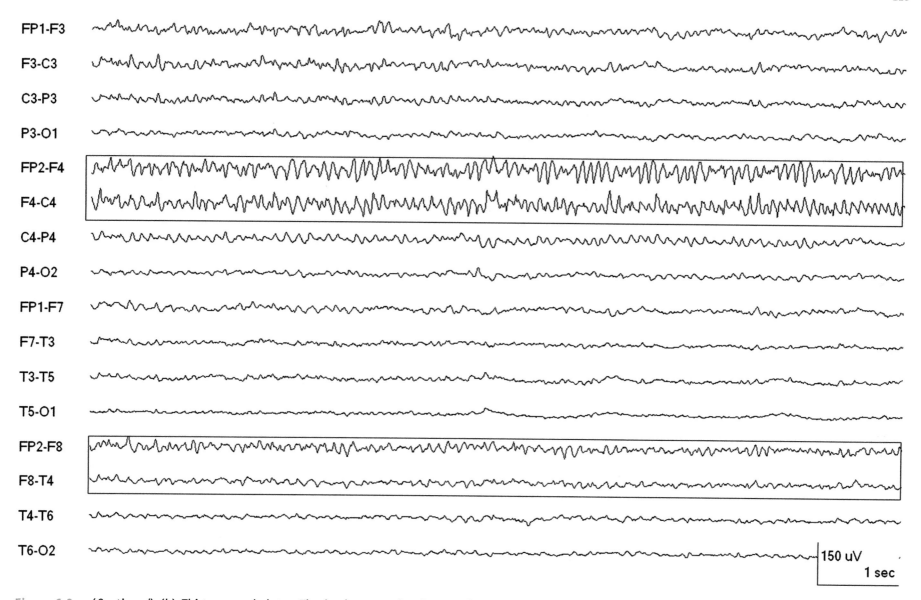

Figure 6.3. (*Continued*) (b) Thirty seconds later. The ictal pattern has become faster, thus demonstrating evolution in frequency and morphology lasting ≥10 seconds and therefore unequivocally ictal. The frequency in this sample is predominantly in the alpha range (box).

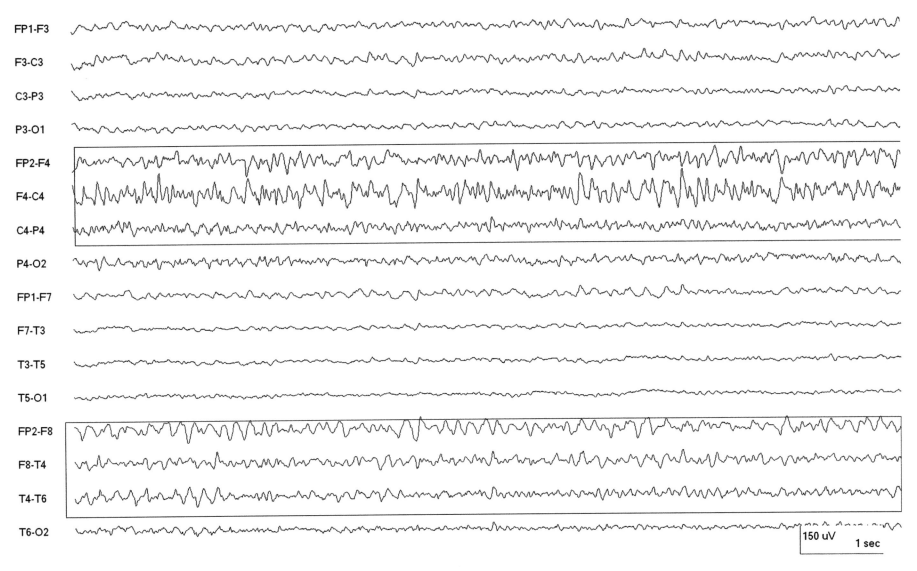

Figure 6.3.   (*Continued*) (c) Four minutes later. The ictal discharges continue, becoming more widespread and slower, thus demonstrating evolution in location and further evolution in frequency and morphology. There were no associated movements.

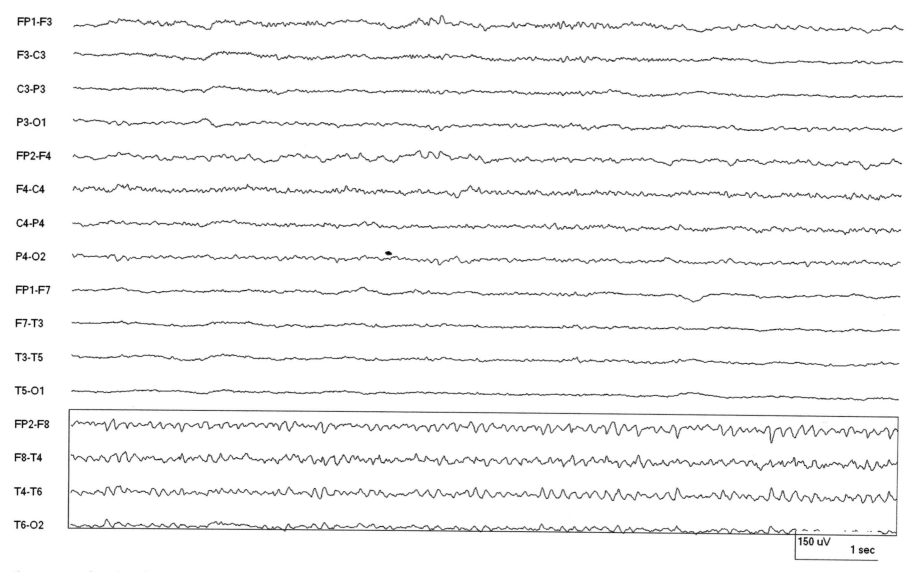

Figure 6.3. (*Continued*) (d) The ictal rhythm is now in the right temporal region only. The patient was given intravenous lorazepam at this point.

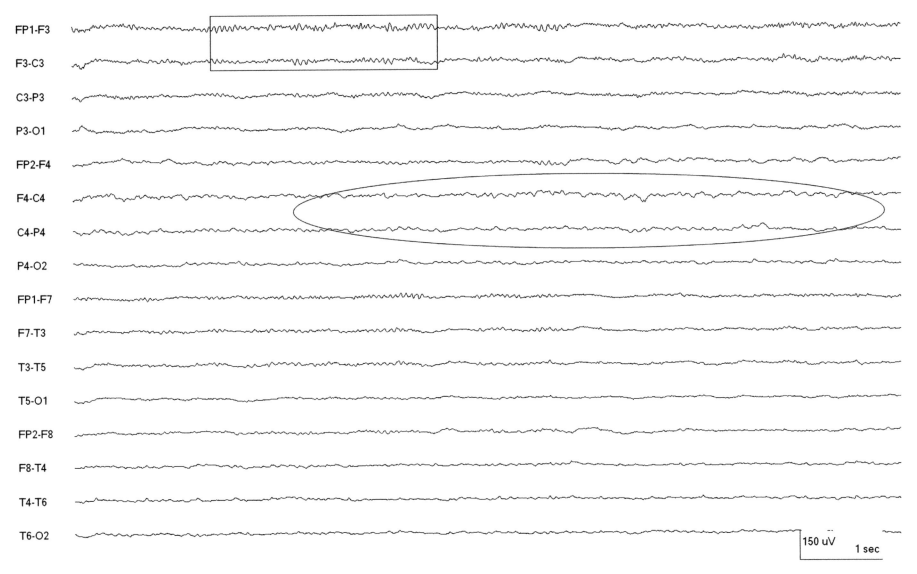

Figure 6.3. (*Continued*) (e) The seizure stopped after the administration of lorazepam. Beta activity (likely from the benzodiazepine) is present, but predominantly over the left hemisphere (box). This is because the more physiologic rhythms are absent (attenuated) in the right hemisphere, suggesting cortical dysfunction on that side postictally. There is also mild focal slowing in the right parasagittal region (ellipse), which additionally suggests dysfunction of subcortical white matter. Both of these findings are commonly seen postictally.

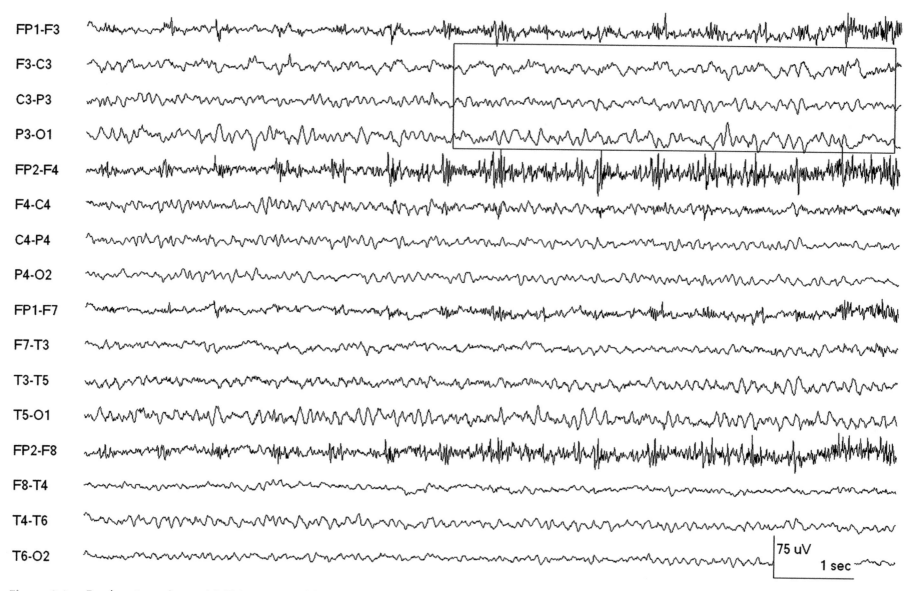

Figure 6.4. Focal motor seizure. (a) This 82-year-old man with a left-sided subdural hematoma developed new onset of twitching of the right thumb. This sample shows subtle rhythmic delta starting to emerge in the left central parietal region near the end of the sample (box). Bifrontal muscle artifact is gradually increasing as well.

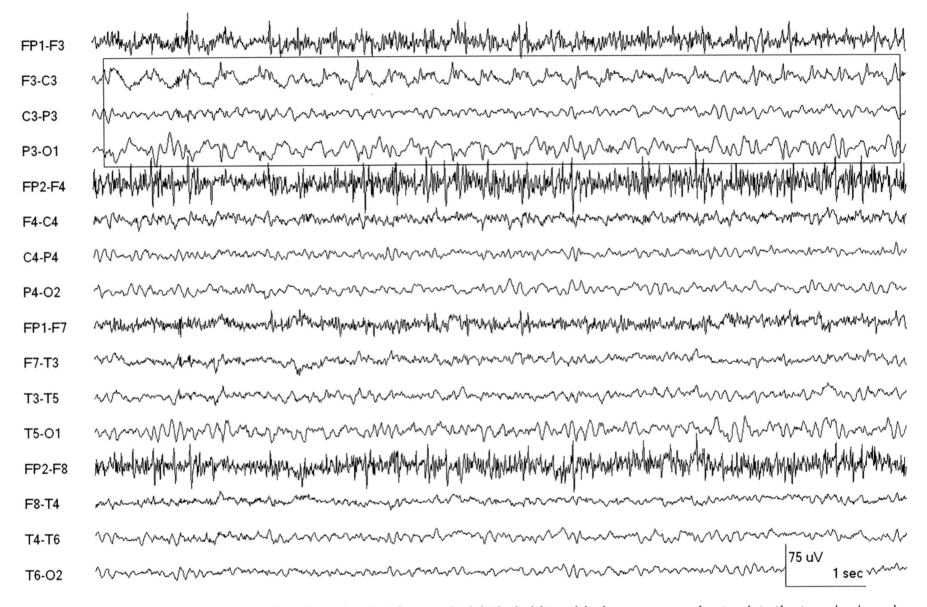

Figure 6.4.   (*Continued*) (b) The next page of EEG shows that the left parasagittal rhythmic delta activity is now more prominent and starting to evolve, becoming faster and lower amplitude, and associated with superimposed spikes. Fp1 and Fp2 show prominent muscle artifact.

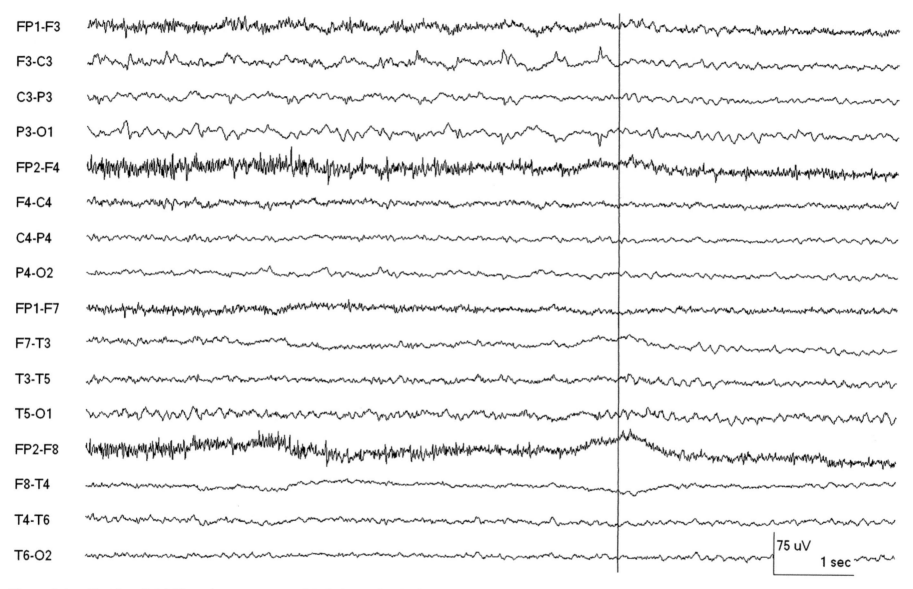

Figure 6.4. (*Continued*) (c) The subsequent page of EEG shows the rhythmic delta ending rather abruptly, and the muscle artifact also subsides. This is a focal seizure that was associated with twitching of the right thumb, but clearly the facial/scalp muscles were involved with prominent EMG activity correlating with the electrographic seizure. This is an example of both an electrographic seizure (fairly subtle but evolving) and an electroclinical seizure with focal motor semiology.

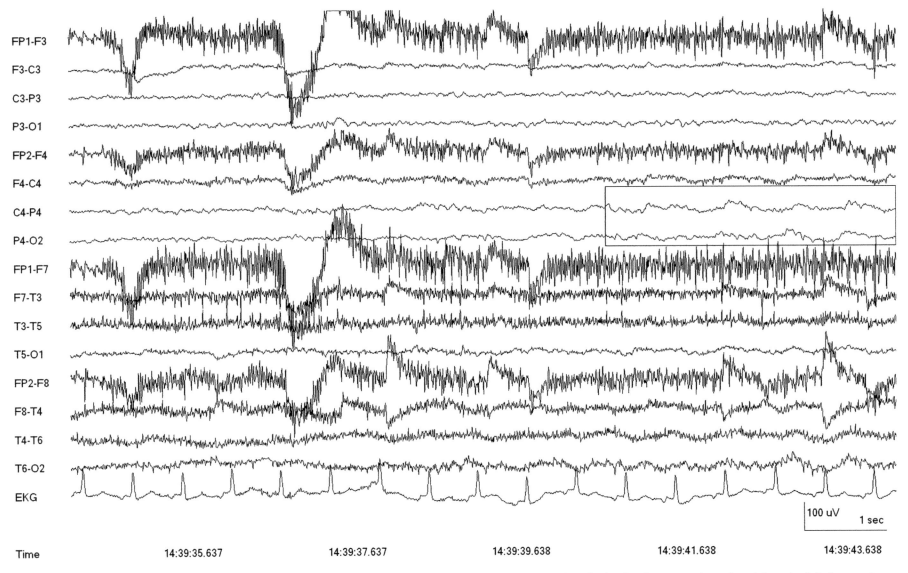

Figure 6.5. Focal electrographic seizure. (a) This EEG is from a 22-year-old man s/p lung and heart transplant. The patient had a right-sided subdural hematoma evacuated 10 days prior to this EEG. One hour before the onset of the recording, the patient had a focal motor seizure involving the left face and eye. At baseline, there is mild focal slowing in the right posterior head region (box).

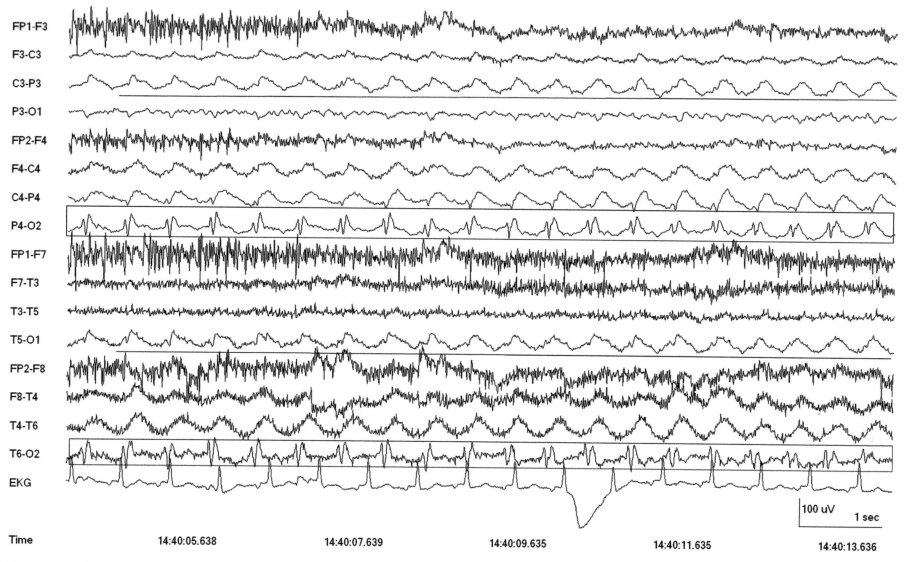

Time   14:40:05.638   14:40:07.639   14:40:09.635   14:40:11.635   14:40:13.636

Figure 6.5.   (*Continued*) (b) Thirty seconds later. Spike-and-wave discharges are present at 2 per second in the right posterior head region (boxed) with synchronous rhythmic delta present over homologous areas on the left (underlined). The EKG channel confirms that this is not EKG or pulse artifact.

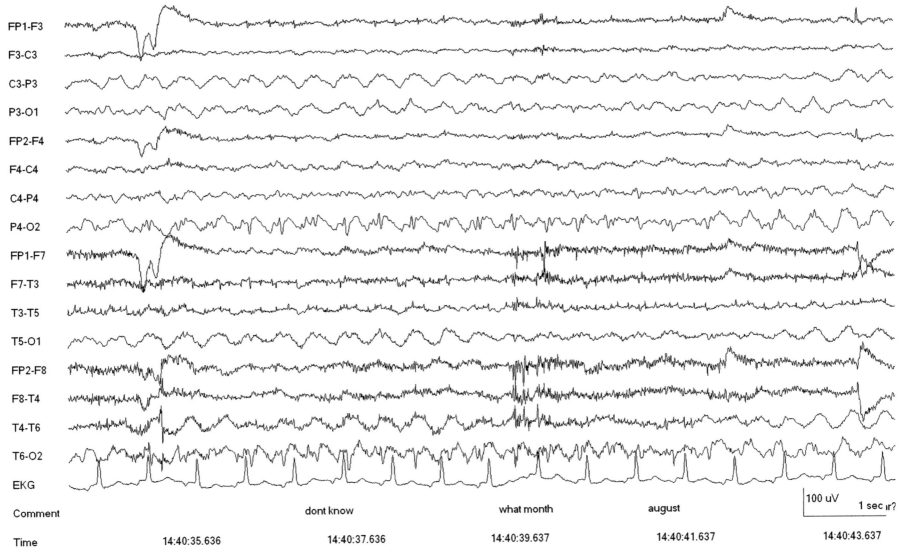

Figure 6.5. (*Continued*) (c) The discharges continue another 30 s later, at which time the patient was answering questions (documented at the bottom of the page). There is clear evolution, with the ictal discharges, still maximal in the right posterior quadrant, becoming lower amplitude and faster, and changing in morphology.

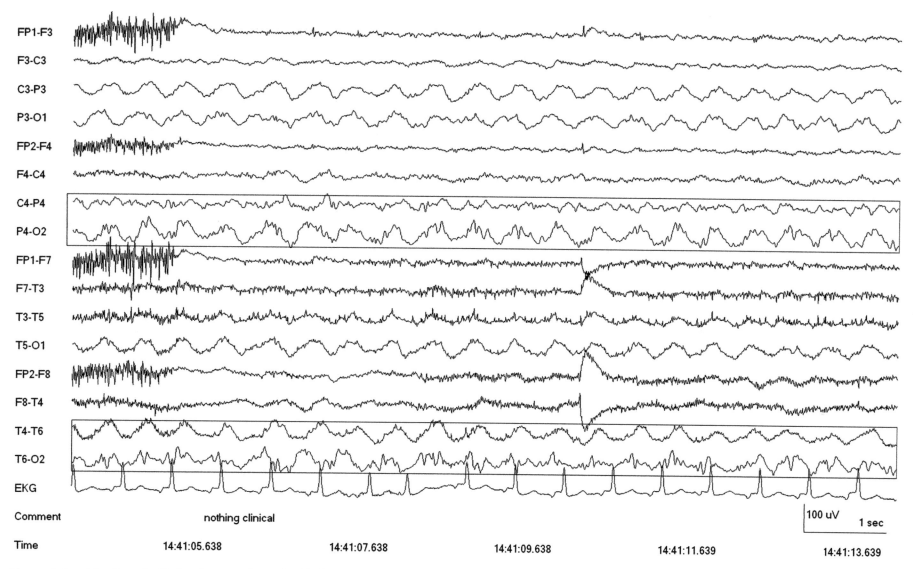

Figure 6.5. (*Continued*) (d) Another 30 s later the discharges are still present, although now becoming slower and again changing somewhat in morphology. The pattern now consists of rhythmic delta with superimposed fast activity (box).

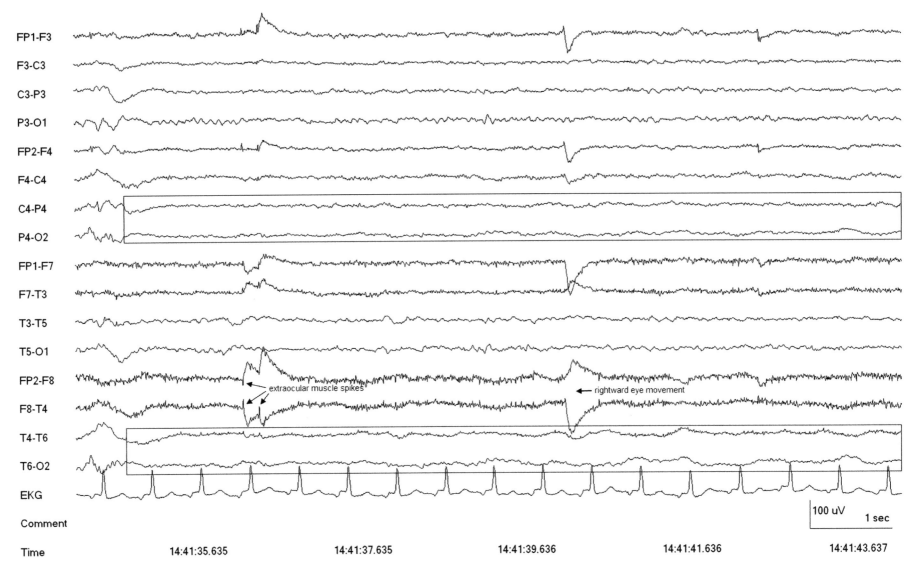

Figure 6.5. (*Continued*) (e) An additional 30 s later. There appears to be attenuation of faster activity in the same area that had the maximal ictal discharge (boxes), likely postictal attenuation of cortical activity, though this should be confirmed in a referential recording. This is an example of an electrographic seizure that was not an electroclinical seizure (i.e., there were no signs or symptoms associated with the seizure). Eye movement artifacts are labeled as well.

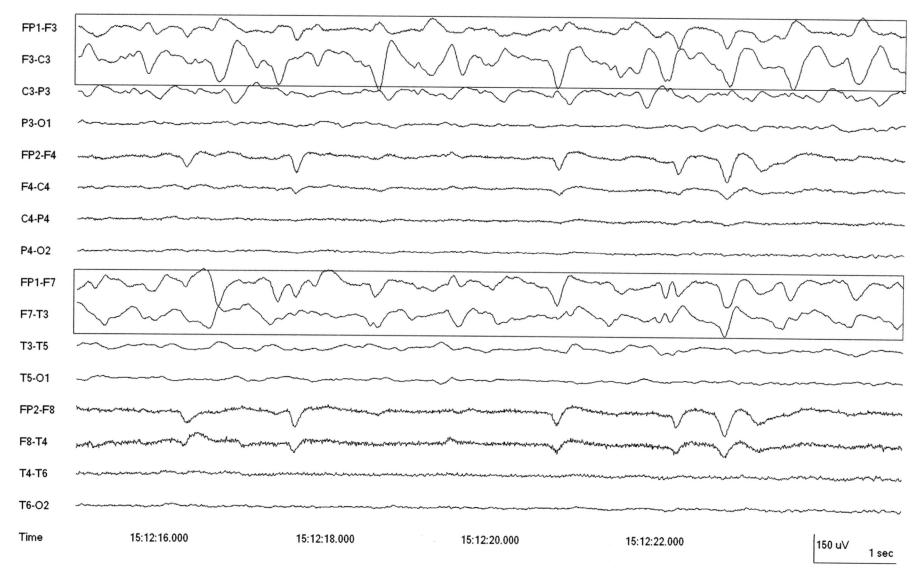

Figure 6.6. Focal electroclinical seizure. (a) The baseline EEG in this 49-year-old woman with a left-sided stroke s/p partial resection of infarcted tissue and cranioplasty shows high voltage irregular delta activity, sometimes sharply contoured (possibly due to breach effect), in the left fronto-temporal region (boxes).

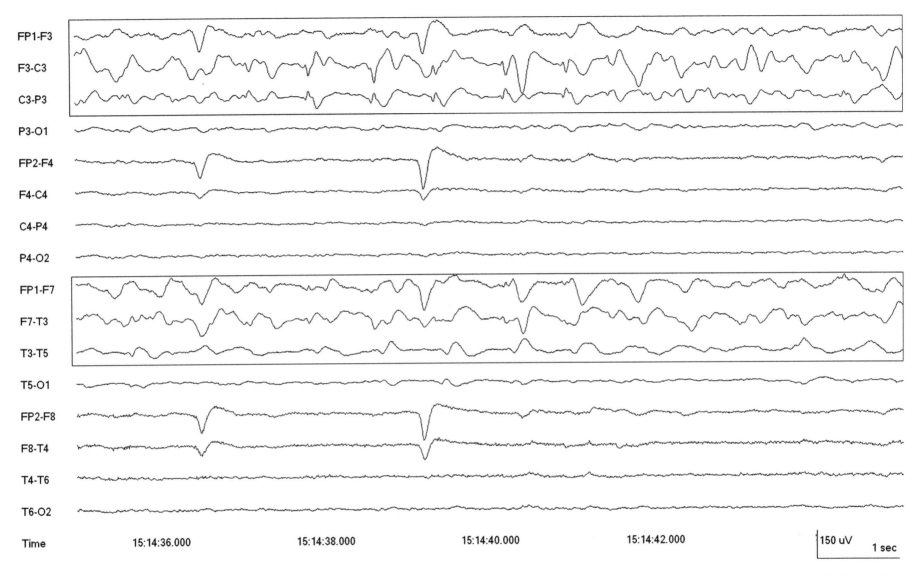

Figure 6.6. (*Continued*) (b) EEG onset. A left-sided seizure begins to emerge but is not yet fully apparent; there is subtle evidence of an increase in fast activity in the boxes, and an increase in sharp waves at C3, almost periodic.

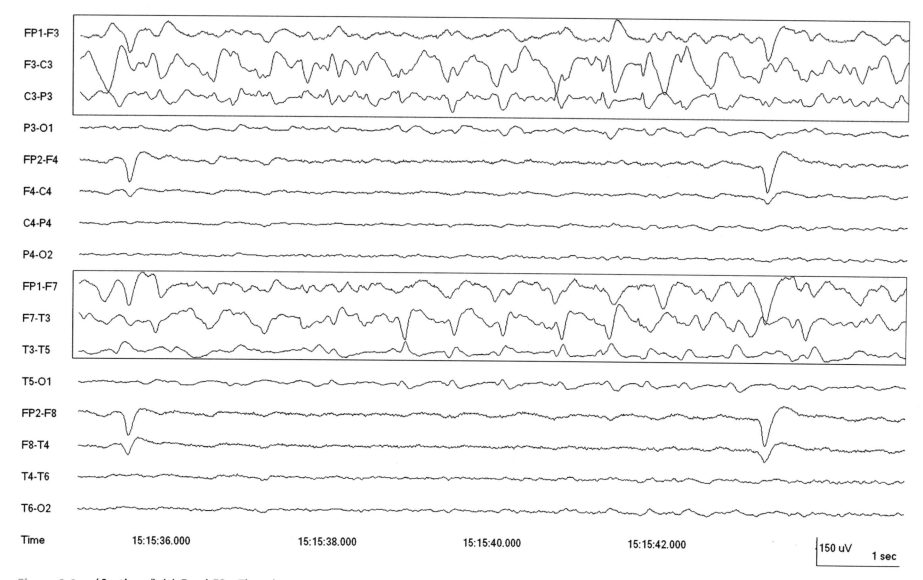

Figure 6.6. (*Continued*) (c) Focal ESz. There is now a greater amount of intermixed fast activity and the periodic epileptiform discharges have spread in location, now well established at T3 with a field into T5.

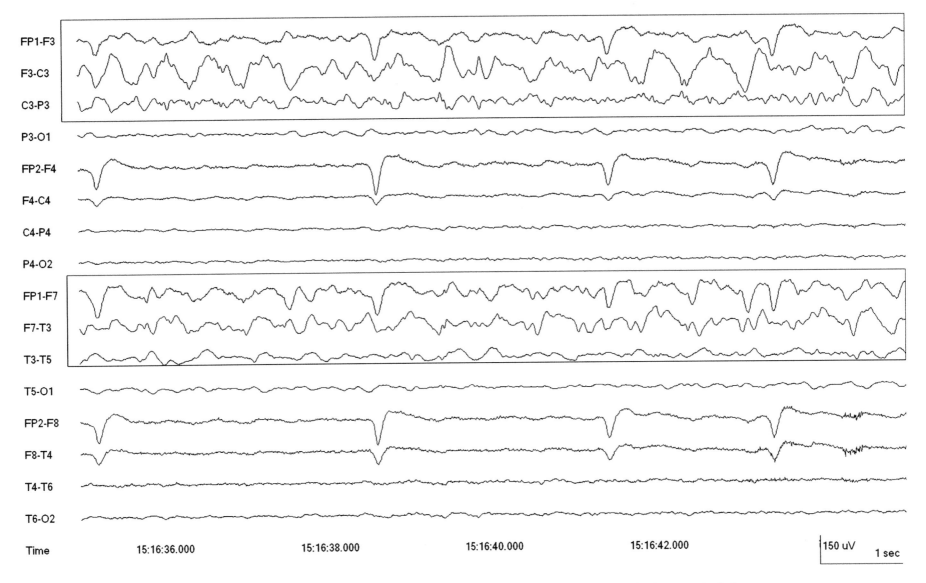

Figure 6.6. (*Continued*) (d) Focal ESz. Further slow evolution with the emergence of lower voltage and faster rhythms on the left.

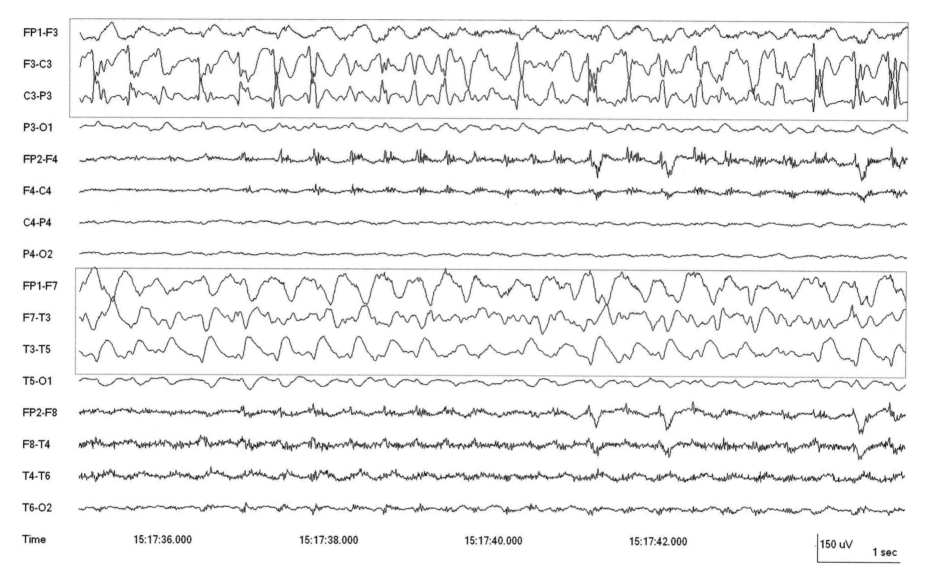

Time

15:17:36.000   15:17:38.000   15:17:40.000   15:17:42.000

150 uV

1 sec

Figure 6.6. (*Continued*) (e) Clinical onset. Now with repetitive medium-high amplitude spikes in the left central area that become more widespread and were associated with head jerking to the right and extension of the right arm and leg (i.e., becoming electroclinical). Low-amplitude right-sided muscle artifact begins to appear, likely due to face/scalp muscle contraction on that side (contralateral to the ictal discharge).

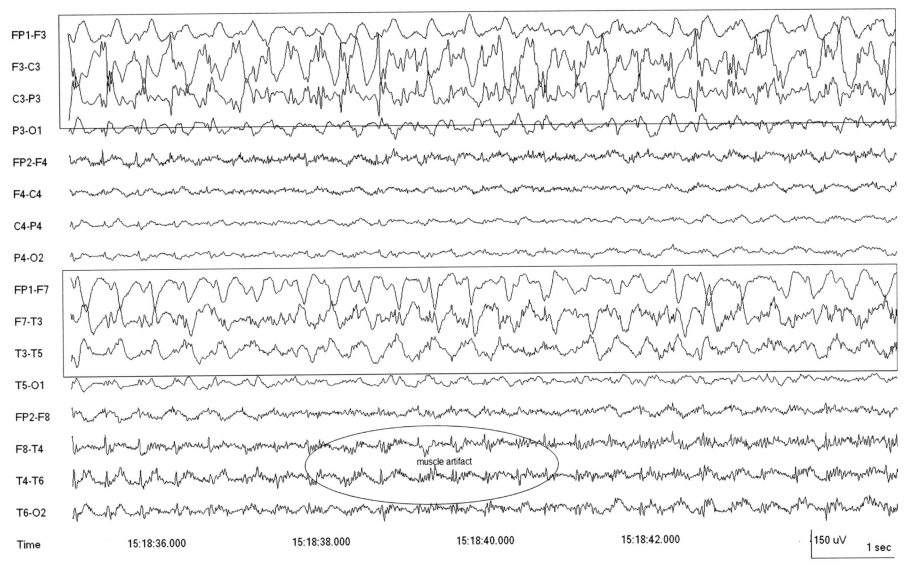

Figure 6.6. (*Continued*) (f) Focal ECSz. Muscle artifact on the right increases, now with repetitive higher amplitude muscle artifact from clonic jerking of the right face and scalp muscles (ellipse). The ictal pattern on the left continues to evolve, higher amplitude, sharper and faster (boxes).

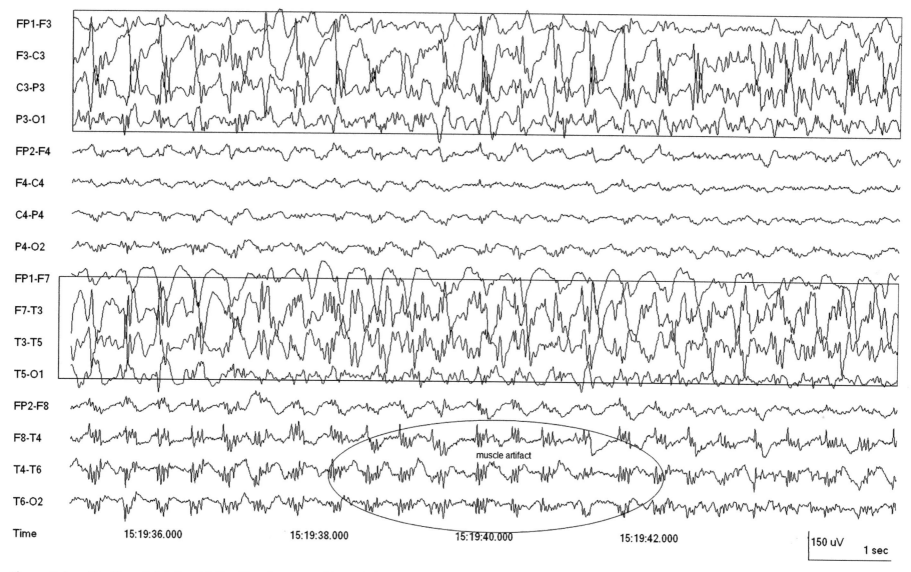

Figure 6.6. (*Continued*) (g) Focal ECSz. The electrographic and electroclinical seizure continues.

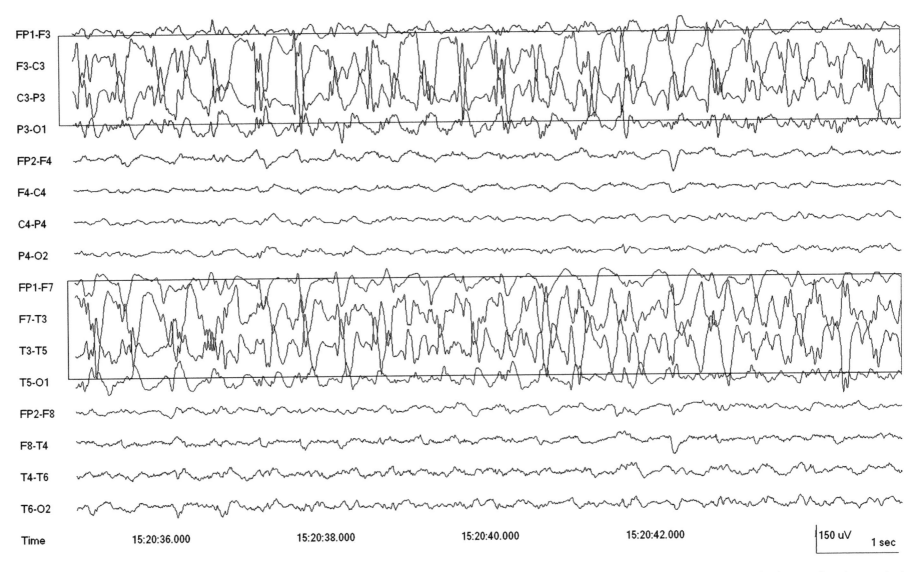

Figure 6.6. (*Continued*) (h) Clinical offset. The electrographic seizure continues, but the clinical component (clonic jerking of the right face and scalp muscles) has subsided (periodic EMG artifact no longer present on the right side of the head).

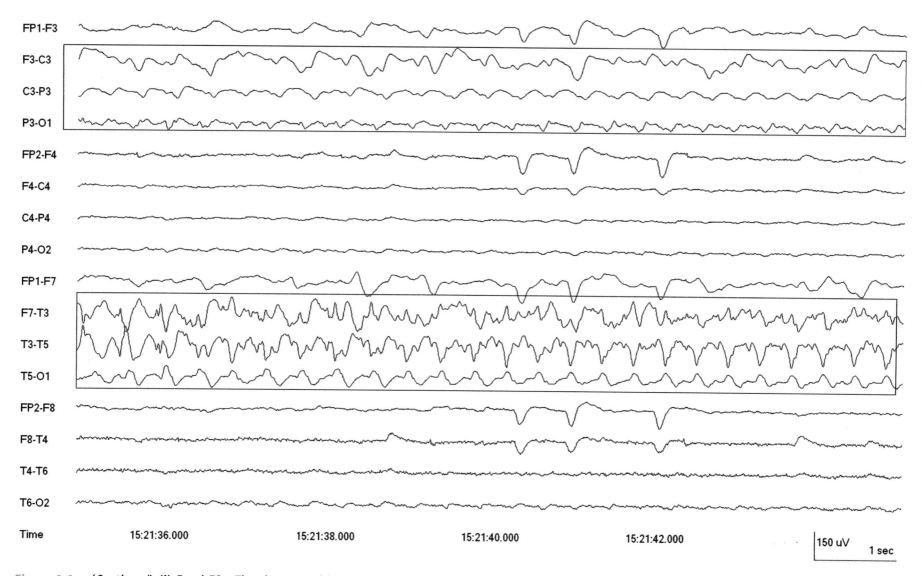

Figure 6.6. (*Continued*) (i) Focal ESz. The electrographic seizure has ceased in the left central region but continues in the left temporal region.

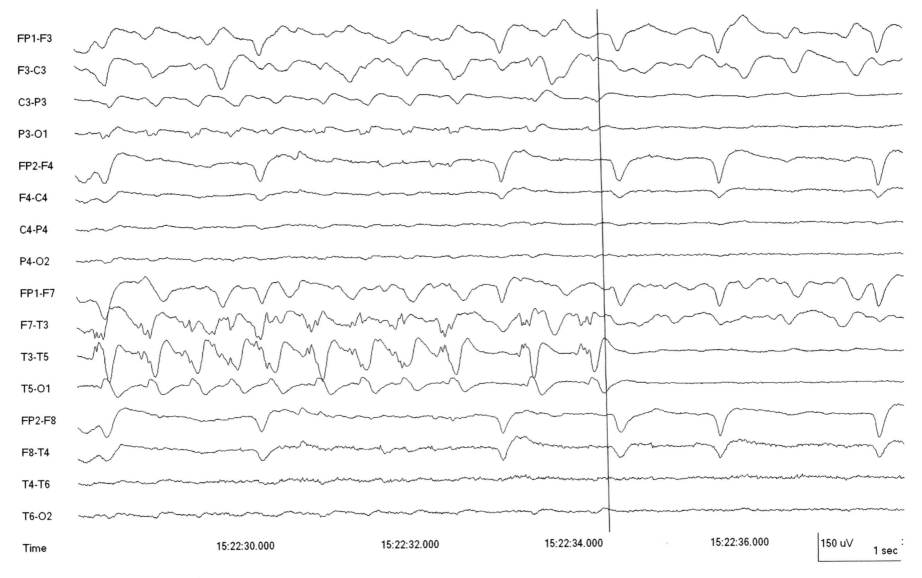

Figure 6.6. (*Continued*) (j) EEG offset. The seizure ends after a total of 8 minutes (vertical line representing seizure offset).

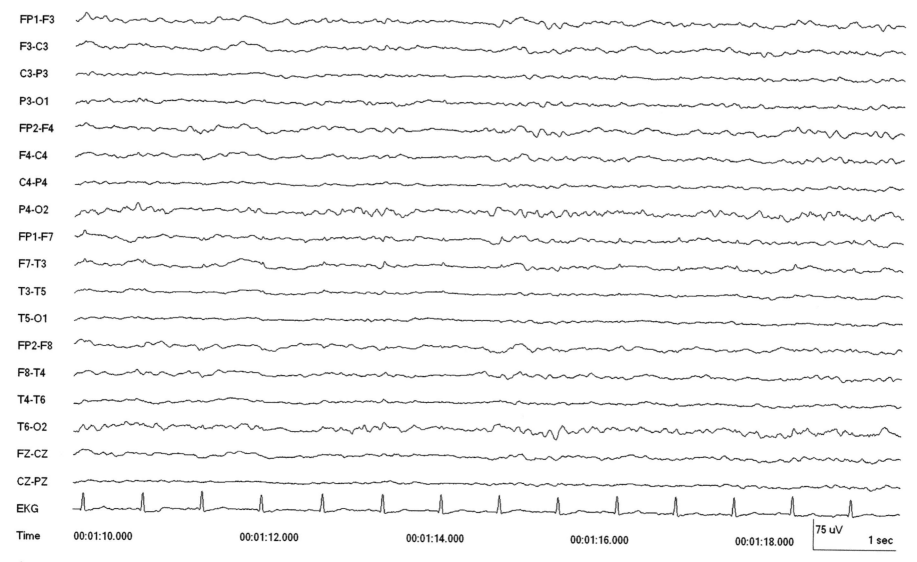

FP1-F3
F3-C3
C3-P3
P3-O1
FP2-F4
F4-C4
C4-P4
P4-O2
FP1-F7
F7-T3
T3-T5
T5-O1
FP2-F8
F8-T4
T4-T6
T6-O2
FZ-CZ
CZ-PZ
EKG

Time   00:01:10.000   00:01:12.000   00:01:14.000   00:01:16.000   00:01:18.000

75 uV
1 sec

Figure 6.7. LPDs evolving into a focal seizure. (a) The baseline EEG in this 82-year-old woman with a history of acute renal failure, being evaluated for seizures, shows diffuse slowing and attenuation of background activity.

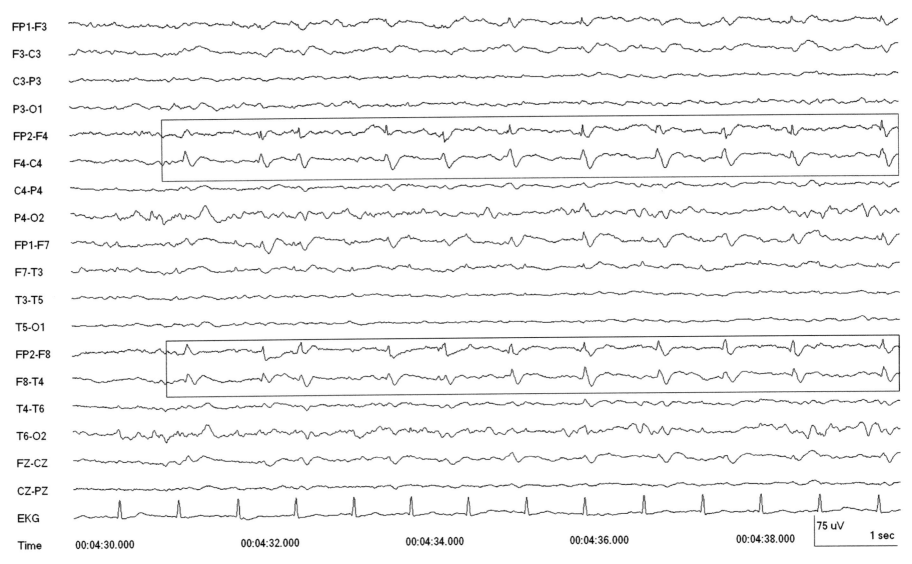

Figure 6.7.   (*Continued*) (b) Right frontal LPDs at ~1 Hz begin to appear, maximal at F4 and F8 (boxes).

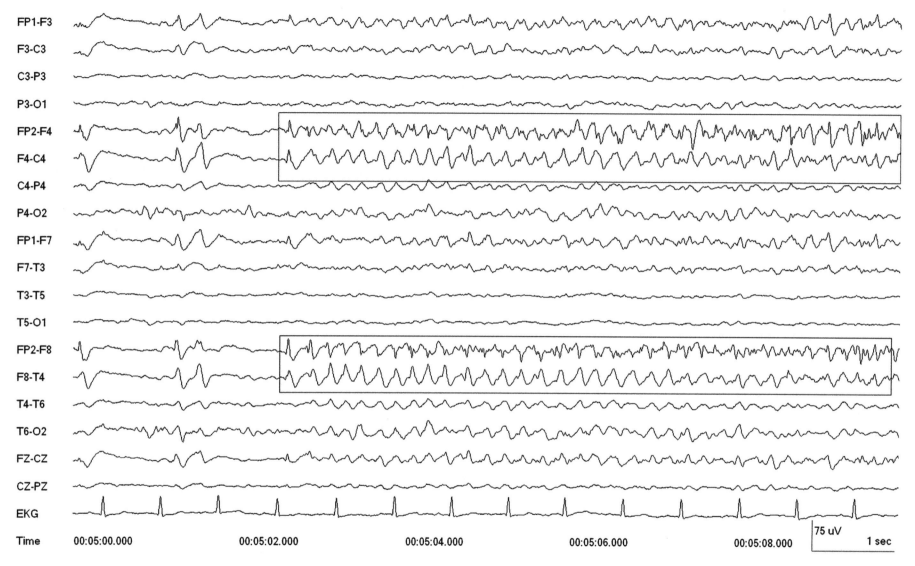

Figure 6.7. (*Continued*) (c) The LPDs are then replaced by an electrographic seizure that begins with rhythmic sharply contoured theta (boxes).

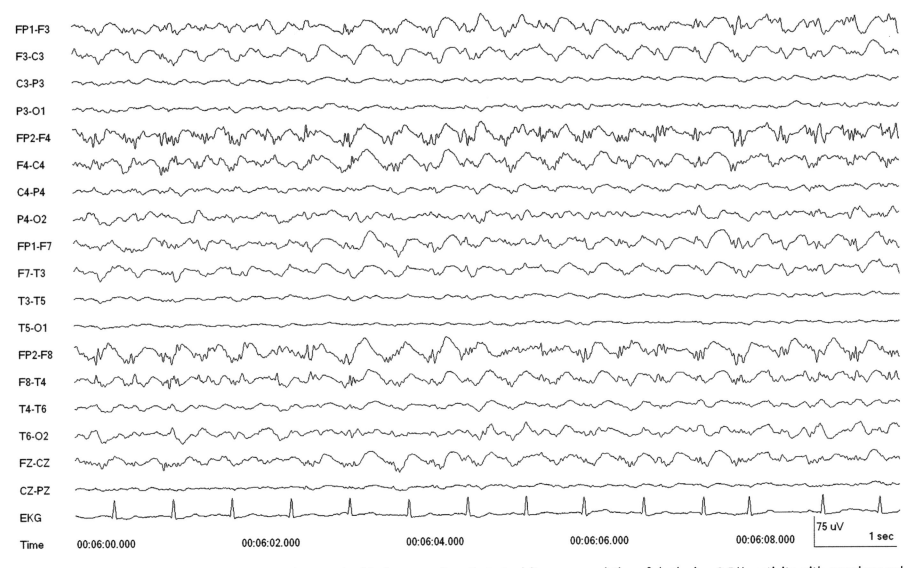

Figure 6.7. (*Continued*) (d) The ictal discharges have evolved in frequency from theta to delta, now consisting of rhythmic ~2.5 Hz activity with superimposed sharply contoured beta at F4 and F8. It has also spread to involve more of the left hemisphere now, though remaining maximal on the right.

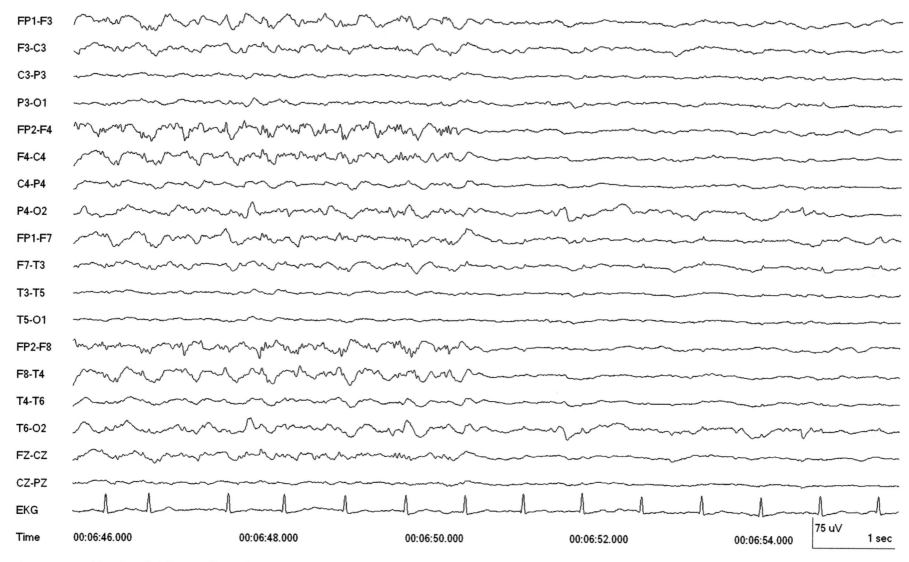

FP1-F3	
F3-C3	
C3-P3	
P3-O1	
FP2-F4	
F4-C4	
C4-P4	
P4-O2	
FP1-F7	
F7-T3	
T3-T5	
T5-O1	
FP2-F8	
F8-T4	
T4-T6	
T6-O2	
FZ-CZ	
CZ-PZ	
EKG	

Time   00:06:46.000   00:06:48.000   00:06:50.000   00:06:52.000   00:06:54.000   75 uV   1 sec

Figure 6.7. (*Continued*) (e) EEG offset. The seizure ends abruptly in the middle of this page.

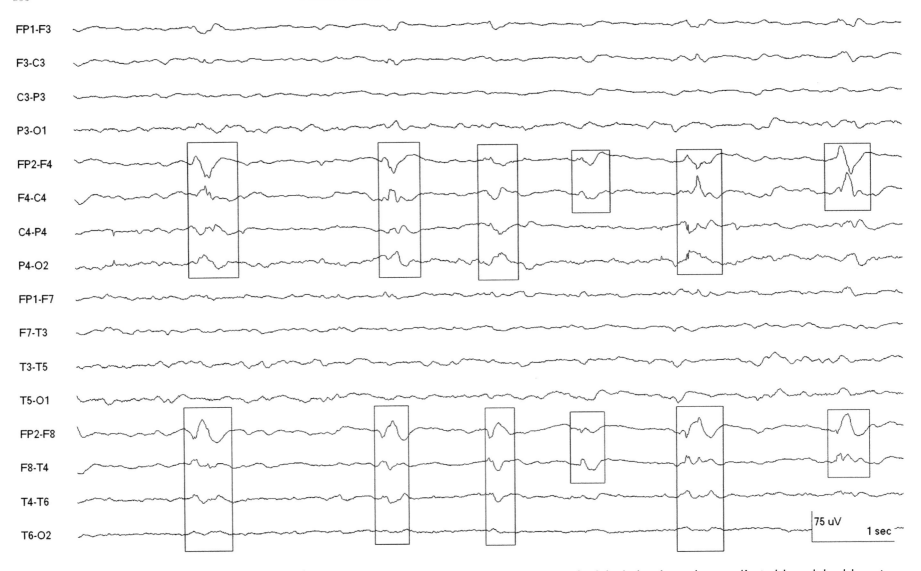

Figure 6.8.   Blunt LPDs evolving into focal seizure (a) These EEGs are from a 57-year-old woman s/p right ischemic stroke complicated by subdural hematoma requiring evacuation. This page shows blunt ~0.5 Hz right-sided LPDs (one or two are sharply contoured, but most are blunt).

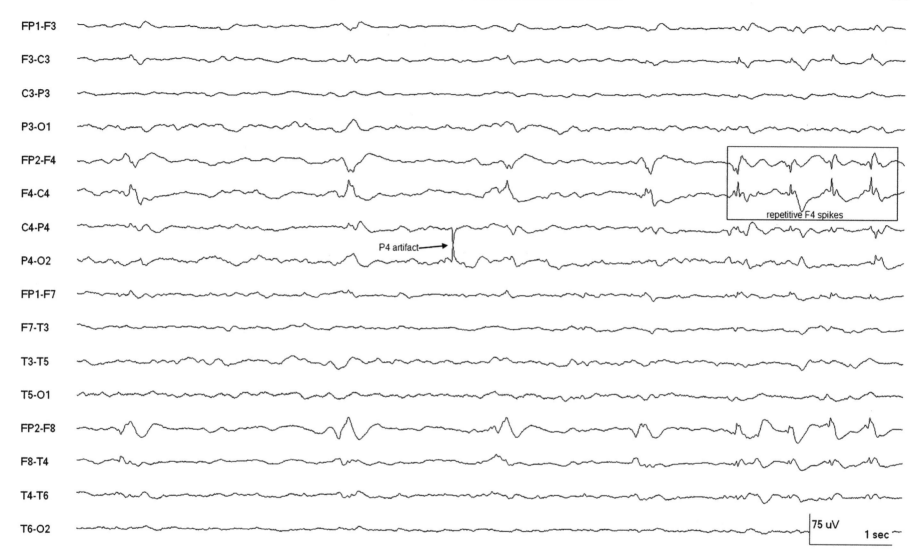

Figure 6.8. (*Continued*) (b) EEG onset. Ten seconds later, the discharges have changed morphologically, particularly toward the end of the sample, now consisting of faster repetitive spikes or polyspikes, maximal at electrode F4 [box]. This represents the beginning of an electrographic seizure. There is also an electrode artifact (sometimes referred to as an electrode 'pop') at P4 (arrow; note the morphology with a purely vertical initial phase and complete lack of field: it only involves P4, so it is visible in the two channels recording from that electrode)

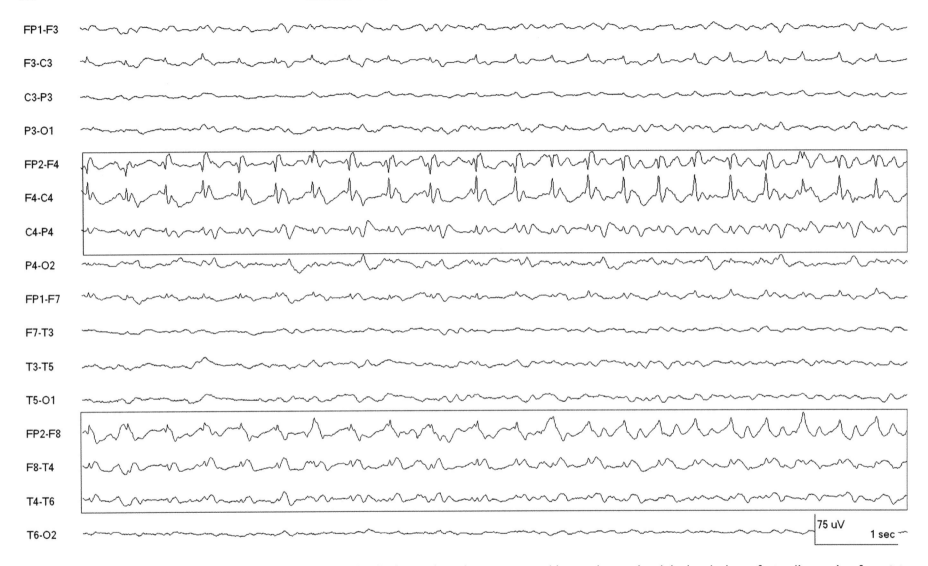

Figure 6.8.   (*Continued*) (c) Focal ESz. Ten seconds later, the discharges have become more widespread over the right hemisphere, faster (increasing from 2 to 2.5 Hz during this page), and with slowly evolving morphology.

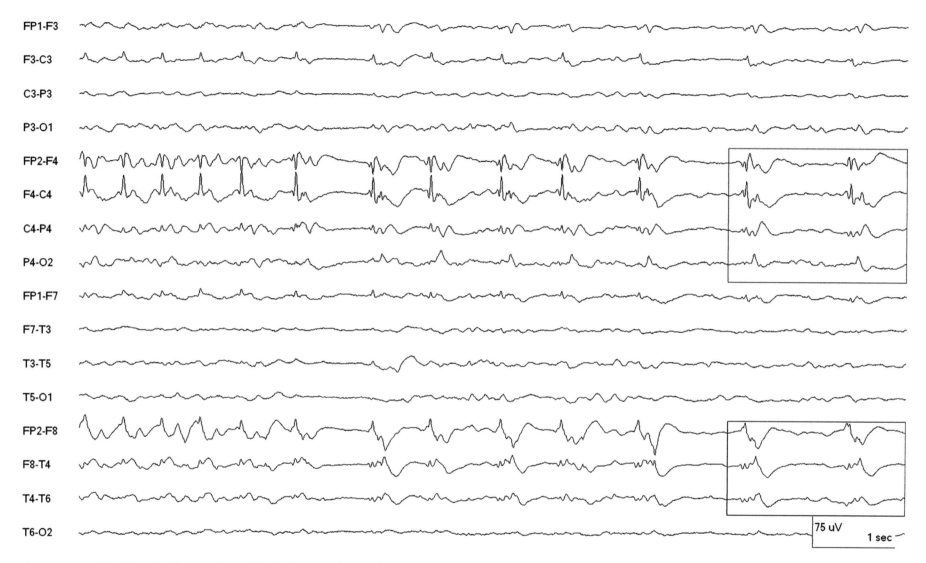

Figure 6.8. (*Continued*) (d) EEG offset. The discharges slow and break up 10 s later, returning to spiky LPDs in the last few seconds of the page (boxes).

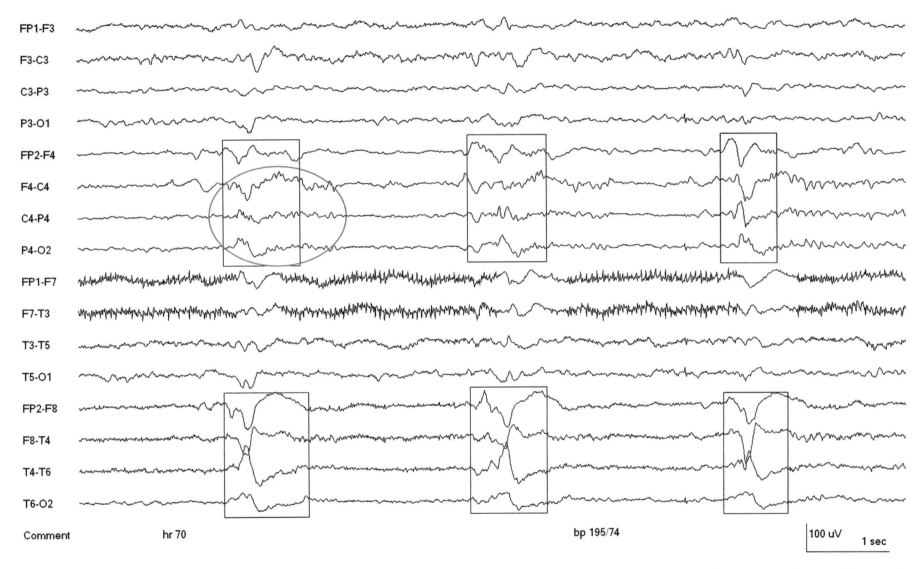

Figure 6.9. LPDs evolving into a focal seizure. (a) Right-sided LPDs (boxes) are present in this 87-year-old woman with herpes simplex encephalitis (HSE). Note that each discharge is not actually epileptiform (i.e., not a spike or sharp wave) but is primarily a delta wave, perhaps sharply contoured at times, with some superimposed fast activity visible in some of the channels (red ellipse); thus, this would be blunt LPD+F. Blunt, long-duration LPDs such as this are typical of HSE and does not change the high correlation with seizures. This example highlights the rationale behind the original change of the nomenclature from periodic epileptiform discharges (e.g., PLEDs or GPEDs) to LPDs and GPDs. Blunt transients or periodic complexes (as demonstrated here) are not in themselves epileptiform, but this does not change their high association with seizures.

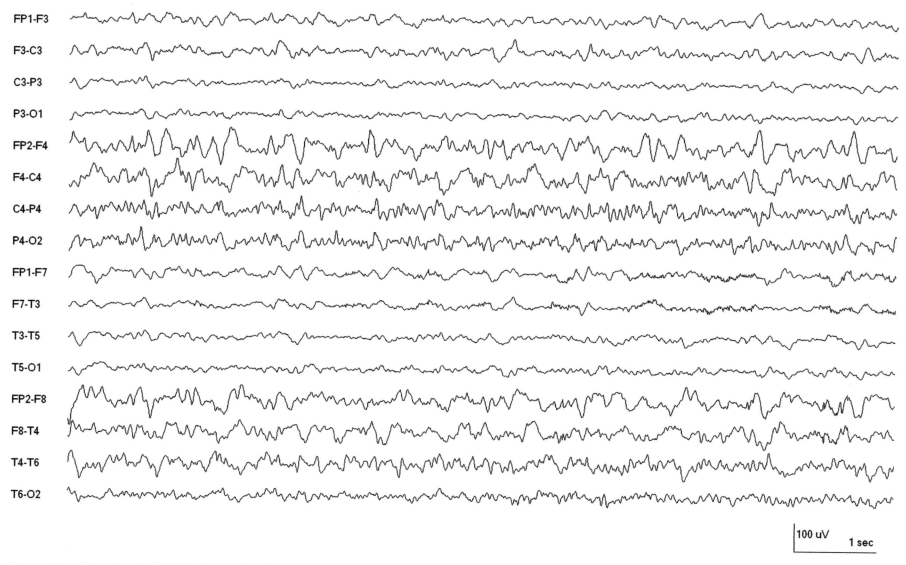

100 uV 1 sec

Figure 6.9. (*Continued*) (b) ESz. A sample taken later in the same recording shows that the LPDs have been replaced by a focal electrographic seizure involving the entire right hemisphere. This rather common occurrence of LPDs being replaced by a completely different seizure pattern has been used to support the widely held impression that LPDs are usually interictal rather than ictal. Only one page in the middle of the seizure is shown; thus, evolution cannot be appreciated in this one page.

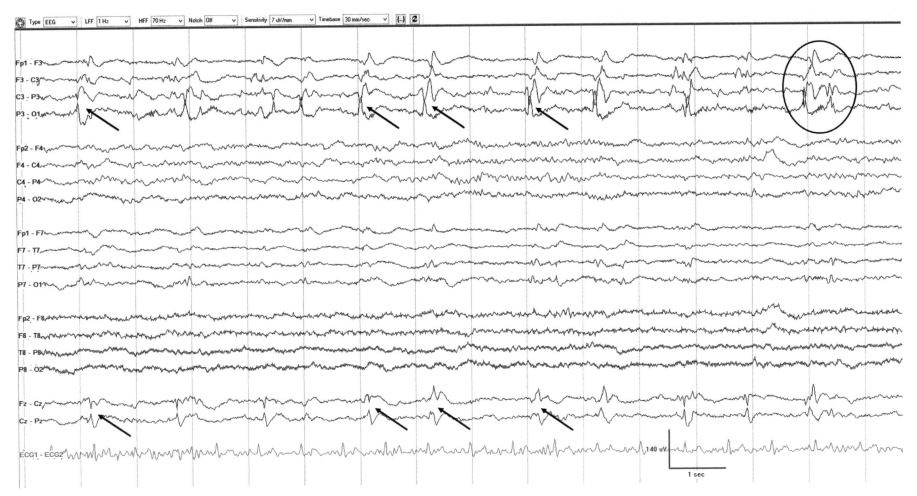

Figure 6.10. LPDs evolving to LPD+F, then seizure. (a) LPDs. The EEG is from a 65-year-old man with a left SDH s/p hemicraniectomy. There are continuous LPDs in the left parieto-central region (maximal at P3 and Cz) (arrows). Several minutes before a focal electrographic seizure there was a change in the character of the LPDs. The discharges became consistently associated with fast activity and often a complex of activity following each discharge. This page highlights this transition to LPDs+F. Note the first several discharges are 'simple' (i.e., it is a single spike-and-wave with no fast activity, so no '+'). Contrast this to the last discharge (ellipse) that is polyspike wave with associated low-amplitude fast activity at P3 and a series of aftergoing irregular theta waves forming a complex lasting about 0.5 s.

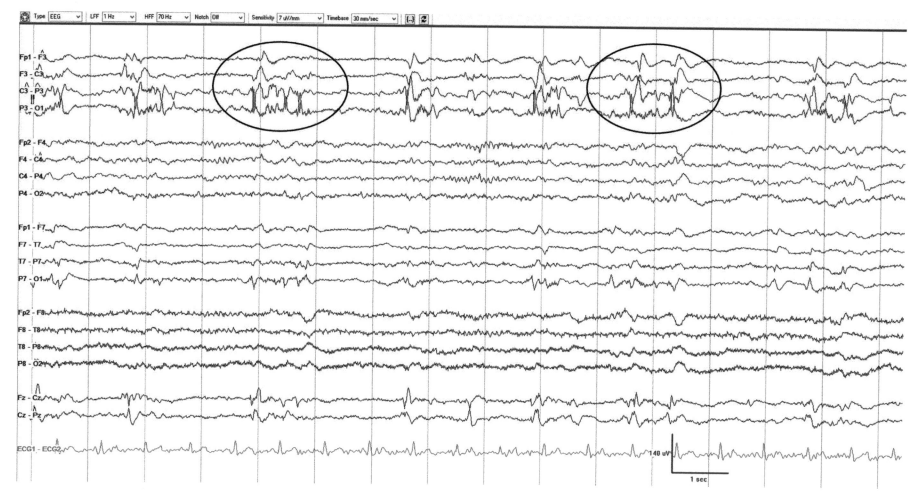

Figure 6.10. (*Continued*) (b) LPDs+F and BIRDs. Following from Figure 6.10a, the LPDs have now changed to LPDs+F and sometimes even repetitive or periodic BIRDs (brief potentially ictal rhythmic discharges) since they last >0.5 seconds. Now each discharge is 'complex' (some highlighted in the ellipses): each discharge is now at least a polyspike with associated low-amplitude fast activity, and when the complexes consist of activity that is >4 Hz and lasting ≥0.5 s, these qualify as BIRDs.

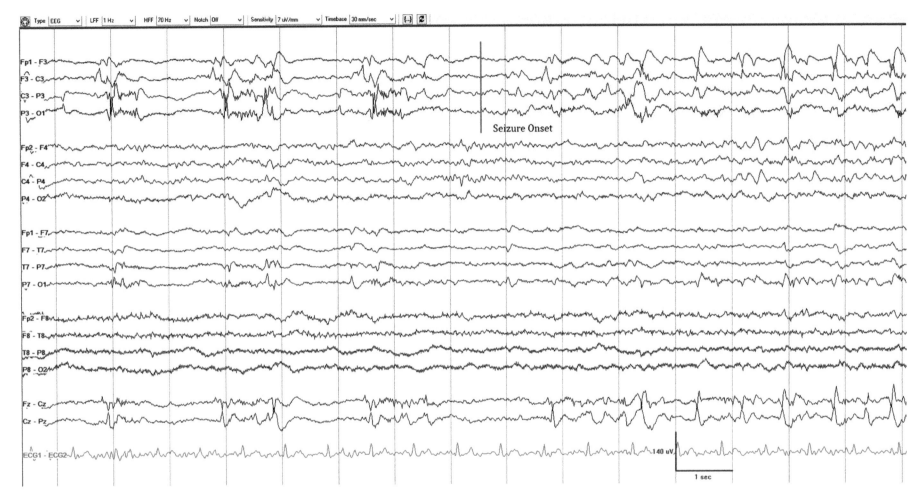

Figure 6.10. (*Continued*) (c) EEG onset, The labeled red line documents the beginning of the electrographic seizure. Before this line there are periodic BIRDs, which, if alternating with periods of attenuation/suppression that occupy 50–99% of the record, can also be classified as lateralized burst suppression with highly epileptiform bursts. After the third complex on the page, theoretically where the fourth complex should be, there is now instead an irregular theta pattern that is continuous (note there are no longer the periods of attenuation between complexes after the seizure has started), and this evolves into irregular sharp waves in this region.

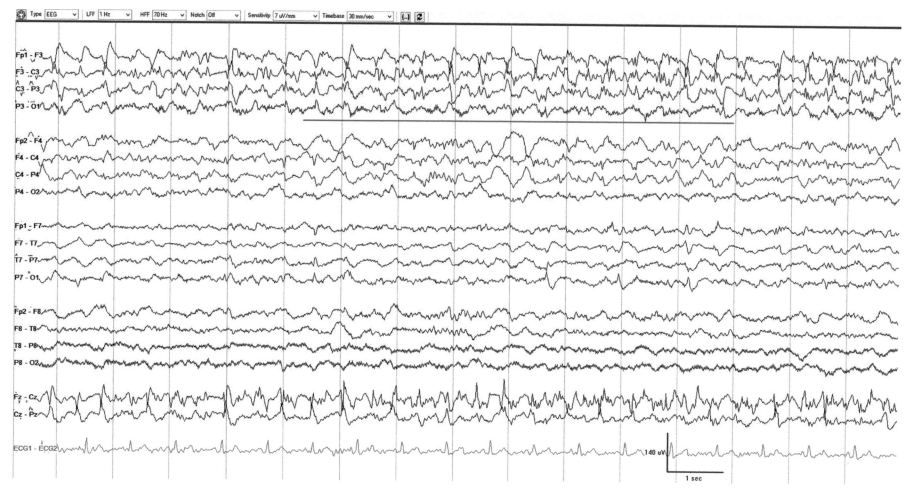

Figure 6.10. (*Continued*) (d) Focal ESz: The next page of EEG demonstrates definite evolution. The continuous activity in the left parasagittal region evolves into 2-Hz spiking with continuous low-amplitude fast activity (red underline). There is additional spread with rhythmic delta activity and discharges becoming apparent in the right central region. Thus, this is evolving in frequency, morphology and location.

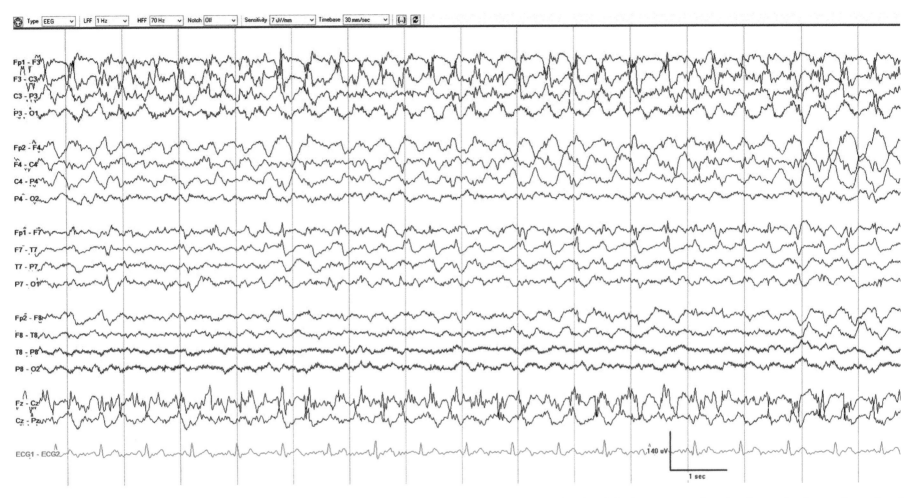

Figure 6.10. (*Continued*) (e) Focal ESz. Further evolution of the seizure with the rhythmic activity in the right fronto-central region becoming better formed and higher voltage. There is also now a broader field of the spike-and-wave, involving much of the left hemisphere (including the left temporal chain of electrodes).

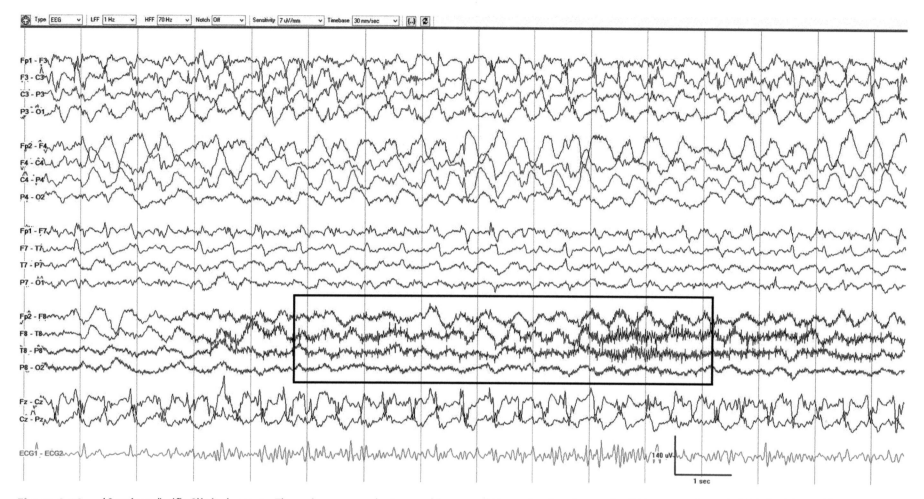

Figure 6.10. *(Continued)* (f) Clinical onset. The seizure was electrographic-only (i.e., nonconvulsive and subclinical: no signs visible clinically). Even though this was not noticed, at the height of the seizure there is some very subtle motor involvement of the contralateral (right) side, evidenced by the onset of scalp EMG artifact (box); this is not necessarily something visible clinically.

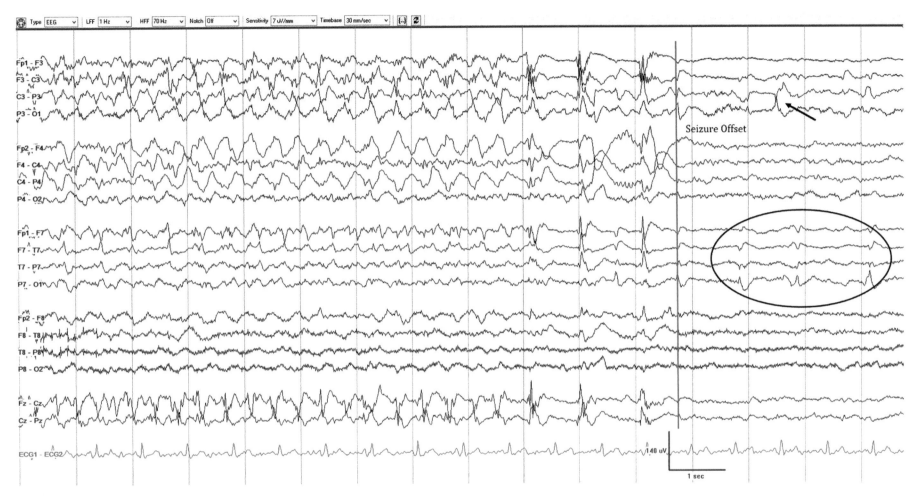

Figure 6.10. (*Continued*) (g) EEG offset. The electrographic seizure ends at the labeled line. There are two interesting phenomena after the seizure ends: 1. The continuous LPDs in the left parietal region have 'reset'. Note the arrowed discharge is only at P3 (versus P3 and C3 at the very beginning) and has returned to being 'simple' with no '+' (i.e., no associated fast activity); and 2. There are now well formed LPDs in the left posterior temporal region (T7/P7 maximal) that were not there before the seizure and appear independent of the PDs at P3 (i.e., UIPDs: unilateral independent PDs). These suggest resetting of the predominant ictal generator in the left parietal region, but the seizure has resulted in at least one additional region of cortical excitability in the same (left) hemisphere.

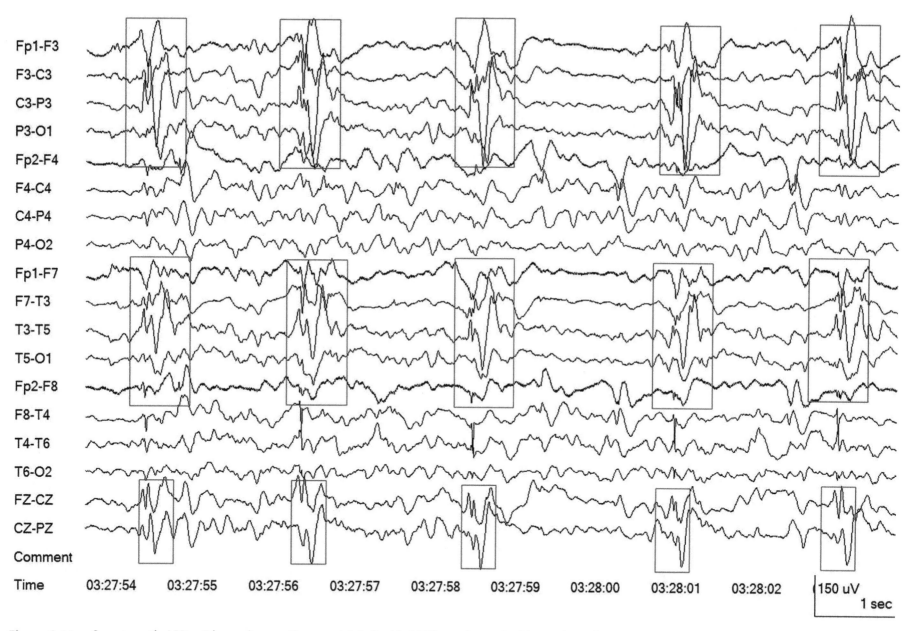

Figure 6.11. Symptomatic LPDs+F becoming continuous. (a) Left-sided LPDs at 0.5 Hz, high voltage and spiky, are present in the EEG of this 28-year-old woman with end-stage renal disease and a blood glucose of 900 ug/ml. There is intermixed low voltage fast activity associated with each discharge making the pattern LPDs+F.

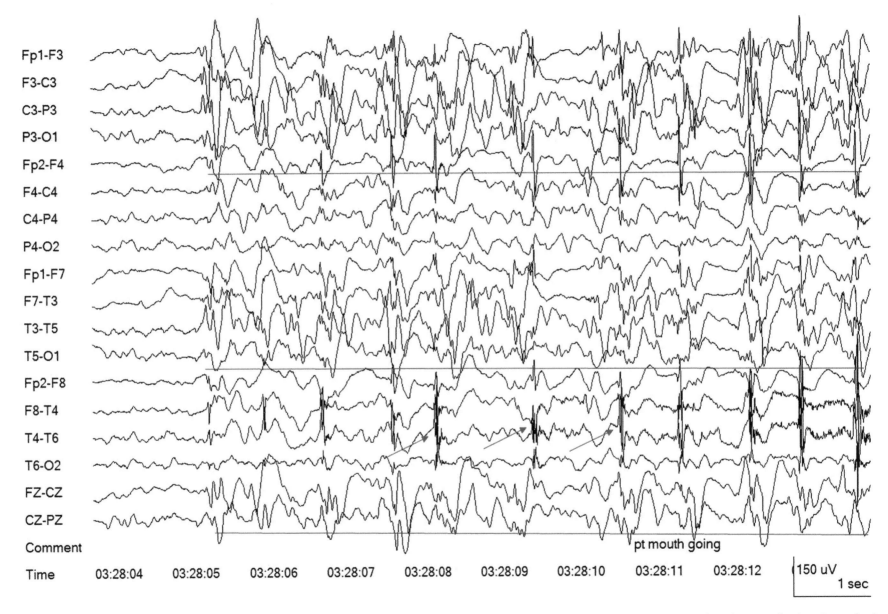

Figure 6.11. (*Continued*) (b) The LPDs+F have evolved into a seizure with the LPDs pattern becoming continuous and then evolving over the next page. This was associated with movements of the right side of the face with prominent muscle artifact over right temporal electrodes that coincides with the discharges (arrows). In retrospect, this EMG artifact was present in a time-locked fashion with the LPDs+F. Looking back on Figure 6.11a each discharge is also associated with a subtle EMG spike in the right temporal region, maximal at T4 and mimicking electrode artifact there (when it is actually EMG artifact; the slight field and the time-locked nature to the LPDs should have been a tipoff that it was not just unrelated artifact). The right head/face muscle involvement could not be clinically appreciated with the LPDs+F, only when the pattern evolved into a seizure did the jerking become clinically apparent in the right face.

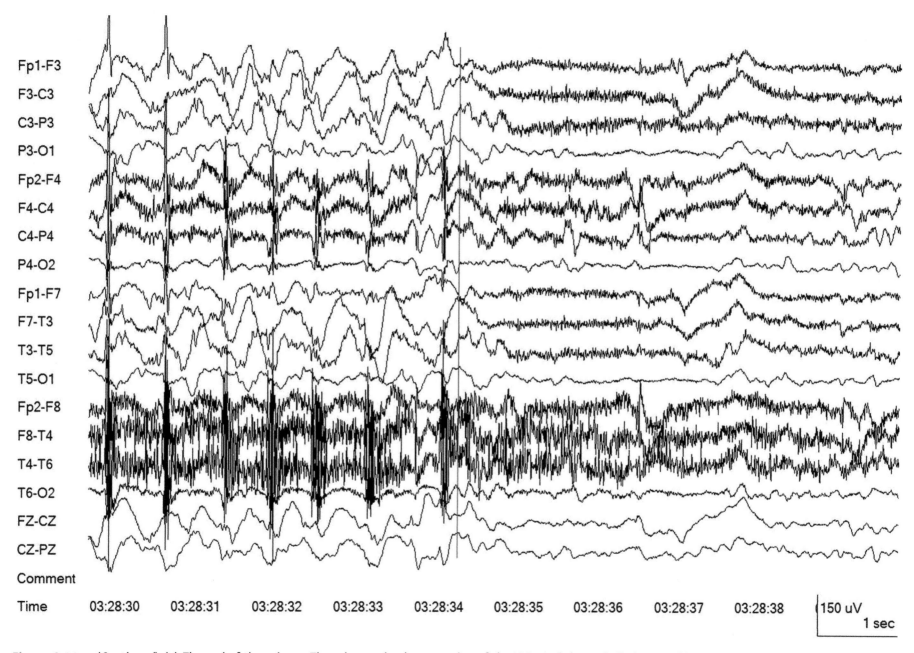

Figure 6.11. (*Continued*) (c) The end of the seizure. There is post ictal attenuation of the LPDs and the periodic bursts of high voltage EMG artifact over the right face stops.

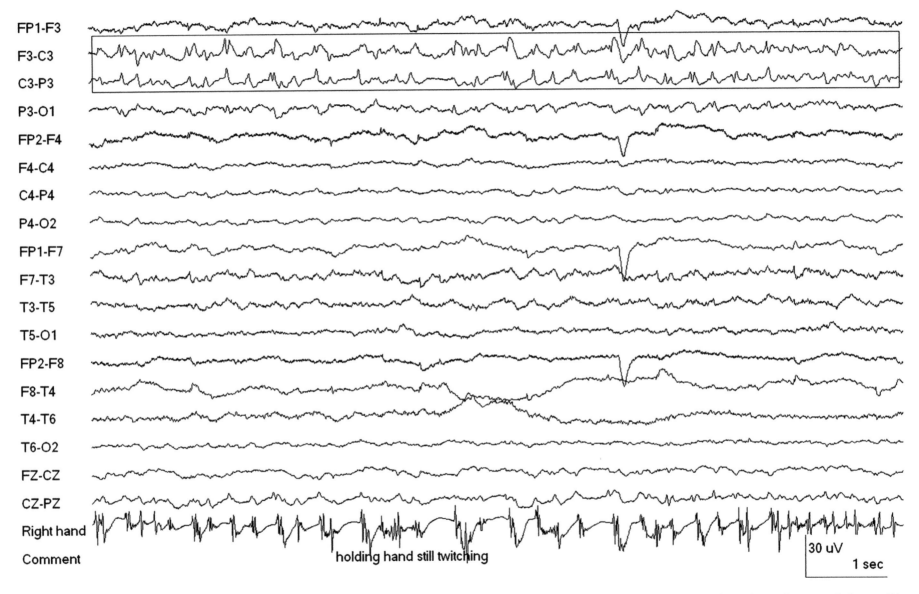

Figure 6.12.   Focal motor seizure. This 33-year-old woman with acute hepatic failure had focal seizures characterized by twitching movements of the right hand; see the last channel, which is an electrode on the right hand and shows the muscle contractions during the twitching. Repetitive spikes and sharp waves are present in the left central area, irregular but recurring at 3–5 per second (box). This is an electroclinical focal seizure from the left Rolandic region. The pattern also meets criteria for an electrographic seizure; however, it is possible (especially for focal motor seizures) to be associated with a pattern that does not. For example, if rhythmic twitching of the right hand were associated with 1-Hz LPDs in the left central region, that would be an electroclinical seizure, but not meet criteria for an electrographic seizure.

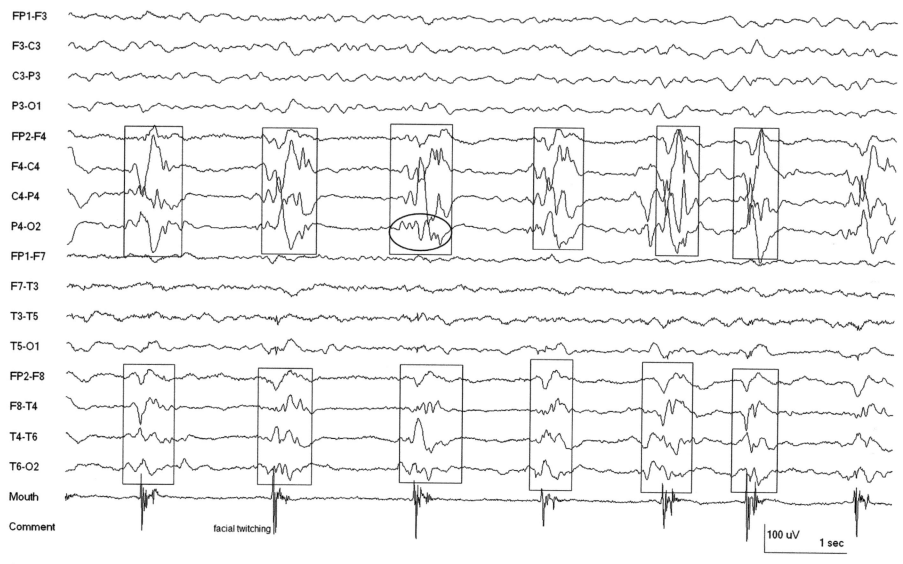

Figure 6.13. Epilepsia partialis continua. The EEG in this 79-year-old man with herpes simplex encephalitis shows lateralized burst suppression (boxes). The right hemispheric complexes consist of 1–2 very high voltage epileptiform discharges with associated polyspike or fast activity (highlighted with an ellipse at O2), with each burst lasting ≥0.5 s. These are therefore either: 1. BIRDs, or 2. Bursts, if occurring as a part of a regularly alternating burst-suppression pattern, as is the case in this example. Each complex is associated with movements of the left side of the face (note EMG channel at the bottom labeled 'mouth' showing the face twitching with each discharge) and is thus ictal by definition. If the patient is fully awake, this is consistent with epilepsia partialis continua (EPC), a form of focal motor status epilepticus, even though the pattern does not qualify as a ESz.

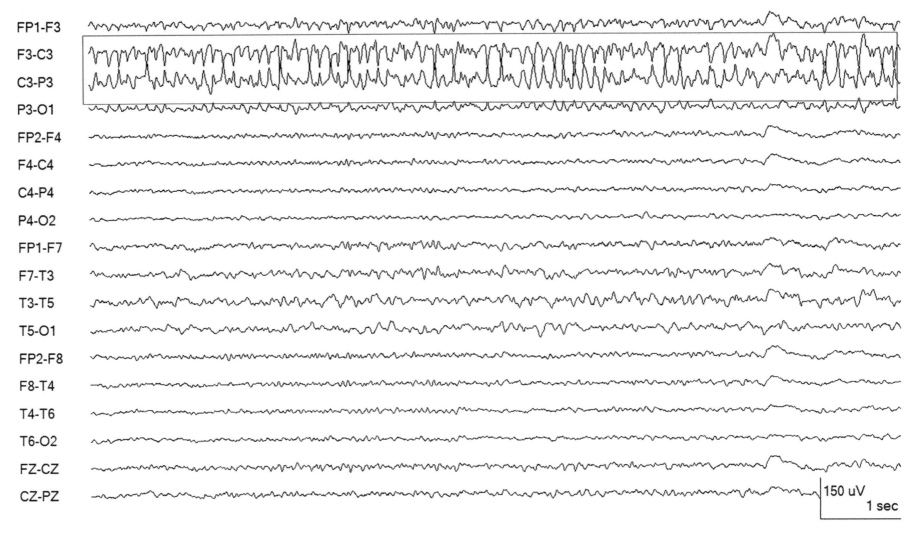

Figure 6.14. Very focal seizure. (a) The EEG in this 58-year-old man with a left-sided glioblastoma multiforme shows a focal seizure that is very prominent at C3, but hardly seen at all at P3 or F3. If not careful this could be mistaken as C3 electrode artifact. The critical point here is that even though subtle, there is a field. The highly restricted field and higher amplitude at C3 are likely due to a skull defect over C3. This page also shows fluctuation and the start of evolution: for most of the page the ictal rhythm consists of 7–8 Hz activity with admixed fast activity making it sharply contoured. By the end of the page this has slowed to 5–6 Hz and some of the faster rhythms are less prominent.

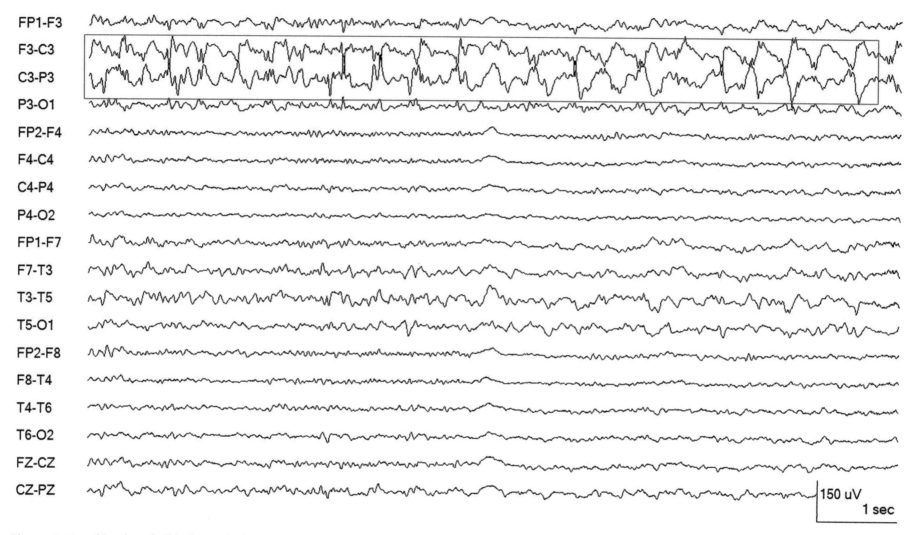

Figure 6.14. *(Continued)* (b) The evolution is even clearer on the next page with the pattern slowing even further in frequency to 2 Hz and the morphology has changed to more rhythmic almost sinusoidal delta activity. In the critical care setting, seizures can at times be very focal, only involving a single electrode in the 10-20 montage. In these cases, it is the physiologic field (albeit subtle), evolution of frequency and morphology that define the pattern as an electrographic seizure.

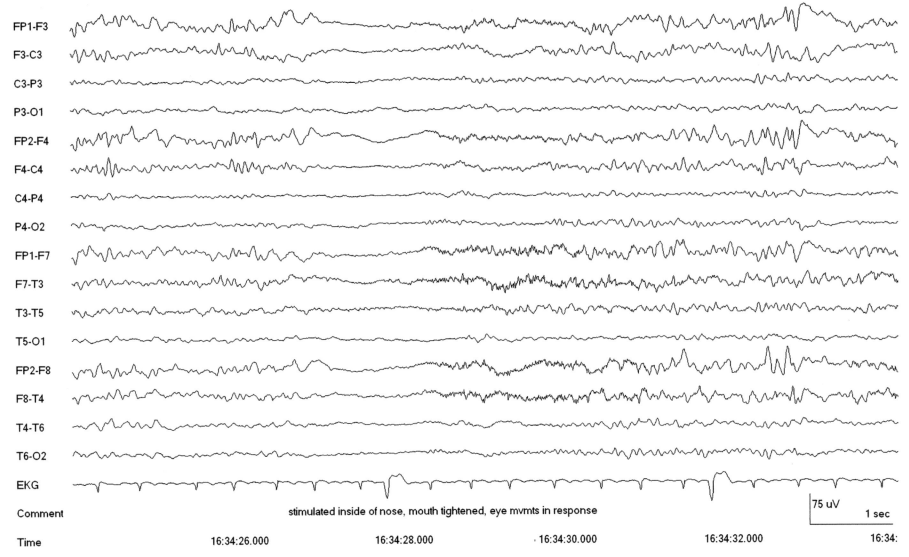

Figure 6.15. Stimulus-induced electroclinical seizure. (a) These four consecutive pages of EEG are from a 73-year-old comatose woman with bilateral watershed infarcts. The patient is stimulated by the EEG technician (nostril tickle, labeled) in the middle of this segment, which results in diffuse attenuation, followed by nondescript continuous low-amplitude alpha and beta activity. At this point it simply appears to be a reactive EEG. However, this turns out to be the subtle onset of a subsequent evolving electrographic, then electroclinical seizure.

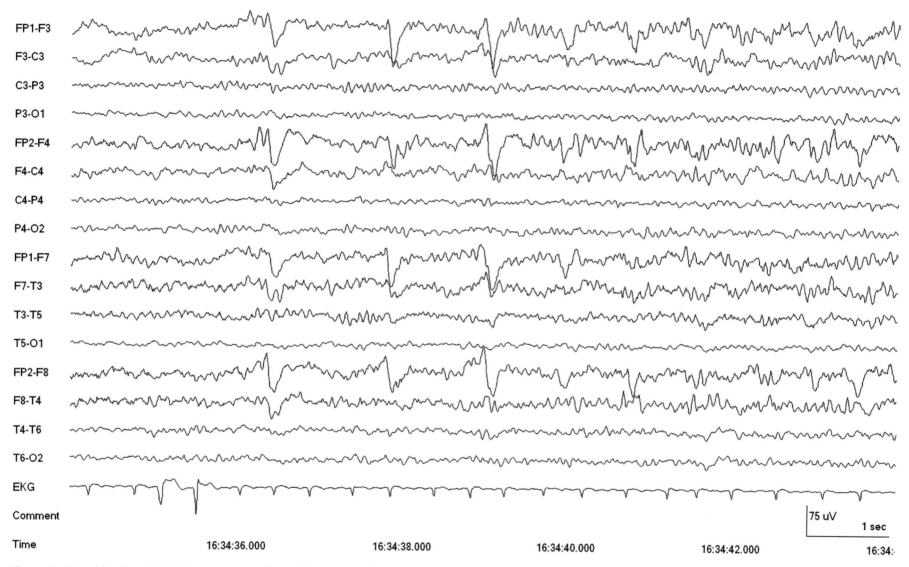

Figure 6.15. (*Continued*) (b) The next 10 s show diffuse fast activity becoming slightly higher in amplitude, though it is still not yet clear that this is a seizure. The patient remained motionless with eyes closed.

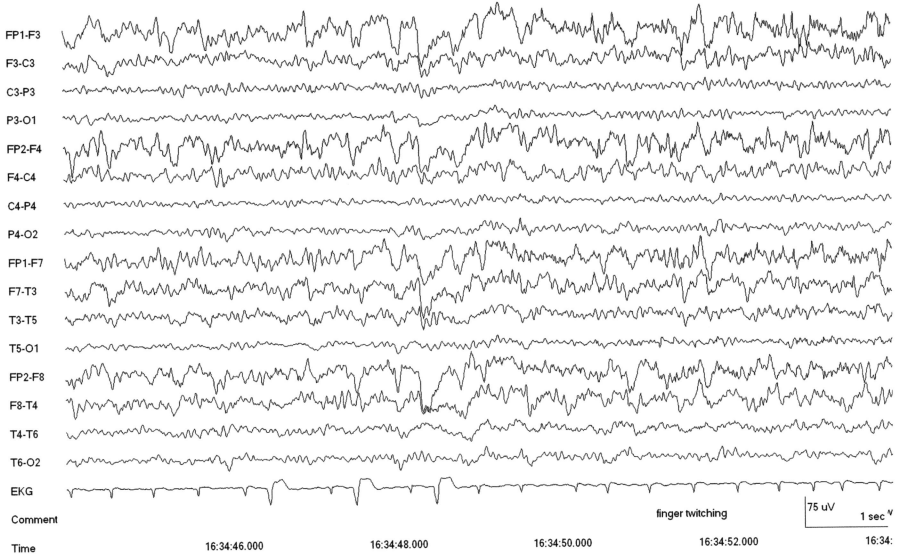

Figure 6.15. (*Continued*) (c) During the subsequent 10 s, this fast activity continues to become more prominent, and now quasi-rhythmic superimposed delta is seen bilaterally, maximal anteriorly. Her eyes opened wide at this point, then left hand finger twitching became visible near the end of this segment, as seen on video and noted by the technician (labeled at the bottom of the page). This is when the seizure also becomes electroclinical.

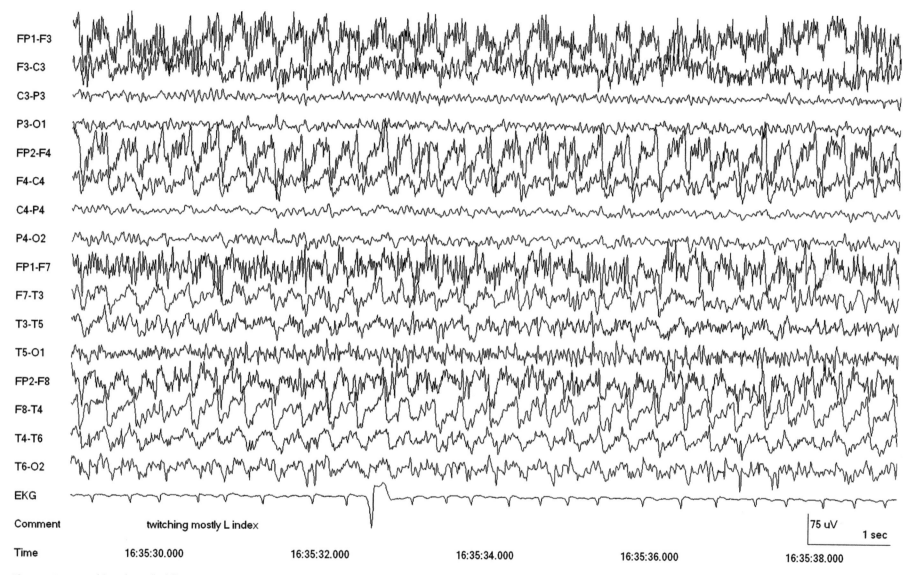

FP1-F3
F3-C3
C3-P3
P3-O1
FP2-F4
F4-C4
C4-P4
P4-O2
FP1-F7
F7-T3
T3-T5
T5-O1
FP2-F8
F8-T4
T4-T6
T6-O2
EKG

Comment   twitching mostly L index   75 uV
                                                                                                                      1 sec

Time   16:35:30.000   16:35:32.000   16:35:34.000   16:35:36.000   16:35:38.000

Figure 6.15. (*Continued*) (d) By 10 s later, the pattern has clearly become ictal, with higher amplitude and rhythmic sharply contoured 3-Hz activity (maximal on the right) with superimposed sharp fast activity. Left hand twitching continued. Thus, this is an electroclinical and electrographic seizure induced by stimulation (stimulus-induced seizure, or SI-seizure). Seizures recurred each time the patient was stimulated that day. This is a form of SIRPIDs, the broader term for stimulus-induced rhythmic, periodic or ictal-appearing patterns.

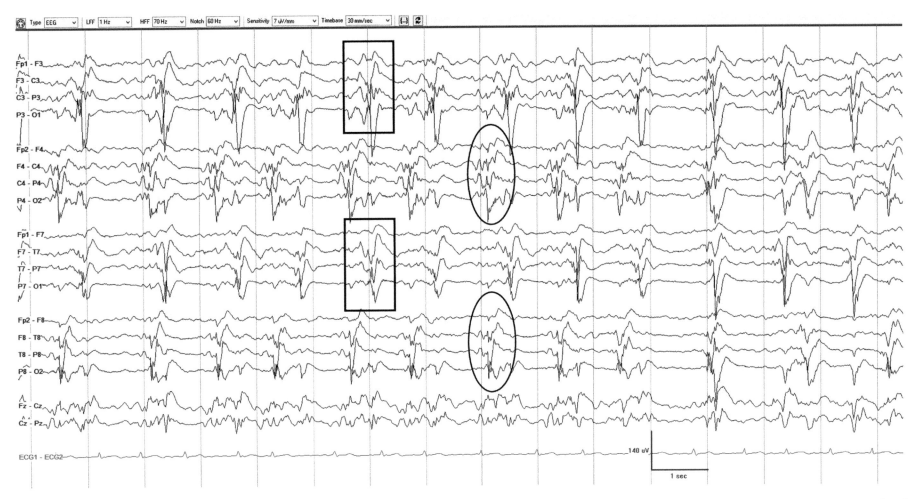

Figure 6.16. BIPDs+F, bilateral independent BIRDs and bilateral independent seizures (a) BIPDs+F. The EEG is from a 77-year-old woman with alcoholic cirrhosis s.p Transjugular, Intrahepatic, Portosystemic Shunt (TIPS). She had an acute onset of decreased mental state that was not explained by her stable hepatic dysfunction.

The 'baseline' EEG consists of continuous ~1 Hz spiky BIPDs+F. An example of the left-sided discharges is highlighted by the boxes and an independent population of periodic discharges in the right hemisphere is highlighted with ellipses. Both populations are associated with low-amplitude fast activity over-riding the periodic discharges (BIPDs+F).

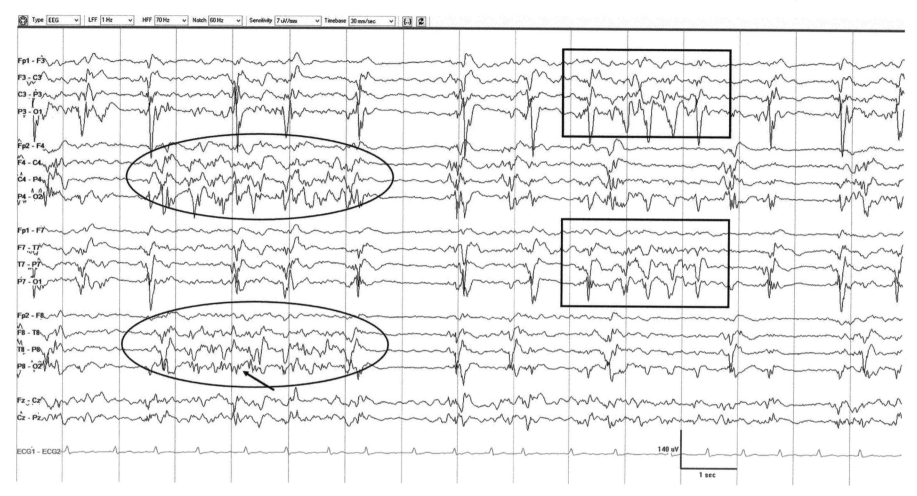

Figure 6.16. (*Continued*) (b) Bilateral independent BIRDs. There were examples where the discharges in either hemisphere became contiguous for 2–5 seconds. These are examples of bilateral independent BIRDs (could be abbreviated as BIBIRDs). This is not specifically defined in the terminology but applies the Main term 1 location descriptor of BI- to describe a pattern consisting of two independent populations of BIRDs overlapping in time (one in each hemisphere). The runs of activity in left and right hemisphere both qualify as definite BIRDs. The activity is ≥0.5 s and consists of low-amplitude high-frequency rhythmic discharges (occurring at approximately 16–20 Hz [best highlighted by the arrow]). In each case the high voltage discharges remain intermixed, but it is the continuous low voltage fast activity that meets criteria for BIRDs (this is because the high voltage discharges are never >4 Hz). Both the left hemispheric BIRDs (boxes) and the right hemispheric BIRDs (ellipses) qualify as definite BIRDs as they share the same morphology and location as independent electrographic seizures arising from their respective hemispheres (shown in the following Figure 6.16c–e and 6.16f–h.

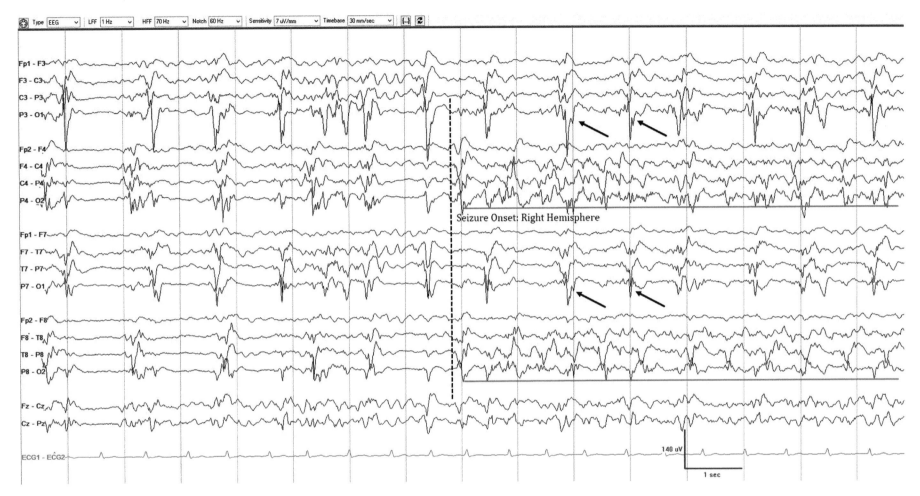

Figure 6.16. (*Continued*) (c) Right hemispheric seizure. The right-sided LPDs and BIRDs are replaced by a continuous evolving ictal rhythm (labeled dashed line for seizure onset/red underline highlighting the evolving seizure). The left hemispheric LPDs continue unchanged (arrows), providing additional evidence that they represent a truly independent population.

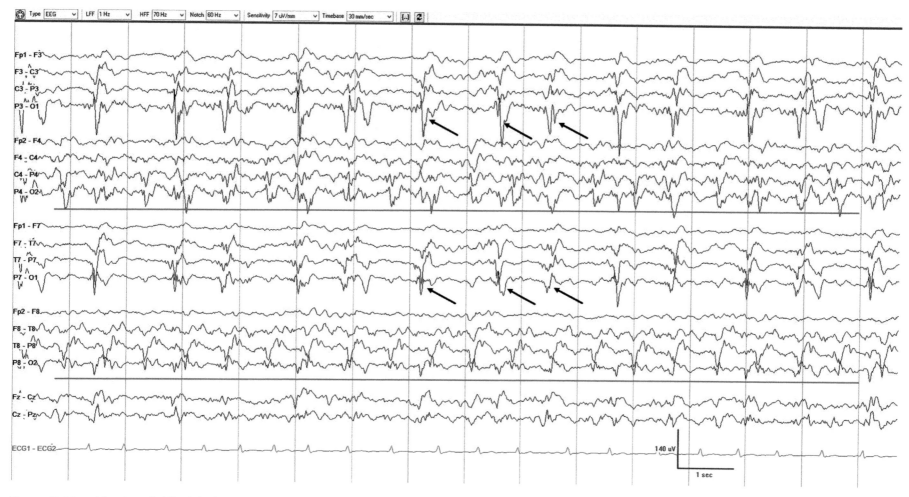

Figure 6.16. *(Continued)* (d) Right hemispheric seizure continues. This page highlights the continued ictal rhythm in the right hemisphere (red underline), while the LPDs in the left hemisphere remain unchanged (arrows).

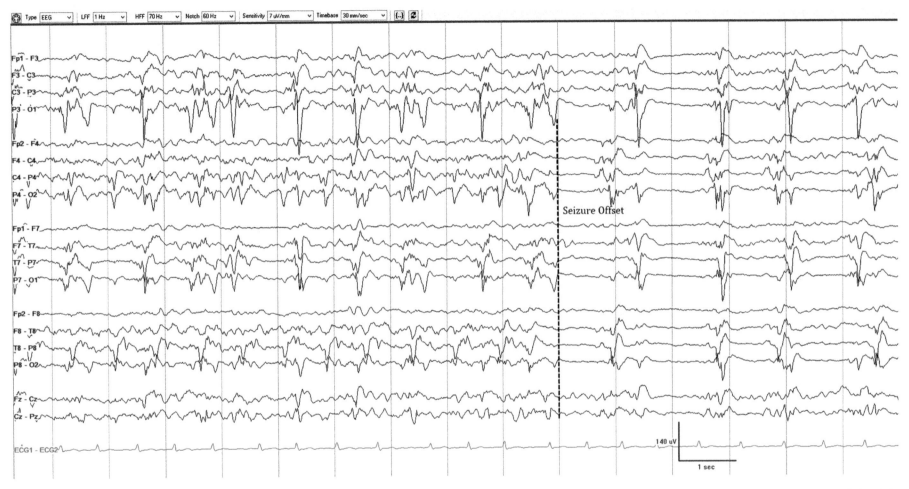

Figure 6.16. (*Continued*) (e) Right hemispheric seizure ends. The right-sided seizure ends (labeled dashed line). There is immediate recommencement of the right LPDs+F, reinstating the pattern of BIPDs+F.

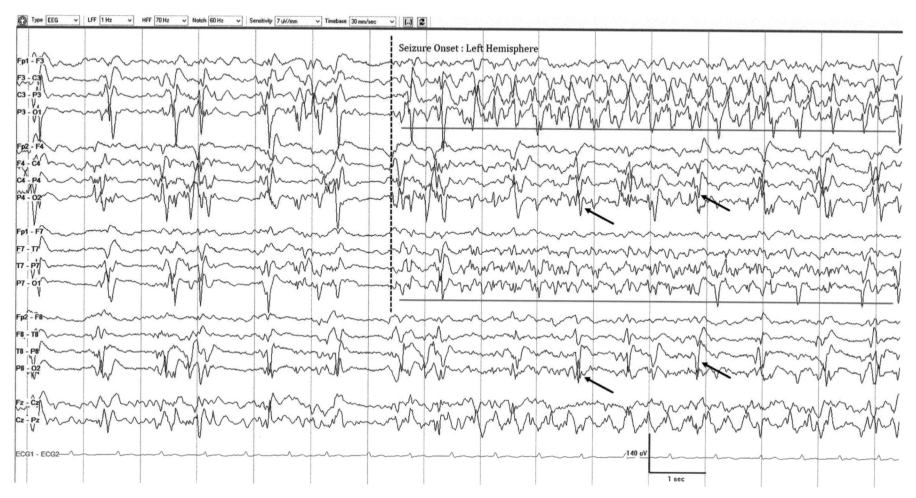

Figure 6.16. *(Continued)* (f) Left hemispheric seizure. This example is of a left hemispheric seizure. This time the left-sided LPDs and BIRDs are replaced by a continuous and evolving ictal rhythm (dashed vertical line for seizure onset/red underline highlighting the ictal rhythm). The direct mirror image to before, now the LPDs+F in the right hemisphere continue, largely unaltered (arrows), though the low voltage fast activity is now more persistent.

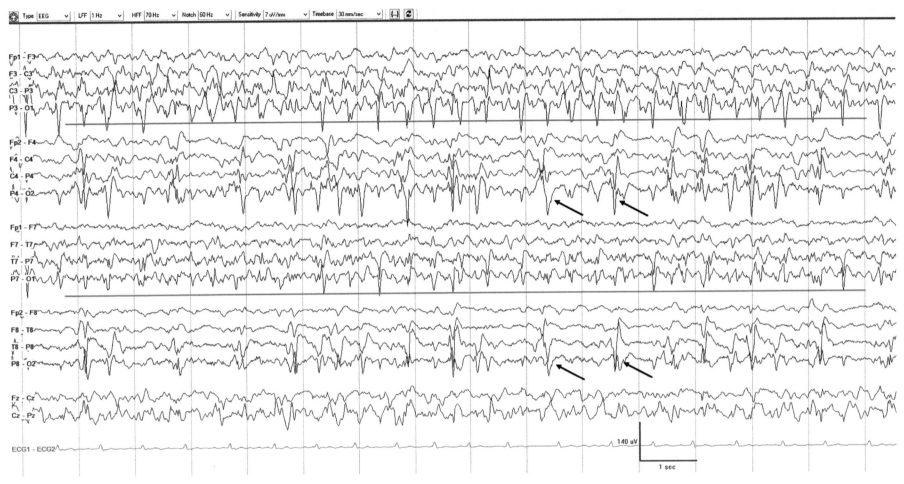

Figure 6.16. (*Continued*) (g) Left hemispheric seizure continues. This page shows the continued ictal rhythm on the left (red underline) and the LPDs on the right (arrows).

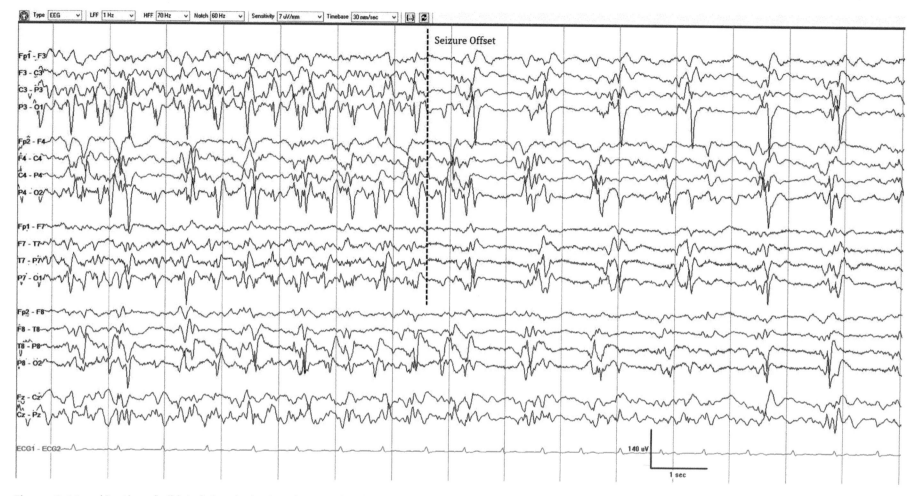

Figure 6.16. (*Continued*) (h) Left hemispheric seizure ends. The left-sided seizure ends (labeled dashed line), again with recommencement of the BIPDs+F.

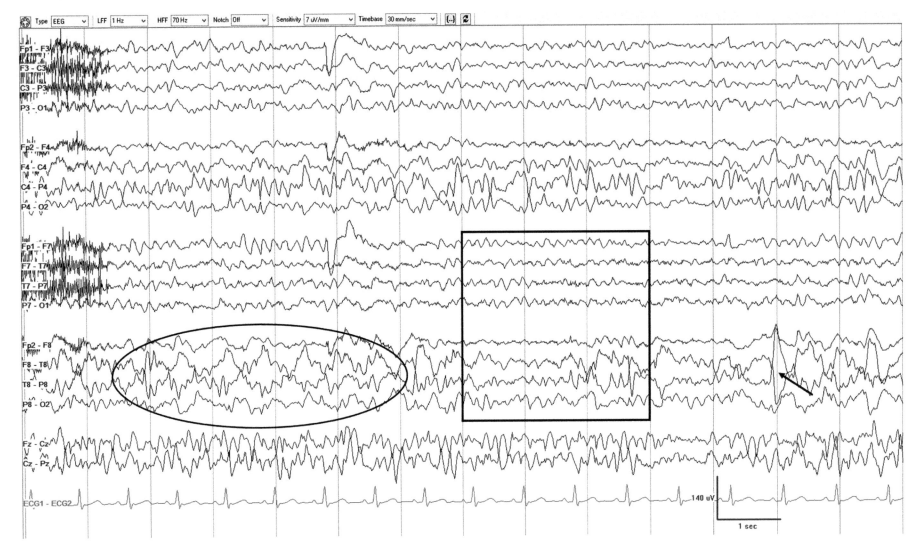

Figure 6.17. Ictal-interictal continuum (IIC), focal. (a) This EEG is from a 69-year-old woman with a remote history of a right frontal arteriovenous malformation (AVM) resection who presented with altered mental status. The background EEG is shown. There is a breach rhythm through the right hemisphere, appreciable with activity on the right being higher voltage and sharper when compared to a homologous region on the left (box). There is also intermittent polymorphic delta slowing of 1.5–2-Hz through the right temporal region (ellipse). There are examples where the activity at T8 is sharply contoured and potentially epileptiform (arrow) but this does not disrupt the background, it does not have a definite field, and in the context of the breach rhythm is not definitely epileptiform (though suspicious).

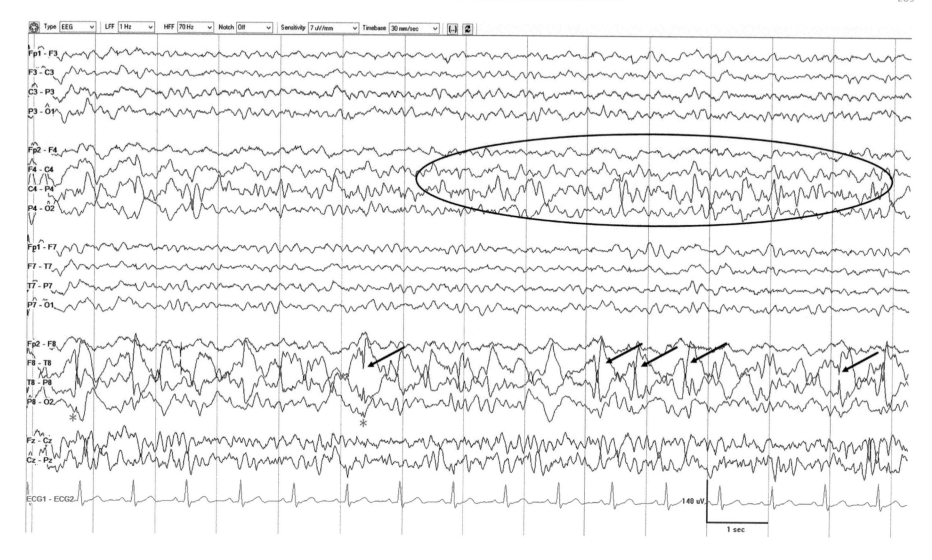

Figure 6.17. (*Continued*) (b) Later in the record the spikes at T8 do become more definitively epileptiform. They start to disrupt the background slowing, are very apiculate, start to develop a field into P8 and O2 (two highlighted with the red asterisks), and become very briefly periodic at times. It is hard to differentiate if some of the associated faster rhythms are associated with the pattern or just present due to the breach, but the pattern at least qualifies as 1.5-Hz LPDs. For the sake of comparing later progression, it is worth noting that there are no epileptiform discharges in the right parasagittal derivations (ellipse).

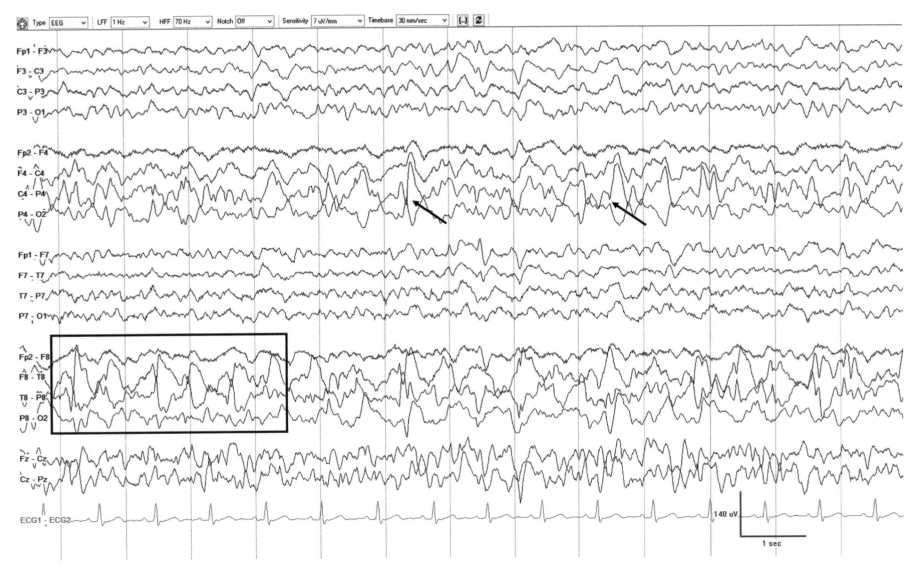

Figure 6.17. (*Continued*) (c) Later again in the record, the LPDs are more prevalent and prominent (box), they often have a field to P4 (arrows), there is now continuous superimposed quasi-rhythmic delta (LPD+R), and there is clear involvement of the right parasagittal chain now, compared to prior (with the slowing in that region potentially due to the expansion of the field of epileptiform activity in the temporal region). The pattern is now on the ictal-interictal continuum. Contrast the three figures. The first there was potentially epileptiform activity but clearly not ictal, the second the establishment of a periodic pattern (LPDs) that remained relatively focal but now possibly ictal (probably not), and then fluctuation in location and morphology, increased prominence of the pattern, and superimposed rhythmicity (+R), becoming more likely to be ictal; given the series of EEGs, we would likely call this last page 'probably ictal' in our impression, though this requires clinical context. The final panel is not definitely ictal (still <2.5 Hz without definite evolution) but is clearly more ictal-appearing than the prior two, and more likely to warrant treatment. This highlights the IIC, forming a continuum of patterns that range from interictal to ictal and often fluctuating between the two (compared to patients who are not critically ill, where the transition between these states is mostly rapid and well defined).

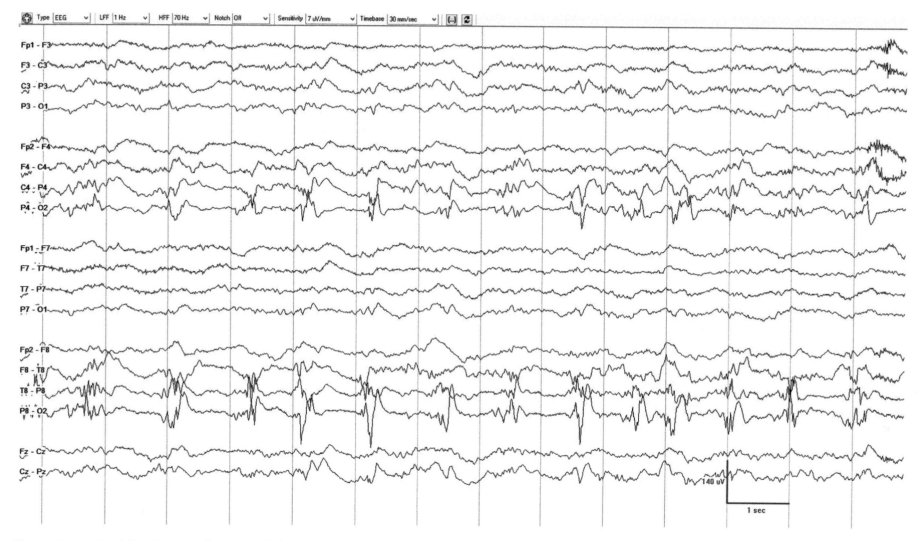

Figure 6.18. Ictal-interictal continuum (IIC), focal. (a) The EEG is from a 75-year-old man with a right SDH s/p hemicraniectomy. Postoperatively his mental state fluctuated. The EEG demonstrates 1-Hz LPDs+F in the right posterior quadrant.

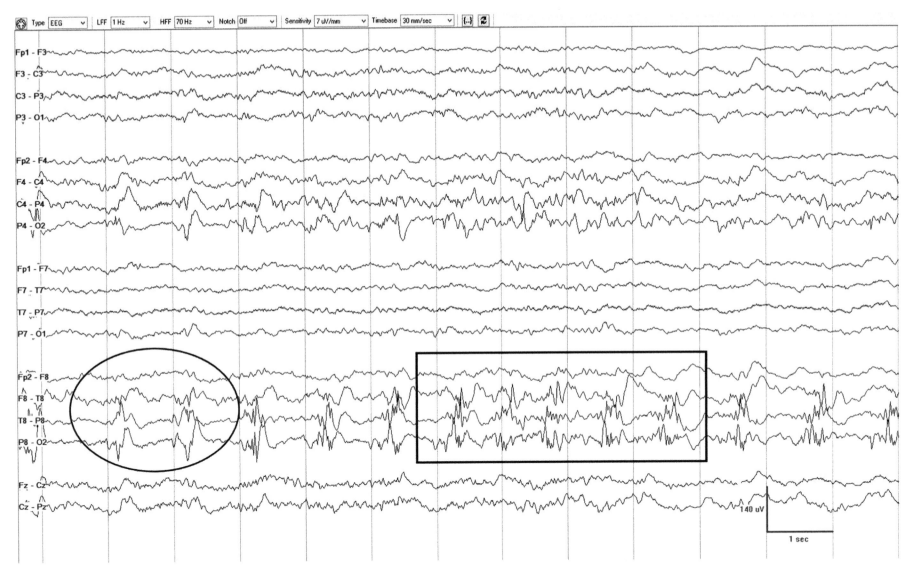

Figure 6.18. (*Continued*) (b) This page demonstrates fluctuation of the pattern. Compare the discharges at the beginning of the page (ellipse) occurring at 1 Hz and a small amount of associated fast activity, then becoming faster (up to 1.5 Hz) with an increase in fast activity or polyspikes, with each discharge being associated with a real buzz of activity. In the middle of the page (highlighted with the box) the buzz of fast activity becomes continuous for 4 seconds. There is no longer a break between polyspike-and-wave complex. The low voltage fast activity of > 4 Hz, lasting ≥0.5 s and <10 s qualifies as definite BIRDs (under the category of having the same field as interictal discharges in the same patient).

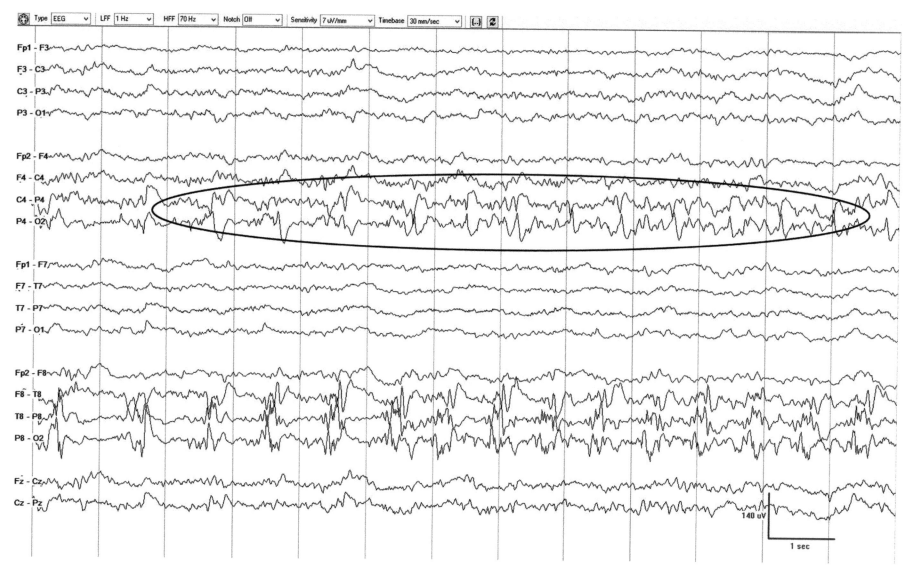

Figure 6.18. (*Continued*) (c) Additional fluctuation of the pattern in location, with the LPDs now involving a field to P4. The activity in the temporal derivations is highly epileptiform and nearly continuous (with only a very small break in between complexes). Again, the pattern is not definitely a seizure, demonstrating fluctuation in all of frequency (1 Hz to 1.5 Hz [but never 2 Hz]), morphology (becoming higher amplitude with greater associated fast, even qualifying as definite BIRDs at times), and location (into P4 [only one standard electrode on the 10-20 montage rather than two sequential locations]), but not definite evolution and never lasting for ≥10 seconds. Again, this demonstrates the principle of the IIC. There are patterns that are clearly not causing additional neuronal injury or clinical signs/symptoms (interictal), but the point at which the pattern could potentially be contributing to these is often not well defined in critically ill patients.

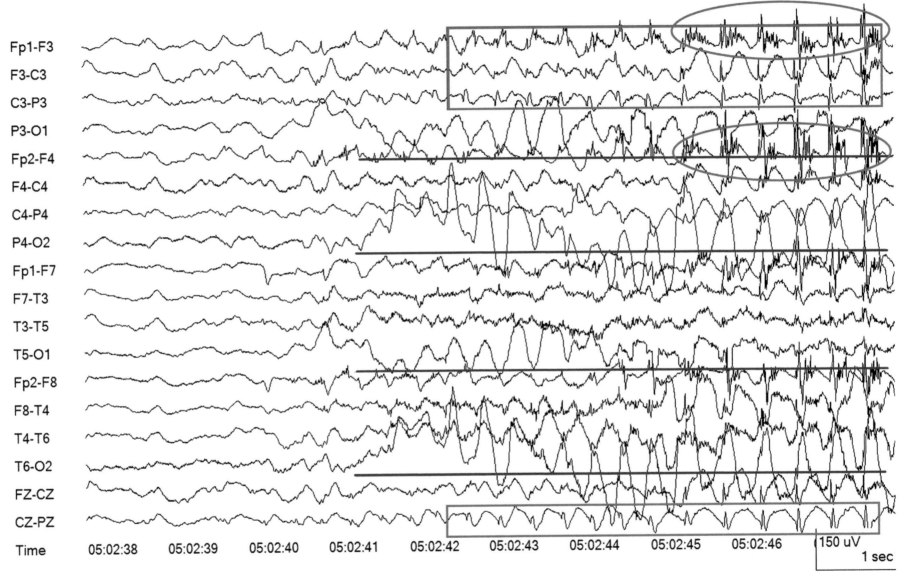

Figure 6.19. Generalized tonic-clonic seizure. (a) The EEG in this 19-year-old recently pregnant woman with seizures following delivery shows a seizure beginning with evolving spike-and-wave complexes through the left central region (red boxes). This is especially evident in the Cz-Pz channel at the bottom of the page. As the pattern evolves, the complexes become associated with EMG artifact (best appreciated in the anterior derivations at the end of the page [red ellipses]). There is also prominent rhythmic movement artifact in the posterior head derivations from the clinical jerking (blue underline).

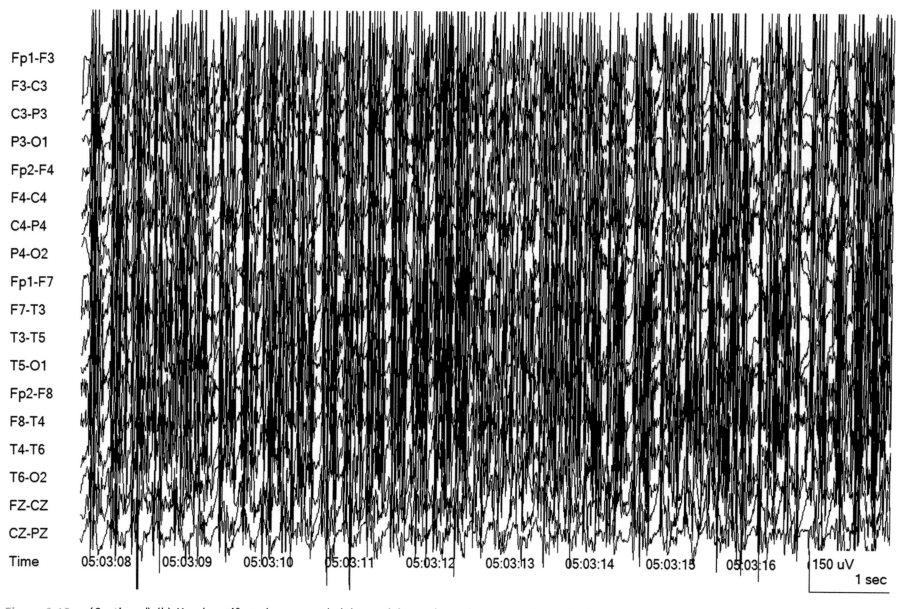

Figure 6.19.   (*Continued*) (b) Muscle artifact obscures underlying activity as the patient enters the tonic phase of a convulsion. Some of this pattern might include rapid spiking from the brain, but it is very difficult to determine that without removing the muscle artifact.

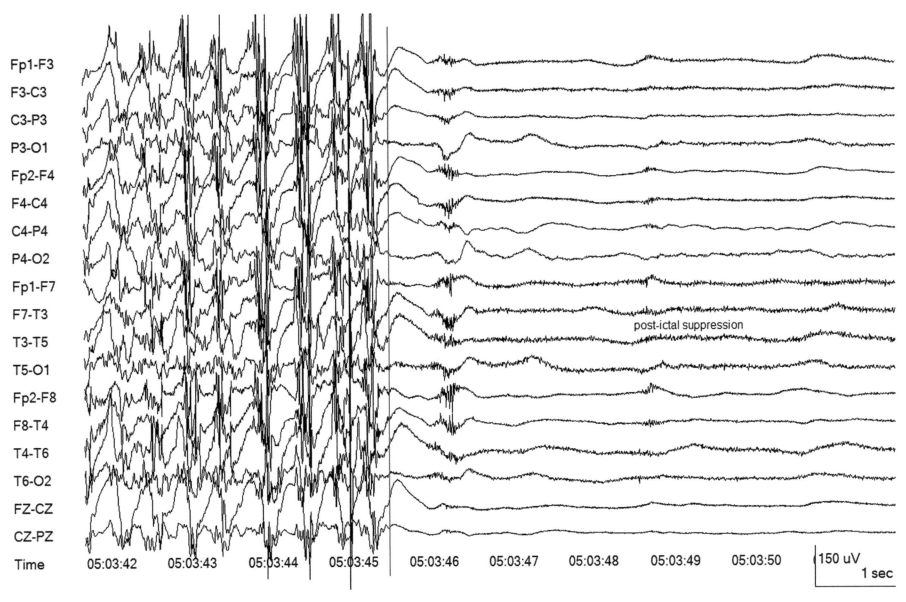

Figure 6.19. (*Continued*) (c) This page shows the clonic phase of the convulsion with periodic bursts of EMG activity (highest amplitude and fastest activity on the page; associated with clonic jerking) as well as polyspike-wave discharges on the EEG. The end of the seizure is highlighted by the line and after this there is prominent postictal suppression, often termed postictal generalized EEG suppression (PGES) when seen in an epilepsy monitoring unit setting.

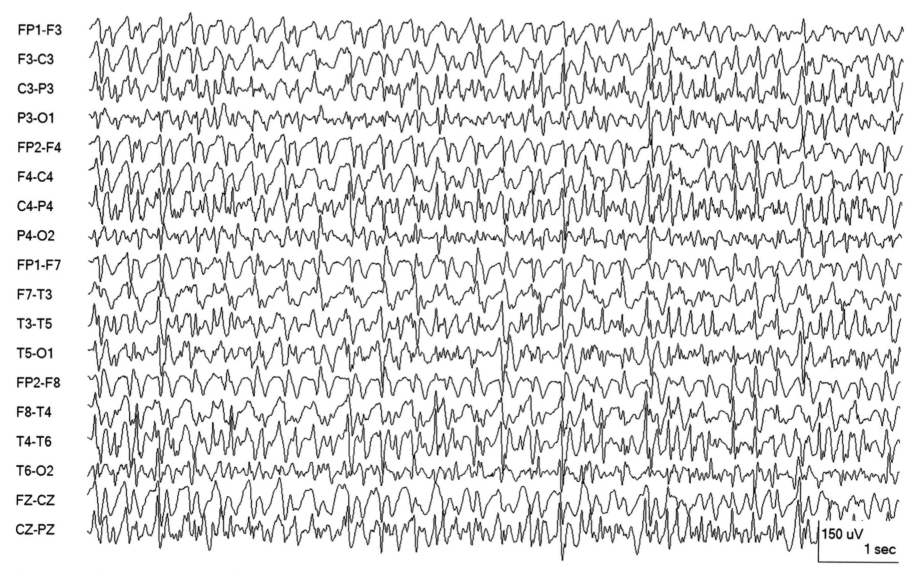

Figure 6.20. Nonconvulsive status epilepticus, generalized. (a) This EEG is from a 56-year-old man being evaluated for encephalopathy and eyelid fluttering. Prior to the onset of this recording, he had received lorazepam and was placed on a propofol infusion. At the start of the recording, as shown here, the patient was in generalized nonconvulsive status epilepticus with continuous generalized spikes and sharp waves at 3–10 Hz, depending which channel.

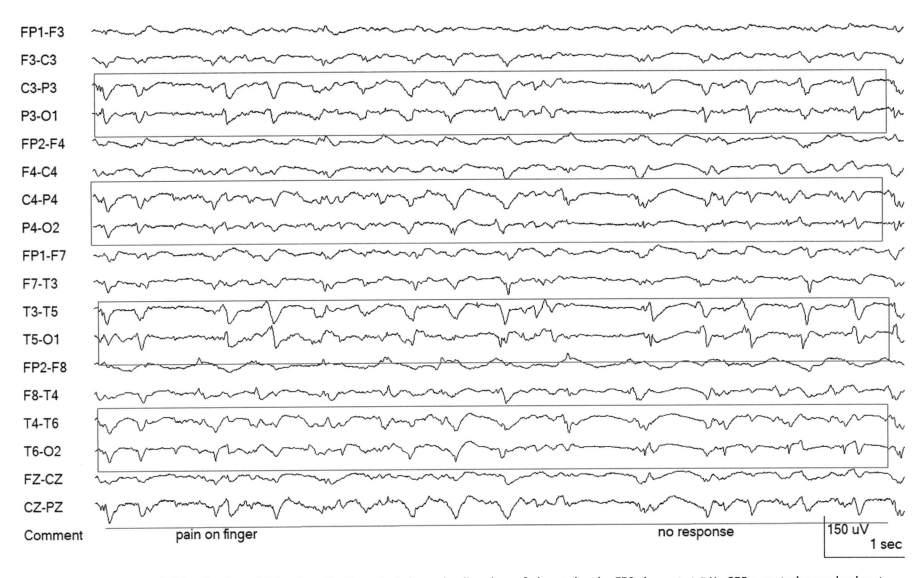

Figure 6.20.   (*Continued*) (b) Following additional medications, including a loading dose of phenytoin, the EEG shows 1–1.5 Hz GPDs, posterior-predominant.

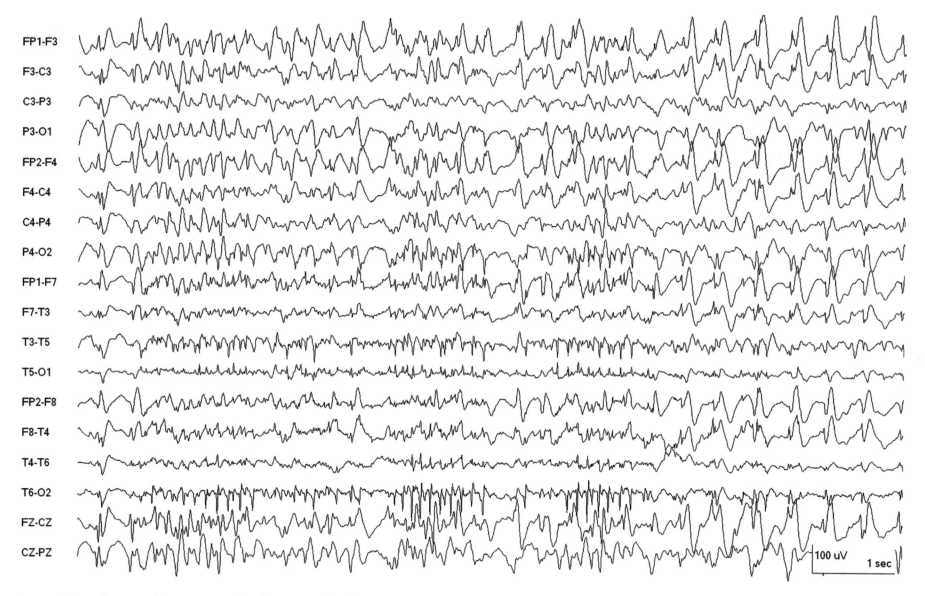

Figure 6.21. Nonconvulsive status epilepticus, generalized. (a) Longitudinal bipolar. This EEG in a 44-year-old man with a history of developmental disability and seizures shows generalized epileptiform abnormalities, irregular and fast (varying from 3 to >8 Hz), slowing down in the last few seconds to 2.5–3 Hz, when it develops a spike-wave morphology. The patient was in nonconvulsive status epilepticus. The diagnosis of NCSE or electroclinical status epilepticus can be difficult in patients with prior known developmental and epileptic encephalopathy. The critical care terminology provides some guidance by defining ECSE in these patients as: a. an increase in prominence or frequency of epileptiform discharges compared to baseline, with an observable decline in clinical state, or b. EEG and clinical improvement with a parenteral (typically IV) anti-seizure medication. In this case the EEG was clearly much more epileptic compared to a baseline EEG.

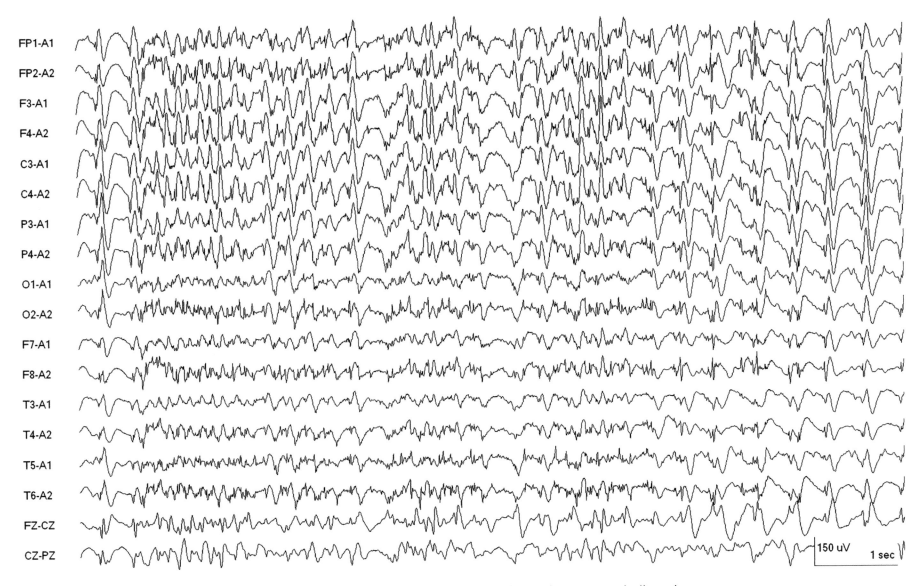

Figure 6.21. (*Continued*) (b) Referential. The epoch has been reformatted utilizing a referential montage to ipsilateral ears.

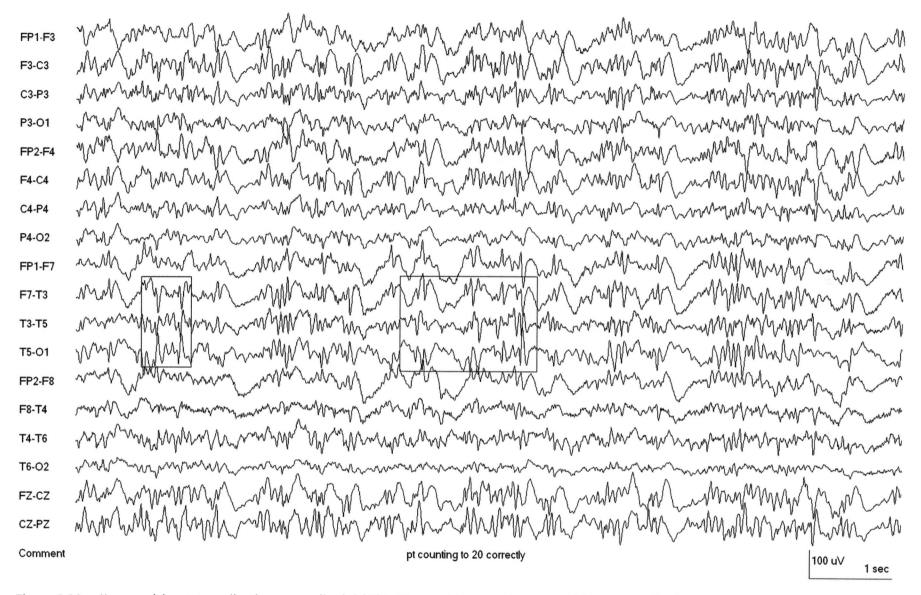

Comment   pt counting to 20 correctly   100 uV
                                                                                                                                    1 sec

Figure 6.22.   Nonconvulsive status epilepticus, generalized. (a) This 20-year-old man was in nonconvulsive status epilepticus associated with continual, widespread ictal activity of mixed frequency, mostly alpha and beta. The patient was able to answer many questions correctly, although he was frequently slow in his responses.

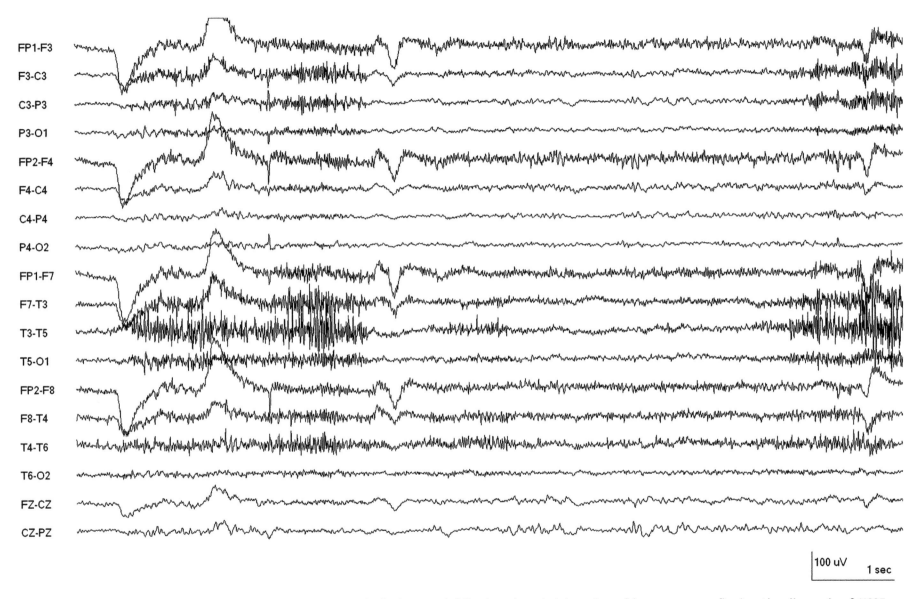

FP1-F3
F3-C3
C3-P3
P3-O1
FP2-F4
F4-C4
C4-P4
P4-O2
FP1-F7
F7-T3
T3-T5
T5-O1
FP2-F8
F8-T4
T4-T6
T6-O2
FZ-CZ
CZ-PZ

100 uV   1 sec

Figure 6.22. (*Continued*) (b) His clinical state and EEG markedly improved following the administration of lorazepam, confirming the diagnosis of NCSE, or electroclinical status epilepticus (ECSE).

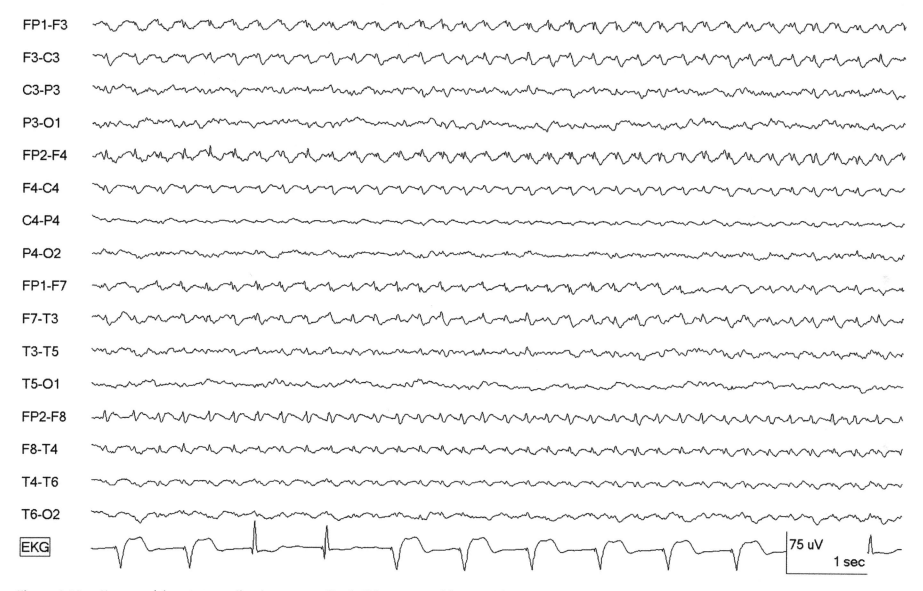

Figure 6.23. Nonconvulsive status epilepticus, generalized. This 82-year-old man with recent head trauma is in generalized nonconvulsive status epilepticus. Rhythmic discharges are present diffusely at 3–4 per second, maximal anteriorly, where there is a spike-and-wave morphology.

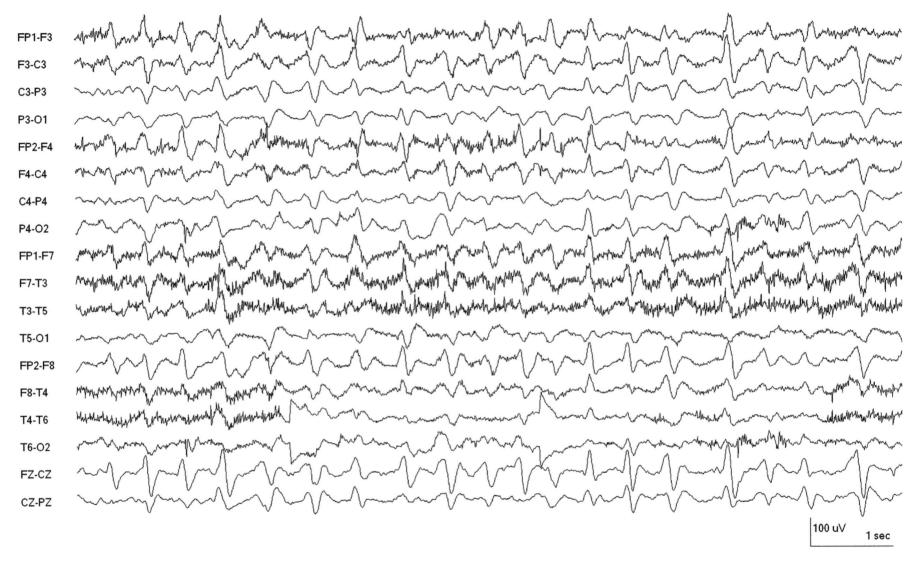

Figure 6.24. NCSE with triphasic waves. (a) This EEG of a 75-year-old man with altered mental status and renal failure shows GPDs at 1.5–2.5–3 Hz, sometimes with triphasic morphology. It was felt that the patient may have been in nonconvulsive status due to taking cefepime.

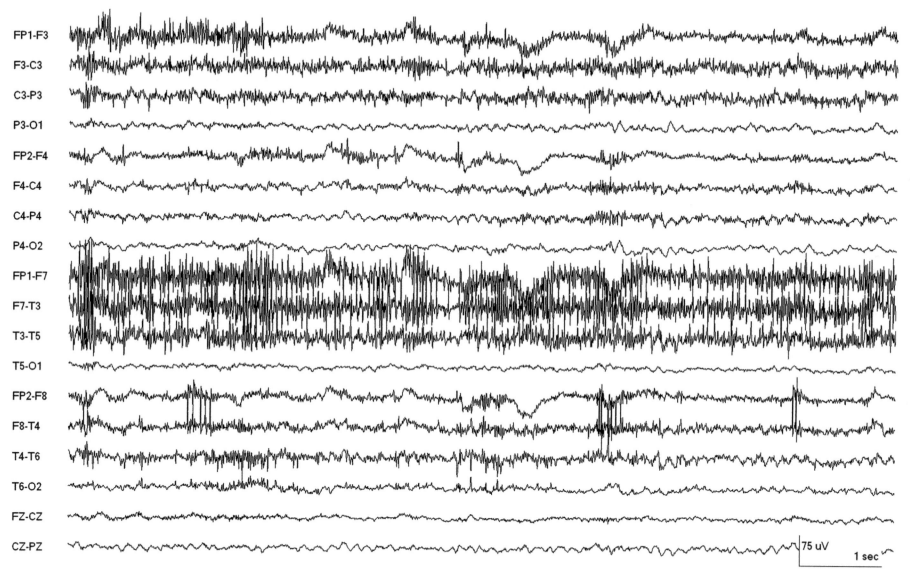

Figure 6.24. (*Continued*) (b) The next day, following treatment and cessation of cefepime, the EEG was considerably improved (only demonstrating mild diffuse dysfunction), as was the patient. The improvement in the EEG AND the clinical state would be diagnostic of NCSE or ECSE if the clinical improvement was immediate or rapid after IV anti-seizure medication; however, in this case it was too slow to be certain what led to her improvement. If the EEG improved, but the patient remained clinically the same this, could be classified as possible NCSE or possible ECSE. His renal function remained unchanged over the period of these EEGs and so reversal of metabolic encephalopathy is not sufficient to explain the improvement in clinical state in this case. We believe this was most likely cefepime-induced nonconvulsive status epilepticus but cannot prove it in this case.

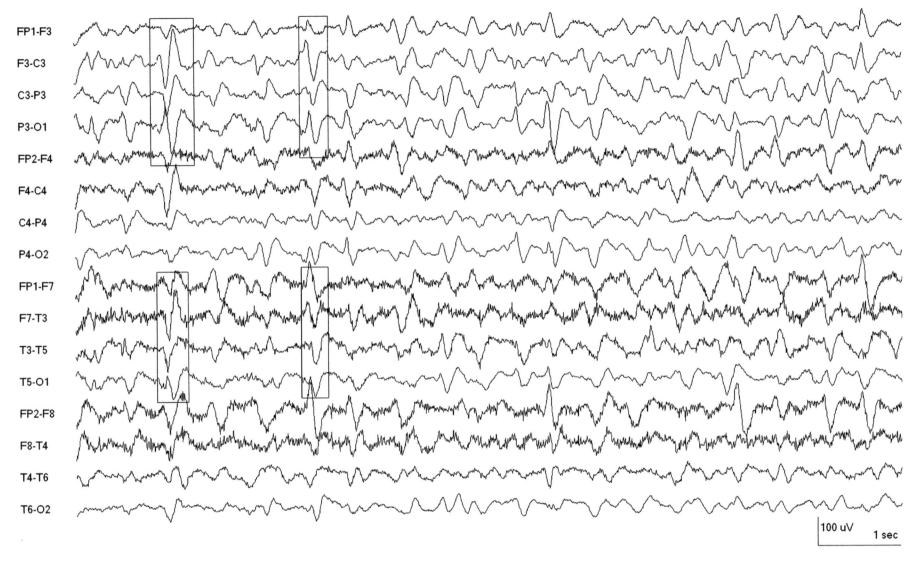

Figure 6.25. NCSE with metabolic encephalopathy and triphasic morphology, based on clinical criteria (electroclinical SE). (a) This EEG is from an 83-year-old woman with acute renal failure who suddenly became unresponsive. It shows high voltage probable sharp waves (some highlighted), often biphasic or triphasic in configuration and frequently of higher voltage on the left, and superimposed on a quasi-rhythmic, slow background. Occasionally, these were periodic with a frequency of 1.5–2 Hz. The discharges did not change following application of auditory or painful stimuli. It was felt that the patient may have been in nonconvulsive status epilepticus, and she was given 2 mg of intravenous lorazepam.

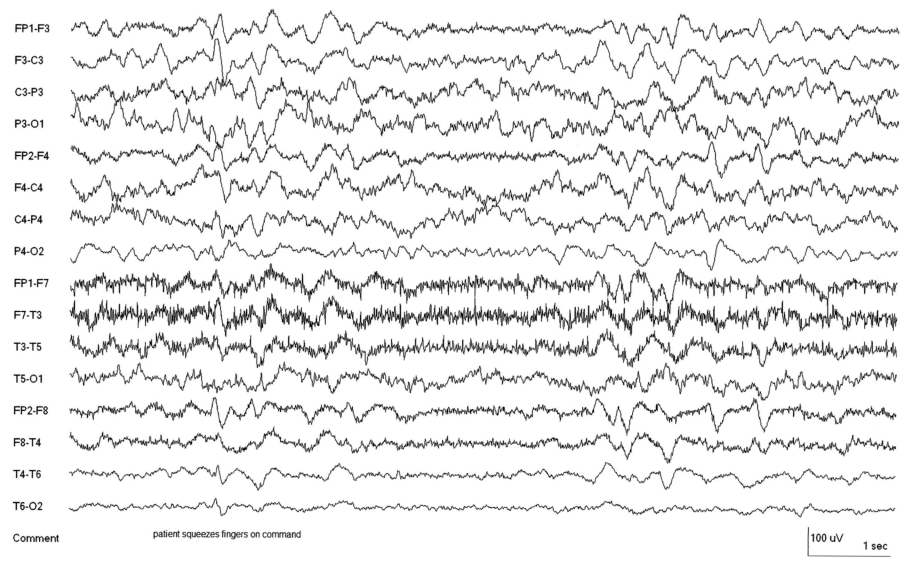

FP1-F3

F3-C3

C3-P3

P3-O1

FP2-F4

F4-C4

C4-P4

P4-O2

FP1-F7

F7-T3

T3-T5

T5-O1

FP2-F8

F8-T4

T4-T6

T6-O2

Comment   patient squeezes fingers on command

100 uV   1 sec

Figure 6.25. (*Continued*) (b) Following treatment the EEG improved. The patient awakened quickly, and later in the recording, was following commands and attempting to speak. The clinical improvement confirmed the diagnosis of nonconvulsive status epilepticus. If the EEG had improved like this but the patient did not improve, no conclusion could have been reached regarding the presence or absence of NCSE, as many patterns resolve with benzodiazepines. EEG improvement but not clinical improvement therefore only qualifies as possible NCSE, or possible ECSE.

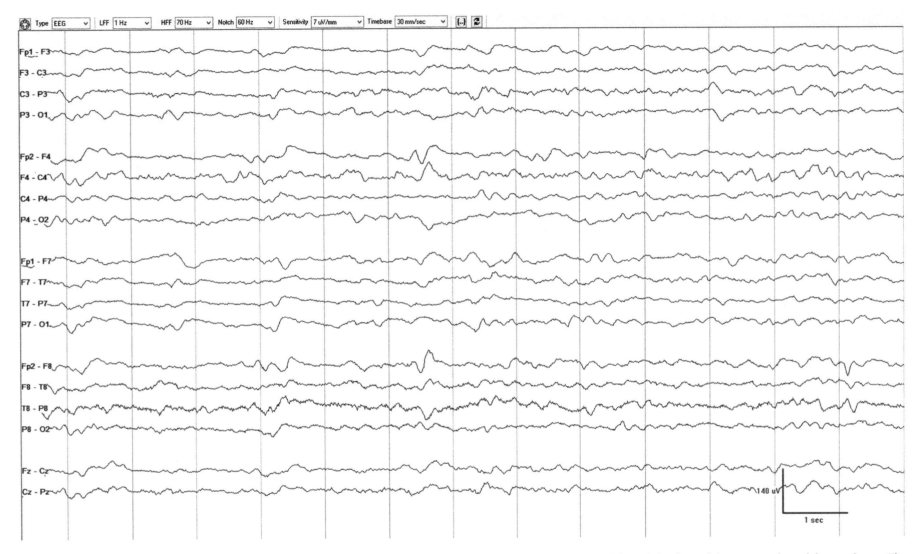

Figure 6.26. Ictal-interictal continuum (IIC), generalized. (a) This EEG is from an 86-year-old woman with a right frontal intraparenchymal hemorrhage. The initial EEG appeared relatively benign, mostly consistent with mild to moderate diffuse dysfunction.

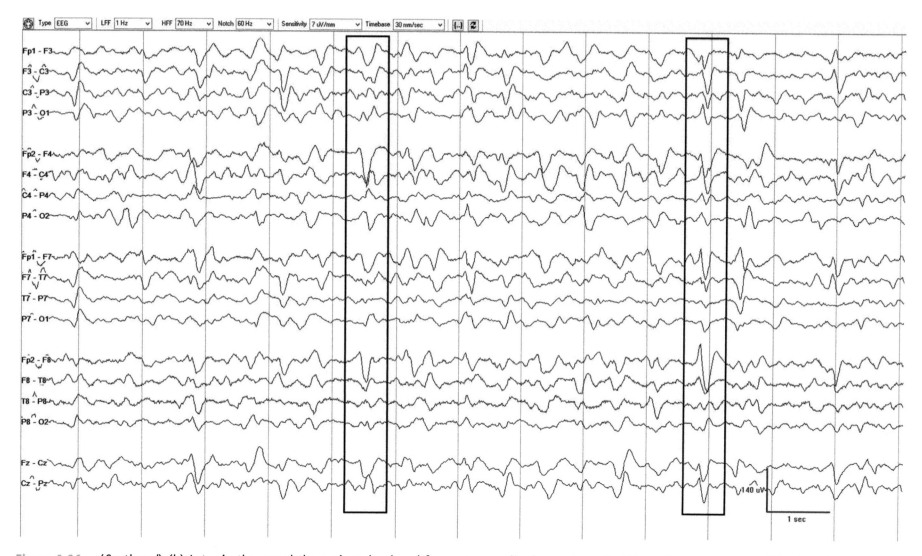

Figure 6.26. (*Continued*) (b) Later in the record the patient developed frequent generalized sporadic epileptiform discharges, often with triphasic morphology (such as those highlighted in the boxes).

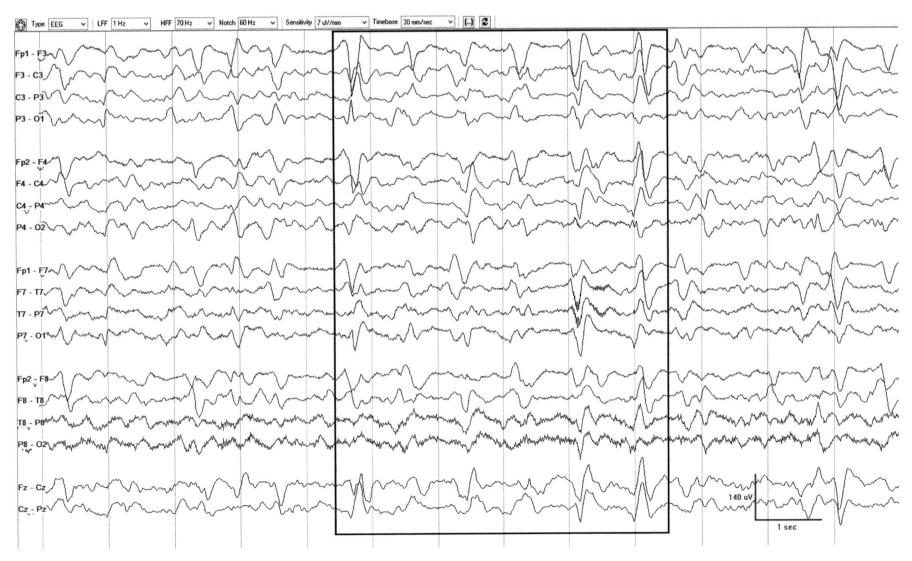

Figure 6.26. (*Continued*) (c) Later again in the record, the generalized discharges have now become more prevalent, higher amplitude and sometimes periodic at ~1 Hz (GPDs with shifting laterality) (box).

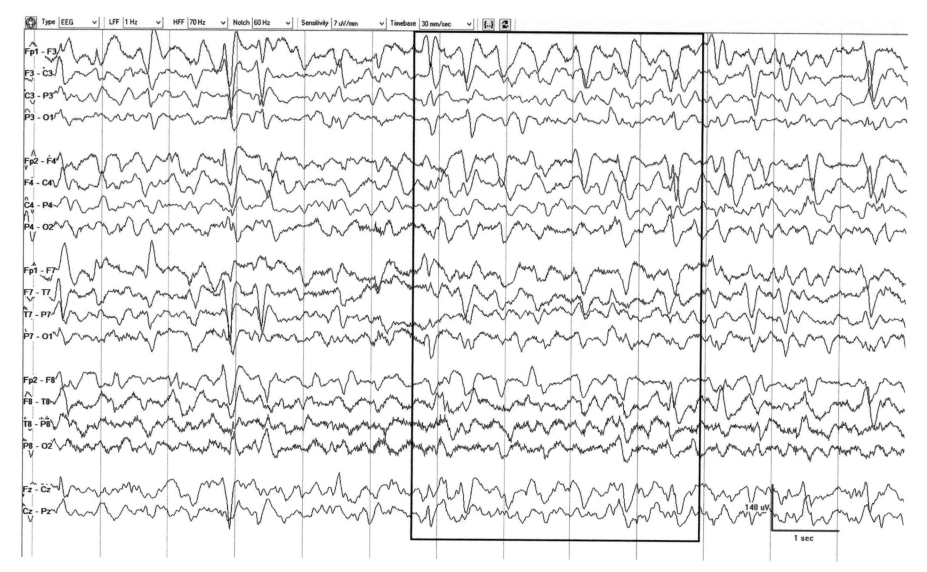

Figure 6.26. (*Continued*) (d) Later again in the record, the GPDs have further increased in prevalence and increased in frequency to 1.5 Hz (box). The pattern does not qualify as an ESz or ESE, but clearly the final panel is more 'ictal-appearing' than the first. In this patient these changes (from Figures 6.26b to 6.26d) occurred over 48 hours, with the EEG very gradually becoming more and more epileptiform.

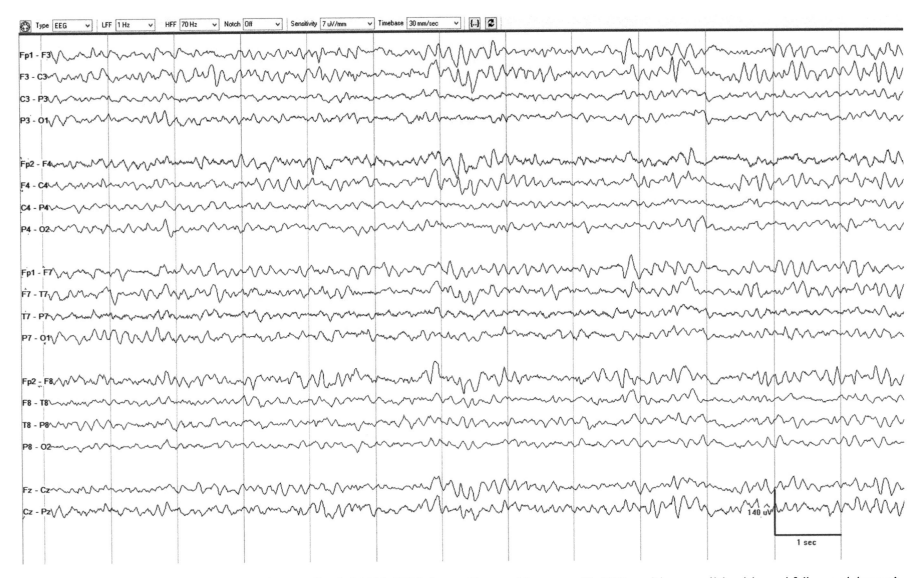

Figure 6.27. Ictal-interictal continuum (IIC), generalized. (a) This EEG is from a 71-year-old woman with ANCA positive vasculitis with renal failure and dementia. Upon commencing the EEG there was mild diffuse dysfunction.

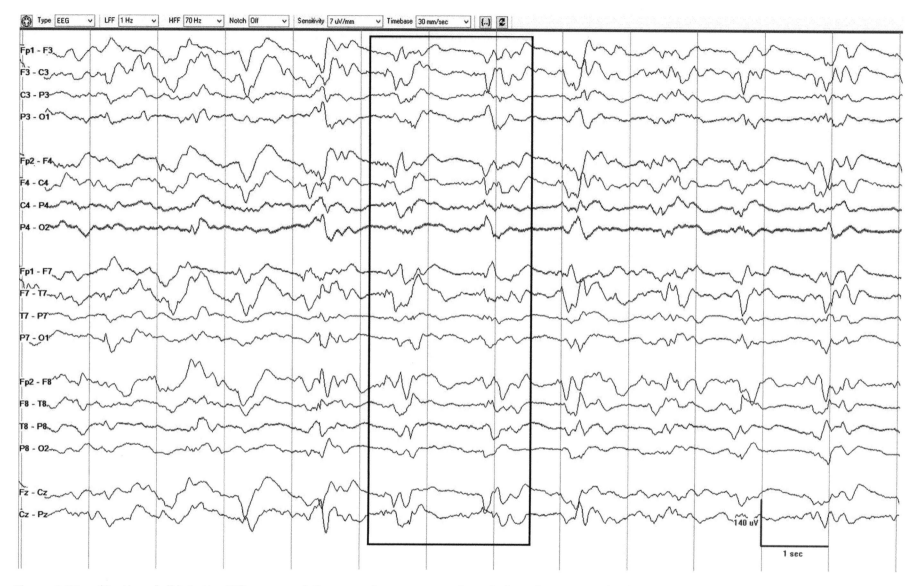

Figure 6.27. (*Continued*) (b) As the EEG progressed there was the emergence of poorly formed 1-Hz GPDs (such as the two highlighted in the box).

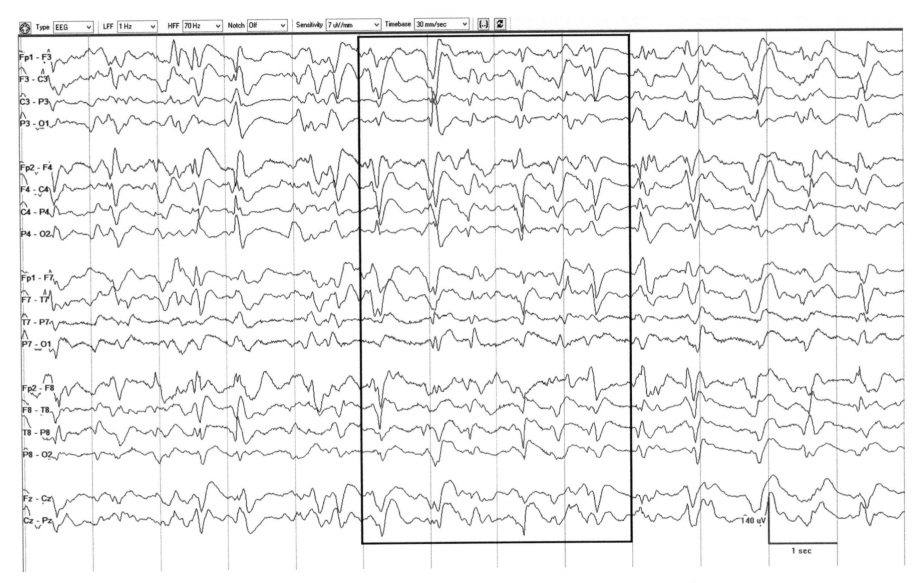

Figure 6.27.   (*Continued*) (c) With stimulation, these GPDs became higher voltage and faster, now mostly 1.5 Hz (SI-GPDs).

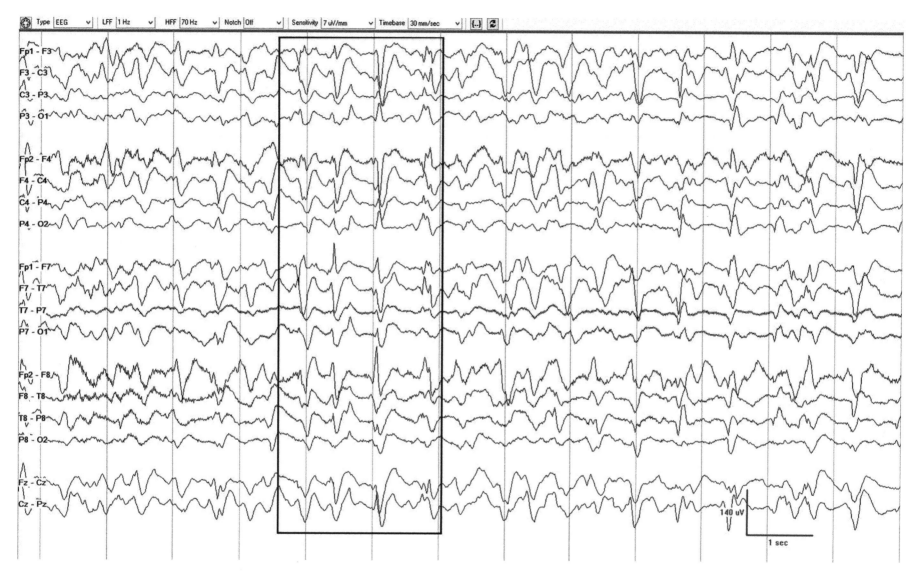

Figure 6.27. *(Continued)* (d) With any stimulation later in the record, there were long periods where the GPDs would consistently reach 2 Hz (such as those in the box [2 discharges per second]). If the pattern was >2.5 Hz for ≥10 seconds then it would qualify as an ESz, and if continuous for ≥10 minutes it would qualify as ESE. However, because this pattern does not reach 2.5 Hz, the pattern cannot be called an electrographic seizure (but is close to being one). There is a real continuum between an EEG that is clearly not ictal (Figure 6.27a) that does not have any epileptiform findings, and this panel, clearly highly epileptiform and potentially ictal, but not qualifying as definite seizure. There is no clear-cut point along this spectrum where it is known that the pattern can be contributing to clinical signs or further neuronal injury, and this concept is defined by the IIC. For patterns such as this one, we usually suggest a non-sedating IV anti-seizure medication trial to see if clinical status improves.

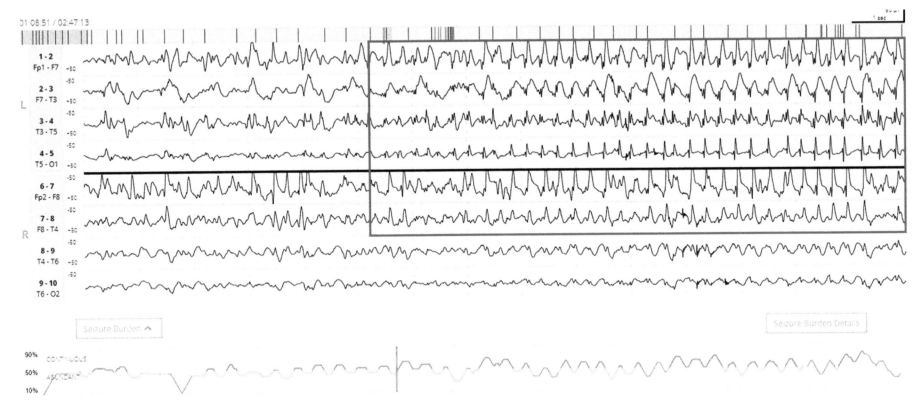

Figure 6.28. Rapid-response EEG. This EEG is from a 71-year-old woman with a meningioma and epilepsy that presented with seizures and persistent encephalopathy. A rapid-response EEG (rrEEG) was placed (a belt-like device placed around the head), taking ~5 minutes to apply and begin EEG recording. The top 4 channels represent the left temporal derivations, and the next 4 channels (below the line) the right temporal chain. At the bottom of the page is an automated seizure burden (% of rolling 5-minute window that consists of potential seizure activity) with the teal vertical line indicating time of the current page of EEG. There is an evolving ictal rhythm that is greatest in the left hemisphere but extending to the anterior channels on the right (all in the red box), and the seizure burden (often above 50%) indicates electrographic status epilepticus (ESE). The limitation of rrEEG in this case is that the seizure is poorly localized; for example, it could have started or could be maximal in the central region (where there are no electrodes), but these limitations are largely overshadowed by the significant benefit of detecting definite seizures and status epilepticus very early, allowing prompt treatment and potentially improving outcomes.

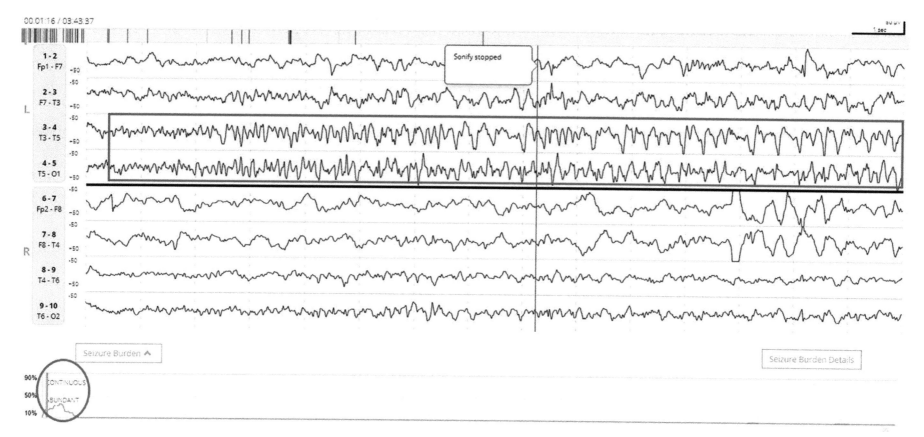

Figure 6.29. Rapid-response EEG. This EEG is from a 69-year-old woman with post-traumatic epilepsy. She presented with convulsive status epilepticus where the convulsion was stopped with lorazepam and levetiracetam loading. The patient remained sedated, and thus an urgent EEG was indicated. A rapid-response EEG was performed at the bedside in the emergency room, and demonstrated 12 seizures in the first 20 minutes, occupying about 1/3 of the record, sufficient to qualify as electrographic status epilepticus (ESE); one seizure captured in the first two minutes is shown here. The evolving seizure in the left posterior quadrant is highlighted (red box). A clinician listened to this page via the sonification feature (conversion of the EEG into sound), as noted in the small box near the top-middle stating when sonification stopped. The seizure burden indicator at the bottom of the page demonstrates that this rapid alerting of clinicians lead to prompt treatment. After the initial seizure burden of up to 40% (red ellipse in lower left of the figure, with the teal vertical line showing the timing of the raw EEG page shown above it), there are no further seizures for the rest of the record; subsequent full montage cEEG demonstrated left LRDA without seizures.

7 Artifacts that can mimic seizures or other physiologic patterns

A major problem in critical care EEG performance and interpretation is the proper identification and elimination, when possible, of artifacts. EEGs performed in the ICU are often contaminated by artifacts arising from monitoring equipment, life support systems and personnel. From the viewpoint of an electroencephalographer or technologist, an artifact may be defined as any recorded signal not originating in the brain. Artifacts are not always undesirable and physiological artifacts frequently provide clinically useful information, such as eye movements, including nystagmus, muscle artifact, tremors, body movements, respiration artifact and EKG.

Artifacts do need to be properly identified. Sherlockian deduction and reasoning are helpful in interpreting EEGs; however, there are many artifacts that may appear identical or very similar to cerebral discharges. The ideal time to answer the question as to whether the activity being recorded is cerebral or artifact is during the recording, though this is often not possible with prolonged monitoring. The use of additional electrodes, the monitoring of the electrocardiogram (EKG), movements (e.g., body, tongue and eye), respiration and the temporary disconnection of other equipment may be needed to identify the non-cerebral origin of such activity. Failure to properly identify artifacts may have serious consequences. For example, misinterpretation of artifact as spikes or seizures may lead to misdiagnosis and inappropriate treatment.

Artifacts may be divided into two groups: (1) physiological and (2) nonphysiological. At times, there is an overlap between these two categories.

Physiological artifacts originate in the body but outside the brain. They include:

(1) Ocular – eye movement, eyelid flutter, nystagmus, electroretinogram (ERG)

(2) Muscle

(3) Sweat

(4) Tongue and mouth – glossokinetic potentials, sobbing, chewing, dissimilar metals, palatal myoclonus

(5) Vascular – EKG, pulse, cardioballistic artifact, pacemaker

(6) Movement – tremor, respiration, facial, extremities, nursing care, physical exams (discussed in the non-physiologic section below)

(7) Skull defect (already discussed in Chapter 4: Focal abnormalities; e.g., Figures 4.13–4.17).

The eyeballs and eyelids are factors in the production of eye movement artifact. The former acts as a dipole with the cornea being positive with respect to the retina. With eye closure or blinking, the eyeball rotates upward (Bell's phenomenon) briefly, and the field of the strong corneal positivity involves the electrodes that are closest on the forehead (Fp1 and Fp2). Hence these electrodes become surface positive. The reverse is true with downward eye

Hirsch and Brenner's Atlas of EEG in Critical Care, Second Edition. Lawrence J. Hirsch, Michael W.K. Fong, and Richard P. Brenner.
© 2023 John Wiley & Sons Ltd. Published 2023 by John Wiley & Sons Ltd.

movement. Vertical eye movements are always maximal in the Fp1 and Fp2 electrodes and, therefore, the voltage gradient of this potential will often indicate its source. That is, if the activity is not greatest in Fp1 and Fp2 it cannot be a vertical eye movement. The converse, however, is not always true; some cerebral potentials may be maximal in the Fp1 and Fp2 electrodes. In order to resolve this difficulty, the simplest solution is to place additional electrodes below the eyes. Vertical eye movements will be out of phase when comparing superior (Fp1 and Fp2) and inferior orbital (LIO and RIO) electrodes referred to ipsilateral ear, while frontal slowing of cerebral origin will be in phase. There are some artifacts, such as a glossokinetic potentials (tongue movements), which can be mistaken for frontal or temporal slowing. This potential will be in phase between the superior and inferior orbital electrodes, and of higher voltage in the inferior orbital electrodes, which are closer to the tongue. Further monitoring of glossokinetic artifact is discussed later. Lateral eye movements are maximal in the F7 and F8 electrodes and are of opposite polarity (assuming conjugate gaze). Additional electrodes placed at the outer canthus of the eyes and referred to ipsilateral ear may help further delineate this activity since these electrodes (LOC, ROC) are closer to the source. It is standard to place eye leads by the right upper canthus and the left lower canthus (RUC, LLC); in that manner, all conjugate eye movements, horizontal or vertical, will be out of phase at those two diagonally-opposite locations (one is above the eyes, the other below; and one is to the left, the other the right). Eye movement artifacts are also discussed in Chapter 1: EEG basics, e.g., Figures 1.7, 1.9 and 1.12.

An electroretinogram (ERG) – low voltage electrical signals generated in the retina – can be seen in some normal individuals if the Fp1 and Fp2 electrodes are used during photic stimulation. However, this artifact is most often seen in patients with cerebral death. In part this is due to the increased sensitivities employed in such recordings, as well as the absence of cerebral potentials. It does not invalidate the diagnosis of electrocerebral inactivity (ECI) or cerebral death, if other criteria are met. Eyelid flutter is also maximal in the Fp1 and Fp2 electrodes and often not well detected with infraorbital electrodes. At times, rapid eyelid flutter or nystagmus can give rise to confusion if not properly identified. In patients with a prosthetic eye or third nerve palsy, unilateral eye movement artifact may be mistaken for focal frontal delta activity. It is not unusual for a unilateral upgaze palsy (sometimes related to dysfunction of cranial nerve III) to be detected by the EEGer via asymmetric blink artifact.

Muscle artifact is common in routine EEG recordings. Getting the patient more relaxed, if possible, is the best way to reduce this artifact. Occasionally the artifact can be unilateral, persist in sleep, and if severe, can obscure underlying cerebral potentials. Shivering artifact during therapeutic hypothermia is a common source of continuous prominent muscle artifact, even when shivering is not obvious on clinical observation (sometimes called 'micro-shivering'). The use of the high-frequency filter (HFF) to reduce this activity can lead to difficulties in interpretation. For example, prominent muscle artifact may appear as beta activity when a HFF of 15 Hz is employed (avoid lowering the HFF that much!), or muscle spikes may be misinterpreted as epileptiform at this filter setting. The same is true of isolated muscle spikes seen with eye movements, particularly in the anterior temporal electrodes (F7 and F8), where lateral rectus spikes are commonly seen. There are commercially available modules, often as part of quantitative EEG measures, which have algorithms in place to assist with digital removal of muscle artifact. When it is critical to know if there is or is not cerebral activity underlying EMG artifact, such as with large myoclonic jerks in postanoxic coma, paralytics are occasionally recommended to allow definitive interpretation of the underlying EEG.

Artifacts from tongue and mouth movements may be misinterpreted. The tongue acts as a dipole with the tip being surface negative and the base positive. Tongue movements in some patients will result in a prominent burst of slow waves, which may have a widespread distribution but are usually maximal anteriorly. If the technologist is aware of this, the artifact can easily be reproduced by having the awake patient say 'Tom Thumb' or 'lilt'. If that is not effective, performing vertical and/or lateral tongue movements may reproduce the pattern. This type of artifact can resemble a 'projected' rhythm or frontal intermittent rhythmic delta activity (FIRDA). Unfortunately, glossokinetic artifact can occur in patients who are confused and lethargic who may also have anterior frontal slowing that is cerebral. To help resolve this, additional electrodes can be placed above and below the mouth and slightly off-center in opposite directions on either side. A bipolar derivation from these perioral electrodes (above the mouth on one side and below the mouth on the other) will display this artifact clearly.

Perspiration or sweat artifact is a long-duration potential (commonly lasting a few seconds) that usually involves several electrodes. Although the use of a short time constant (i.e., a higher low frequency filter [LFF] setting) will eliminate this artifact, it will also affect slow frequency cerebral activity. Therefore, this is not recommended, but rather one should try to decrease the sweating by cooling the head, applying alcohol or an antiperspirant to the area and having adequate air conditioning.

EKG artifact is usually recognized by its regular, stereotyped appearance, and by comparing to a dedicated channel for chest recording. It is best seen on montages employing the ipsilateral ear as a reference and is less noticeable in bipolar montages or in referential recordings using Cz as a reference. Occasionally, irregular beats may be mistaken for cerebral potentials, or the coincidental coupling of an EKG artifact and a slow wave may give rise to the appearance of a spike-and-wave complex. Cardiac activity is best monitored by placing two additional electrodes on the chest and recording between them (to record cardiac potentials only, not a combination of cerebral and cardiac). The ear electrodes should not be used because they may record temporal spikes as well as the EKG. Occasionally EKG complexes may be mistaken for lambda waves.

Pulse artifact can be mistaken for focal delta activity. This artifact is due to the movement of an electrode due to pulsation of an artery under it and is time-locked to the QRS complex. It usually occurs approximately 200 msec after the R wave (the estimated time taken for a systolic contraction of the heart to send a pulse of blood to a scalp vessel). Another way of thinking of it is that it usually aligns roughly with the T wave. A similar but more widespread artifact is seen in comatose patients, including cerebral death recordings, which is due to movement of electrodes, electrode wires, or the head from the mechanical 'recoil' effect of the beating heart (cardioballistic artifact). A pacemaker artifact is cardiac-related and results in 'spikes' that will be intermittent or regular, depending on the type of pacemaker.

There are a wide variety of movement artifacts affecting the EEG. These include head tremors, body tremors that passively move the head, and body movements. The tremor can often be monitored with additional electrodes.

Muscle and movement artifact are often prominent in patients having psychogenic nonepileptic seizures. Rhythmic activity in the occipital regions due to head movement can be eliminated by raising the patient's head from the bed. Facial movement, such as during a focal motor seizure, hemifacial spasm, facial myokymia or facial synkinesias, can result in muscle artifact.

Nonphysiological artifacts include:

(1) electrodes – disc, wire, connection, jackbox, placement

(2) external sources – 60 Hz, electrostatic, ICU equipment

(3) instrumentation – amplifier, settings, cables

(4) patient care – chest percussion, cleaning patient, suctioning

An electrode 'pop' is a common occurrence in any recording and will appear in all channels of the montage in which that electrode is present, but no others. An electrode pop occurs when there is an abrupt change in the electrical potential between the electrode and the scalp, which results in a sudden-onset, high voltage, usually positive (but occasionally negative) discharge, similar to the potential when a capacitor is discharged. An electrode artifact can occur intermittently or occasionally can be regular or even seemingly evolving (e.g., as an electrode is falling off the scalp). Findings limited to a single electrode should be viewed with suspicion and assumed to be artifact until proven otherwise. The use of an additional electrode placed next to the one in question can indicate whether the discharge is cerebral or artifact, if simple measures such as filling or replacing the electrode, etc., has not eliminated it. Electrodes with high impedance, usually due to poor electrical contact with the scalp, are more prone to show artifact, and unequal resistances frequently result in 60 Hz artifact. The electrode problem may be with the disc itself, but can also involve the wire, its connections or the jackbox into which the wire is plugged. Occasionally, one can get a ground electrode recording artifact without 60 Hz interference. The type of artifact seen will depend on the location of the ground electrode. In addition to ensuring low (<10 kohms) and relatively equal impedances (never >5 kohms difference between any two electrodes), accurate placement of electrodes is crucial to good recording technique, and a spurious asymmetry may result from inaccurate placement.

Of the external sources of artifacts, 60 Hz is the most common. Although often encountered routinely in the laboratory, it can become a difficult problem in the ICU. Here, judicious disconnection of various equipment is often required to eliminate the artifact. Sixty Hz artifact is not necessarily bad since it often indicates electrode problems. Furthermore, the indiscriminate use of 60 Hz 'notch' filter will make recognition of electrode artifact more difficult; one should read without a notch filter on whenever possible. Artifacts may result from electrostatic interference. This often occurs with movement of persons in the vicinity of the patient and is most common in the ICU. Another artifact, which is rare, is due to an intravenous infusion and is also probably electrostatic in origin. There are a variety of instrumentation artifacts and include those due to an amplifier, settings (filters, sensitivity) and cables.

During prolonged EEG monitoring when a technologist is not present throughout the recording, there are many other artifacts. The most troublesome are those that cause rhythmic artifact that can mimic seizures, such as patting and chest percussion by respiratory therapists or bed oscillators. Recording video is very helpful for the quick and accurate identification of these artifacts.

Thus, there are multiple causes of artifact, both of a physiological and non-physiological nature, and these need to be recognized by both the technologist and the electroencephalographer. They may not always be able to be eliminated, but they must be properly identified and proven, when in doubt, at the time of the recording.

Figure list

Figure 7.1 Facial twitching artifact mimicking LPDs.

Figure 7.2 Widespread muscle artifact.

Figure 7.3 Muscle artifact from shivering.

Figure 7.4 Muscle artifact mimicking cerebral activity.

Figure 7.5 Muscle artifact vs. cerebral activity.

Figure 7.6 Artifact from shivering and myoclonus (effect of filtering and artifact reduction algorithms).

Figure 7.7 Muscle artifact misinterpreted due to over-filtering.

Figure 7.8 Muscle artifact obscuring epileptiform discharges (effect of artifact reduction algorithms).

Figure 7.9 Chewing artifact.

Figure 7.10 Sweat artifact.

Figure 7.11 Electrode artifact.

Figure 7.12 Snore artifact.

Figure 7.13 Dialysis artifact.

Figure 7.14 Pulse artifact and electrode artifact.

Figure 7.15 Cardioballistic artifact.

Figure 7.16 Ocular bobbing.

Figure 7.17 Vertical nystagmus.

Figure 7.18 Ventilator artifact.

Figure 7.19 Ventilator artifact.

Figure 7.20 Chest percussion artifact.

Figure 7.21 Chest percussion artifact mimicking seizure.

Figure 7.22 'Pseudoalpha' from oscillator artifact.

Figure 7.23 Stimulus-induced electroclinical seizure (SI-ECSz) from oscillator artifact.

Figure 7.24 Glossokinetic artifact.

Figure 7.25 Glossokinetic artifact.

Figure 7.26 Glossokinetic artifact mimicking GRDA.

Figure 7.27 'Virtual' or disconnected patient.

Figure 7.28 'Virtual' or disconnected patient.

EEGs throughout this atlas have been shown with the following standard recording parameters unless otherwise specified: LFF 1 Hz, HFF 70 Hz, notch filter off.

Suggested reading

Barlow JS. Automatic elimination of electrode-pop artifacts in EEGs. *IEEE Trans Biomed Eng.* 1986;**33**(5):517–521.

Cobb WA, Guiloff RJ, Cast J. Breach rhythm: the EEG related to skull defects. *Electroencephalogr Clin Neurophysiol* 1979;**47**:251–271.

Gaspard N, Hirsch LJ. Pitfalls in ictal EEG interpretation: critical care and intracranial recordings. *Neurology.* 2013 Jan 1;**80**(1 Suppl 1):S26–S42

Klass DW. The continuing challenge of artifacts in the EEG. *Am J EEG Technol* 1995;**35**:239–269.

Rampal N, Maciel CM, Hirsch LJ. EEG and artifact in the intensive care unit. In: Tatum WO, ed. *Atlas of Artifact in Clinical Neurophysiology.* Springer Publishing Company, 2019;59–94.

Reilly EL. EEG recording and operation of the apparatus. In: Niedermeyer E, Lopes de Silva F, eds. *Electroencephalography: Basic principles, clinical applications and related fields.* Philadelphia: Lippincott, Williams and Wilkins, 2005; 167–192.

Tyner FS, Knott JR, Mayer WB Jr., Artifacts. In: *Fundamentals of EEG Technology*, Volume 1, New York, Raven Press, 1983:280–311.

Westmoreland BF, Espinosa RE, Klass DW. Significant prosopo-glossopharyyngeal movements affecting the electroencephalogram. *Am J EEG Technol* 1973;**13**:59–70

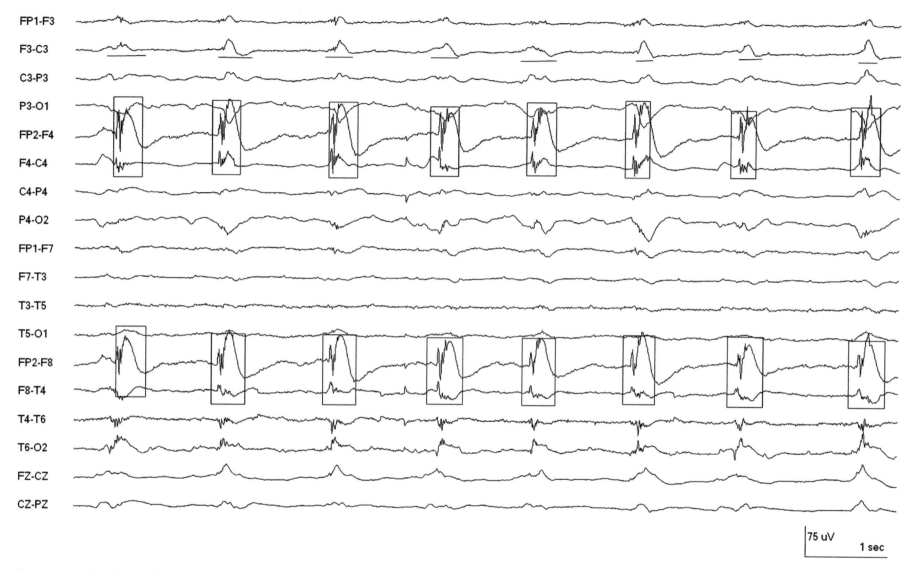

Figure 7.1. Facial twitching artifact mimicking LPDs. (a) The EEG in this 39-year-old woman shows periodic spike-wave- or polyspike-wave-like potentials over the right hemisphere (boxes). Lower voltage periodic slow waves (blunt LPDs) are present on the left (underlined).

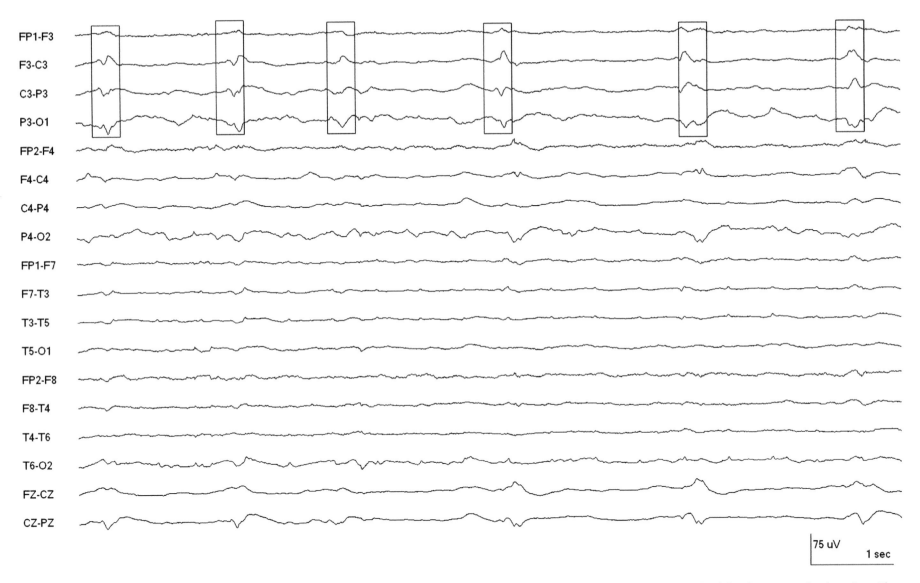

Figure 7.1. (*Continued*) (b) Following the administration of vecuronium (a paralytic), the right-sided 'spikes' are no longer present. They were due to muscle artifact associated with twitching movements on the right side of the face. The movements were associated with the low voltage LPDs present over the left hemisphere (now in boxes), maximal in the parasagittal region. Thus, the left LPDs were cerebral in origin, and ictal in this case (even though they have a blunt morphology), representing focal motor status epilepticus, but the right 'LPDs' were muscle artifact.

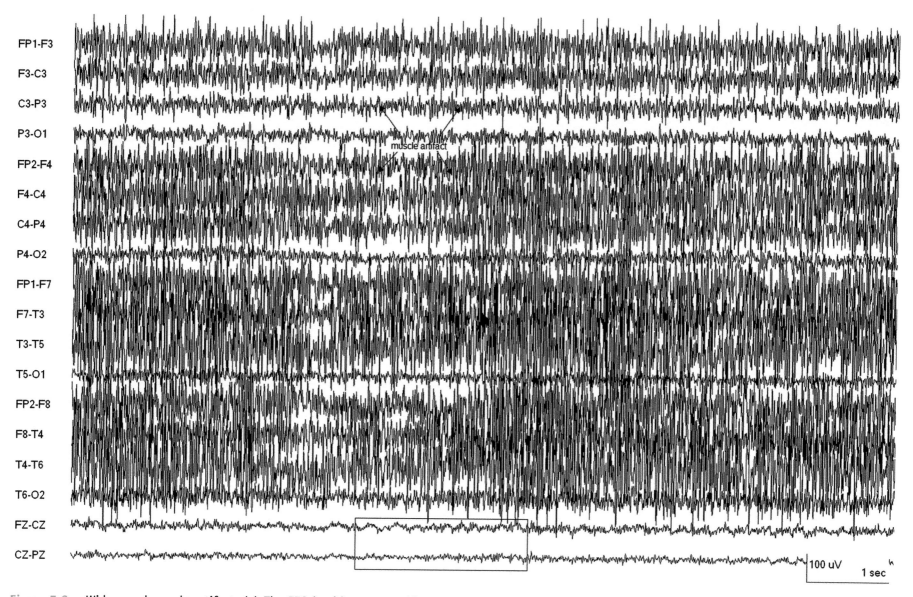

Figure 7.2. Widespread muscle artifact. (a) The EEG in this 25-year-old woman s/p cardiac arrest shows muscle artifact in a widespread distribution. Note the relative sparing of this activity in the midline derivations, the channels least likely to show muscle artifact.

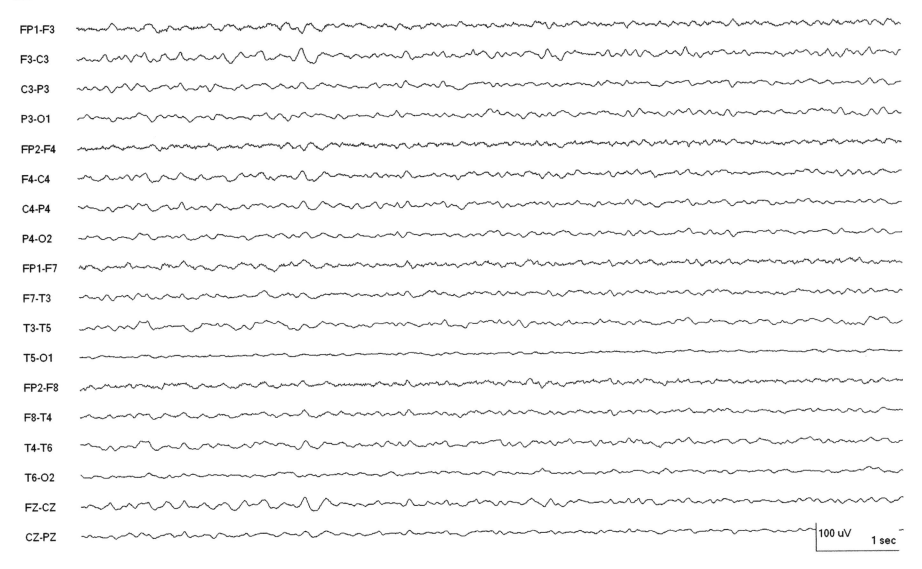

Figure 7.2.   (*Continued*) (b) Following the administration of vecuronium, muscle artifact disappears. Background EEG can now be seen, predominantly in the theta and alpha range in a widespread distribution.

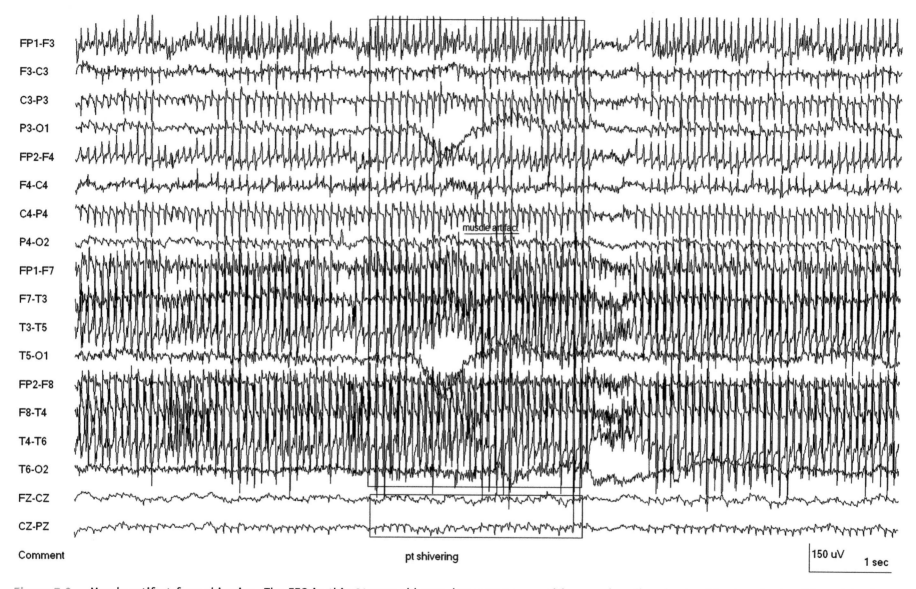

Figure 7.3. Muscle artifact from shivering. The EEG in this 61-year-old man demonstrates repetitive muscle spikes due to shivering. Again, this activity is not well represented in the midline derivations, as is typical of muscle artifact.

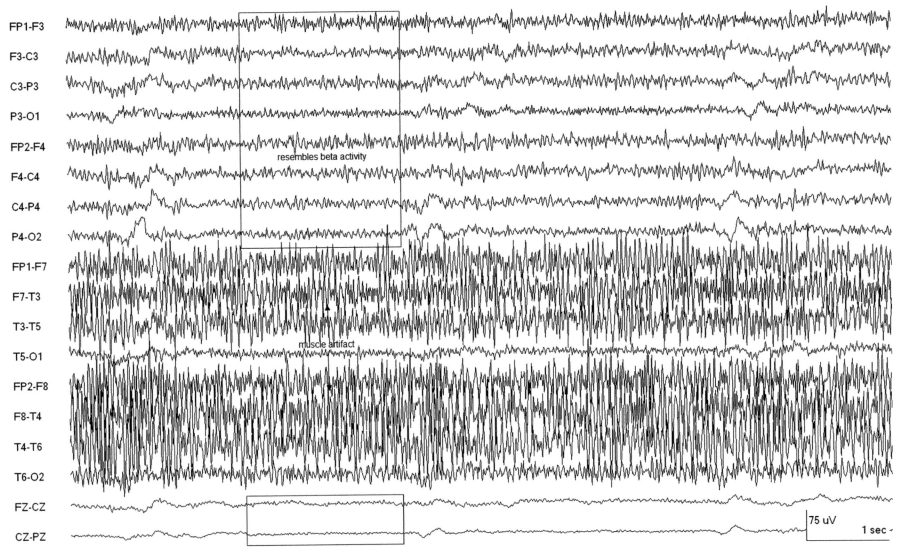

Figure 7.4.   Muscle artifact mimicking cerebral activity. (a) The EEG in this 77-year-old woman s/p revision of a right frontal craniotomy shows muscle artifact that is prominent in the temporal areas. There appears to be beta activity (the high-frequency filter was 70 Hz) in the parasagittal regions. However, this activity is not well seen in the midline derivations (Fz-Cz and Cz-Pz), suggesting that it is more likely to be muscle artifact, rather than beta activity.

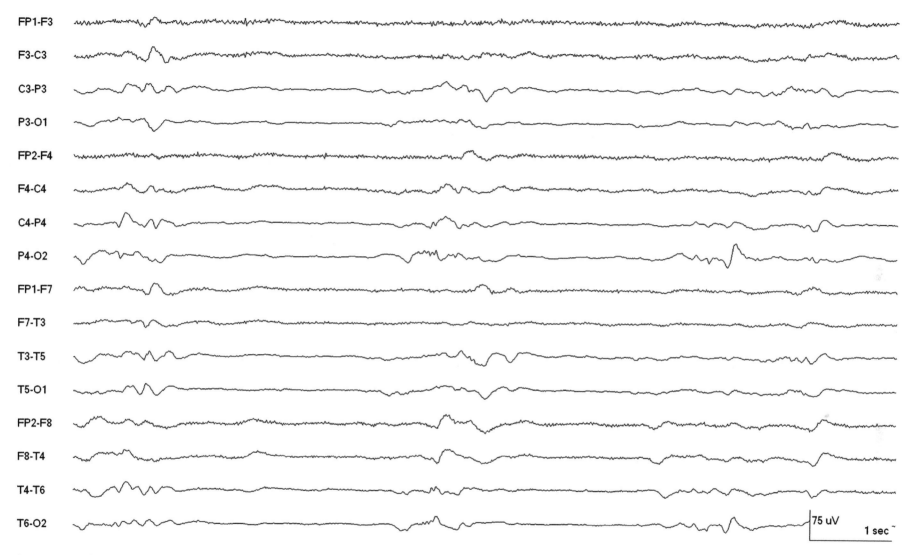

Figure 7.4. (*Continued*) (b) Following the administration of vecuronium, a low voltage burst-suppression pattern, previously largely obscured by muscle artifact, is now much more apparent.

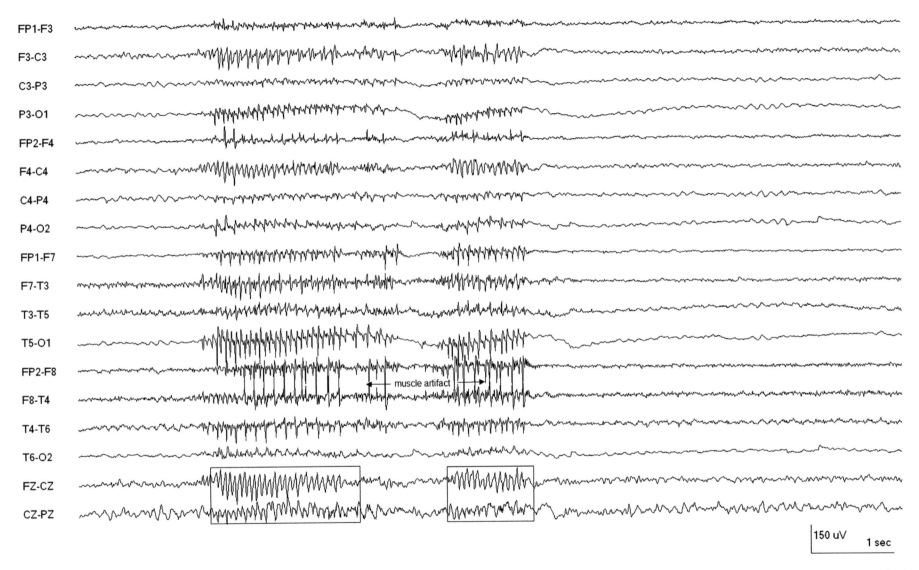

Figure 7.5. Muscle artifact vs. cerebral activity. The EEG in this 60-year-old man, being evaluated for a confusional state, shows muscle artifact, most marked in the right temporal region. However, there is also fast activity best represented in the midline derivations (boxes), strongly suggesting that there is a cerebral discharge as well. In fact, he was having tonic seizures with paroxysmal fast activity as the ictal EEG correlate (a rare seizure type at this age).

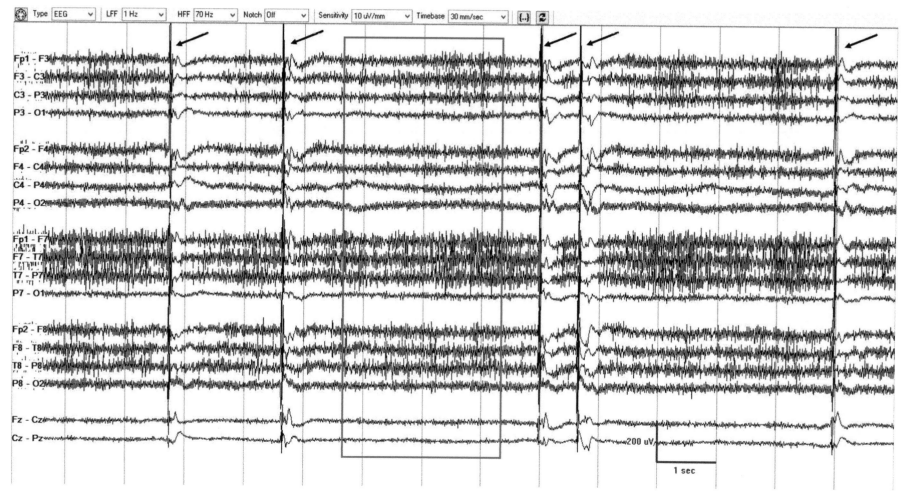

Figure 7.6. Artifact from shivering and myoclonus (effect of filtering and artifact reduction algorithms). (a) This EEG is from a 59-year-old man post cardiac arrest with clinical myoclonus receiving targeted temperature management (TTM) causing shivering. At commencement of the EEG there is prominent EMG activity from shivering (red box). In addition, there are also discrete very high voltage (note the sensitivity of 10 μV/mm) spikes of EMG activity from repetitive face, head and upper torso myoclonic jerking (arrows).

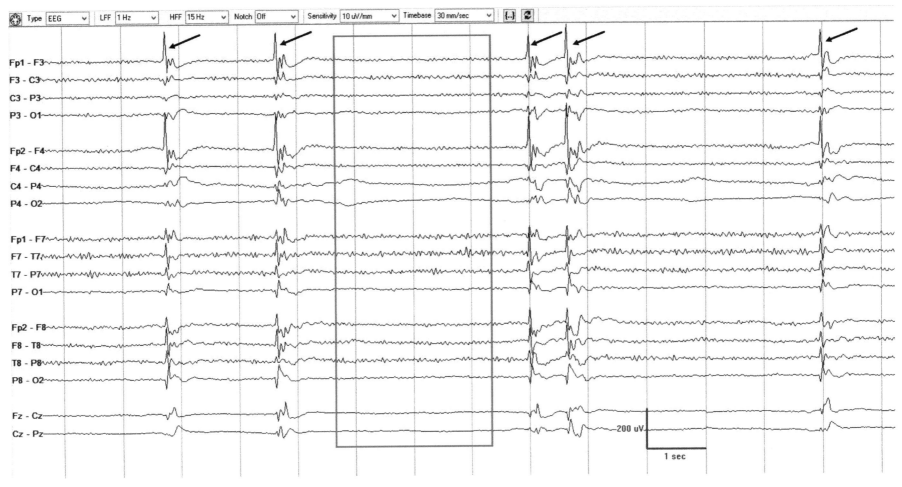

Figure 7.6. (*Continued*) (b) The same page of EEG with the high-frequency filter inappropriately reduced aggressively to 15 Hz. The effect is important to recognize. The EEG looks too clean and if this is not recognized it is possible to mistake heavily filtered artifact as cerebral (red box). The result of the 15-Hz HFF on the spikes are that they now appear cerebral and epileptiform (the filter removed much of the very fast muscle artifact and made it less sharp). In addition, the background appears to consist of beta activity from the brain, when is really just filtered muscle activity.

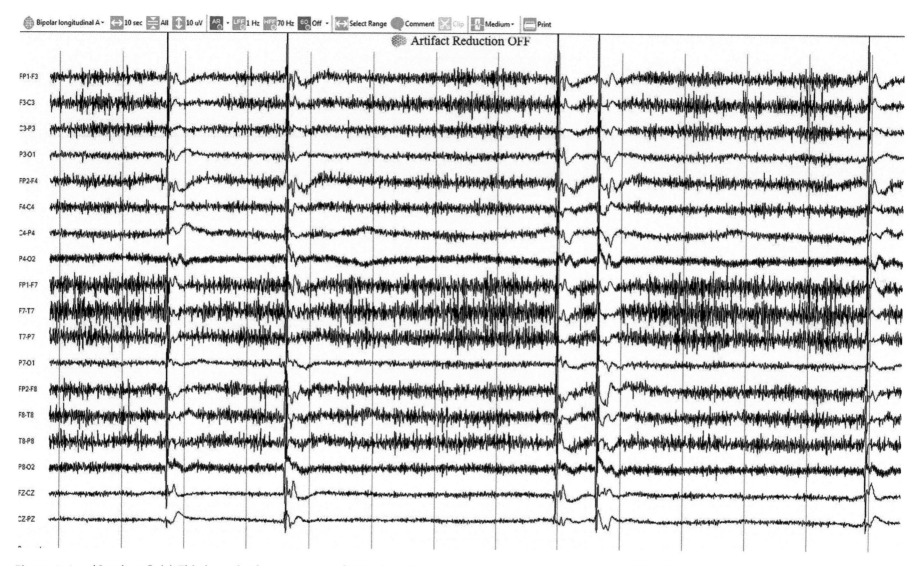

Figure 7.6. (*Continued*) (c) This is again the same page of EEG when the raw trace is viewed in a quantitative EEG software package. Note the 'artifact reduction' is off (labeled at the top of the page as AR with a red dot).

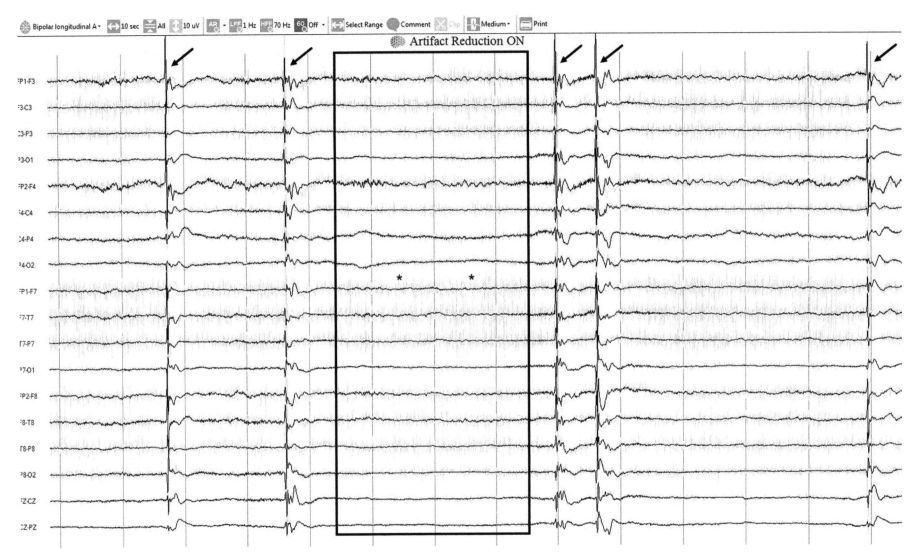

Figure 7.6. (*Continued*) (d) The same page of EEG with the artifact reduction turned on (AR with green dot). There are now a few commercially available algorithms that are designed to eliminate artifact (especially muscle and EKG artifact). The result of applying such an artifact reduction algorithm to this page of EEG is that it is better at determining muscle artifact and reducing it. The box highlights that artifact reduction has eliminated the EMG and suggests that there is no cerebral activity in between the high amplitude spiky discharges. The asterisks highlight the activity that has been 'rejected' in light or shaded out gray. Note the discharges still appear spiky even with the artifact reduction on, which suggests a possible cortical potential underlying the clinical myoclonus.

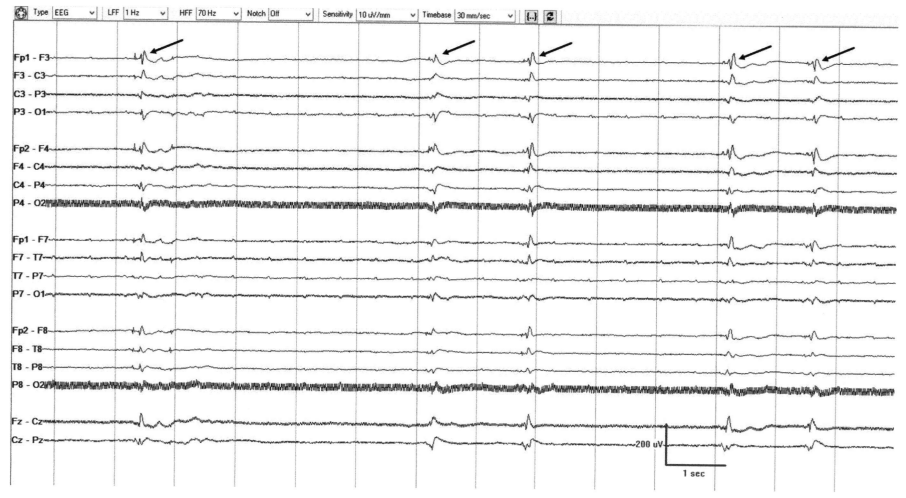

Figure 7.6. (*Continued*) (e) The 'true' EEG in patients with high amplitude muscle artifact (common with myoclonus) can only be seen with neuromuscular blockade, in this case following rocuronium. There is now 60 Hz (electrical) artifact at electrode O2. Neuromuscular blockade (given without sedation) confirms that the background EEG is suppressed. It also confirms a cerebral correlate to the myoclonus and demonstrates the true morphology of this cerebral activity. It was likely that clinical jerking was associated with medium voltage spiky GPDs, but most of the very high amplitude activity was actually from the EMG artifact associated with the myoclonus. This example highlights that there are several ways of attempting to see through artifact on an EEG (e.g., commonly with filters or artifact reduction software), but no method is perfect (all with potential pitfalls that need to be understood when applying these techniques) and none is a replacement for acquiring a high-quality recording at the time of recording.

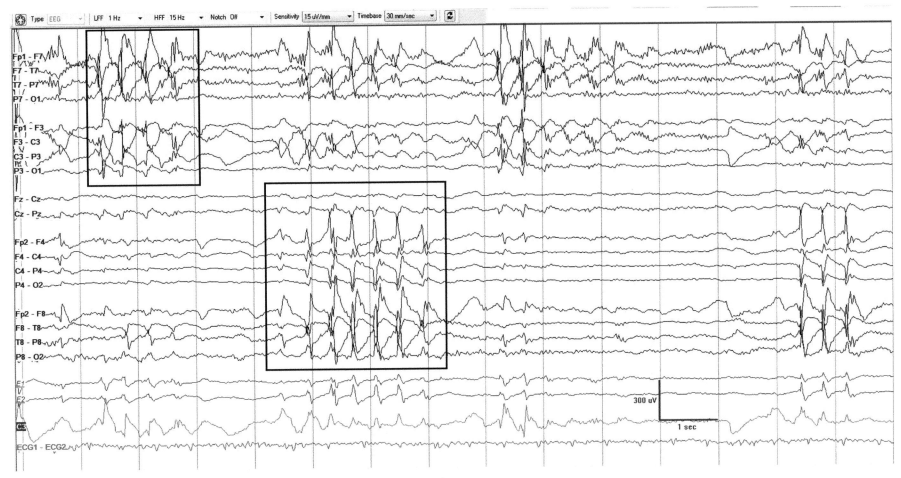

Figure 7.7. Muscle artifact misinterpreted due to over-filtering. (a) longitudinal bipolar, hemispheric left over right: This page of EEG appears to have runs of high voltage spikes occurring at ~2.5 Hz in left and right hemispheres (boxes).

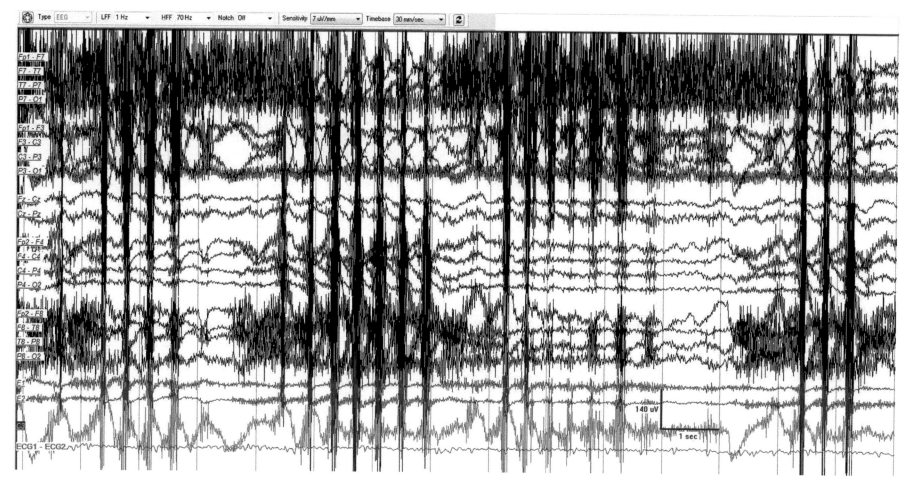

Figure 7.7. *(Continued)* (b) longitudinal bipolar, hemispheric left over right: The activity in Figure 7.7a was actually due to muscle artifact. The HFF had been erroneously set at 15 Hz, which mislead the EEGer. This is the same page with conventional filter settings (HFF 70 Hz).

Reproduced from Rampal N, Maciel CM, Hirsch LJ. EEG and Artifact in the Intensive Care Unit. In: Tatum WO, ed. Atlas of Artifact in Clinical Neurophysiology. Springer Publishing Company, 2019:59–94, with permission.

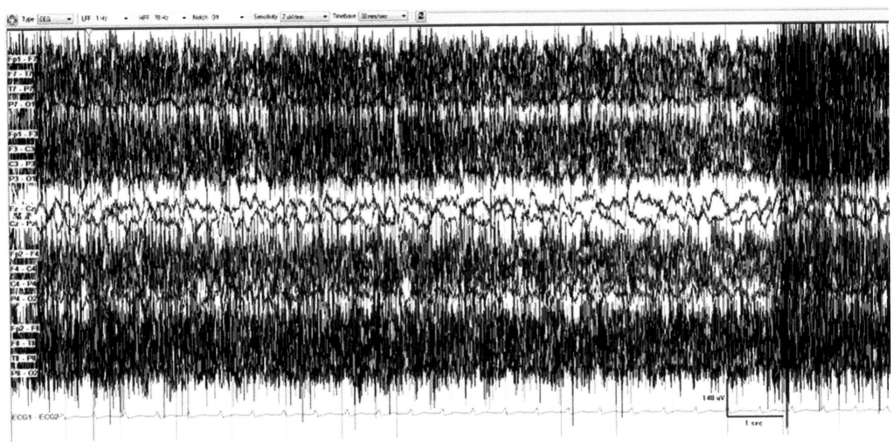

Figure 7.8. Muscle artifact obscuring epileptiform discharges (effect of artifact reduction algorithms). (a) longitudinal bipolar, hemispheric left over right: There is significant EMG artifact on this page that obscured most of the underlying cerebral rhythms.

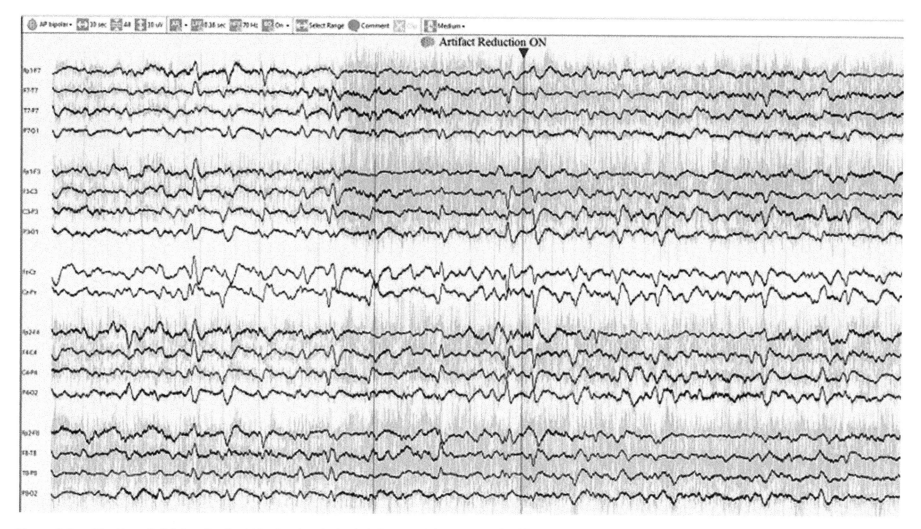

Figure 7.8. (*Continued*) (b) longitudinal bipolar, hemispheric left over right: The same page of EEG has undergone automated artifact reduction (labeled as artifact reduction ON at the top of the page). The EMG artifact has been removed and the EEG reveals moderate diffuse slowing with abundant (perhaps periodic) generalized epileptiform discharges, previously obscured by muscle artifact.

Reproduced from Rampal N, Maciel CM, Hirsch LJ. EEG and Artifact in the Intensive Care Unit. In: Tatum WO, ed. Atlas of Artifact in Clinical Neurophysiology. Springer Publishing Company, 2019:59–94. with permission.

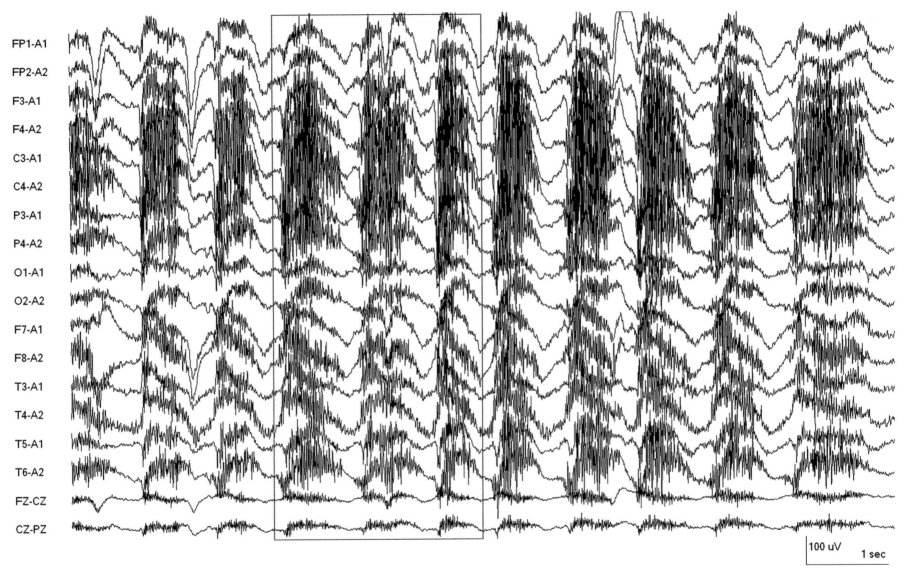

Figure 7.9. Chewing artifact. The EEG in this 41-year-old woman demonstrates repetitive muscle artifact that was due to chewing movements. Note the relative sparing of the midline derivations (bottom 2 channels).

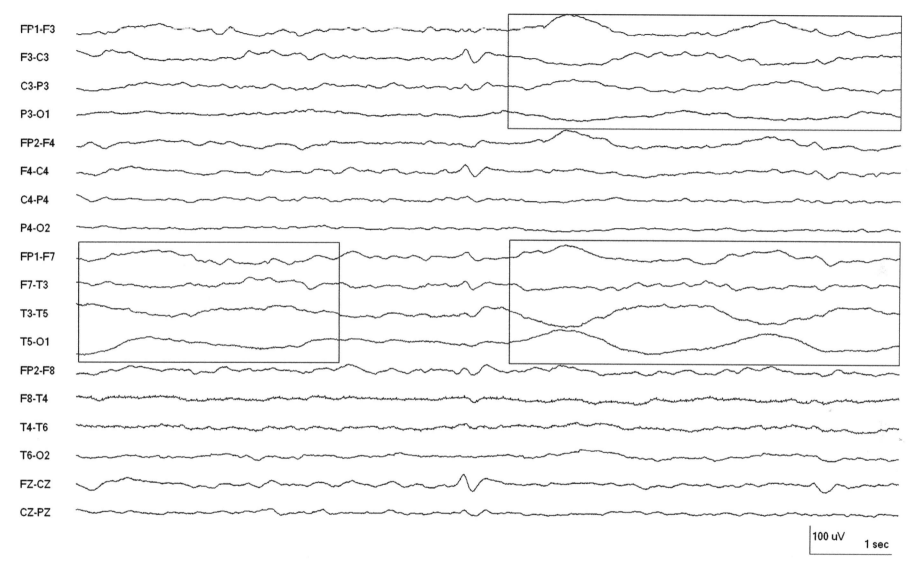

Figure 7.10. Sweat artifact. The EEG in this 66-year-old woman with possible metastatic carcinoma shows prominent slowing, particularly over the left hemisphere (boxes). This represents sweat artifact. Sweat artifact usually involves several electrodes and consists of very slow, irregular, delta activity, appearing as a wandering baseline. Delta slower than 1 Hz such as this is often either sweat artifact or slow roving horizontal eye movements seen during drowsiness.

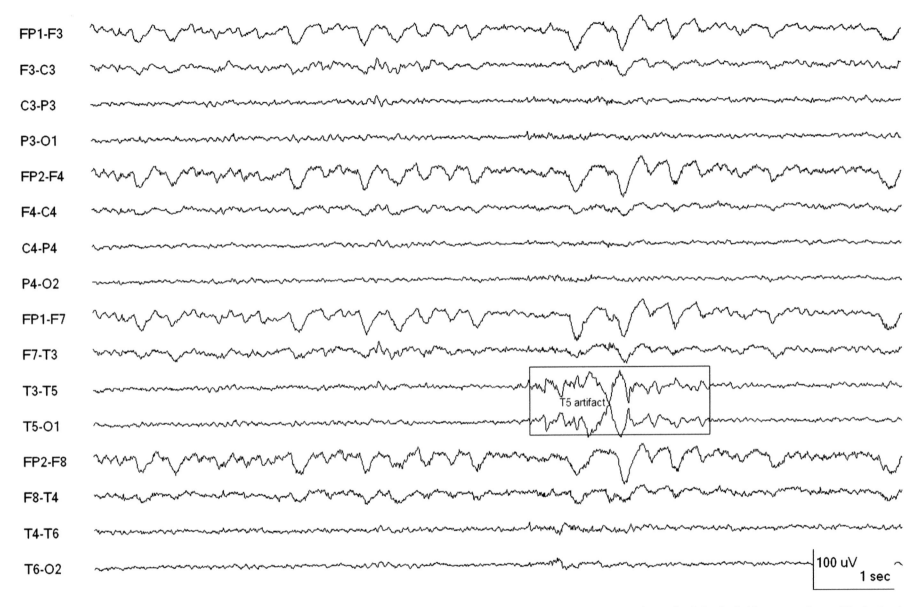

Figure 7.11. Electrode artifact. (a) Longitudinal bipolar. Eye blink or eye flutter artifact is prominent in Fp1 and Fp2 in this 24-year-old man (present in Fp1 and Fp2 derivations). In addition, in the seventh second, a sharp wave admixed with slow waves is present in the T3-T5 and T5-01 derivations (box). This has a mirror image appearance and no physiologic field, suggesting a T5 electrode artifact. There is no involvement at T3 or 01. Thus, the deflections are a mirror image of one another since the activity is purely at T5; it is mirrored because T5 is input 2 in the T3-T5 derivation but input 1 in the T5-01 derivation.

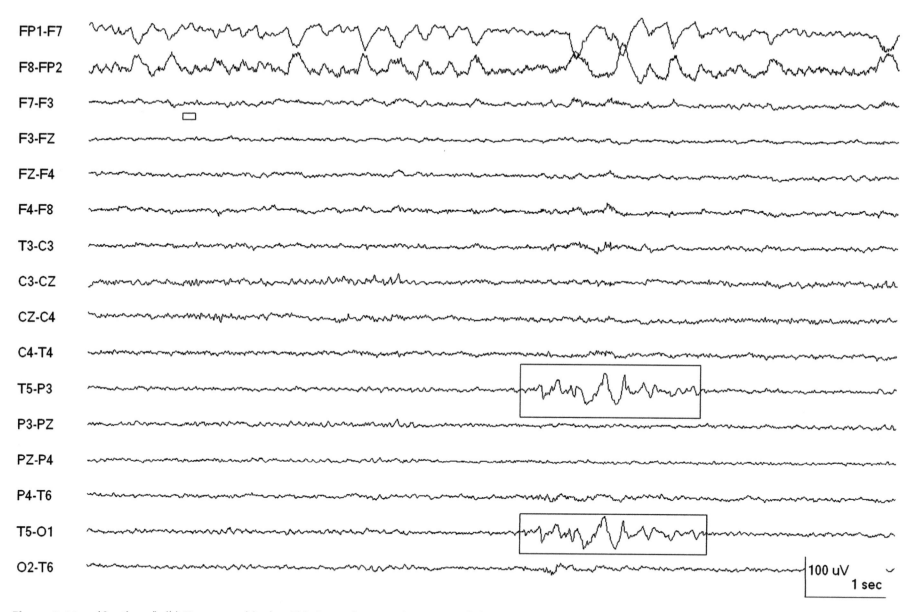

Figure 7.11. (*Continued*) (b) Transverse bipolar. This is a reformatted montage of the same epoch. Notice that the artifact (boxes) appears in all channels, and only those channels, which have electrode T5. The vertical eye movement artifacts from eye flutter are now at the top of the page, in the channels containing Fp1 and Fp2.

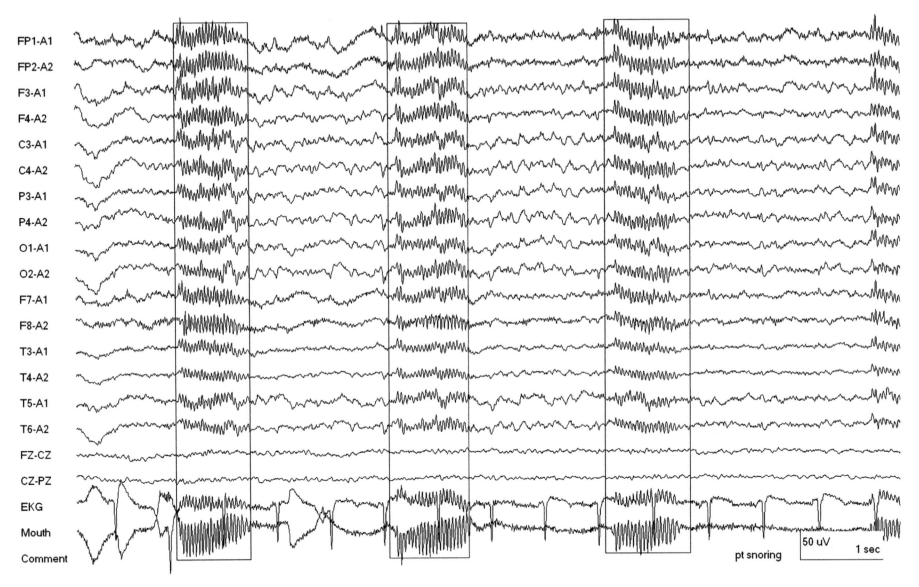

Figure 7.12. Snore artifact. The EEG in this 72-year-old man shows bursts of fast activity (approximately 25 Hz), present in a widespread distribution. The discharges, however, are not present in the midline electrodes, which usually are relatively free of artifact, are most prominent near the mouth, and seen in the EKG channel. This is an artifact and was due to snoring.

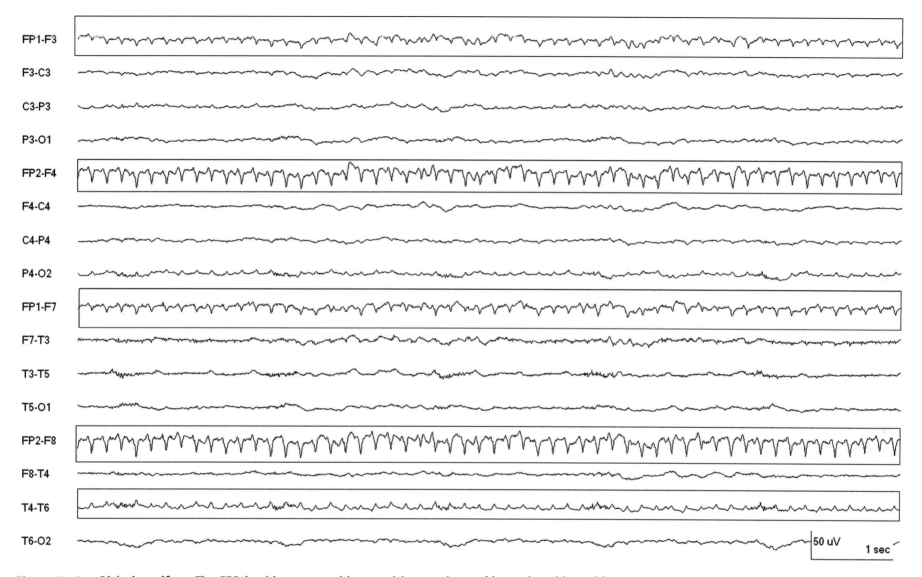

Figure 7.13. Dialysis artifact. The EEG in this 92-year-old man with mental status changes and renal failure shows rhythmic artifact (boxes), predominantly involving the anterior head regions, (electrodes Fp1 and Fp2), more marked on the right. The discharges are also present in the T4-T6 derivation, which provides evidence that this could not represent eye movement artifact. The patient was being dialyzed utilizing slow continuous ultra filtration (SCUF) that resulted in this artifact.

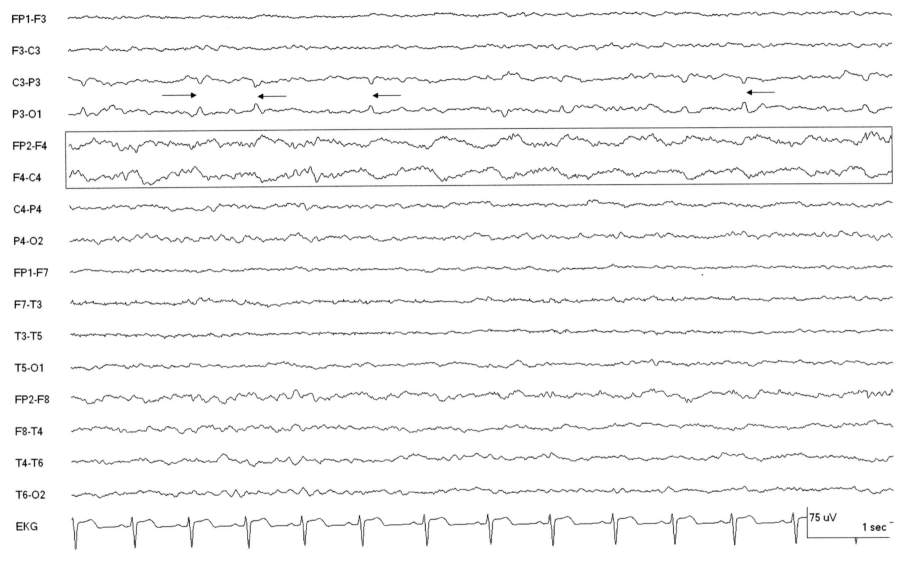

Figure 7.14. Pulse artifact and electrode artifact. Rhythmic slowing is present in the F4 electrode (box) and has a mirror image appearance in derivations FP2-F4 and F4-C4. In addition, intermittent, repetitive, low voltage sharp potentials are present in electrode P3 (arrows). The slowing at F4 is due to a pulse artifact; it is time-locked to the EKG trace, with the slow wave following the QRS complex by approximately 200 msec. Pulse artifact is a mechanical/physical artifact versus EKG artifact that is an electrical artifact. EKG artifact is the conduction of the very high voltage QRS complex to an EEG derivation. Thus, EKG artifact takes the form of small repetitive spikes that coincide (precisely) with the QRS complexes of the EKG, most commonly seen in the temporal chains. Pulse artifact is due to the physical displacement of an electrode by a nearby or underlying scalp vessel; therefore, the artifacts are repetitive slow waves (mimicking the pulse) and occur roughly 200 msec after each QRS complex (the time taken from cardiac ventricular systole to propagate a wave [pulse] of blood to a scalp vessel). The sharp activity in the P3 electrode was due to a P3 electrode artifact; Note the lack of a field (only seen in P3).

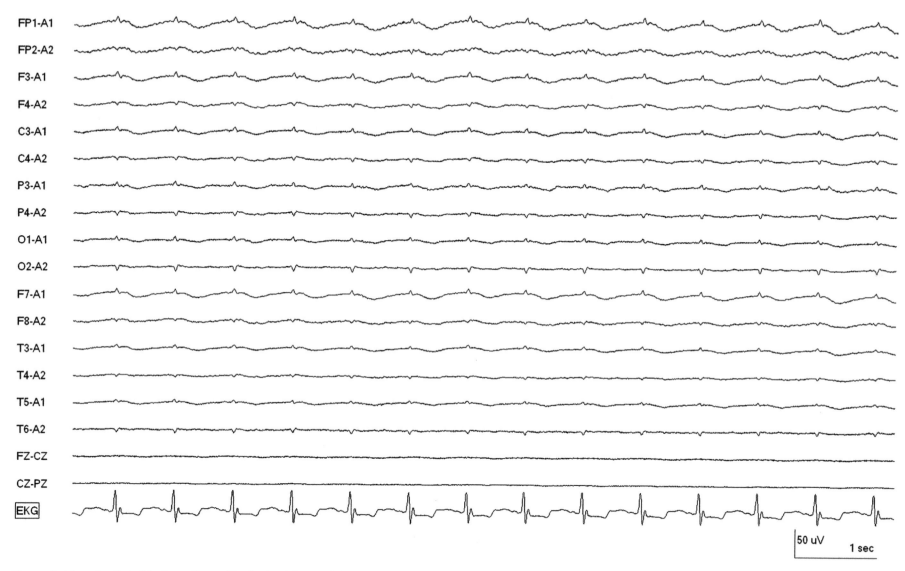

Figure 7.15. Cardioballistic artifact. Rhythmic delta activity is present in a widespread distribution. This represents a cardioballistic artifact (head movement with each pulse) in a 62-year-old man being evaluated for brain death. The slow waves have a fixed relationship to the QRS complex

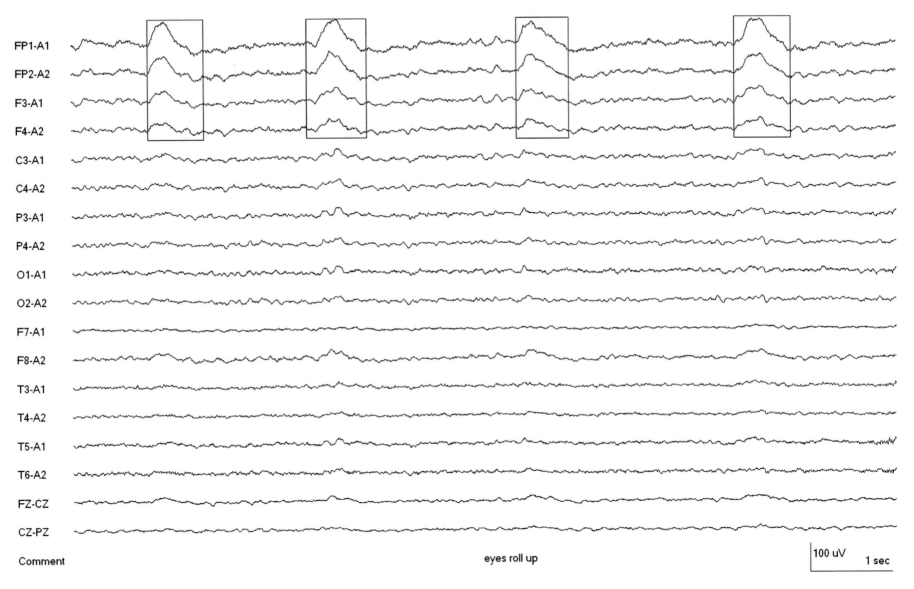

Figure 7.16. Ocular bobbing. The EEG shows repetitive slow waves present in the frontal regions, maximal at electrodes Fp1 and Fp2. The ascending portion of the waveform in the Fp1 and Fp2 electrodes is more rapid than its descending portion, that is, it has a steeper slope. This is because the upward deflection is due to the fact that the eyes are quickly moving down and then coming up more slowly. Examination revealed ocular bobbing corresponding with the bifrontal slow waves in this 75-year-old man with a brainstem stroke.

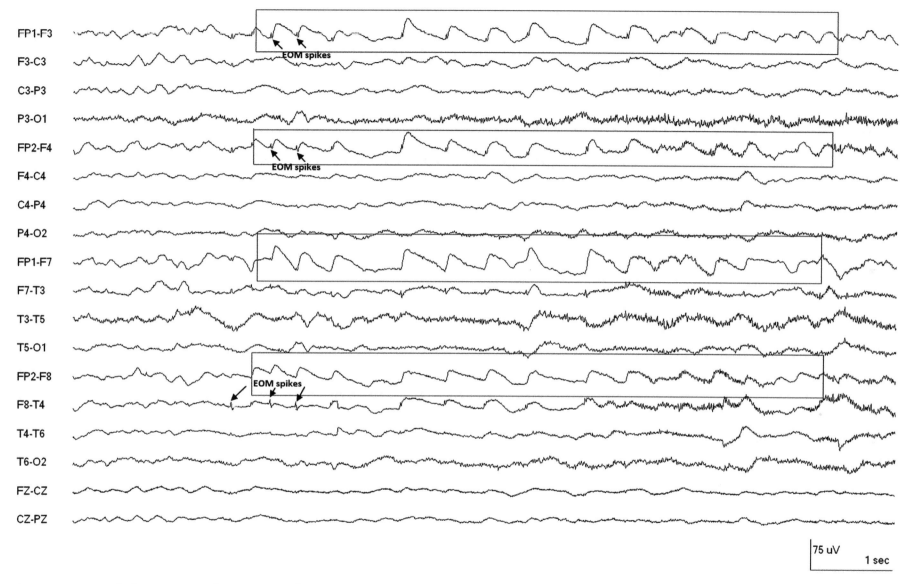

Figure 7.17. Vertical nystagmus. The prominent feature in this 65-year-old man with an intracerebral hemorrhage is the slowing in the frontal electrodes. This activity has a very steep field (i.e., high amplitude at Fp1/Fp2, but rapidly drops off at F3/F4) and is consistent with vertical eye movement, although rarely cerebral activity may have a similar field. In this case, the eye movements have a quick phase, at which time electrodes Fp1 and Fp2 become relatively surface negative, indicating a downward eye deflection (the positive cornea moving away from Fp1 and Fp2). Following this, there is a slower return. In addition, small extraocular muscle spikes (arrows) can be seen at the start of most of these discharges. These movements represent downbeat nystagmus.

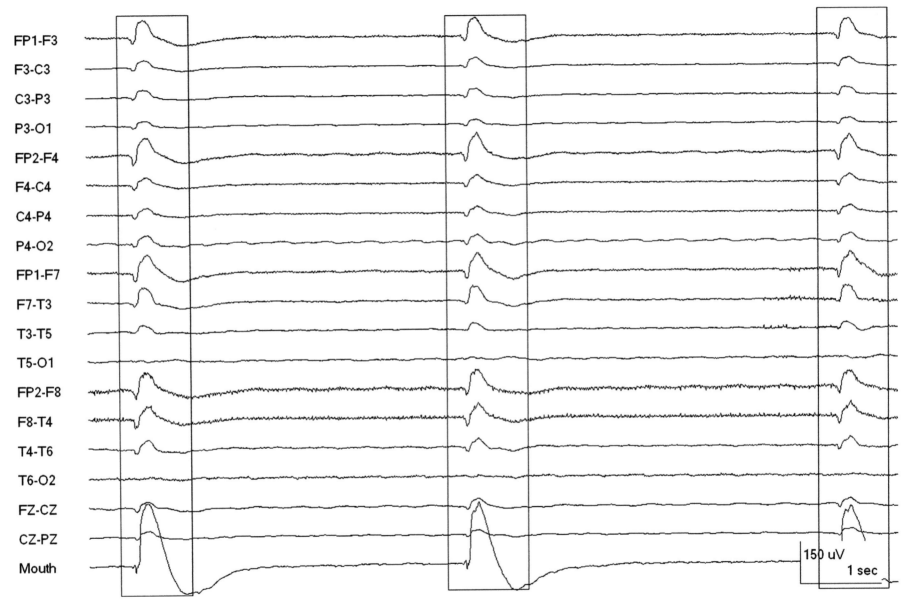

Figure 7.18. Ventilator artifact. The EEG in this 84-year-old woman shows regular repetitive slow waves. This activity does not represent widely spaced periodic discharges but was due to ventilator artifact, as demonstrated in the electrodes placed about the mouth. One should always consider this possibility in intubated patients with artifact repeating every 2–6 seconds.

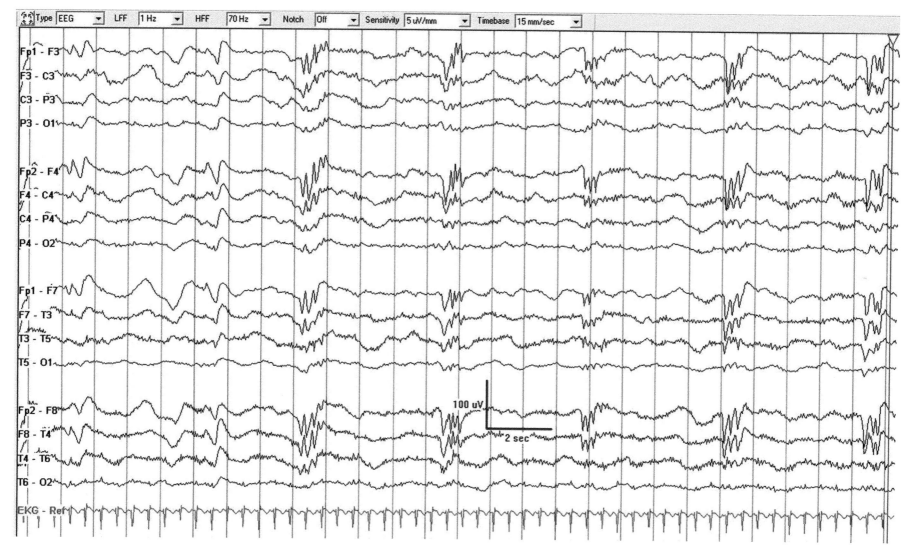

Figure 7.19. Ventilator artifact. This EEG is from a young HIV-positive woman with a left hemisphere infarct and right hemisphere abscess. EEG (shown compressed, at 15 mm/s rather than the usual 30 mm/s) shows generalized, frontally predominant, polyspike-like discharges every 4–5 seconds. Review of video showed that this corresponded with ventilator-delivered breaths and resolved after clearing fluid from the ventilator tubing.

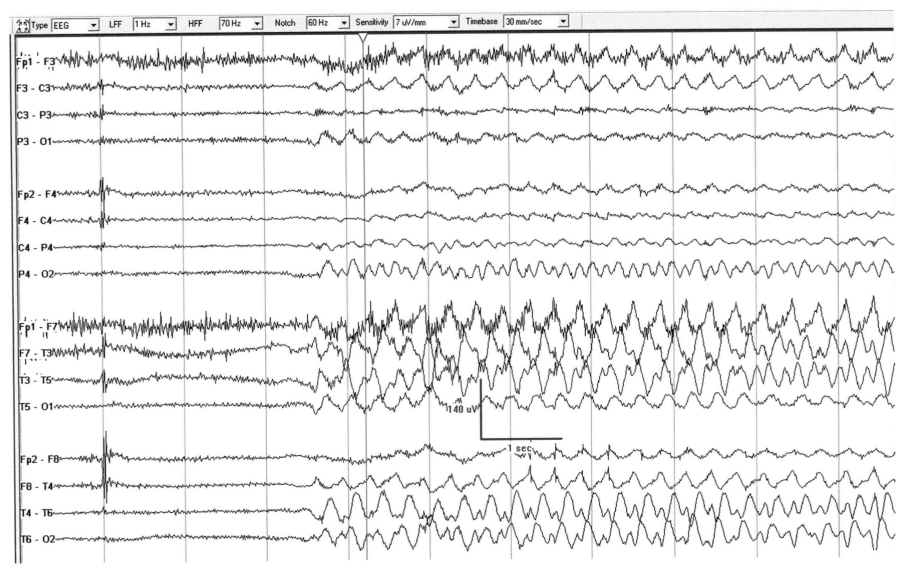

Figure 7.20. Chest percussion artifact. Paroxysmal rhythmic pattern due to chest percussion by a respiratory therapist in a 34-year-old with AIDS, end-stage renal disease and seizures. Recording video allows rapid confirmation of the artifactual nature of this pattern. This is a common rhythmic artifact in the ICU, and even more common in neonates and infants, and can mimic seizures quite effectively at times.

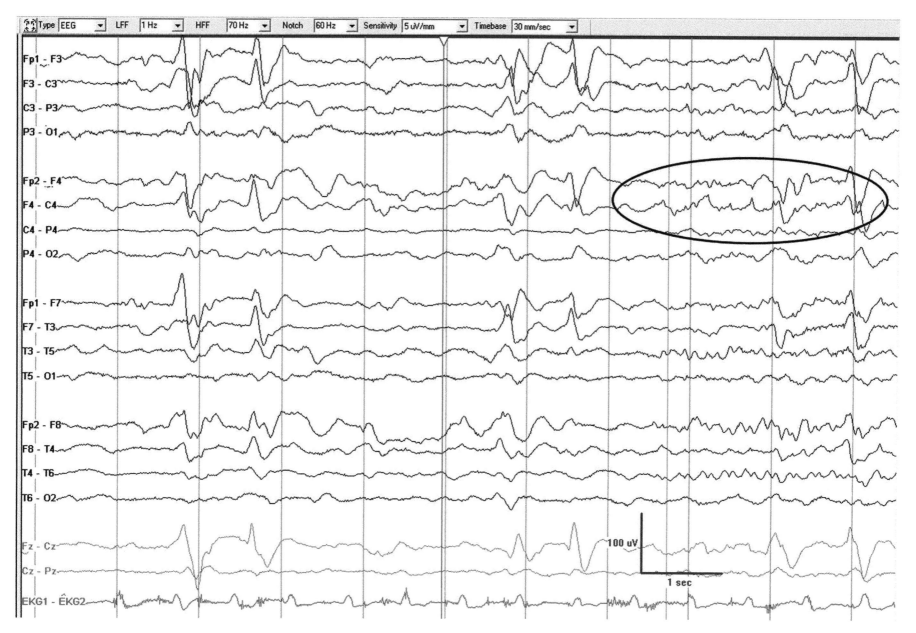

Figure 7.21. Chest percussion artifact mimicking seizure. (a) Four consecutive pages of EEG in an elderly woman s/p meningioma resection with postoperative convulsive seizure and impaired mental status. The beginning of the page demonstrates abundant generalized sporadic epileptiform discharges. In the last few seconds of the page there is the beginning of medium voltage rhythmic activity with a wide field that appears to have small, intermixed spikes at F4 (ellipse).

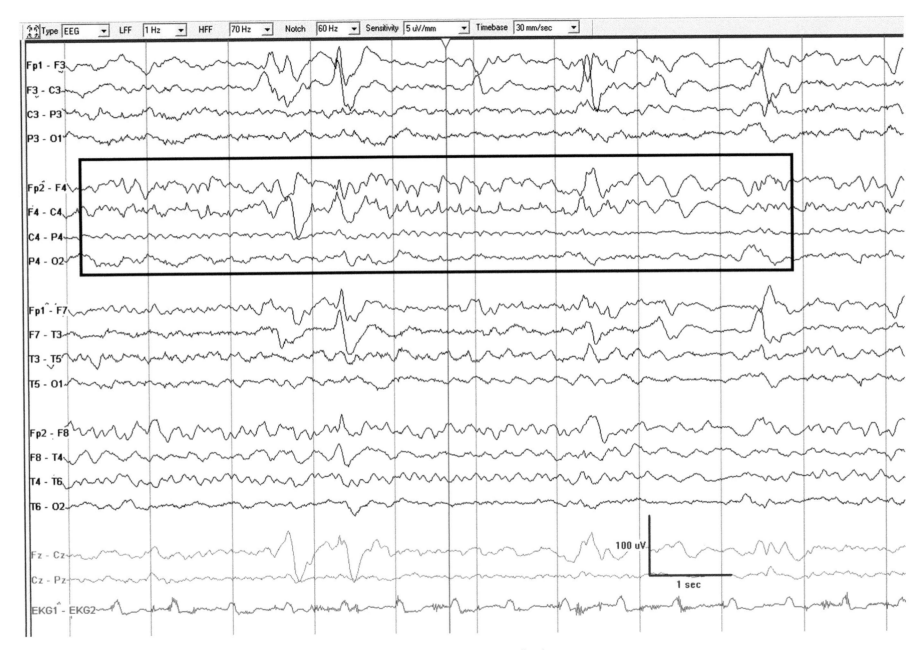

Figure 7.21. (*Continued*) (b) The small spikes at F4 evolve in morphology and frequency (box).

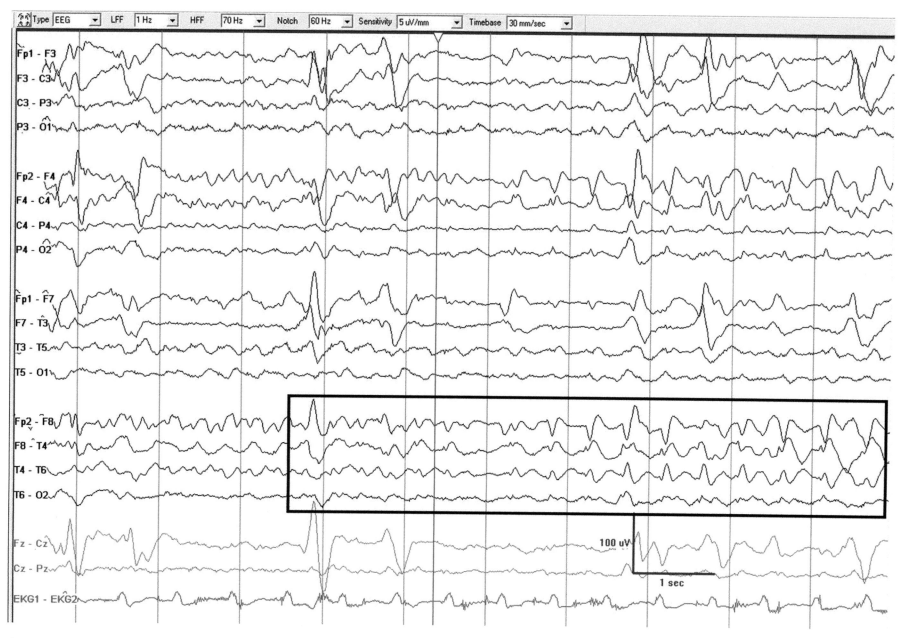

Figure 7.21. (*Continued*) (c) Additional evolution with a physiological field, appearing to spread from the right frontal region into the right temporal region (box).

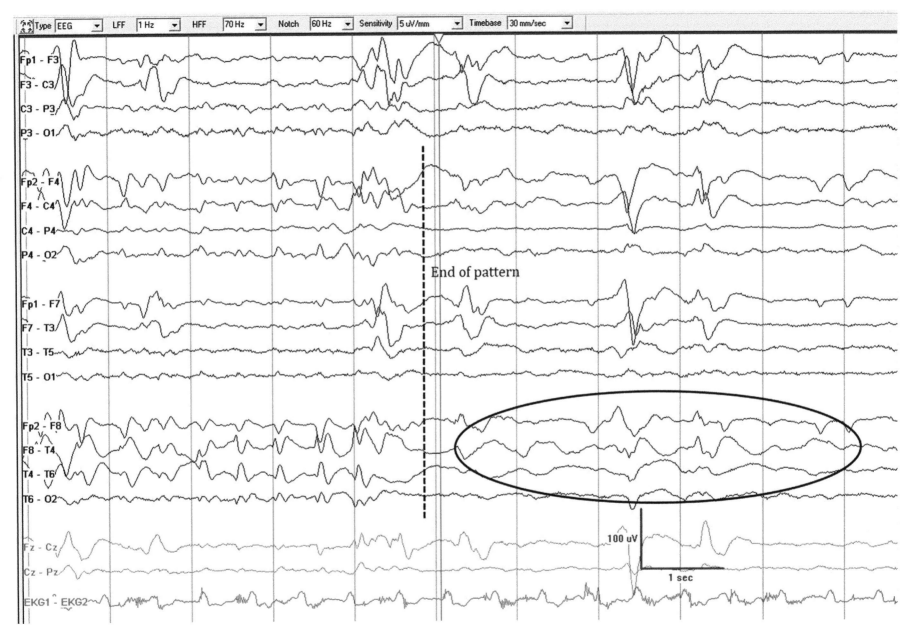

Figure 7.21. (*Continued*) (d) The pattern abruptly stops (labeled dashed line) and there appears like there is possible post ictal right temporal slowing (ellipse). Review of video showed that this was due to chest percussion and was artifact, not seizure. The patient was rolled onto her right side during the respiratory therapy; this explained the physiologic field on the right side. Without video this pattern is likely to be misinterpreted as a seizure.

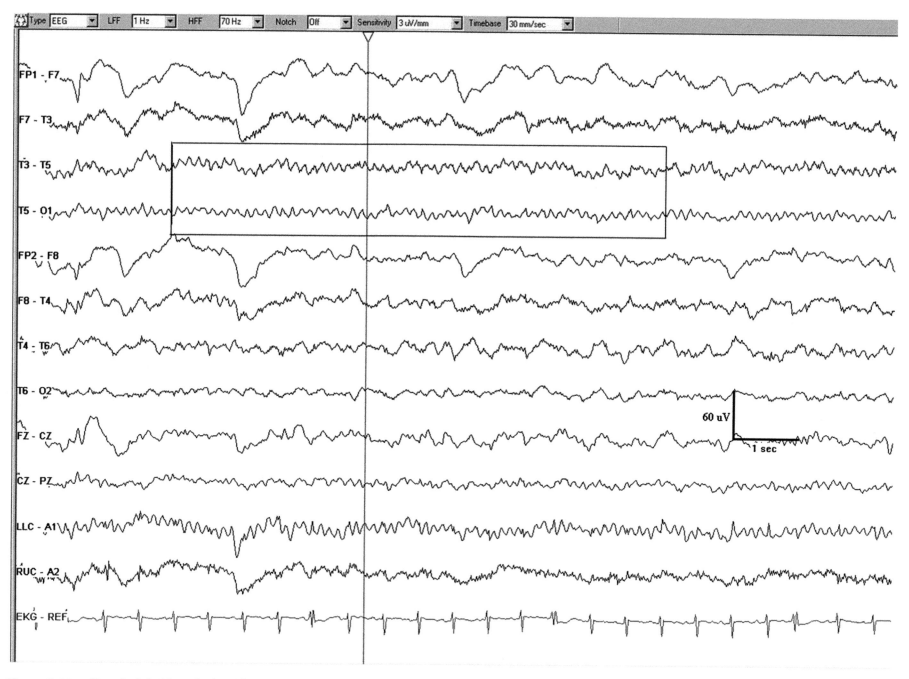

Figure 7.22. 'Pseudoalpha' from bed oscillator artifact. There appears to be a well-developed posterior dominant 'alpha' rhythm on the left (box) in this comatose patient. However, this was due to a bed oscillator, with the patient's head turned somewhat to the left (so that O2 was not touching the bed).

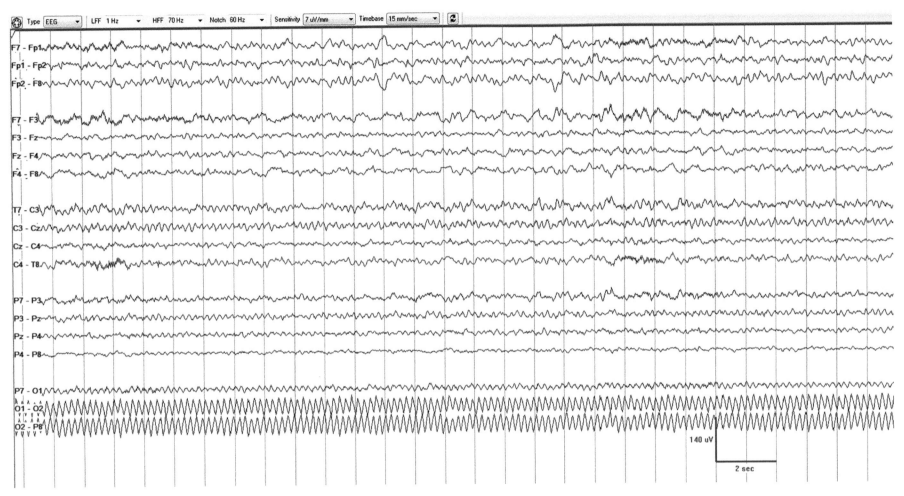

Figure 7.23. Stimulus-induced electroclinical seizure from bed oscillator. (a) Oscillator artifact, transverse bipolar (compressed timescale of 15mm/s instead of conventional 30 mm/s): These EEGs are from a 69-year-old man with hypoxemic respiratory failure and septic shock. The EEG demonstrates mild diffuse dysfunction. In the posterior head regions (at the bottom of the page) there is an exquisitely monomorphic sinusoidal pattern occurring at exactly 5 Hz. This was due to bed oscillator artifact (and is too monomorphic and unchanging to be cerebral).

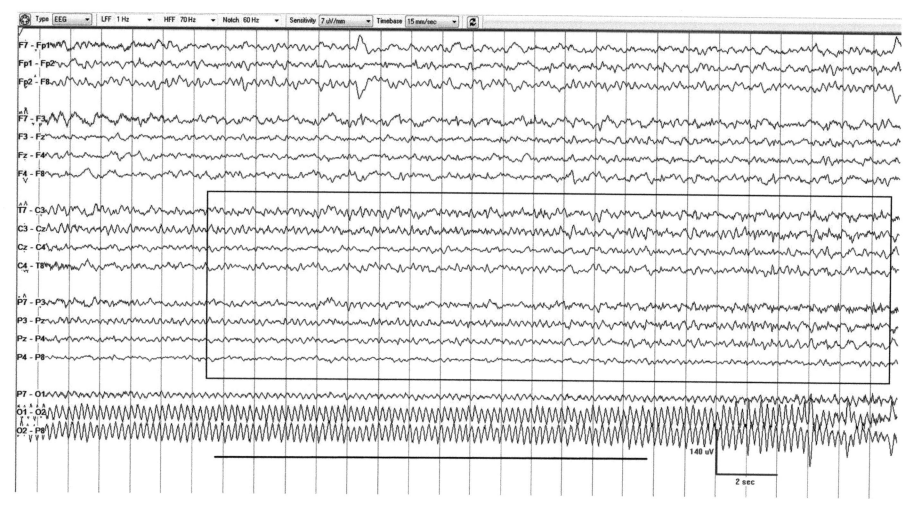

Figure 7.23. (*Continued*) (b) Seizure onset, transverse bipolar montage, still with a compressed timescale of 15 mm/s. The oscillator appeared to trigger an electroclinical seizure (by acting as an alerting stimulus, a form of SIRPIDs; see Figures 5.41, 5.42 and 5.43). On this compressed timescale there is slow evolution of low voltage spiking in the midline (Cz/Pz). The absolute onset is difficult to appreciate, but taking the parietal derivations, the EEG at the end of the page is clearly different from the beginning.

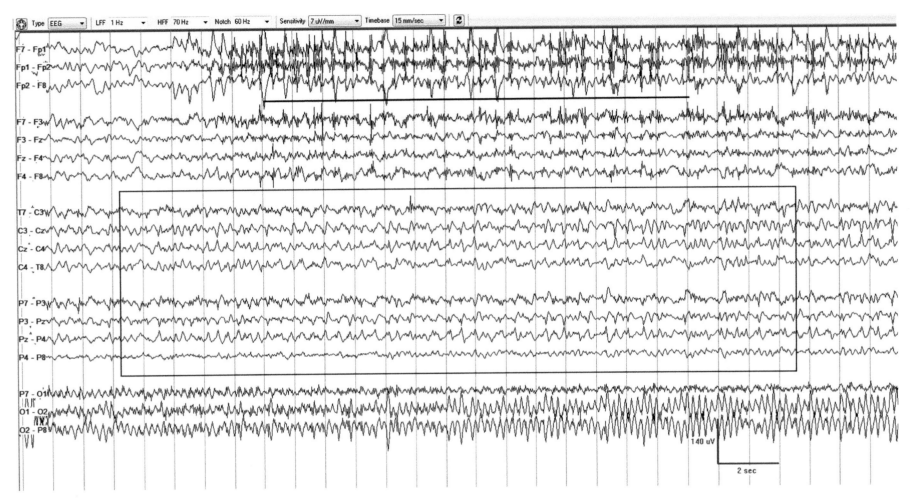

Figure 7.23. (*Continued*) (c) Electroclinical seizure, transverse bipolar montage, still with a compressed timescale of 15 mm/s. On this next page, it is much easier to appreciate that there is a seizure with irregular 2–4-Hz spikes in the midline with a wide field over central and parietal derivations. A clinical seizure begins at this point, with repetitive twitching of the face muscles (evidenced by the beginning of EMG activity in the frontal electrodes [underlined]). Note the bed oscillator artifact at the bottom of the page: it remains unchanged at 5 Hz despite the start of a ECSz.

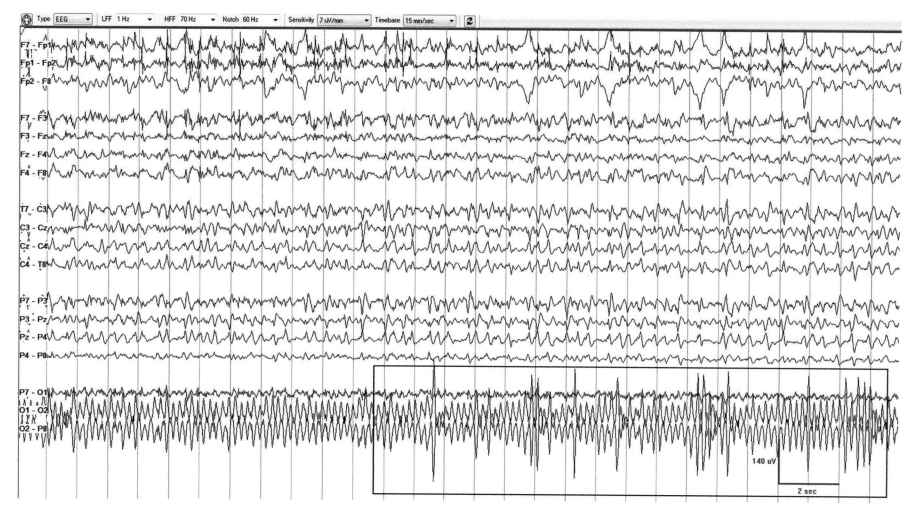

Figure 7.23. (*Continued*) (d) Electroclinical seizure, transverse bipolar montage, still with a compressed timescale of 15 mm/s. Further evolution of the seizure with greater involvement of the posterior head regions (where the oscillator artifact is evident). The result of this is the spikes and slowing from the seizure disrupts the oscillator artifact as the patterns are superimposed on one another (box). Note the frequency of the oscillator artifact still remains absolutely unchanged at 5 Hz

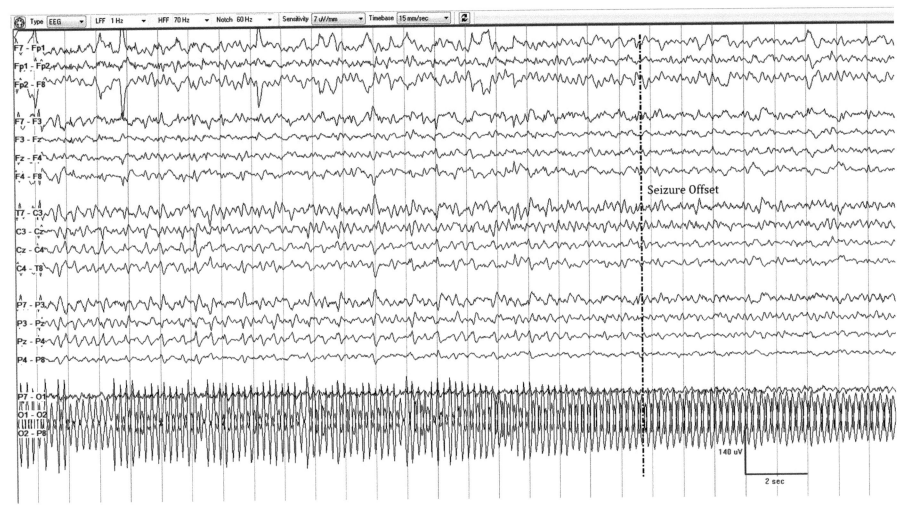

Figure 7.23. (*Continued*) (e) Seizure offset, transverse bipolar montage with a compressed timescale of 15 mm/s. As the seizure stops (labeled dashed line) the oscillator artifact continues on, resuming its monomorphic pattern.

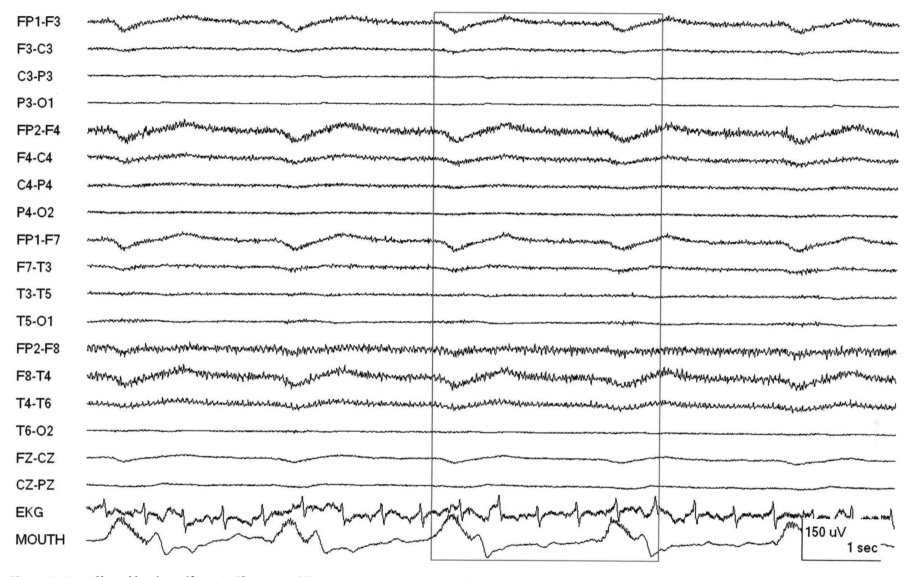

Figure 7.24. Glossokinetic artifact. Artifact resembling eye movements in a 70-year-old comatose woman. The derivation at the bottom of the page labeled 'mouth', is recording from an electrode placed below the mouth. The theory of a mouth electrode is similar to an eye electrode to determine vertical eye movement artifact. An electrode that is placed below the source will display the opposite polarity to electrodes placed above it. Here we see negative deflections in the mouth channel resulting in positive deflections at Fp1 and Fp2 on the scalp EEG. The tip of the tongue is relatively negative compared to the base (this can be thought of as the opposite to the eye, where the cornea is positive compared to the retina). Note that glossokinetic artifact will appear 'in phase' in EOG and scalp electrodes, as they are all above the mouth. This artifact was from repetitive primarily downward tongue movements.

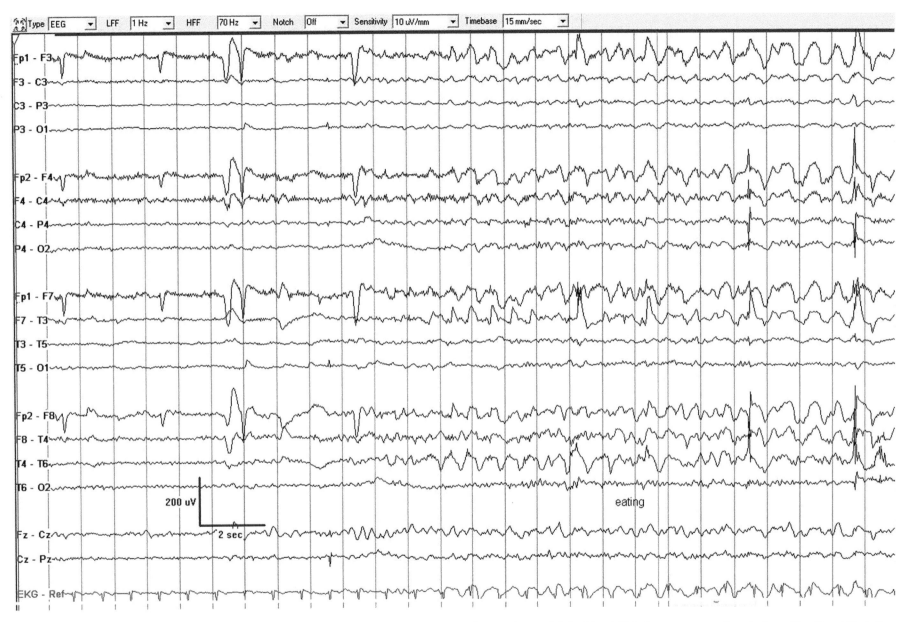

Figure 7.25. Glossokinetic artifact. This EEG (compressed, with recording at 15 mm/s rather than the usual 30 mm/s) in a man in his 70s with seizures s/p evacuation of a left subdural hematoma, shows a bilateral rhythmic pattern, maximal in the right temporal lobe, and possibly evolving (slowing and changing morphology). Video revealed that this was due to chewing and was reproduced after each mouthful of food. This is a more prominent glossokinetic artifact than is typically seen, but again shows the importance of video for avoiding misinterpretation of rhythmic artifacts. Note that the pattern is absent at the vertex (Cz), typical of most artifacts.

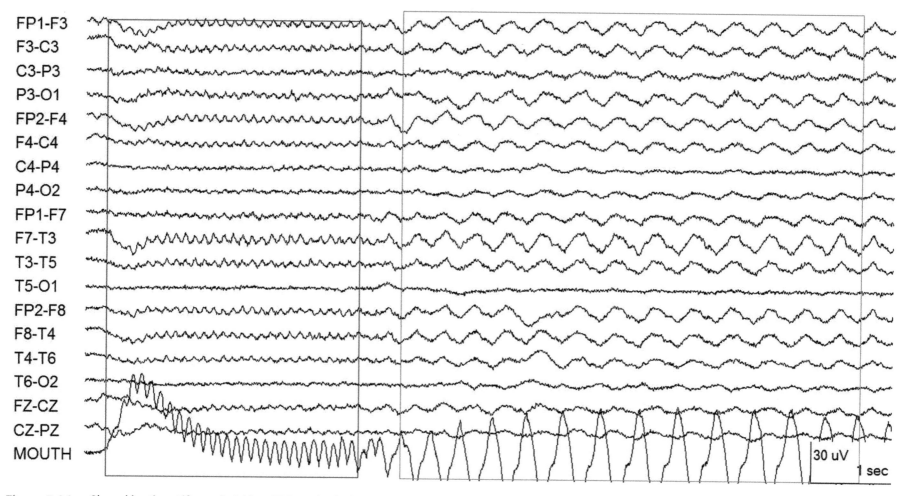

Figure 7.26.   Glossokinetic artifact mimicking GRDA. Rhythmic tongue movement artifact resembling GRDA in a this 72-year-old comatose man, post arrest. Note the very high gain (sensitivity at 2 uV/mm, the setting used for determination of electrocerebral inactivity). The faster activity (red box) does not exceed 5 μV and is also artifact, while the higher voltage slower activity (blue box) is less than 10 μV and correlated with rhythmic tongue movements. Note that this cannot be chewing artifact since there is no muscle activity.

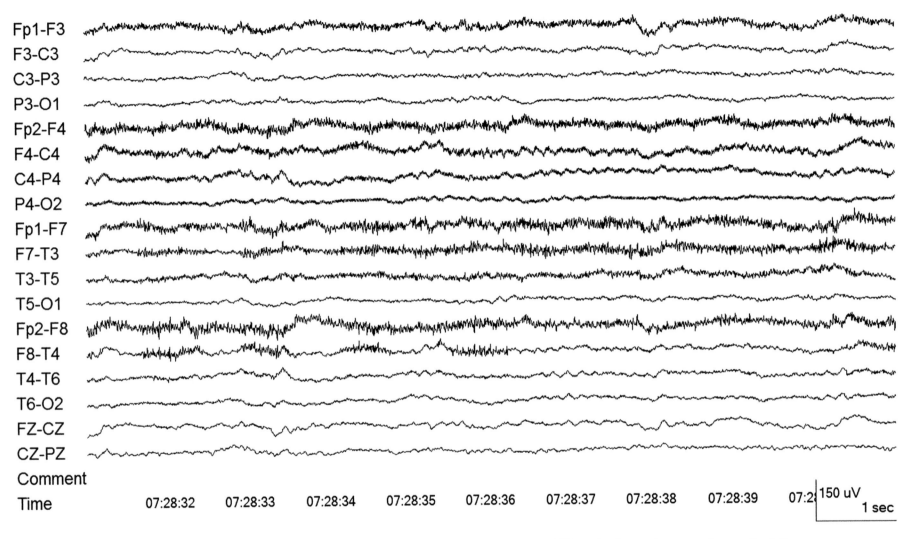

Figure 7.27. 'Virtual' or disconnected patient. (a) The initial EEG in this 66-year-old man shows diffuse slowing and attenuation on the left.

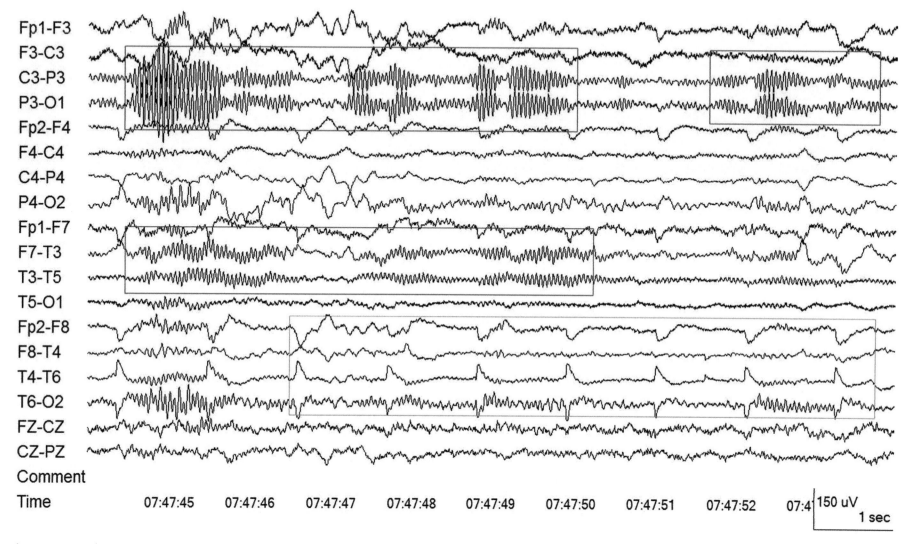

Figure 7.27. (*Continued*) (b) Shortly afterwards the EEG showed marked changes with bursts of rapid activity present, particularly over the left hemisphere (red) and periodic complexes in the right temporal region (blue).

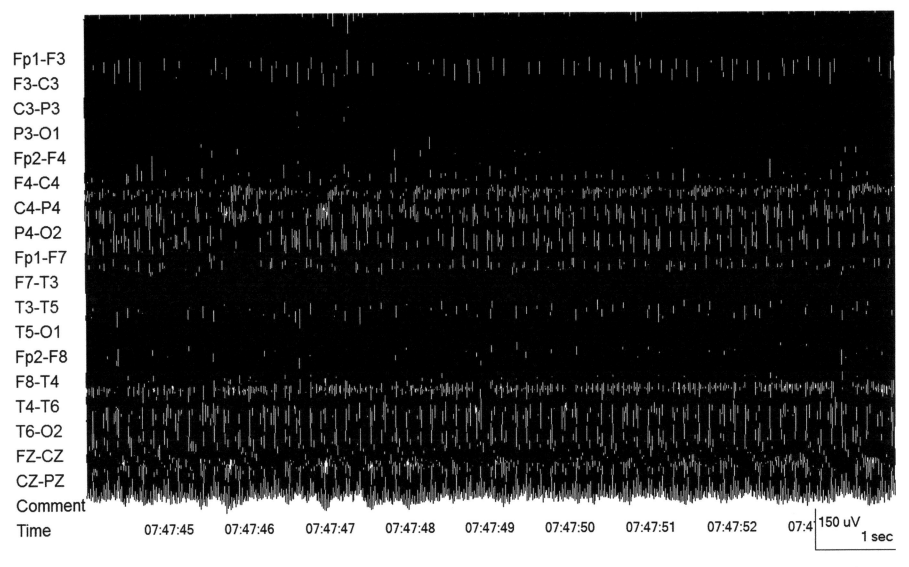

Figure 7.27.   (*Continued*) (c) The reason for this marked change was because many (or all) electrodes had become disconnected. This is obvious when the same epoch is viewed with the 60 Hz filter off (It was on in Figure 7.27b).

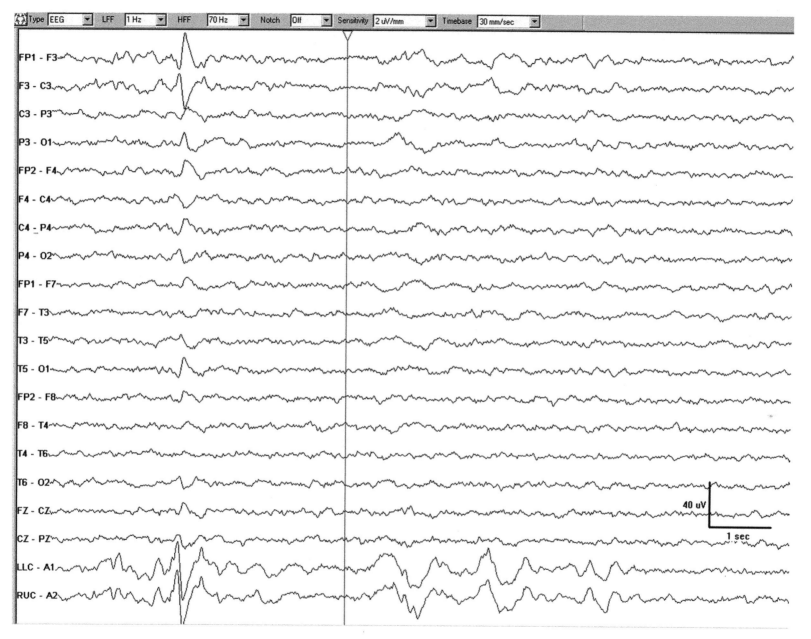

Figure 7.28. 'Virtual' or disconnected patient. There appears to be diffuse attenuation and slowing, but there is actually no patient in the room as the patient was rushed to an emergency scan in the middle of the night. This is the pattern seen when no electrodes are plugged into the headbox (jackbox). Note the very high gain of 2 μV/mm (but the 60 Hz, or notch filter, is not on, as electrical noise is not recorded when nothing is connected to the headbox). Video confirmed the lack of a patient in the room.

8 Post cardiac arrest patterns

Cardiac arrest and hypoxic brain injury can cause encephalopathy, coma and seizures. There are several clinical and electrographic considerations that are fairly specific to the post cardiac arrest EEG. After cardiac arrest, patients can be in myoclonic status epilepticus. This is a clinical syndrome that is associated with significant hypoxic brain injury and for the most part holds a poor outcome (although not universally). In the post cardiac arrest setting, one thing EEGers are asked frequently is to make some estimate on prognosis based on the EEG. This chapter will introduce patterns that are more specific to the post cardiac arrest setting that are associated with a poor (or good) prognosis. It should be noted, however, that none of these are absolute (although some reportedly close) and a discussion of prognosis must be integrated with the remainder of the clinical features, and other electrophysiologic information, including somatosensory evoked potentials (SSEPs).

8.1 Myoclonic status epilepticus

Myoclonic status epilepticus is the syndrome whereby there is continuous or near continuous myoclonus after cardiac arrest. Myoclonus is often proximal with jerking of the eyes, face, shoulders or trunk/abdomen. Although often dramatic the state can also be fairly subtle, limited to just the eyelids and eyes for example. The EEG correlate of myoclonic status epilepticus is often suppression-burst or generalized periodic discharges, with the clinical jerk associated with the beginning of the burst or the discharge.

Myoclonic status epilepticus is said to carry a grave prognosis; however, many of the studies that concluded this preceded the era of therapeutic hypothermia or targeted temperature management (TTM) and are retrospective. This raises the possibility of a self-fulfilling prophecy whereby a common practice was to withdraw care based on the clinical and EEG finding. This has been questioned in more recent times with the emergence of an increasing number of reported cases that have had myoclonic status epilepticus and have gone on to have a good clinical outcome; this is usually in patients with a better (continuous) EEG background and no other indicators of poor prognosis (e.g., loss of brainstem reflexes or bilaterally absent SSEPs).

8.2 Prognostication

Prognostication after cardiac arrest is a complex integration of clinical history, patient examination, neuroimaging and neurophysiologic measures. The EEG is merely one of these factors and the electrographic patterns should be weighted in conjunction with the remainder of the patient's findings. A patient whose EEG demonstrates reactive slowing with clear physiologic sleep states has a much better chance of good outcome than a patient with no clear cerebral rhythms, including after stimulation. However, these points are never absolute (i.e., a patient with reactive slowing still has a reasonable chance of succumbing to death). The patients who fall in between these end points can be more challenging, and there are a number of patterns emerging that sway

Hirsch and Brenner's Atlas of EEG in Critical Care, Second Edition. Lawrence J. Hirsch, Michael W.K. Fong, and Richard P. Brenner.
© 2023 John Wiley & Sons Ltd. Published 2023 by John Wiley & Sons Ltd.

prognosis toward one end of the spectrum versus the other. In general, the background EEG is the most important prognosticator, and the EEG around 24 h after arrest may be the most useful timepoint (though the trajectory may be important as well).

There are many features of the EEG that have demonstrated prognostic significance in post cardiac arrest patients. The background voltage and continuity, the theta spectral content within burst suppression (i.e., the amount of relative power in the theta range), the time taken to recovery of a normal-voltage continuous background, and reactivity have all shown to have prognostic implications. Negative prognostic indicators have included the presence of SIRPIDs, a shorter time to the emergence of epileptiform activity, and electrographic and electroclinical seizures (usually myoclonic status epilepticus); again, none of these are absolute indicators of poor outcome, but they are associated with worse outcomes overall.

A pattern with a great degree of emerging dichotomy is burst suppression. Burst suppression is defined as 50–99% of the record being suppressed, but the amount of inherent brain dysfunction in a patient with 98% of their record suppressed is clearly greater than a patient with 50% of their record attenuated.

Burst suppression actually consists of a wide variety of patterns. Bursts can consist of fairly benign appearing admixed theta and delta range frequencies, or bursts can appear highly epileptiform (with a significant component of epileptiform activity). Two concepts have emerged to further refine the group of burst suppression.

Highly epileptiform bursts are defined as either:

(1) two or more epileptiform discharges (spikes or sharp waves) seen within the majority (>50%) of bursts and occurring at an average of 1 Hz or faster within a single burst (frequency is calculated as the inverse of the typical interpeak latency of consecutive epileptiform discharges within a single burst), or

(2) arhythmic, potentially ictal-appearing pattern occurring within the majority (>50%) of bursts.

Highly epileptiform bursts (HEBs) were initially described (in the non-cardiac arrest setting) as a differentiating factor for seizure recurrence if highly sedating ASMs used to control refractory status epilepticus were withdrawn. For example, in one study, in patients with HEBs at the time of sedative withdrawal, they had a 65% chance of seizure recurrence in the next 24 hours, vs. 0% if the EEG did not demonstrate HEBs at the time of medication withdrawal. It was subsequently established that the presence of HEBs in post cardiac arrets patients also inferred an independent poor prognostic factor. It should be noted that unequivocal seizure also pertains a poor prognostic factor in this setting, but the majority of these refer to the emergence of myoclonic status epilepticus; other forms of postanoxic status epilepticus seem to have a better chance of favorable outcome.

The other prognostic feature is 'identical' vs 'non-identical' bursts. Non-identical bursts are more physiologic, with the content of bursts varying between each other. Identical bursts on the flip side can be viewed as an extreme form of invariance, where the brain is so dysfunctional that it is only capable of generating the exact same group of rhythms over and over again.

Identical bursts are defined as follows:

(1) present if the first 0.5 s or longer of each burst appears visually similar in all channels in the vast majority (>90%) of bursts, or

(2) present if the first 0.5 s or longer of each stereotyped cluster of 2 or more bursts appears visually similar in all channels in the vast majority (>90%) of bursts.

The presence of identical bursts in the post cardiac arrest setting may have a nearly universal poor outcome, though there are limited data on this to date. In addition, there is an important caveat that although the prognosis of many of the above patterns are termed dire, there are examples in the literature whereby patients with these patterns have a good outcome. There are even descriptions of patterns that are associated with good outcome in patients with postanoxic myoclonus, such as narrow vertex-maximal spikes time-locked to the jerks. It must be stressed that the clinical scenario is critical for prognostication and these life-or-death decisions should not be based on one test alone.

The EEG is not usually helpful in patients in a vegetative or minimally conscious state as it can show a wide variety of degrees of diffuse dysfunction. EEG records cortical activity, not brainstem activity. Thus, in patients with primary brainstem injury, the EEG can appear remarkably 'healthy'. A completely flat EEG (electrocerebral inactivity) is seen with severe diffuse injury, with or without loss of brainstem function, which must be determined by other means (primarily examination, including apnea testing). There are detailed, formal guidelines for performing an EEG in order to document electrocerebral inactivity, though now these are only used on rare occasions as part of the determination of brain death due to the limitations just mentioned.

Figure list

Figure 8.1 Myoclonic status epilepticus.

Figure 8.2 Myoclonic status epilepticus.

Figure 8.3 Myoclonic status epilepticus.

Figure 8.4 Subtle myoclonic SE.

Figure 8.5 Burst suppression (non-identical, non-HEBs).

Figure 8.6 Progression from burst suppression to GPDs.

Figure 8.7 Progression of burst suppression to moderate slowing.

Figure 8.8 Ictal-interictal continuum.

Figure 8.9 Stimulus-induced post-hypoxic myoclonus.

Figure 8.10 Burst suppression with highly epileptiform bursts (HEBs).

Figure 8.11 Highly epileptiform bursts, ESz and ESE.

Figure 8.12 Nonconvulsive status epilepticus.

Figure 8.13 Emergence of NCSE post rewarming.

Figure 8.14 Central spikes leading to myoclonic status epilepticus.

Figure 8.15 Discrete myoclonic seizures (i.e., not myoclonic status epilepticus).

EEGs throughout this atlas have been shown with the following standard recording filters unless otherwise specified: LFF 1 Hz, HFF 70 Hz, notch filter off.

Suggested reading

Alvarez V, Oddo M, Rossetti AO. Stimulus-induced rhythmic, periodic or ictal discharges (SIRPIDs) in comatose survivors of cardiac arrest: Characteristics and prognostic value. *Clinical Neurophysiology.* 2013;**124**(1):204–208.

Backman S, Cronberg T, Friberg H, et al. Highly malignant routine EEG predicts poor prognosis after cardiac arrest in the Target Temperature Management trial. *Resuscitation.* 2018;**131**:24–28.

Beretta S, Coppo A, Bianchi E, et al. Neurologic outcome of postanoxic refractory status epilepticus after aggressive treatment. *Neurology.* 2018;**91**(23):e2153–e2162.

Dhakar MB, Sivaraju A, Maciel CB, et al. Electro-clinical characteristics and prognostic significance of post anoxic myoclonus. *Resuscitation.* 2018;**131**:114–120.

Elmer J, Rittenberger JC, Faro J, et al. Clinically distinct electroencephalographic phenotypes of early myoclonus after cardiac arrest. *Ann Neurol.* 2016;**80**(2):175–184.

Geocadin RG, Callaway CW, Fink EL, et al. Standards for studies of neurological prognostication in comatose survivors of cardiac arrest: a scientific statement from the American Heart Association. *Circulation.* 2019;**140**(9).

Hofmeijer J, Tjepkema-Cloostermans MC, van Putten MJ. Burst-suppression with identical bursts: a distinct EEG pattern with poor outcome in postanoxic coma. *Clin Neurophysiol.* 2014;**125**(5):947–954.

Hofmeijer J, Beernink TMJ, Bosch FH, Beishuizen A, Tjepkema-Cloostermans MC, Van Putten MJAM. Early EEG contributes to multimodal outcome prediction of postanoxic coma. *Neurology.* 2015;**85**(2):137–143.

Lamartine Monteiro M, Taccone FS, Depondt C, et al. The prognostic value of 48-h continuous EEG during therapeutic hypothermia after cardiac arrest. *Neurocrit Care.* 2016;**24**(2):153–162.

Rossetti AO, Tovar Quiroga DF, Juan E, et al. Electroencephalography predicts poor and good outcomes after cardiac arrest: a two-center study. *Crit Care Med.* 2017;**45**(7):e674-e682.

Ruijter BJ, Hofmeijer J, Tjepkema-Cloostermans MC, van Putten M. The prognostic value of discontinuous EEG patterns in postanoxic coma. *Clin Neurophysiol.* 2018;**129**(8):1534–1543.

Ruijter BJ, Tjepkema-Cloostermans MC, Tromp SC, et al. Early electroencephalography for outcome prediction of postanoxic coma: A prospective cohort study. *Annals of Neurology.* 2019;**86**(2):203–214.

Sandroni C, D'Arrigo S, Cacciola S, et al. Prediction of poor neurological outcome in comatose survivors of cardiac arrest: a systematic review. *Intensive Care Medicine.* 2020;**46**(10):1803–1851.

Sandroni C, Cariou A, Cavallaro F, et al. Prognostication in comatose survivors of cardiac arrest: An advisory statement from the European Resuscitation Council and the European Society of Intensive Care Medicine. *Intensive Care Medicine.* 2014;**40**(12):1816–1831.

Seder DB, Sunde K, Rubertsson S, et al. Neurologic outcomes and postresuscitation care of patients with myoclonus following cardiac arrest. *Crit Care Med.* 2015;**43**(5):965–972.

Sekar K, Schiff ND, Labar D, Forgacs PB. Spectral content of electroencephalographic burst-suppression patterns may reflect neuronal recovery in comatose post-cardiac arrest patients. *J Clin Neurophysiol.* 2019;**36**(2):119–126.

Sivaraju A, Gilmore EJ, Wira CR, et al. Prognostication of post-cardiac arrest coma: early clinical and electroencephalographic predictors of outcome. *Intensive Care Medicine.* 2015;**41**(7):1264–1272.

Spalletti M, Carraia R, Scarpino M, et al. 34. Burst-suppression with highly epileptiform bursts and with identical bursts: two subtypes within burst-suppression pattern. *Clinical Neurophysiology.* 2016;**127**(12):e331.

Thompson SA, Hantus S. Highly epileptiform bursts are associated with seizure recurrence. *J Clin Neurophysiol.* 2016;**33**(1):66–71.

Westhall E, Rosén I, Rundgren M, et al. Time to epileptiform activity and EEG background recovery are independent predictors after cardiac arrest. *Clin Neurophysiol.* 2018;**129**(8):1660–1668.

Westhall E, Rossetti AO, Van Rootselaar A-F, et al. Standardized EEG interpretation accurately predicts prognosis after cardiac arrest. *Neurology.* 2016;**86**(16):1482–1490.

Wijdicks EFM, Parisi JE, Sharbrough FW. Prognostic value of myoclonus status in comatose survivors of cardiac arrest. *Ann Neurol* 1994;**35**:239–243.

Yamashita S, Morinaga T, Ohgo S, et al. Prognostic value of electroencephalogram (EEG) in anoxic encephalopathy after cardiopulmonary resuscitation: relationship among anoxic period, *EEG grading and outcome. Intern Med* 1995;**34**:71–76.

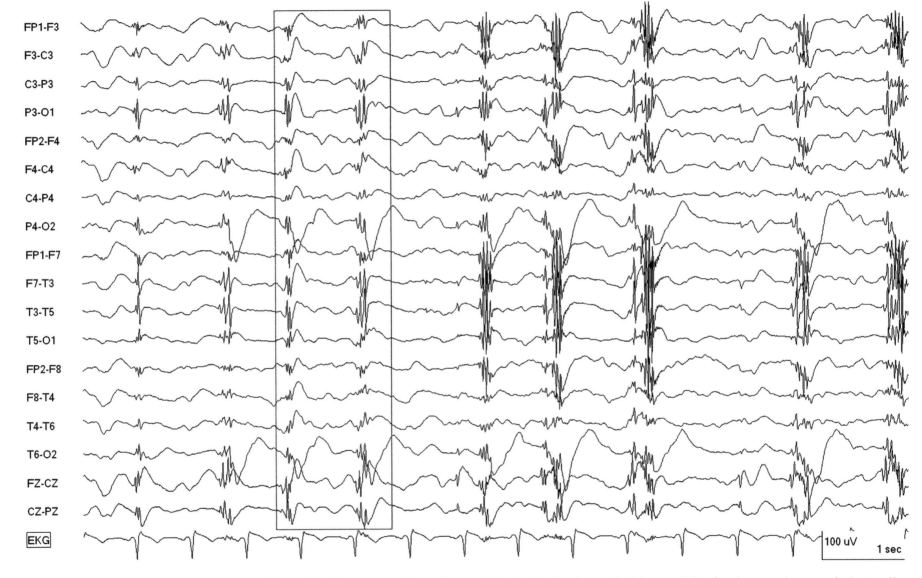

Figure 8.1. Myoclonic status epilepticus. The EEG in this 65-year-old man in myoclonic status epilepticus following a cardiac arrest shows repetitive generalized polyspikes (two examples are inside the box), maximal on the left, on a diffusely slow background. This was right after he was given paralytics to allow review of the EEG, as muscle artifact obscured the EEG during each myoclonic jerk.

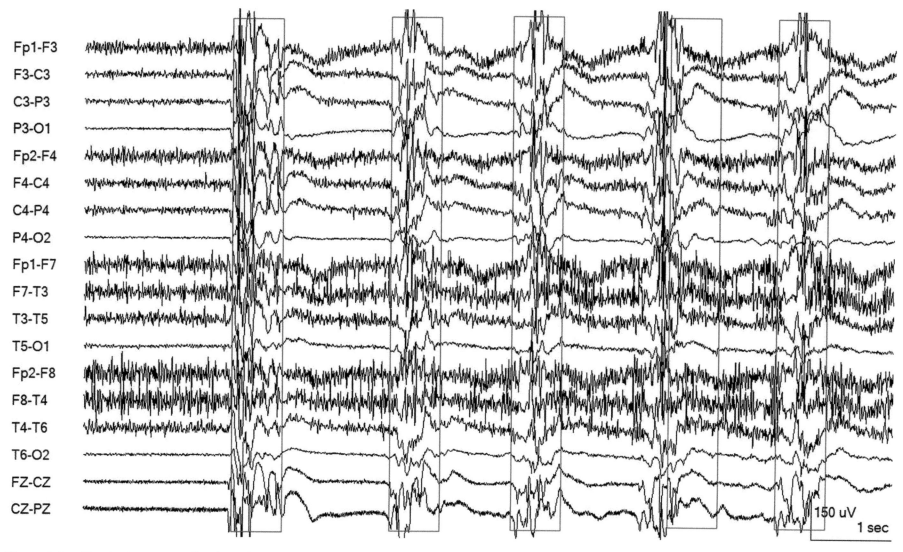

Fp1-F3
F3-C3
C3-P3
P3-O1
Fp2-F4
F4-C4
C4-P4
P4-O2
Fp1-F7
F7-T3
T3-T5
T5-O1
Fp2-F8
F8-T4
T4-T6
T6-O2
FZ-CZ
CZ-PZ

150 uV

1 sec

Figure 8.2.   Myoclonic status epilepticus. (a) The initial recording in this 71-year-old man status post cardiac arrest shows bursts of polyspikes associated with generalized myoclonus (red boxes).

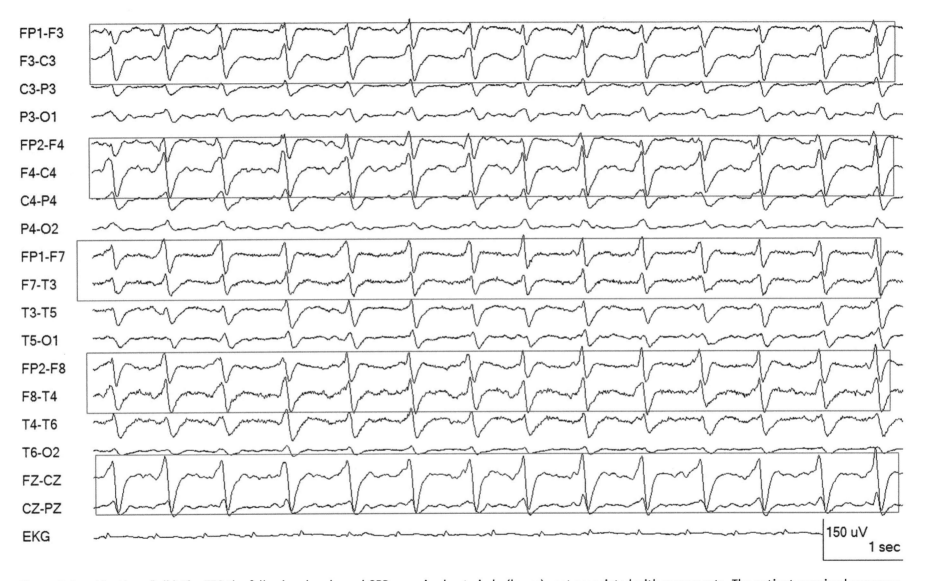

Figure 8.2. (*Continued*) (b) The EEG the following day showed GPDs, maximal anteriorly (boxes), not associated with movements. The patient remained unresponsive.

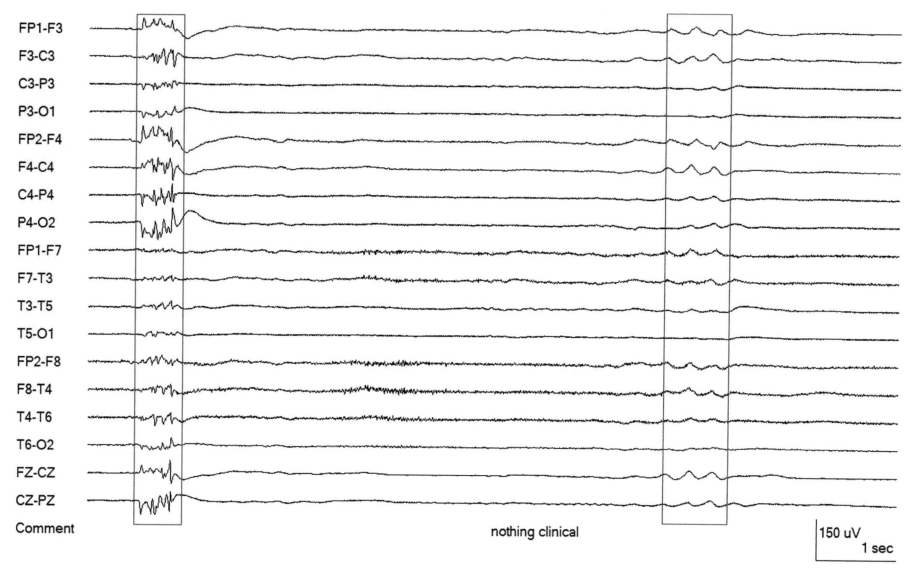

Figure 8.3. Myoclonic status epilepticus. (a) Burst-suppression pattern (with non-identical bursts). The EEG in this 40-year-old woman status post cardiac arrest being treated with hypothermia and receiving propofol shows a burst-suppression pattern. There are 10–15 s of suppression with bursts that look very different from each other (non-identical). The second burst on this page consists of a 1–2 s run of delta and theta rhythms (non-highly epileptiform burst, or HEB). The first burst on this page does qualify as a HEB (i.e., ≥2 epileptiform discharges occurring at >1 Hz); if this burst type (HEB) was seen in the 'majority' of bursts, then the pattern overall would be considered burst suppression with non-identical, highly epileptiform bursts. If the blunt burst on the right was more common than the HEB, then this would be burst suppression with non-identical, non-highly-epileptiform bursts.

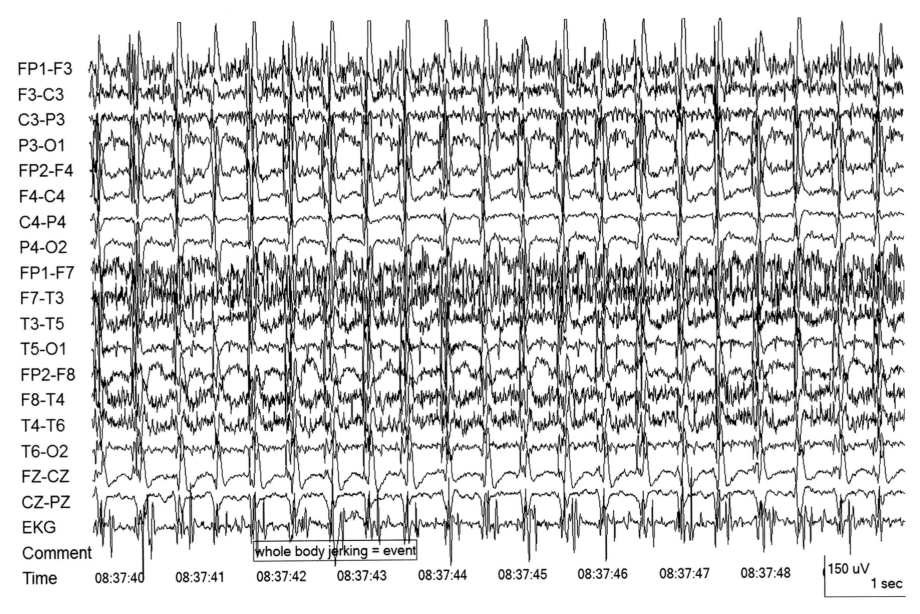

Figure 8.3. (*Continued*) (b) The following day the patient was in myoclonic status epilepticus and the EEG showed generalized periodic spikes and polyspikes.

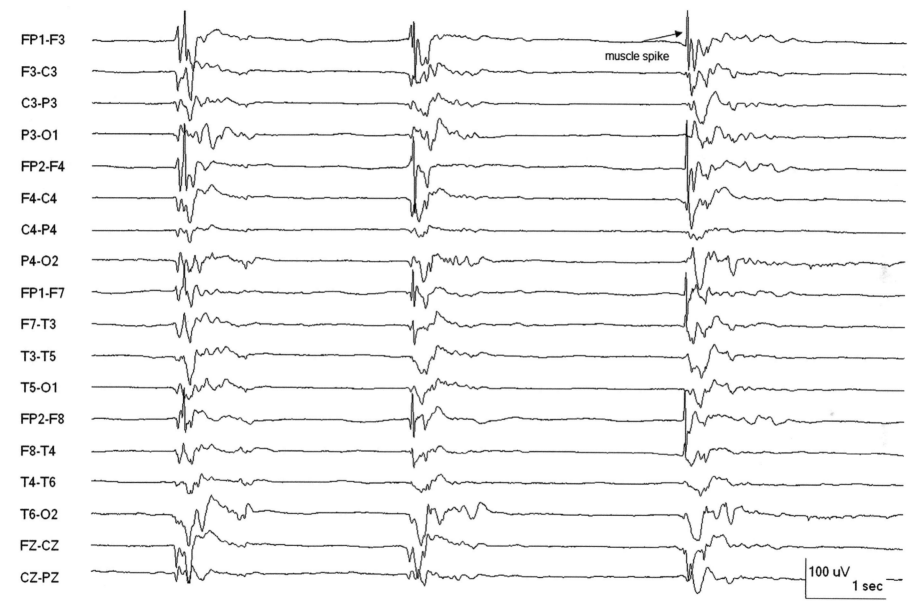

Figure 8.4. Subtle myoclonic SE. (a) The EEG in this 66-year-old woman status post cardiac arrest shows a burst-suppression pattern with superimposed muscle spikes (arrow). The latter are prominent in the Fp1 and Fp2 electrodes but not in the midline electrodes (Fz, Cz and Pz), which are usually free of muscle artifact. The patient was in subtle myoclonic status epilepticus.

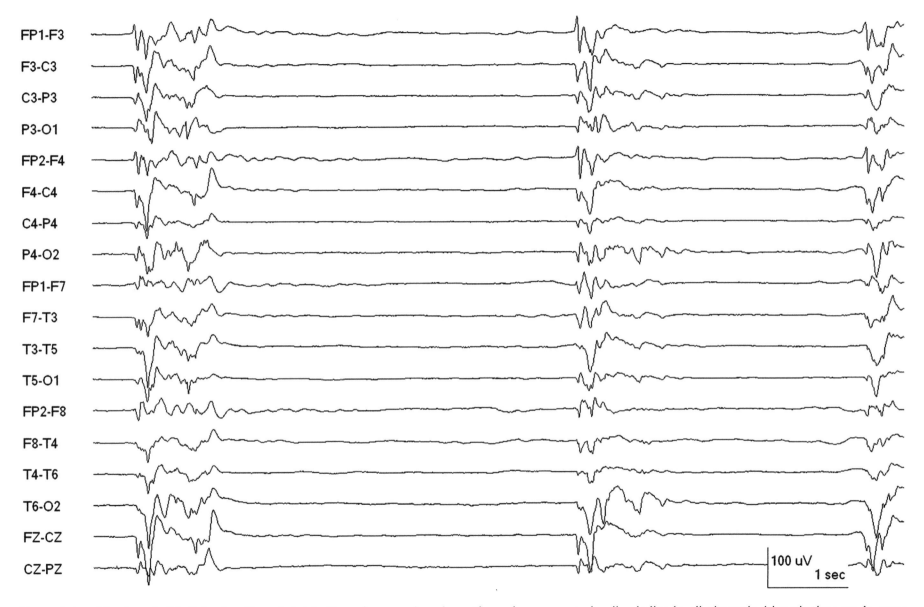

Figure 8.4. (*Continued*) (b) Following the administration of vecuronium (a paralytic) the pattern persists confirming that these bursts represent brain activity; but the small spikes of muscle artifact are no longer present. Note the bursts themselves are not visually similar in all channels (though they are in some channels) (i.e., non-identical).

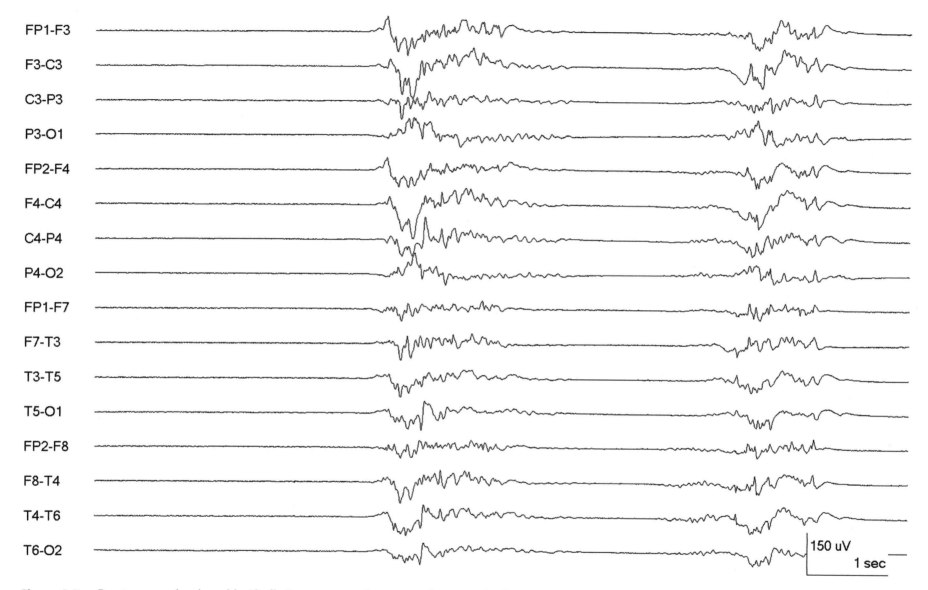

FP1-F3

F3-C3

C3-P3

P3-O1

FP2-F4

F4-C4

C4-P4

P4-O2

FP1-F7

F7-T3

T3-T5

T5-O1

FP2-F8

F8-T4

T4-T6

T6-O2

150 uV

1 sec

Figure 8.5.   Burst suppression (non-identical). Burst-suppression pattern is present in this 55-year-old man status post cardiac arrest. The bursts are non-identical.

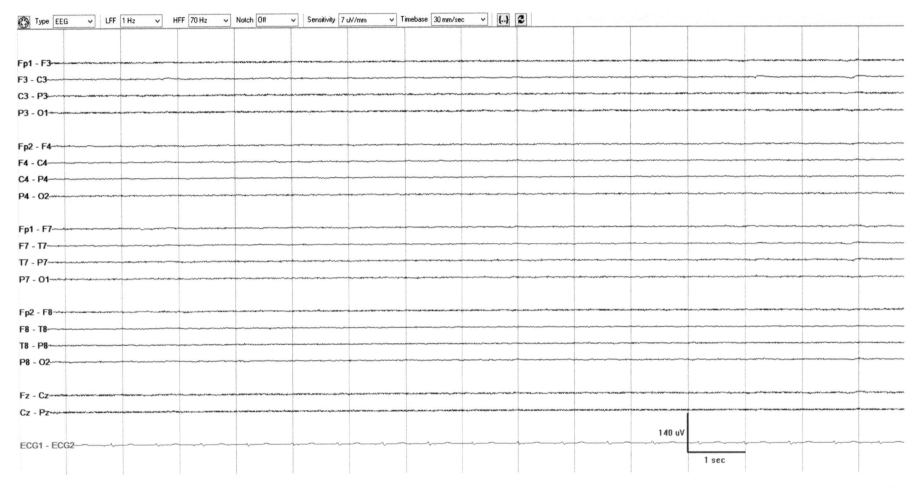

Figure 8.6. Progression from suppression to burst suppression with identical bursts to GPDs. (a) The initial EEG from a 69-year-old woman status post cardiac arrest is suppressed.

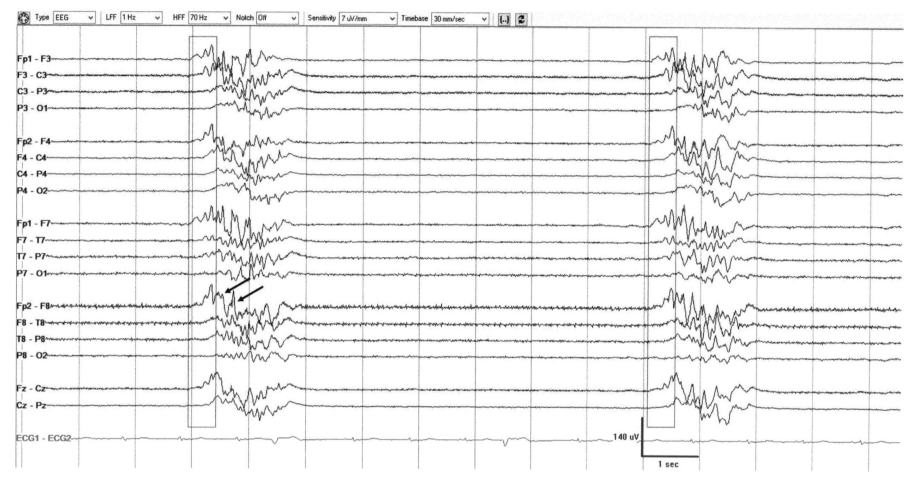

Figure 8.6. (*Continued*) (b) Later in the record the patient enters burst suppression with identical highly epileptiform bursts. The first ≥0.5 s of each burst are visually similar (this is highlighted with the boxes, each of 0.5 s duration). Note that after the first 0.5 s the bursts are not absolutely the same. These however still qualify as identical bursts as only the first 0.5 s are required for this by definition. The bursts also have ≥2 epileptiform discharges (some highlighted with arrows) occurring at an average of ≥1 Hz within a single burst for the majority (>50%) of bursts. This is therefore burst suppression with identical and highly epileptiform bursts (identical HEBs).

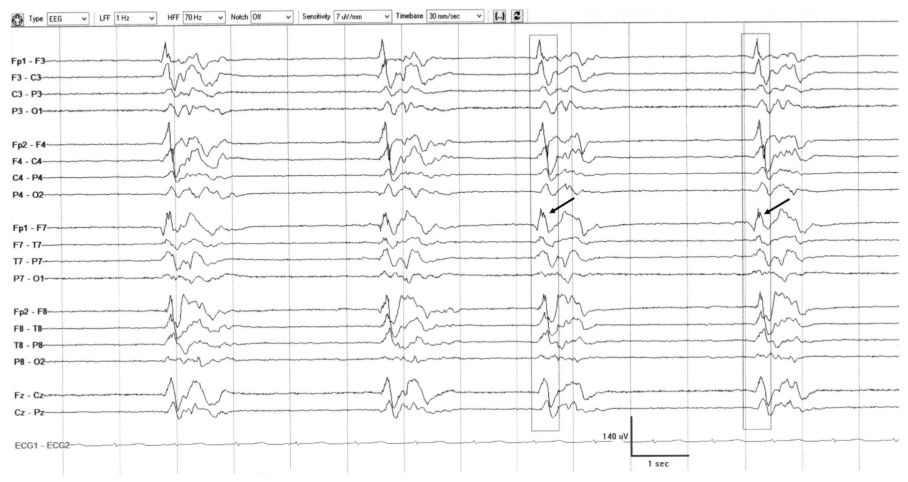

Figure 8.6. (*Continued*) (c) Later again in the record, the bursts of burst suppression have changed to identical non-HEBs. The first ≥0.5 s remains visually similar in the majority of bursts (boxes), but the bursts now consist of a single epileptiform discharge (arrows) followed by a high voltage slow wave and some faster rhythms mixed in. Even though there are epileptiform discharges within each burst, they are not occurring at ≥2 discharges at a rate of ≥1Hz within each burst, and therefore these are not HEBs. The pattern is burst suppression with identical, non-highly epileptiform bursts (identical non-HEBs).

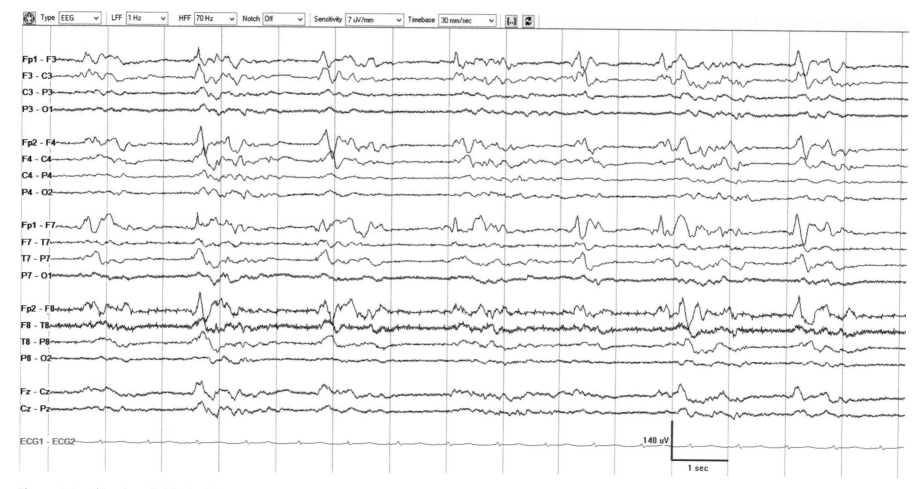

Figure 8.6. (*Continued*) (d) The following day the burst pattern remained the same; however, the interburst interval is significantly reduced. Even though the pattern remains the same, technically this page of EEG is no longer burst suppressed but discontinuous. This is because the activity (lasting approximately 1.5 s) alternates with attenuation lasting approximately 1 s. The suppression percentage in this case (1/[1+1.5] or 1/2.5 s) is 40%. Burst suppression only applies if the suppression percentage is 50–99%. This is now a discontinuous record with GPDs+F at ~0.5 Hz.

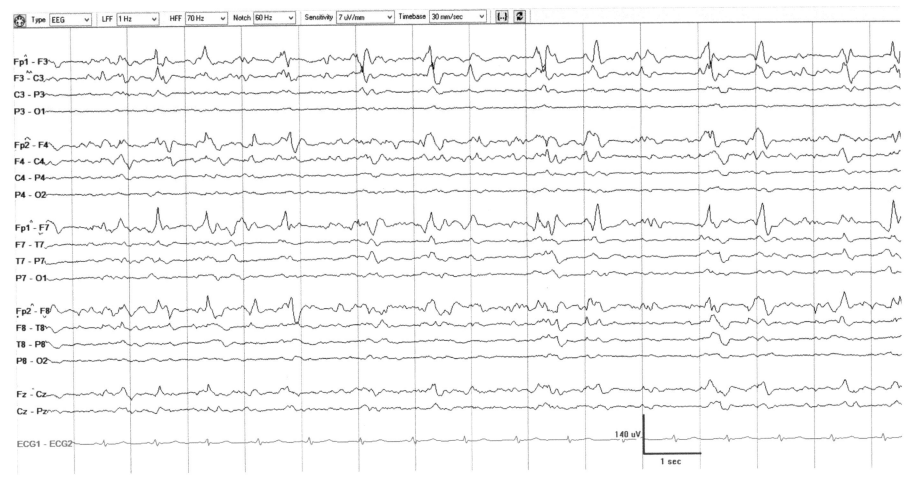

Figure 8.6. (*Continued*) (e) The background EEG actually became nearly continuous (with a couple of 1–2 s periods of attenuation [e.g., where the scale legend is], but not suppression, on this page) with GPDs at 1 Hz, frontally predominant. Although a few of the sharp waves in a row are more prominent on the left, the majority are symmetric, so GPDs is a better fit than LPDs on this page.

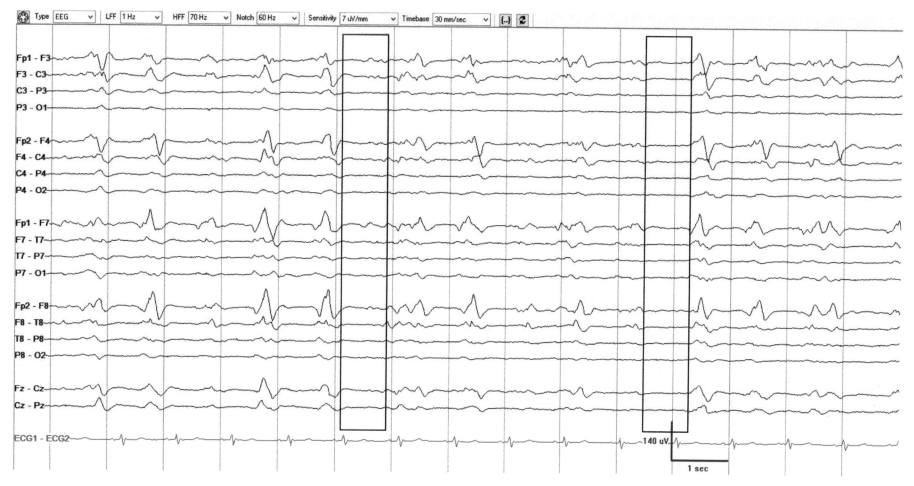

Figure 8.6. *(Continued)* (f) Unfortunately, the background activity worsened, becoming lower amplitude and slower, with the boxes highlighting that there is now suppression (<10 uV; not just attenuation) in between some of the GPDs.

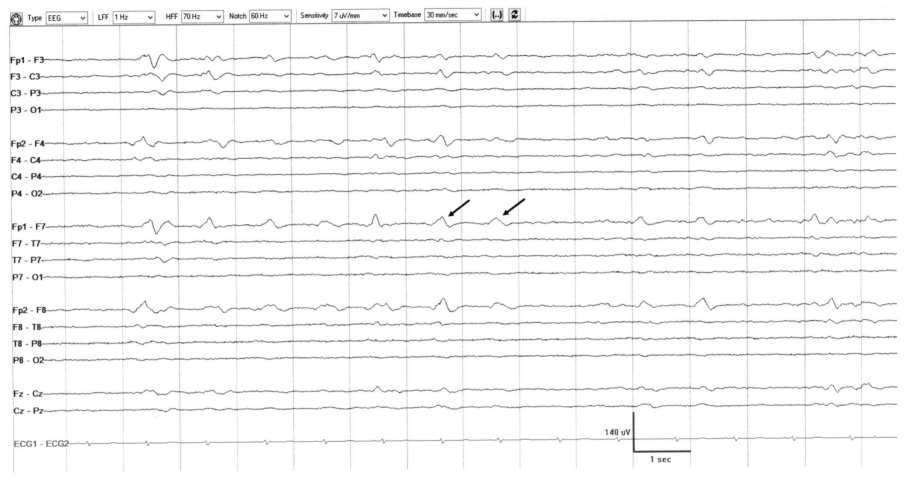

Figure 8.6. (*Continued*) (g) The background became suppressed and the GPDs then became lower voltage and poorly formed (only sharply contoured since >200 msec in duration at the EEG baseline [arrows]). Assuming this is not due to sedative medications, this worsening is a poor prognostic indicator.

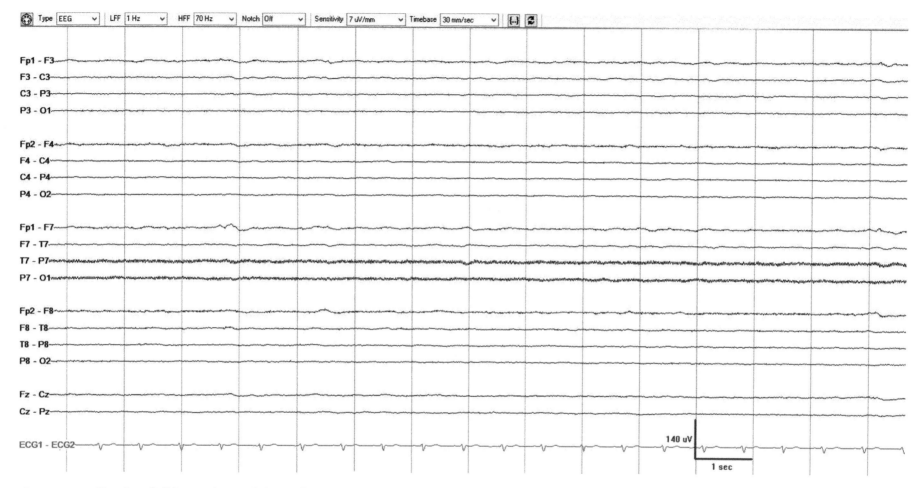

Figure 8.6. (*Continued*) (h) Less than 12 h later, the EEG was completely suppressed. This sequence of EEGs demonstrates the change in patterns over time in the post cardiac arrest setting and helps to highlight an important point: the trajectory is often more important than a specific timepoint, and the EEG should never be used alone for decisions on withdrawal of life-sustaining treatment.

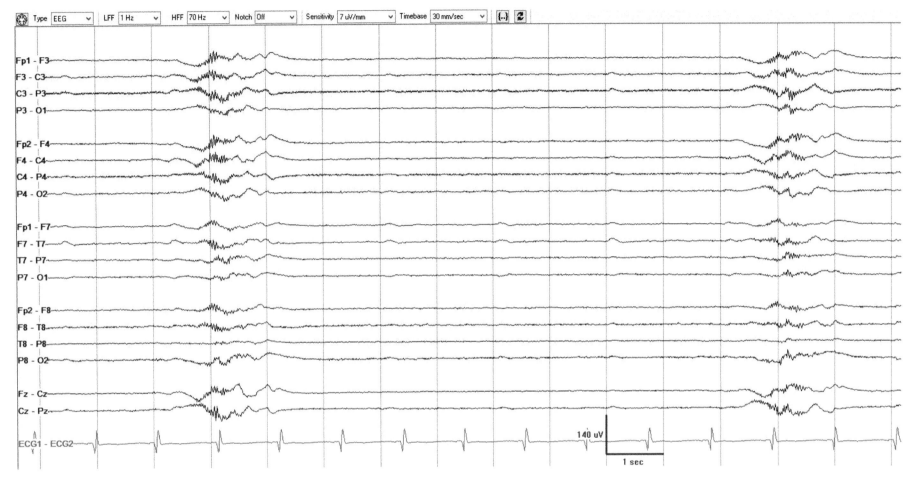

Figure 8.7. Progression of burst suppression to moderate slowing. (a) This EEG is taken from a 33-year-old woman who presented following an intentional polypharmacy overdose, with three bilateral tonic-clonic seizures, and subsequent cardiac arrest, with return of spontaneous circulation (ROSC) after one round of cardiopulmonary resuscitation. The EEG demonstrates burst suppression where the bursts are visually similar in all channels (identical bursts), consisting of a slow wave and fast gamma range activity. These bursts are non-highly epileptiform.

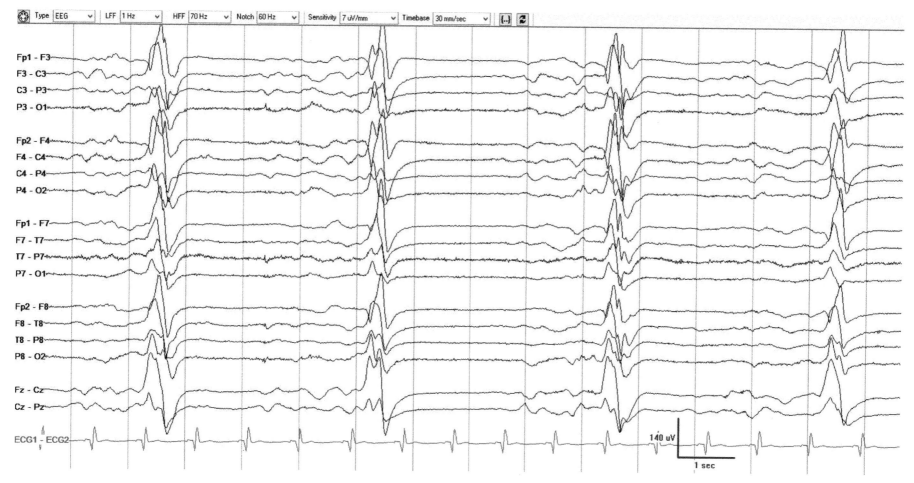

Figure 8.7. (*Continued*) (b) Six hours later the bursts have changed to now include a very high voltage sharp wave at the end of each burst, and with some variability in the earlier portions of the bursts (the low voltage, slower portion). Thus, these are now non-identical bursts.

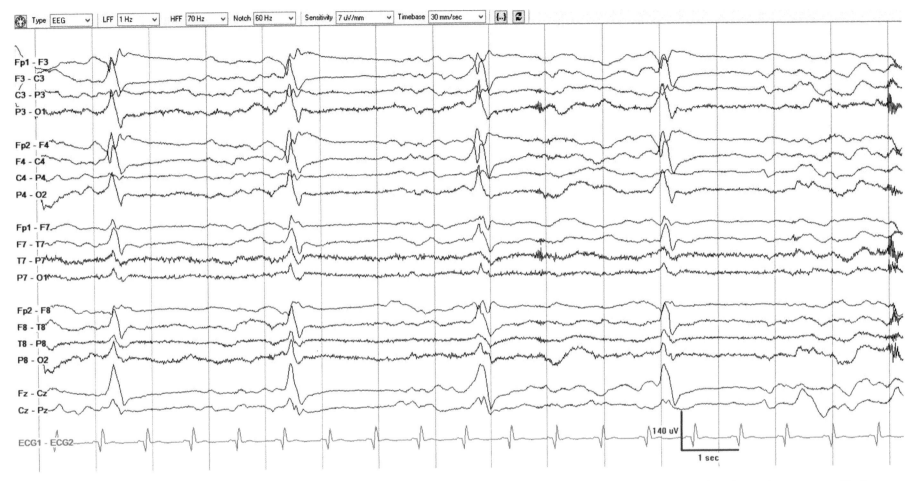

Figure 8.7.   (*Continued*) (c) Twelve hours later, the record is now discontinuous (no longer in burst suppression) with high voltage GPDs at 0.33 Hz (1 every 3 seconds).

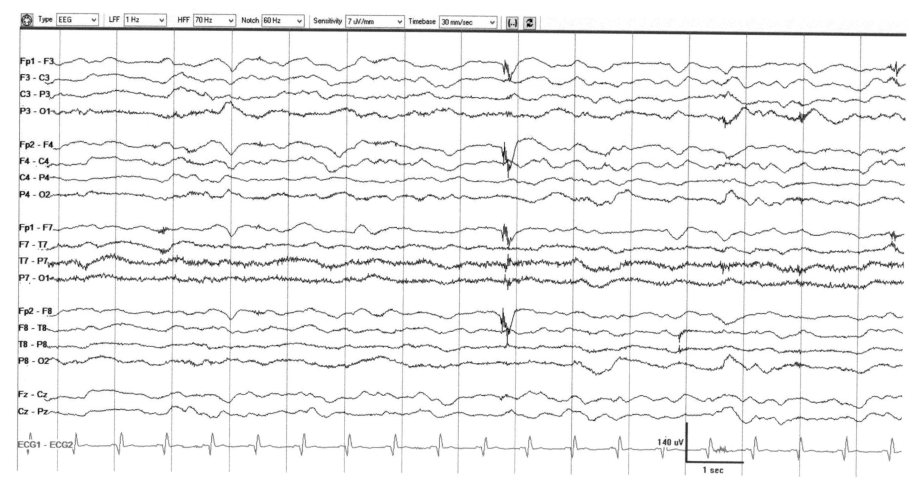

Figure 8.7. (*Continued*) (d) Twenty-four hours later, the record became continuous with resolution of the GPDs (without the addition of anti-seizure medication). The patient did very well and made a complete neurological recovery. This series of EEGs highlights an important point. The literature describing the prognostic implications of specific patterns within burst suppression is mostly limited to single center studies with a relatively small number of patients in each group. For example, identical bursts in the post cardiac arrest setting have been reported to be universally fatal; however, it may be possible for a patient that has strong protective factors (i.e., young age, rapidly reversible cause [polypharmacy], short duration of cardiac arrest) to do well. The caveat remains that the EEG is just one part of the prognostic discussion.

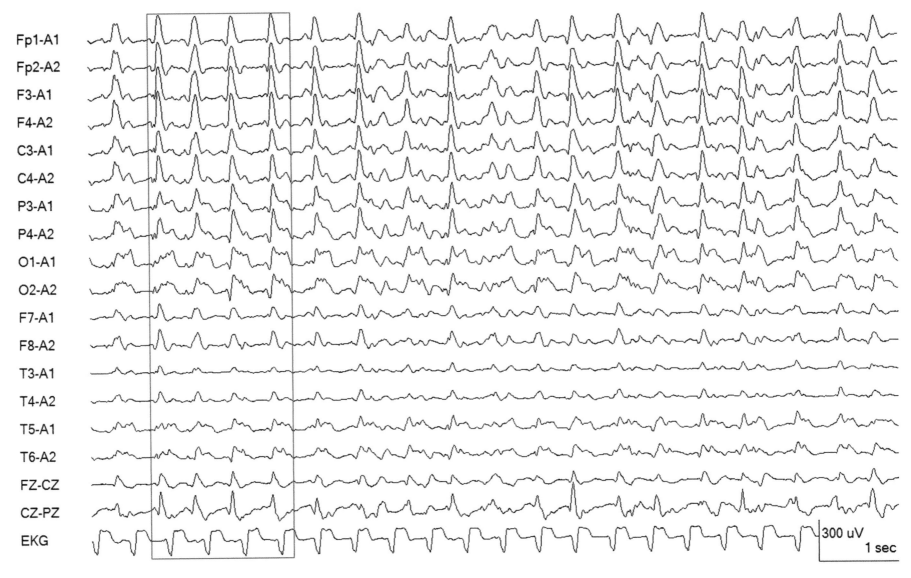

Figure 8.8. Ictal-interictal continuum. This 86-year-old man was being therapeutically cooled following cardiac arrest. He was initially in myoclonic SE. After the clinical myoclonus was controlled, there were continuous GPDs at a rate of 1.5–2 per second. This is not definitely ictal, however significantly abnormal and on the ictal/interictal continuum (IIC). It becomes difficult in this case to know if the pattern is just a result of the hypoxic injury and not harmful, or if the pattern itself is injurious to the hypoxic brain and warrants escalation of anti-seizure medications.

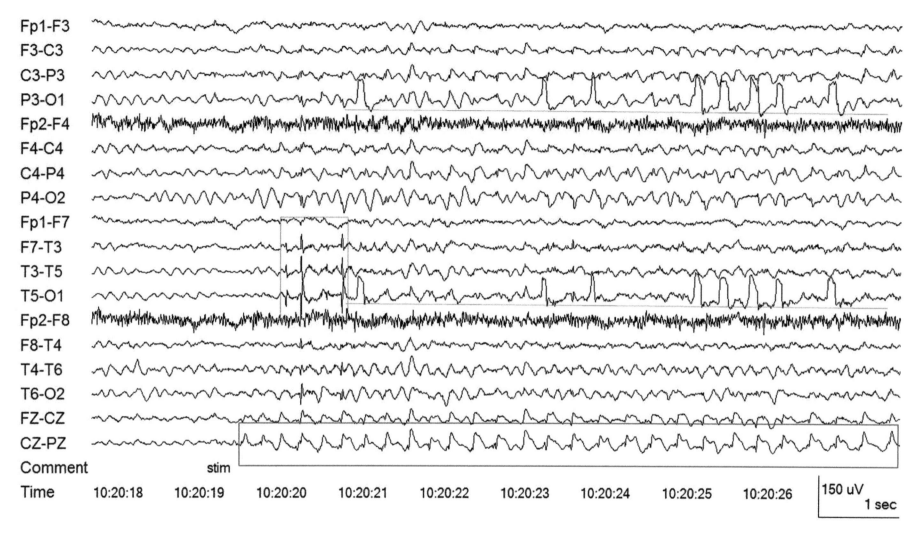

Figure 8.9. Stimulus-induced post-hypoxic myoclonus.
Following stimulation, repetitive spike-and-wave discharges present in the posterior head region (best seen in the Cz-Pz derivation), at times associated with myoclonic head jerks, are present in this 48-year-old woman with a recent hypoxic episode. Background activity is only mildly slow. There is also an O1 artifact (blue underline), as well as muscle spikes from the jerking (green box). The patient was following verbal commands and responsive to questioning. This patient had stimulus-induced post-hypoxic myoclonus that is presumably mostly subcortical given the lack of time-locked EEG correlate with each jerk, and given his awake state, yet there is clearly cortical excitability given the spike-wave discharges brought out with alerting stimuli (a form of SIRPIDs). This situation is not the same as myoclonic SE and may represent a different process, more akin to Lance-Adams syndrome of delayed postanoxic action myoclonus, a presumably subcortical process.

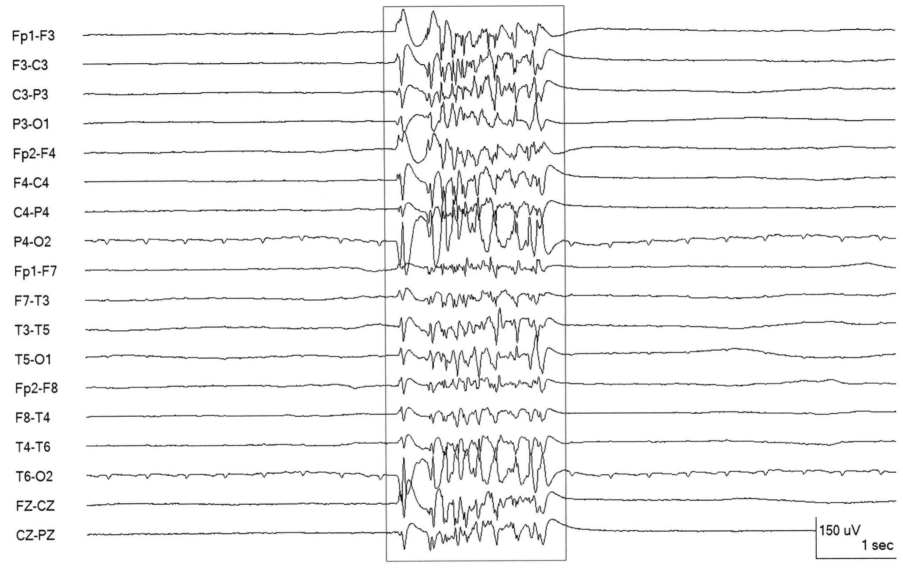

Figure 8.10.   Burst suppression with highly epileptiform bursts (HEBs). (a) The EEG in this 63-year-old woman status post cardiac arrest being treated with hypothermia frequently showed a burst-suppression pattern. The bursts were usually associated with brief eye opening (a variant of myoclonic seizures/status epilepticus). The bursts consist of 2–3 s runs of 5–6 Hz spike-wave-complexes with low-amplitude polyspike activity mixed in (highly epileptiform bursts [HEBs]). Although only one burst is shown due to prolonged periods of suppression, the bursts were not identical.

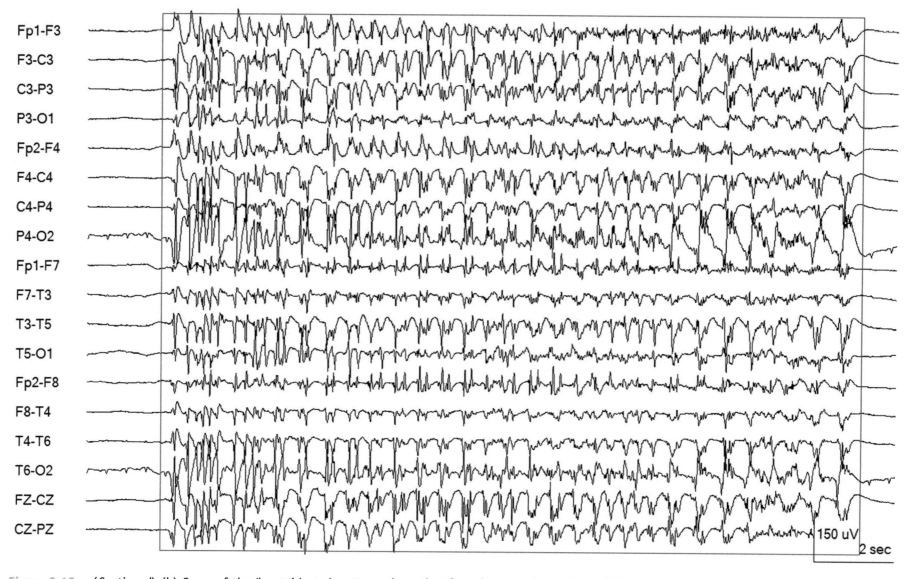

Figure 8.10. (*Continued*) (b) Some of the 'bursts' lasted >10 s and are therefore electrographic seizures (this one is ~15 s and shows evolution in frequency [slows down] and morphology [gets blunter over time]). Note the paper speed has been compressed for this figure.

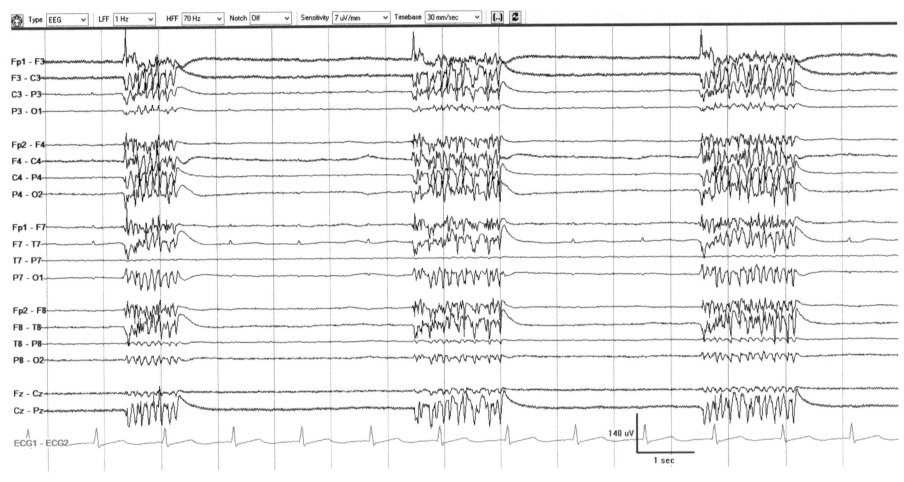

Figure 8.11. Highly epileptiform bursts, ESz and ESE. (a) This EEG is from a 47-year-old woman post cardiac arrest. The initial EEG demonstrates burst suppression with identical, highly epileptiform bursts HEBs.

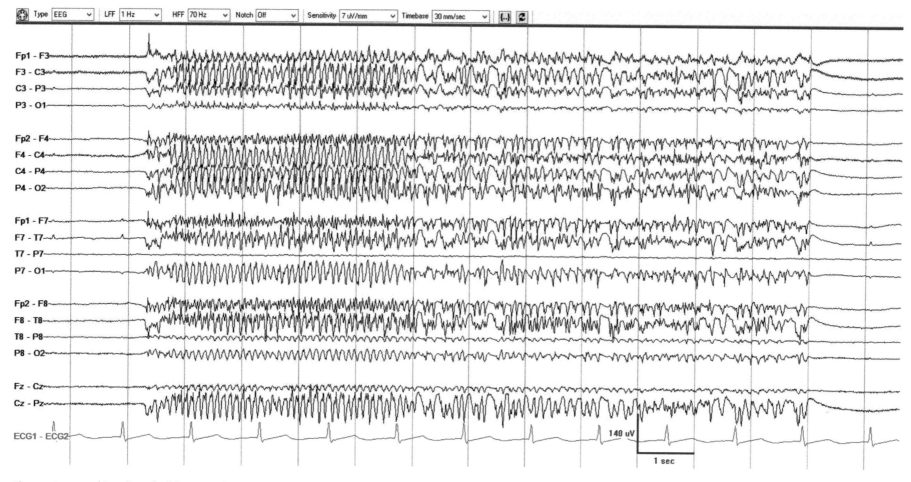

Figure 8.11. *(Continued)* (b) Later that day the patient started having clear electrographic seizures (ESz) lasting ≥10 s (11.5 s in this case), with epileptiform discharges >2.5 Hz (8–9 Hz here), with clear evolution in frequency and morphology.

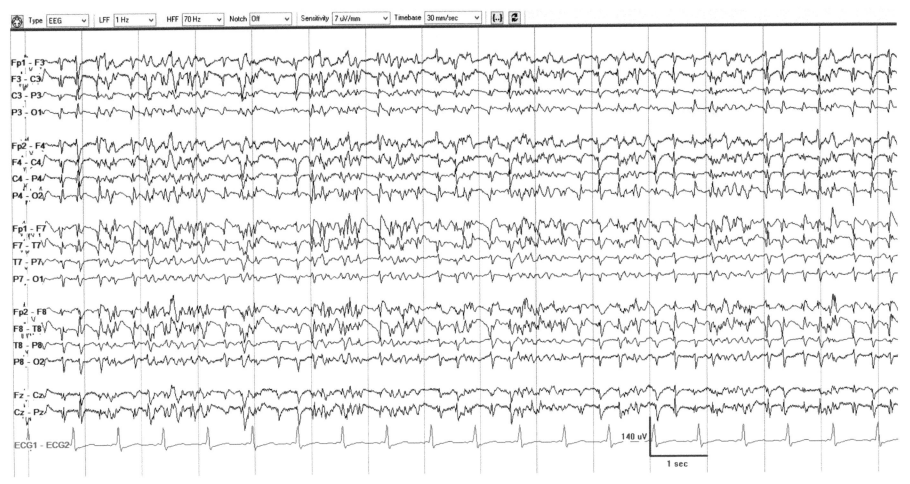

Figure 8.11. *(Continued)* (c) Despite increasing anti-seizure medications the patient developed electrographic status epilepticus (ESE) or NCSE. There was no clinical myoclonus (or other visible clinical correlate) associated with this state.

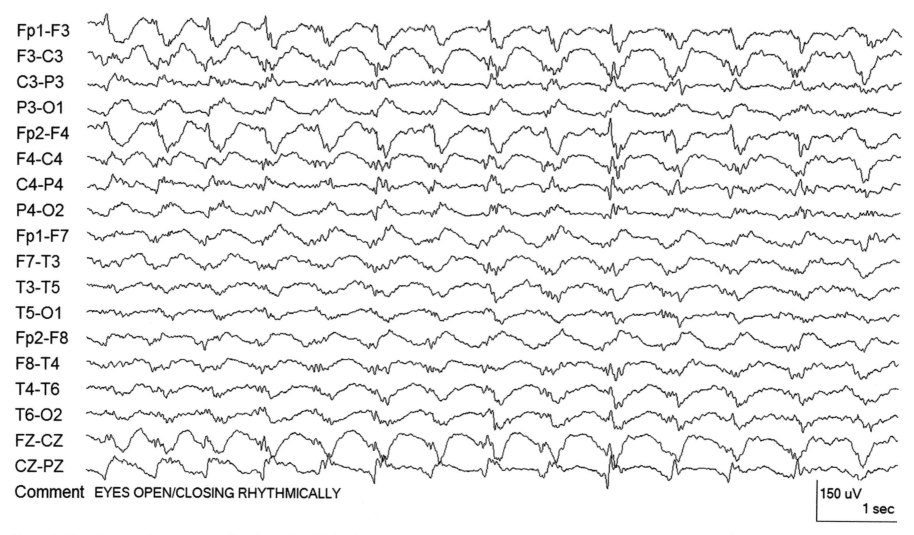

Comment EYES OPEN/CLOSING RHYTHMICALLY

150 uV

1 sec

Figure 8.12. Nonconvulsive status epilepticus. The EEG in this unresponsive 80-year-old woman status post cardiac arrest shows her to be in generalized electroclinical status epilepticus with rhythmic eye opening and closure associated with generalized poly-spike-and-wave (GSW). This also qualifies as nonconvulsive SE due to the subtle and nonconvulsive nature of the clinical correlate. Note that although this is electroclinical status epilepticus (ECSE), it does not qualify as electrographic status epilepticus (ESE). This example makes the point that the term NCSE still applies, but this is not entirely synonymous (although close) to the definitions of ESE and ECSE. For example, NCSE can include patients that have ESE alone, or ECSE where the clinical correlate is not prominent motor activity. In this case the patient has repetitive eye opening associated with GSW, but the GSW alone does not meet criteria for ESz/ESE (too slow). Thus, if there was no clinical correlate, this would not be considered a seizure.

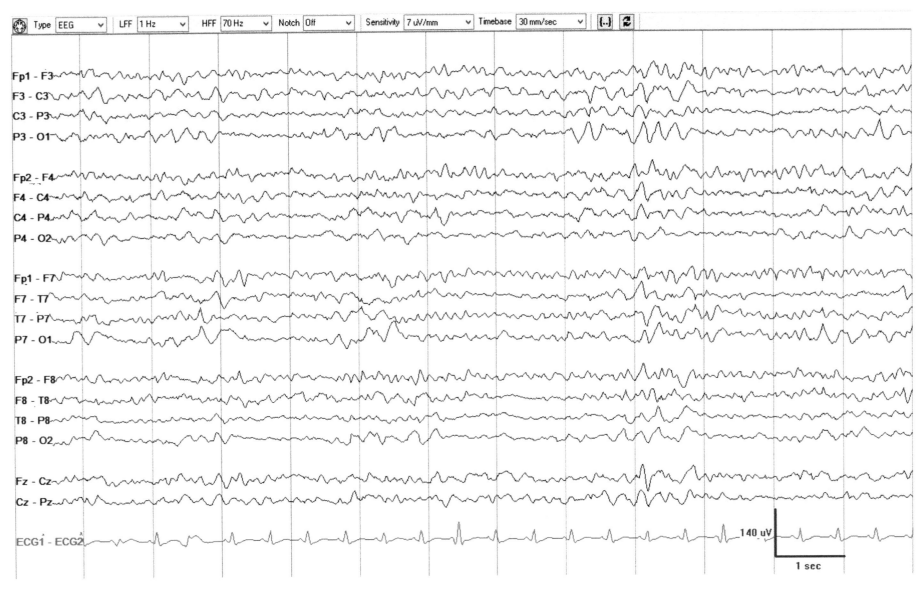

Figure 8.13.   Emergence of NCSE, post rewarming. (a) This EEG is from a 64-year-old woman status post cardiac arrest. The patient underwent TTM for 48 hours post cardiac arrest and for that time the EEG demonstrated reactive near continuous mild to moderate diffuse dysfunction, suggesting a good prognosis.

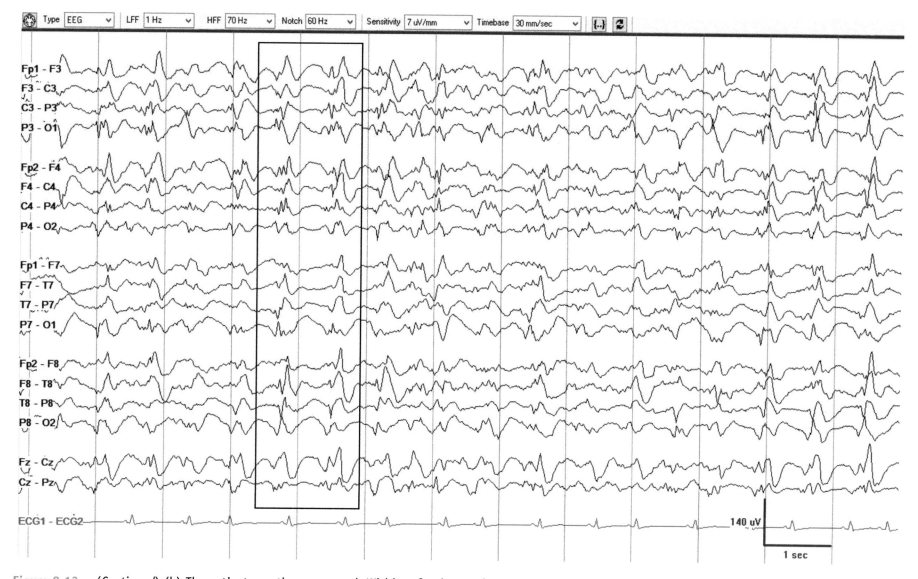

Figure 8.13. (*Continued*) (b) The patient was then rewarmed. Within a few hours of rewarming, the patient developed spiky 1–1.5 Hz GPDs+R (two highlighted in the box).

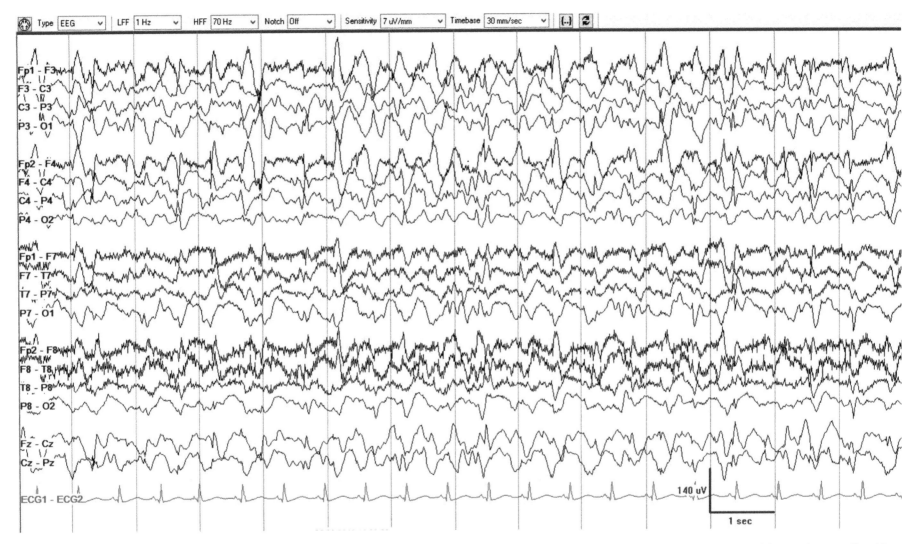

Figure 8.13. (*Continued*) (c) Later that day the patient developed long periods of fluctuating 2–2.5 Hz GPD+F, higher amplitude, felt to be consistent with NCSE (though technically on the ictal end of the ictal-interictal continuum, as mostly <2.5 Hz). This was successfully treated with anti-seizure medication. When a pattern is sustained at ≥2 Hz (even more so with prominent epileptiform discharges, fluctuation and medium-high amplitude), we usually treat them as probable seizures, or at least give an IV anti-seizure medication trial

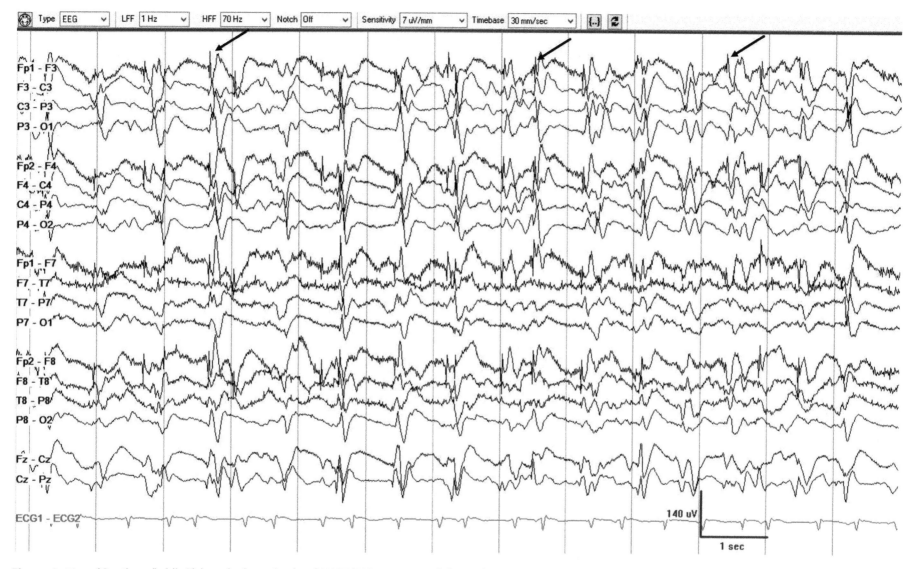

Figure 8.13. *(Continued)* (d) Although the episode of NCSE/ESE was treated, later that day the patient developed myoclonic status epilepticus. The EEG pattern here is of 1 Hz GPDs; however, there is now myoclonic jerking of her face (evidenced by the presence of EMG spikes with many discharges [arrows]).

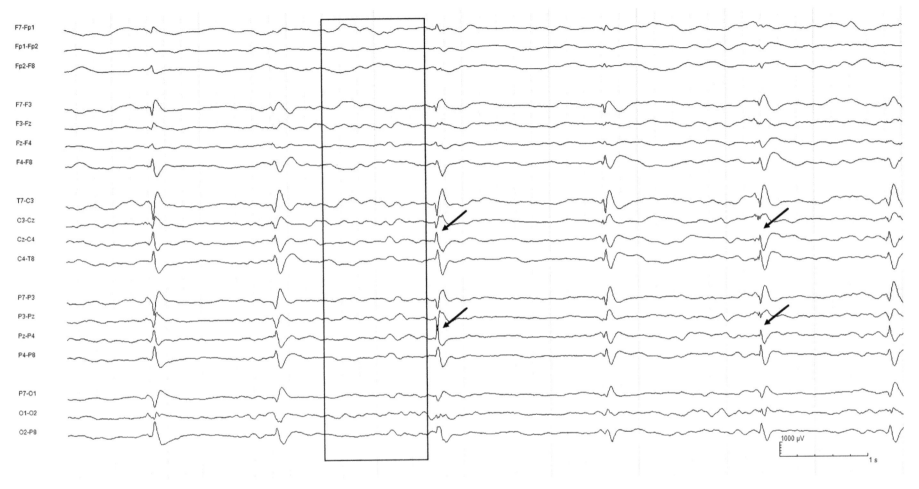

Figure 8.14. Postanoxic midline spikes leading to myoclonic status epilepticus, with good outcome. (a) Bipolar transverse. This series of EEGs is from a 43-year-old woman status post out-of-hospital cardiac arrest after smoking crack, with bystander CPR followed by five rounds of CPR administered by paramedics (return of spontaneous circulation [ROSC] ≈30 mins). The patient was intubated, and therapeutic temperature management (TTM) was commenced. On day 0, the EEG demonstrated moderate to severe generalized slowing with no epileptiform findings (not shown). As the patient was rewarmed on day 2 there was the emergence of vertex-maximal GPDs (phase reversal over Cz and Pz [arrows]) at 0.5 Hz. The other point to make is that there is not complete suppression of background rhythms (box).

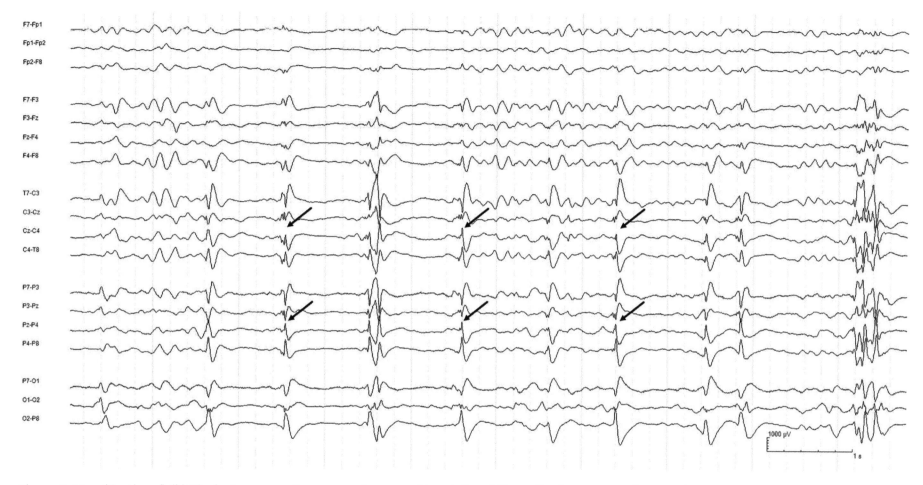

Figure 8.14. *(Continued)* (b) Bipolar transverse. Once rewarming was achieved, the midline spikes became more frequent (now 1 Hz) but also much spikier (arrows), sometimes polyspikes (see the last second of this page). There is still some background activity at times.

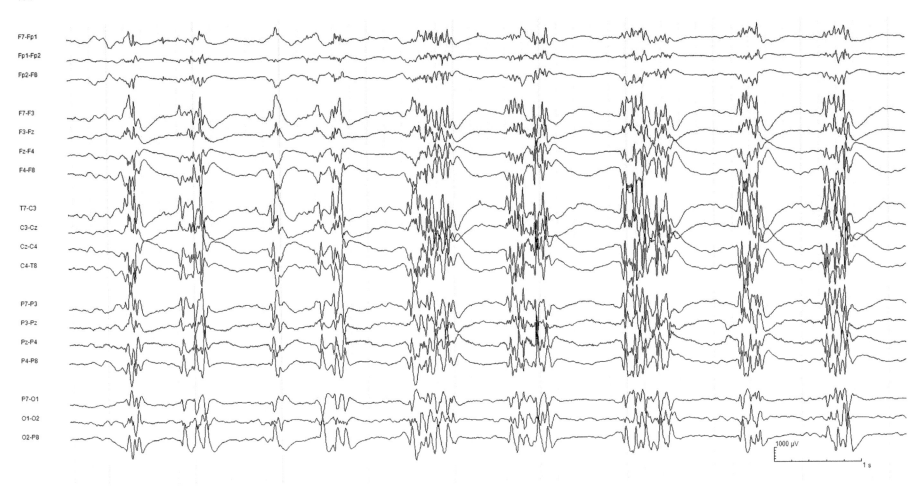

Figure 8.14. (*Continued*) (c) Bipolar transverse. The following day (day 3), the EEG changed to burst attenuation/suppression with highly epileptiform bursts (HEBs). There was subtle jerking associated with this activity at times, consistent with myoclonic status epilepticus.

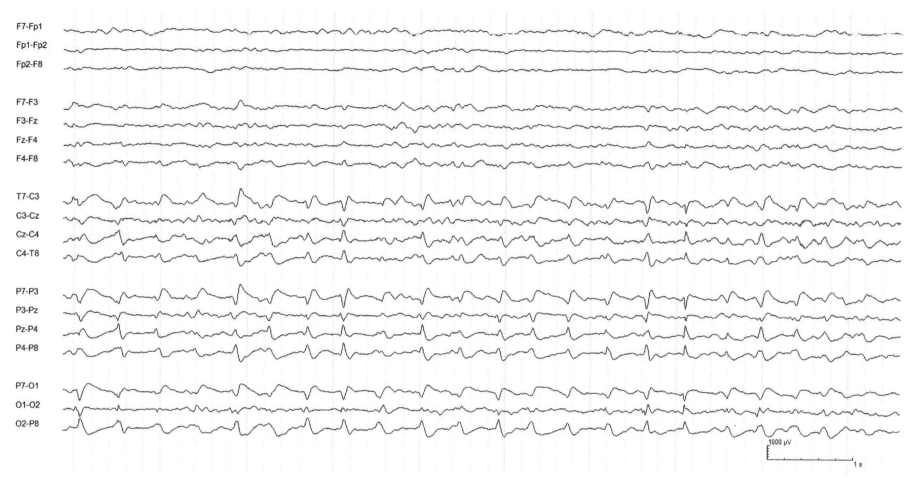

Figure 8.14. (*Continued*) (d) Bipolar transverse. The patient had refractory myoclonic status epilepticus, despite adequate trials of levetiracetam, phenytoin, lacosamide and phenobarbital. The patient was then started on midazolam and subsequently ketamine infusions. At that stage, the clinical jerking stopped, and the EEG pattern returned to midline predominant GPDs at 2–2.5 Hz, still on the ictal-interictal continuum (also with return of the background rhythms in between discharges).

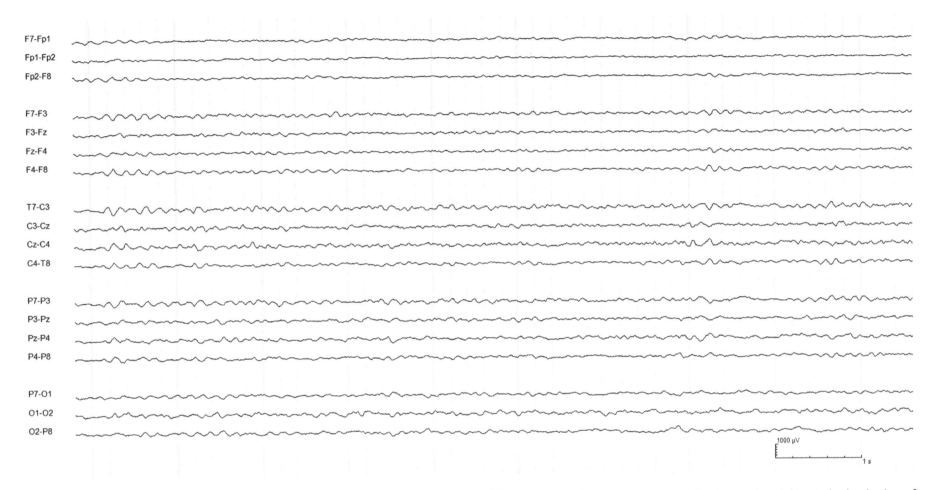

Figure 8.14. (*Continued*) (e) Bipolar transverse. Twenty-four hours later (day 4), with additional adjustment of ASMs, the GPDs resolved and the recovery of background rhythms continued. An MRI on day 10 did not demonstrate any acute abnormalities. Several months after discharge, she was walking and talking, alert and oriented × 3, recalled 1/3 objects after delay but 3/3 with multiple choice, and had a mildly spastic gait. The two points to make with this series of figures are: 1. there was continuous background activity at the beginning of the record and later in between GPDs; and 2. central/midline spikes associated with myoclonic status epilepticus have been reported in at least two small studies to be associated with much better outcome than other forms of myoclonic status epilepticus, including significant potential for good functional neurologic outcome, as seen in this case.

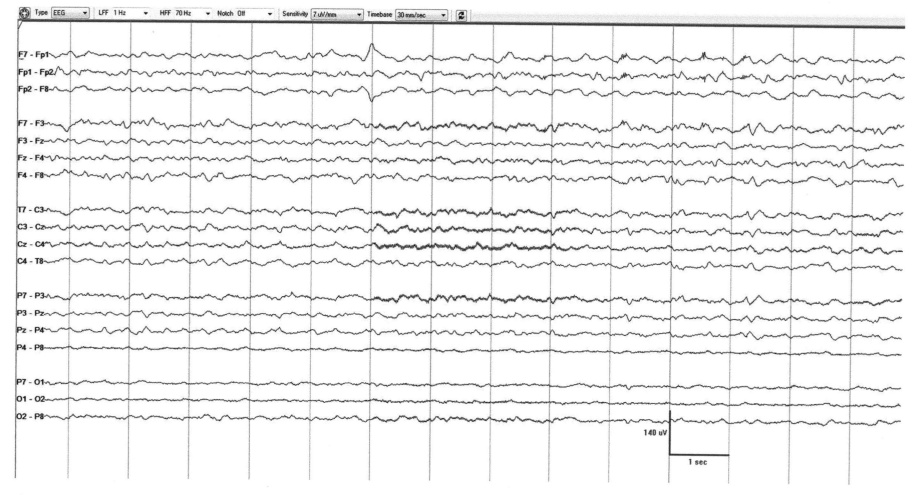

Figure 8.15. Discrete myoclonic seizures (i.e., not myoclonic status epilepticus). (a) Transverse bipolar. This EEG is from a 68-year-old man status post cardiac arrest. The initial EEG demonstrates moderate generalized slowing.

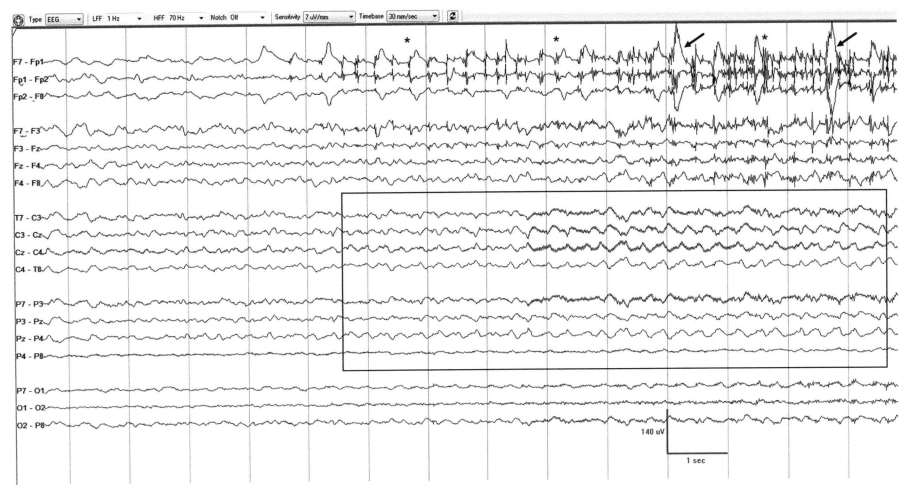

Figure 8.15. (*Continued*) (b) Transverse bipolar. The run of myoclonic seizures begins with an evolving 3–3.5 Hz rhythm in the midline Cz/Pz (box). This is associated with repeated very irregular myoclonic jerking of the head and face, evidenced by the bursts of EMG activity (asterisks) and blink artifacts (arrows) in the anterior electrode derivations.

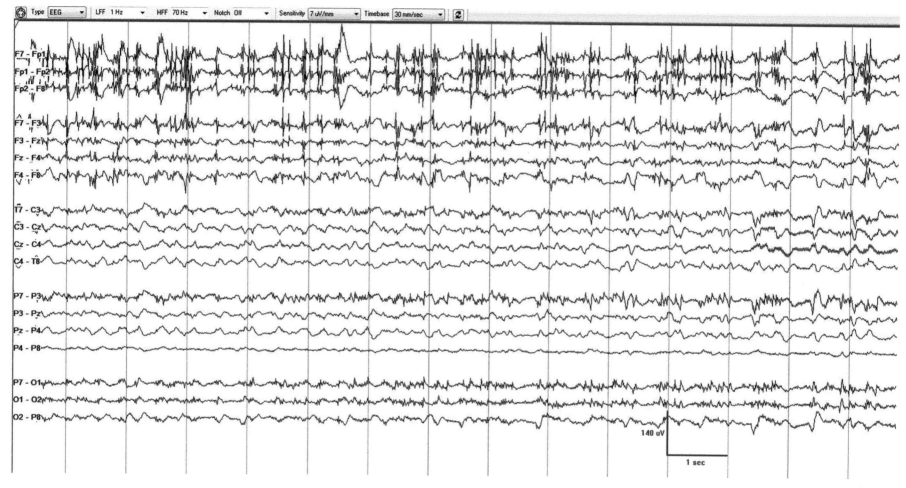

Figure 8.15. (*Continued*) (c) Transverse bipolar. Further evolution of the seizure with increased prominence of myoclonic jerking, yet still with only a subtle EEG correlate, slowing down a bit on this page.

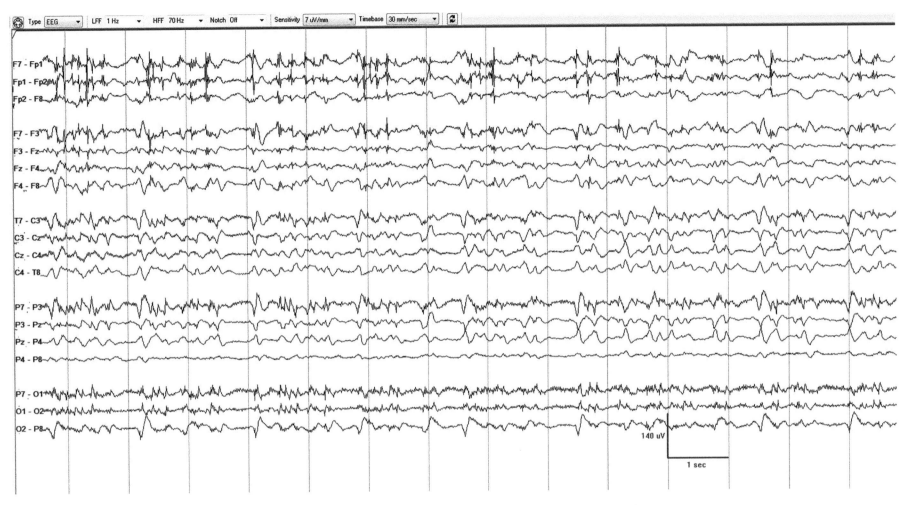

Figure 8.15. (*Continued*) (d) Transverse bipolar. As the seizure started to break up, the myoclonic jerking subsides.

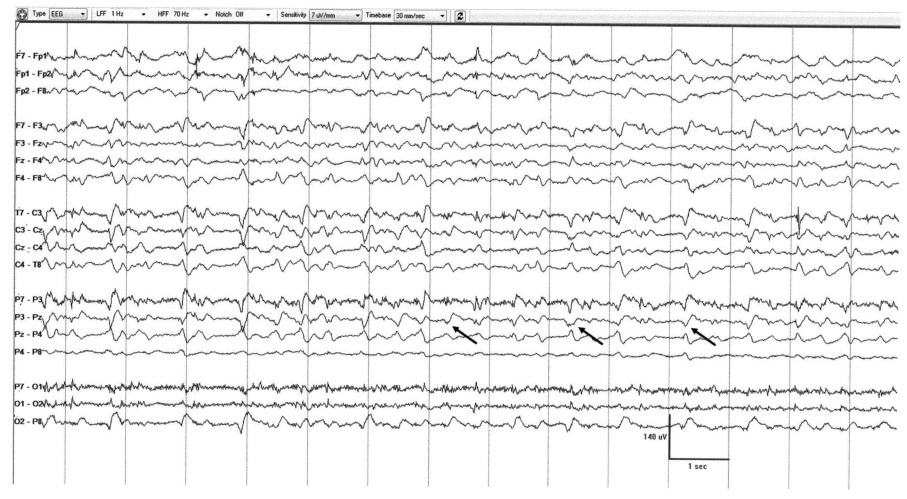

Figure 8.15. (*Continued*) (e) Transverse bipolar. De-evolution of the electrographic seizure with slowing down of the activity at Cz/Pz (arrows).

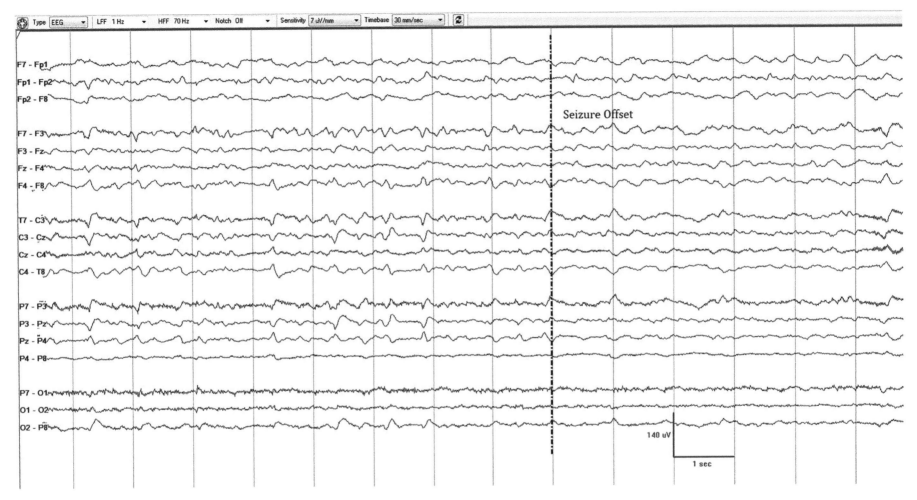

Figure 8.15. (*Continued*) (f) Transverse bipolar. Seizure offset (labeled dashed line). Once the electrographic seizure ends the EEG returns to moderate diffuse slowing. This patient had discrete periods consisting of repetitive myoclonus, but was not in myoclonic SE (i.e., the seizures were not continuous for ≥5 minutes [the time required for a convulsive seizure or seizure with prominent motor activity to qualify as SE], and the total duration of the ESz never exceeded 20% of the record [i.e., 12 minutes in any given hour]). Although rare, this can sometimes be seen following stimulation in the post-cardiac arrest setting.

9 Quantitative EEG: basics, seizure detection and avoiding pitfalls

Due to technical advances and increased awareness of the high prevalence of nonconvulsive seizures, prolonged EEG recording in the critically ill is standard of care in many centers. It is clear that the majority of seizures in the intensive care unit are nonconvulsive and can only be recognized with EEG. It is also clear that it is labor-intensive to review these studies. Quantitative EEG techniques have helped immensely in speeding this up. Although many are intimidated by these techniques, they are actually quite simple in principle and easy to learn. As software programs have improved, QEEG has become more and more useful. Not only can seizures be detected, but other acute brain events as well, such as ischemia, hydrocephalus, hemorrhage and so on. Several existing software programs will enable one to set alarms and, theoretically, to do true real-time monitoring once the infrastructure has been put in place and someone is available to respond to the alarms and interpret the study (currently only possible in a small percent of institutions). In the not-too-distant future, this type of real-time monitoring, or 'neurotelemetry', will be available in many centers, akin to cardiac telemetry today. This chapter covers the initial basics of quantitative EEG with some of the special indications and uses outlined in a subsequent chapter.

Perhaps the simplest way to consider QEEG is to think of it as an additional montage. As introduced in the very first chapter of this book, selecting a different montage does not change the content of the EEG, but rather how this content is displayed. QEEG merely has the advantage of being able to display hours and even days of EEG on a single page. As previously introduced, different montages (or 'trends', the term commonly used with QEEG) have strengths and weaknesses, and this concept also applies to the use of QEEG. The QEEG can be thought of as a Swiss army knife. As a whole it is immensely versatile. However, the ability to apply it to every situation depends on the understanding of the range of unique tools that it contains. This chapter aims to introduce the abilities of QEEG, demonstrate certain limitations, and most importantly demonstrate how these limitations can often be overcome by knowledge-based selection of a trend best suited to the task.

Quantitative EEG is excellent for detecting seizures, rhythmic and periodic patterns, asymmetries, and for following long-term trends, as discussed in this chapter. The use of QEEG can reduce review times by up to 80% compared to manual screening of the raw EEG, while maintaining good (but not perfect) sensitivity. This can be achieved with appropriate training at a resident level and is easy to incorporate into regular EEG review. Automated seizure detection algorithms have also improved over time and are now at the stage of demonstrating non-inferiority compared to expert review in some studies. The gold standard remains review of the raw EEG; however, QEEG can drastically reduce the time this takes, can highlight subtle features such as asymmetries that can be hard to appreciate, and can easily demonstrate long-term trends, which are often hard to register if looking at the EEG page

Hirsch and Brenner's Atlas of EEG in Critical Care, Second Edition. Lawrence J. Hirsch, Michael W.K. Fong, and Richard P. Brenner.

by page. In addition, it allows detailed, focused review of times of interest (especially times of changing EEG patterns or automated detections) rather than superficial review of all times (as occurs with rapid review of the entire raw EEG). QEEG is particularly useful in monitoring for ischemia; such special applications will be covered in Chapter 10.

Figure list

9.1 Spectrogram basics

Figure 9.1 Spectrogram basics: state changes and alpha rhythm.

Figure 9.2 Spectrogram basics: mechanical artifact – bed oscillator.

Figure 9.3 Spectrogram basics: drug-induced beta and asymmetry.

Figure 9.4 Spectrogram basics: multiple seizures.

Figure 9.5 Spectrogram basics: multiple seizures arising from complete suppression.

Figure 9.6 Spectrogram basics: cyclic nonconvulsive seizures.

Figure 9.7 Spectrogram basics: muscle artifact.

Figure 9.8 Spectrogram basics, long-term trends: NCSE culminating with convulsion.

Figure 9.9 Spectrogram basics, long-term trends: slow worsening ictal-interictal continuum (IIC) progressing to electrographic status epilepticus (ESE).

Figure 9.10 Spectrogram basics, long-term trends: gradual resolution of ESE, IIC and BIPDs.

Figure 9.11 Spectrogram basics, long-term trends: wearing off of pentobarbital.

Figure 9.12 Spectrogram basics, long-term trends: glucose load effect in glucose transporter deficiency.

Figure 9.13 Spectrogram basics, long-term trends: CO_2 retention, acidosis and resolution of nonconvulsive seizures.

9.2 Quantitative EEG: basics

Figure 9.14 QEEG basics, suppression percent: wearing off of neuromuscular blockade and return of shivering artifact.

Figure 9.15 QEEG basics, amplitude-integrated EEG and suppression percent: patient death.

Figure 9.16 QEEG basics, amplitude-integrated EEG and asymmetry measures: normal study with state changes.

Figure 9.17 QEEG basics, asymmetry measures and rhythmicity spectrogram: subdural hematoma and breach effect, and aEEG 'false positives'.

Figure 9.18 QEEG basics, asymmetry measures including alpha/delta ratio: left hemispheric ischemia.

Figure 9.19 QEEG basics, artifact detection, spike detection, and artifact reduction: myoclonic status epilepticus, targeted temperature management and neuromuscular blockade.

Figure 9.20 QEEG basics, typical bedside display.

9.3 Quantitative EEG: detection of seizures and rhythmic and periodic patterns

Figure 9.21 QEEG, detection of seizures: evolving nonconvulsive seizures.

Figure 9.22 QEEG, detection of seizures: de-evolving nonconvulsive seizures.

Figure 9.23 QEEG, detection of rhythmic delta activity: bilateral independent rhythmic delta activity (BIRDA).

Figure 9.24 QEEG, spike detector to detect typical frequency of GPDs: ictal-interictal continuum (IIC) monitoring.

Figure 9.25 QEEG long-term trends, spike detector, rhythmic delta detector: gradual development of nonconvulsive status epilepticus, treatment and recurrence.

Figure 9.26 QEEG long-term trends, spike detection, amplitude-integrated EEG, and suppression percent: suppression to GPDs to myoclonic status epilepticus.

Figure 9.27 QEEG, cyclic patterns: Cyclic Alternating Pattern of Encephalopathy (CAPE).

Figure 9.28 QEEG, cyclic patterns: CAPE with cyclic LPDs.

Figure 9.29 Cyclic patterns: CAPE, with abundant generalized sharp waves in the more awake state.

Figure 9.30 QEEG, cyclic patterns: cyclic 'ping-pong' seizures,

9.4   Quantitative EEG: pitfalls and solutions

Figure 9.31 QEEG pitfalls and solutions: artifact obscuring highly focal nonconvulsive seizures.

Figure 9.32 QEEG pitfalls and solutions: artifact mimicking seizures on amplitude-integrated EEG (aEEG).

Figure 9.33 QEEG pitfalls and solutions: multiple seizures and identical-appearing false positives on amplitude-integrated EEG (aEEG).

Figure 9.34 QEEG pitfalls and solutions: brief right and left hemispheric seizures in the context of GPDs and muscle artifact.

Figure 9.35 QEEG pitfalls and solutions: very focal seizures within breach effect.

Figure 9.36 QEEG pitfalls and solutions: very focal unilateral independent seizures and regional rhythmicity.

Figure 9.37 QEEG pitfalls and solutions: bilateral independent BIRDs and seizures.

EEGs throughout this atlas have been shown with the following standard recording filters unless otherwise specified: LFF 1 Hz, HFF 70 Hz, notch filter off.

Suggested reading

Abend NS, Dlugos D, Herman S. Neonatal seizure detection using multichannel display of envelope trend. *Epilepsia.* 2008 Feb;**49**(2):349–352.

Din F, Lalgudi Ganesan S, Akiyama T, et al. Seizure detection algorithms in critically ill children: a comparative evaluation. *Crit Care Med.* 2020;**48**(4):545–552.

Friedman DE, Schevon C, Emerson RG, Hirsch LJ. Cyclic electrographic seizures in critically ill patients. *Epilepsia* 2008 Feb;**49**(2):281–287.

Haider HA, Esteller R, Hahn CD, et al. Sensitivity of quantitative EEG for seizure identification in the intensive care unit. *Neurology.* 2016;**87**(9):935–944.

Koren J, Hafner S, Feigl M, Baumgartner C. Systematic analysis and comparison of commercial seizure-detection software. *Epilepsia.* 2021;**62**(2):426–438.

Kramer AH, Kromm J. Quantitative Continuous EEG: Bridging the Gap Between the ICU Bedside and the EEG Interpreter. *Neurocrit Care.* 2019;**30**(3):499–504.

Moura LM, Shafi MM, Ng M, et al. Spectrogram screening of adult EEGs is sensitive and efficient. *Neurology.* 2014;**83**(1):56–64.

Ng MC, Jing J, Westover MB. *Atlas of Intensive Care Quantitative EEG.* 1 ed. New York, Springer Publishing Company; 2019.

Ng MC, Jing J, Westover MB. A primer on EEG spectrograms. *J Clin Neurophysiol.* 2021.

Scheuer ML, Wilson SB. Data analysis for continuous EEG monitoring in the ICU: seeing the forest and the trees. *J Clin Neurophysiol.* 2004 Sep–Oct;**21**(5):353–378.

Scheuer ML, Wilson SB, Antony A, Ghearing G, Urban A, Bagic AI. Seizure detection: interreader agreement and detection algorithm assessments using a large dataset. *J Clin Neurophysiol.* 2021;**38**(5):439–447.

Shah DK, Mackay MT, Lavery EEG at B S, Watson S, Harvey AS, Zempel J, Mathur A, Inder TE. Accuracy of bedside electroencephalographic monitoring in comparison with simultaneous continuous conventional electroencephalography for seizure detection in term infants. *Pediatrics.* 2008 Jun;**121**(6):1146–1154.

Shellhaas RA, Soaita AI, Clancy RR. Sensitivity of amplitude-integrated electroencephalography for neonatal seizure detection. *Pediatrics.* 2007 Oct;**120**(4): 770–777.

Toet MC, van der Meij W, de Vries LS, Uiterwaal CS, van Huffelen KC. Comparison between simultaneously recorded amplitude integrated electroencephalogram (cerebral function monitor) and standard electroencephalogram in neonates. *Pediatrics.* 2002 May;**109**(5):772–779.

Williamson CA, Wahlster S, Shafi MM, Westover MB. Sensitivity of compressed spectral arrays for detecting seizures in acutely ill adults. *Neurocrit Care.* 2014;**20**(1):32–39.

Zafar SF, Amorim E, Williamsom CA, et al. A standardized nomenclature for spectrogram EEG patterns: Inter-rater agreement and correspondence with common intensive care unit EEG patterns. *Clin Neurophysiol.* 2020;**131**(9):2298–2306.

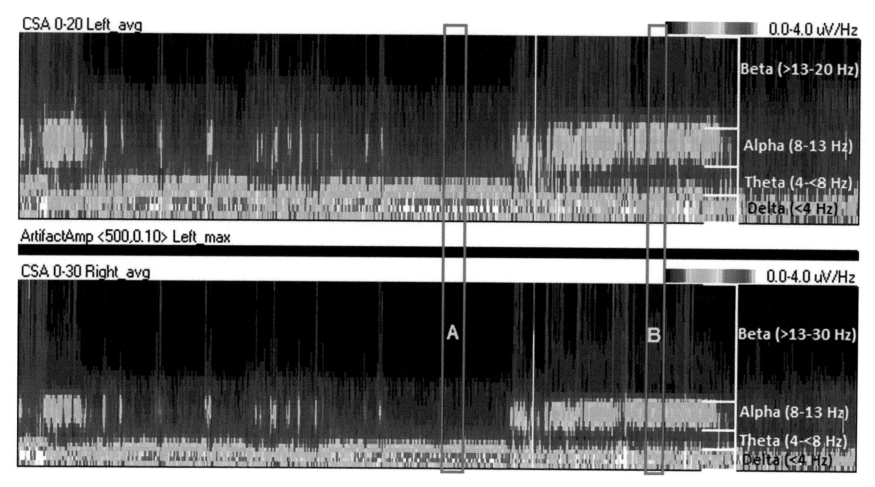

Figure 9.1. Spectrogram basics: state changes and alpha rhythm

Figure 9.1main Four hours of normal EEG. A basic and very useful quantitative EEG (QEEG) trend is the Compressed Spectral Array (CSA), which is also referred to as the Fast Fourier transform (FFT), density spectral array (or even compressed density spectral array), or power spectrogram ('spectrogram' for short). The premise of the CSA or FFT is that the raw EEG is made up of a series of superimposed rhythms of varying frequencies (delta, theta, alpha, beta, etc.). A Fourier transform can assist with breaking down that EEG into its products. It does this by matching how much of a specific frequency is present at any given time and represents this absolute amount on a color scale. The color scale can be seen at the top right of each row. On the left of the scale, black represents no activity, green the middle and red a high amount of activity. This 'amount of activity' is termed 'power', and it is akin to area under the curve for activity in that frequency (a combination of amplitude and duration). Within each row, frequency is mapped on the y axis, and time on the x axis. The bottom of the y axis is zero or 1 Hz, and the top of the y axis is typically set between 20–30 Hz (i.e., beta range activity). The scale for the y axis has been superimposed to the right of both rows. The top panel on this page is the CSA for the left hemisphere and the bottom panel the CSA for the right hemisphere.

(A)

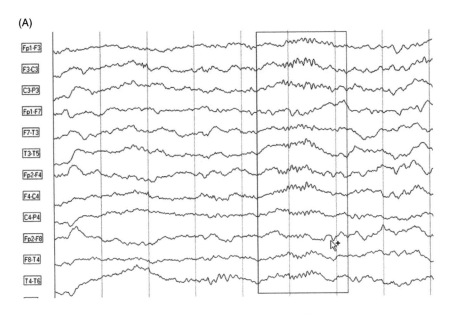

(B)

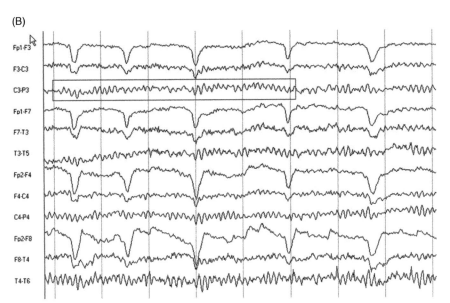

Figure 9.1.   (*Continued*) While the patient is asleep (A), most power is in the delta frequency (near the bottom). While awake (B), there is less delta (the white and red are no longer seen at the bottom of the tracings, and there is a prominent horizontal green band at ~10 Hz. The 10 Hz activity is due to the alpha rhythm (see raw EEG). Note, to demonstrate the effect of altering the scale of the y axis, the top row [left hemisphere] is displaying 0–20 Hz and the bottom row [right hemisphere] is displaying 0–30 Hz (therefore there is more black at the top of the lower row because there is little activity in the 20–30 Hz range that has been omitted from the top row). In practice the y scales of the left and right hemisphere should be equal so a comparison can be easily made between hemispheres. (A) EEG at A: normal stage N2 sleep with a sleep spindle shown in the box. (B) EEG at B: normal awake EEG with a 9.5–10 Hz posterior dominant (alpha) rhythm (box).

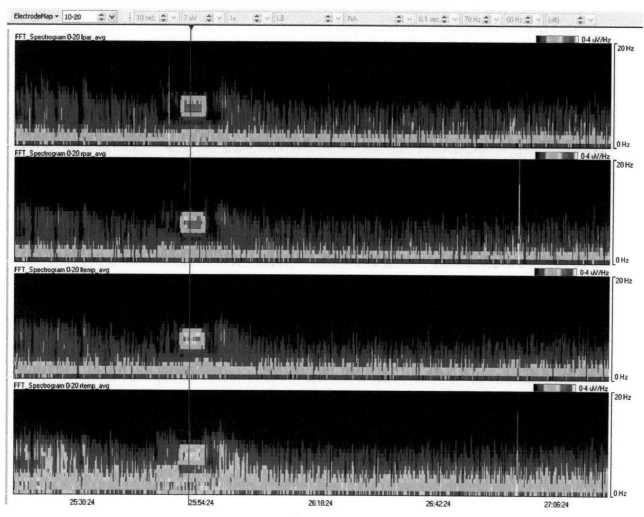

Figure 9.2. Spectrogram basics: mechanical artifact – bed oscillator

Figure 9.2main Spectrogram showing 3 hours of QEEG. The concept of the CSA is highlighted by this example. A pair of CSA rows usually comprises of homologous brain regions (in order to make direct comparison). In Figure 9.1, the left and right hemispheres were being compared. In this example, the top two rows are the left and right parasagittal regions (labels in the top left of each row) and the bottom pair of rows are the left and right temporal regions. Throughout this 3-hour period, the EEG demonstrates diffuse slow activity (with mostly delta, especially <2 Hz, and some theta range power) with no faster frequencies (no power above 10 Hz here, and little above 5–6 Hz). There is then a period lasting several minutes with sudden appearance of activity between 5 and 10 Hz, remaining constant, then stopping suddenly (cursor line is during this activity). This causes a square shape on the spectrogram. Raw EEG at that time shows widespread 7 Hz activity. This was caused by the bed vibrating at 7 Hz due to a mechanical oscillator. Sharp edges on a spectrogram (sudden on, sudden off) and a constant frequency activity (perfectly flat tops and bottoms) with little change should raise suspicion of mechanical artifact. The example highlights the concept of the CSA: when a 7 Hz activity is suddenly introduced into the EEG, there is a high amount of power seen at this specific frequency. The activity is unchanging, and therefore the red band remains as long as the artifact is present. As soon as it is turned off, there is very little power in this frequency, and therefore the band instantly disappears.

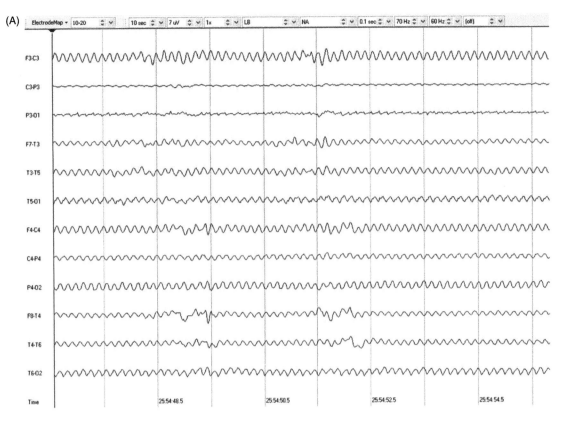

Figure 9.2.   (A) EEG at line showing a monomorphic sinusoidal 7-Hz activity from a bed oscillator.

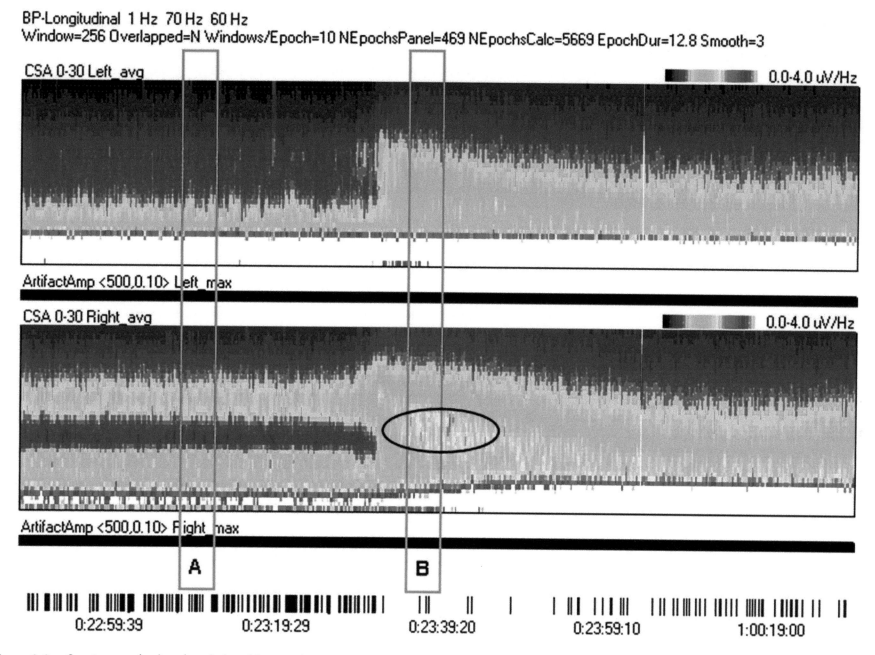

BP-Longitudinal 1 Hz 70 Hz 60 Hz
Window=256 Overlapped=N Windows/Epoch=10 NEpochsPanel=469 NEpochsCalc=5669 EpochDur=12.8 Smooth=3

CSA 0-30 Left_avg 0.0-4.0 uV/Hz

ArtifactAmp <500,0.10> Left_max

CSA 0-30 Right_avg 0.0-4.0 uV/Hz

ArtifactAmp <500,0.10> Right_max

A   B

0:22:59:39   0:23:19:29   0:23:39:20   0:23:59:10   1:00:19:00

Figure 9.3. Spectrogram basics: drug-induced beta and asymmetry
Figure 9.3main Two hours of QEEG demonstrating the spectrogram between
1–30 Hz in a 4-year-old with status epilepticus (with right body twitching at
times), treated with midazolam infusion. The case demonstrates the benefit of
viewing homologous brain regions.

(A)

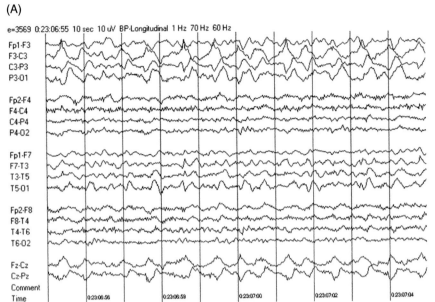

(B)

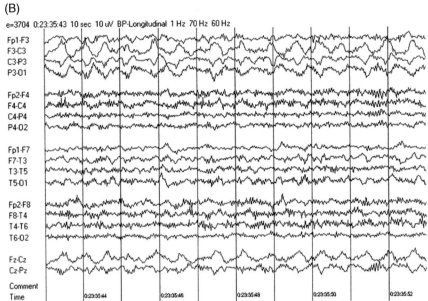

Figure 9.3. (*Continued*) At the beginning of the record there is a clear asymmetry with slowing (more delta power) and attenuation (less power in alpha/beta ranges) on the left (A). A benzodiazepine bolus (midazolam) is then administered, and a marked increase in fast activity can be seen (B), still somewhat greater on the right (where the power in the alpha band reaches yellow and even red at times; ellipse) (the healthier side). There is also an increase in the delta power on the right side, matching the left (white band at the bottom) as the patient becomes sedated. (A) EEG at A: marked left-sided slowing, maximal parasagittally, consisting of high amplitude, continuous 1–2 Hz delta (this explains the very high delta power at the beginning of the record: continuous and high amplitude = very high power). There is attenuation of normal faster activity on the left as well, but faster frequencies are fairly prominent on the healthier right side. (B) EEG at B: much more fast activity (enhanced beta), a common effect of benzodiazepines and barbiturates; this is increased on both sides, but still asymmetric (more on the right). Note the left hemisphere is very slow (high delta power); because of this it is difficult to appreciate an increase/change in the delta power in that hemisphere following benzodiazepine. What is appreciated is that the right hemisphere has become proportionately much slower when compared to before benzodiazepine. This difference can be easily appreciated on the spectrogram, and the delta power at the end of the epoch looks fairly similar to that in the left.

Figure 9.4. Spectrogram basics: multiple seizures.

Figure 9.4main Four hours of EEG in a young woman with an unusual leukodystrophy (ovarioleukodystrophy) and intractable nonconvulsive seizures. This quantitative EEG (QEEG) sample shows time along the x axis (4 hours shown), frequency on the y axis (0–20 Hz, which can be found in the top left of each row), and power in the z axis, with power shown on a color scale where the highest power is white, followed by pink and red (see color scales in the upper right of each panel). There are four rows shown in this QEEG panel, representing different electrode chains (left parasagittal, right parasagittal, left temporal, right temporal).

Most power is near the bottom in the delta range for most of the tracing. There are intermittent bursts of power in higher frequencies on the right, usually maximal in the temporal region; one example is shown in B. These represent seizures, although review of the raw EEG at that point is necessary to confirm this. QEEG should never be interpreted without reviewing portions of the original waveforms as well. Ictal patterns have this characteristic shape on a spectrogram with the sudden increase of power through higher frequencies and then sudden decline to baseline; this appearance is sometimes called 'flames'. Additional examples of flames with a full QEEG panel can be found in figures 9.21 and 9.22.

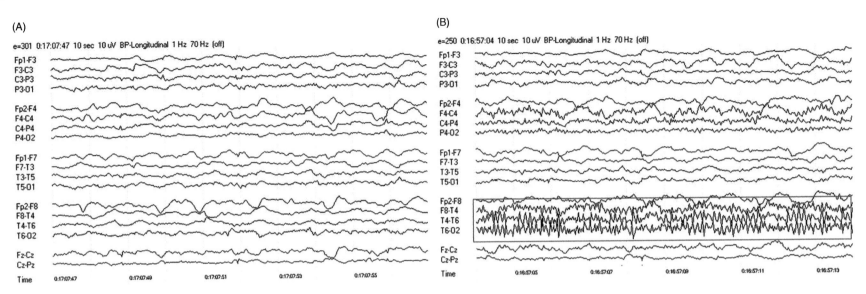

Figure 9.4.   (*Continued*) (A) EEG at A: baseline, showing diffuse delta activity. (B) EEG at B: right temporal seizure (box).

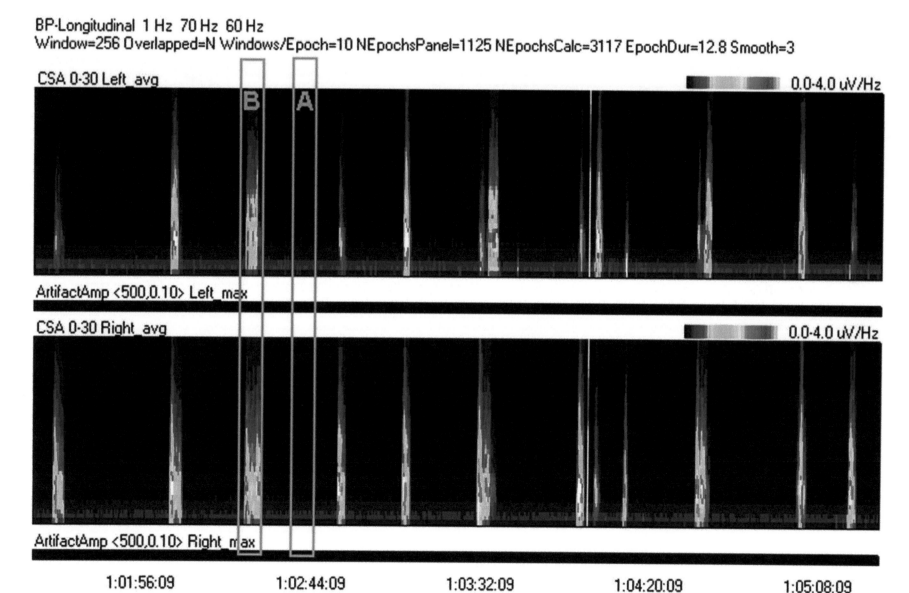

Figure 9.5. Spectrogram basics: multiple seizures arising from complete suppression

Figure 9.5main Six hours of QEEG in a 12-year-old boy with refractory status epilepticus being treated with pentobarbital coma. The background was completely suppressed (A) with no bursts, yet well-developed seizures still occurred about twice per hour (B). Note, at point A the spectrogram is mostly black apart from a very faint signal in the low delta band. This is typical of complete suppression, i.e., there is no power in any frequency, with some delta power being registered due to artifact. This example demonstrates the limitations of intermittent short EEGs for monitoring barbiturate-induced coma, which would miss seizures if a short EEG was done at the time of suppression.

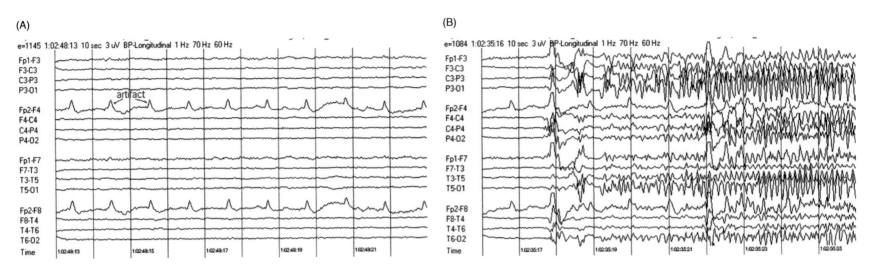

Figure 9.5. (*Continued*) (A) EEG at A: interictal, showing complete suppression and Fp2 artifact. Sensitivity 3 uV/mm (high gain). (B) EEG at B: start of a seizure, beginning maximally on the left, but rapidly becoming bilateral.

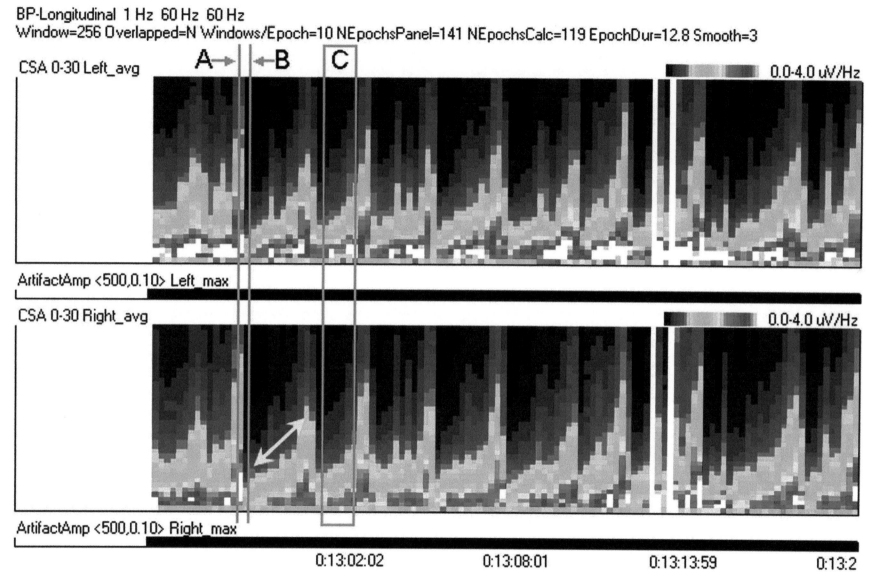

BP-Longitudinal 1 Hz 60 Hz 60 Hz
Window=256 Overlapped=N Windows/Epoch=10 NEpochsPanel=141 NEpochsCalc=119 EpochDur=12.8 Smooth=3

CSA 0-30 Left_avg

0.0-4.0 uV/Hz

ArtifactAmp <500,0.10> Left_max

CSA 0-30 Right_avg

0.0-4.0 uV/Hz

ArtifactAmp <500,0.10> Right_max

0:13:02:02   0:13:08:01   0:13:13:59   0:13:2

Figure 9.6. Spectrogram basics: cyclic nonconvulsive seizures. Figure 9.6main ~30 minutes of QEEG in a middle-aged woman with encephalitis, seizures and brief cardiac arrest. Brief nonconvulsive seizures were occurring every ~3 minutes in a very stable pattern of seizure (A), postictal attenuation (B), then gradual buildup of epileptiform activity (yellow arrow and C) until another seizure occurs.

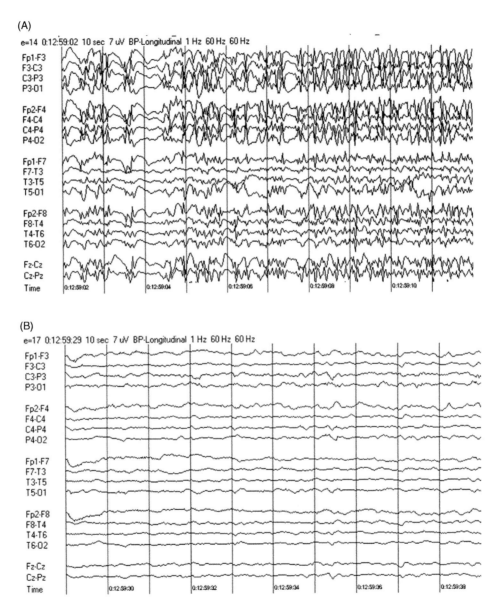

Figure 9.6. (*Continued*) (A) EEG at A: definite electrographic seizure, maximal in bilateral parasagittal chains. (B) EEG at B: postictal, with marked diffuse attenuation.

(C)

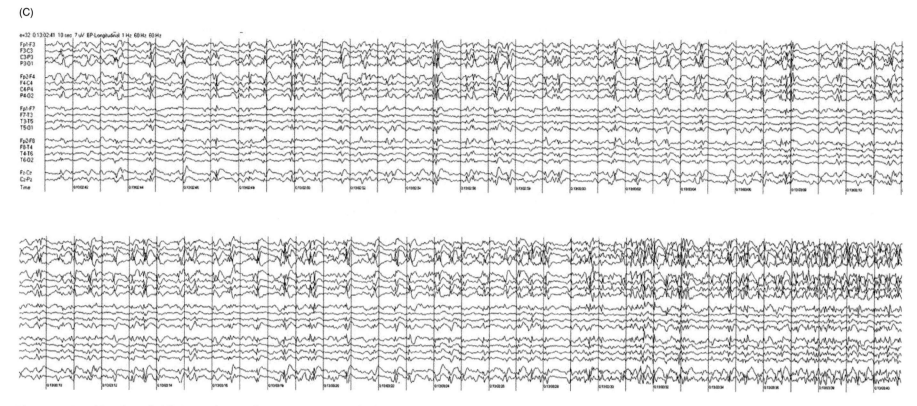

Figure 9.6. (*Continued*) (C) One minute of raw EEG at C: gradual buildup of epileptiform activity between seizures.

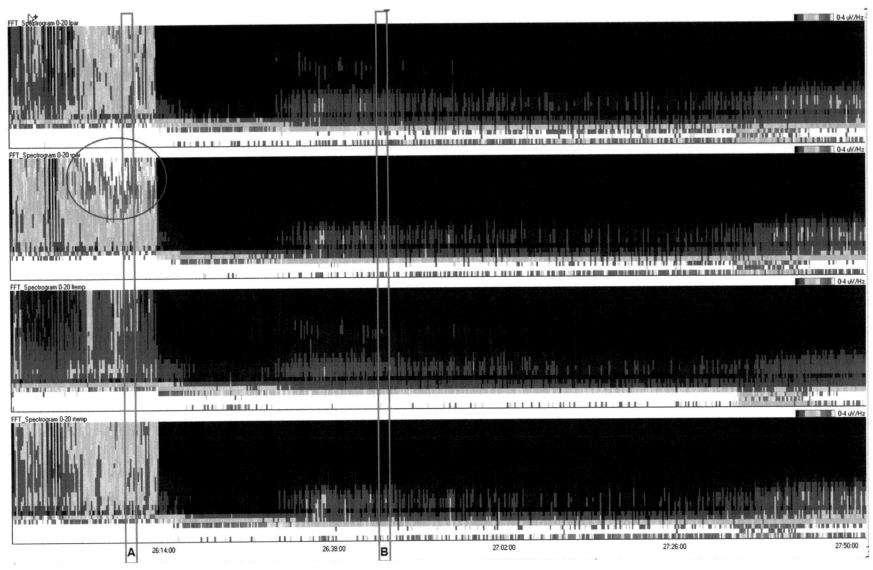

Figure 9.7. Spectrogram basics: muscle artifact

Figure 9.7main Two hours of EEG showing an initial period with prominent muscle artifact, maximal in the right parasagittal region (blue ellipse). Muscle artifact on a spectrogram tends to appear as if it is coming down from the top (stalactites) of the tracing (as in this example). This is because EMG artifact is usually composed primarily of frequencies greater than those being displayed (>20 Hz in this example). A sample of EEG during this time period is shown at point A. There is then a period with no muscle artifact and with most power in the lower frequencies, corresponding to sleep (point B).

(A)

(B)

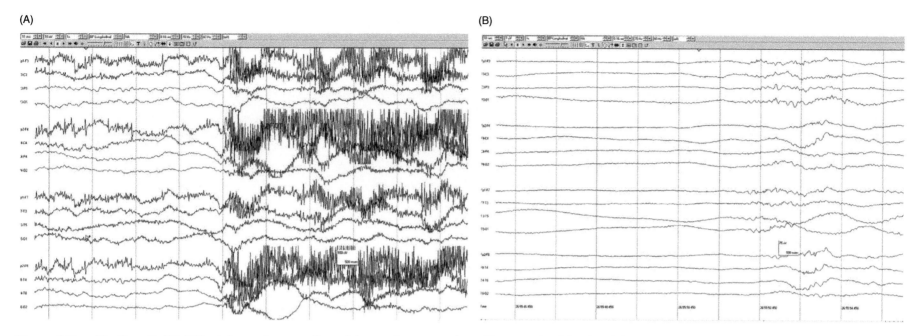

Figure 9.7. (*Continued*) (A) EEG at A: awake recording with prominent muscle artifact, maximal in the right parasagittal region as seen on the spectrogram. (B) EEG at B: sleep recording with no muscle artifact.

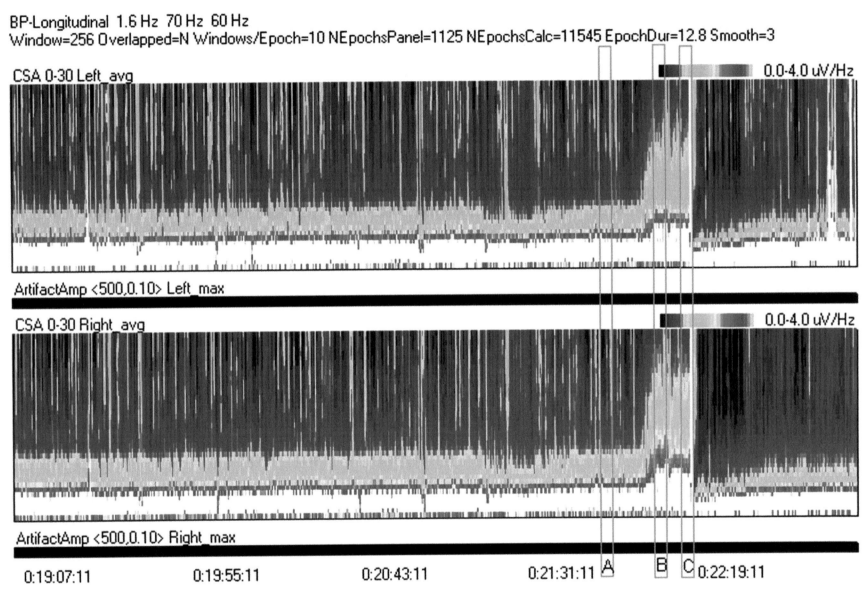

Figure 9.8. Spectrogram basics, long-term trends: NCSE culminating with convulsion

Figure 9.8main Four hours of QEEG power spectrograms (CSA) from a middle-aged man with genetic generalized epilepsy and seizures since age 9, now admitted with intermittent confusion. Baseline EEG (point A) shows diffuse slowing. He then develops nonconvulsive status epilepticus for 15–20 minutes (point B), which continues until he develops a generalized tonic-clonic seizure (point C). There is brief post ictal attenuation after this point.

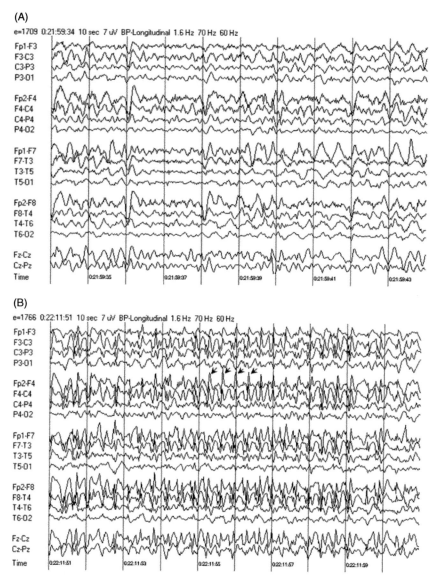

Figure 9.8. (*Continued*) (A) EEG at A: diffuse slowing with no definite ictal activity. (B) EEG at B: nonconvulsive status epilepticus (NCSE), with irregular, ~3 Hz generalized spike-wave. Arrows highlight a few of the spikes.

(C)

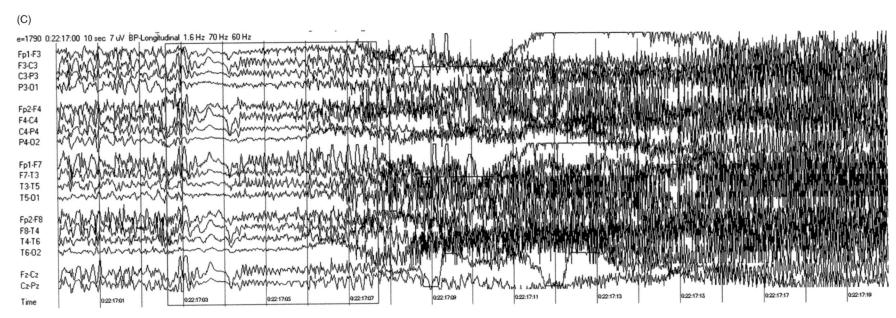

Figure 9.8.   (*Continued*) (C) EEG at C: transition from NCSE (first few seconds) into a typical generalized tonic-clonic seizure.

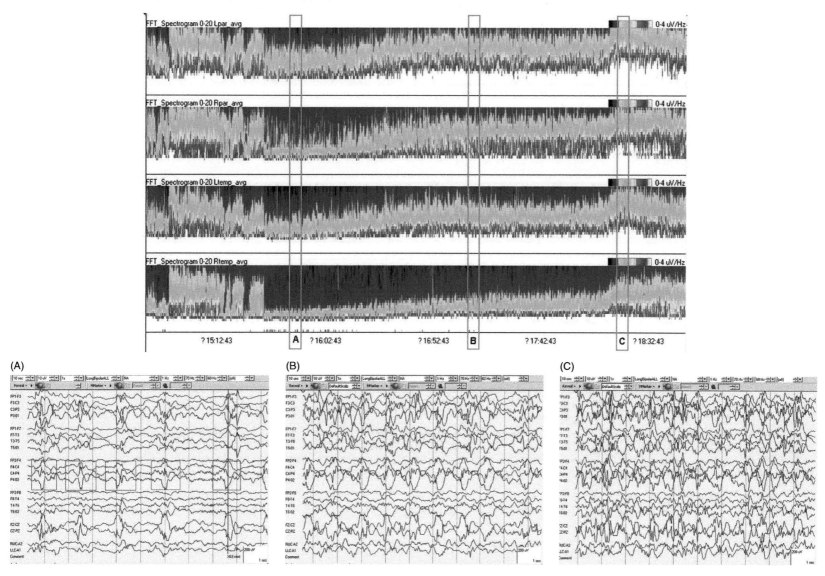

Figure 9.9. Spectrogram basics, long-term trends: slow worsening ictal-interictal continuum (IIC) progressing to electrographic status epilepticus (ESE).

Figure 9.9main Power spectrogram showing 4 hours of EEG in a 4-month-old boy with refractory nonconvulsive seizures. Although treatment had stopped NCSE just prior to point A, the ictal pattern gradually resumed and worsened over the next several hours. This is a good example of the IIC. There is no clear demarcation and no clear and abrupt transition from interictal to ictal states. Instead (as is often the case in critically ill patients) there is a gradual, smooth transition from one to the other. (A) EEG at A: periodic complexes every 1.5–2 seconds (boxes), bisynchronous and maximal in the parietal regions (LPDs, bilateral asymmetric). This is most likely not an ictal pattern. (B) EEG at B: higher amplitude complexes (sensitivity is at 10 uV/mm), more epileptiform and faster, now at 1 Hz and with more superimposed fast frequencies (LPDs+F, high amplitude). This is not definite electrographic seizure activity (but on the ictal end of the ictal-interictal continuum), but we would consider this to be probably ictal at this point, though the exact point that interictal became ictal is not well defined. (C) EEG at C: even higher amplitude and continuous epileptiform activity including fast frequencies, which is unequivocally an ictal EEG pattern at this point. There was no clear clinical correlate (electrographic status epilepticus [ESE]).

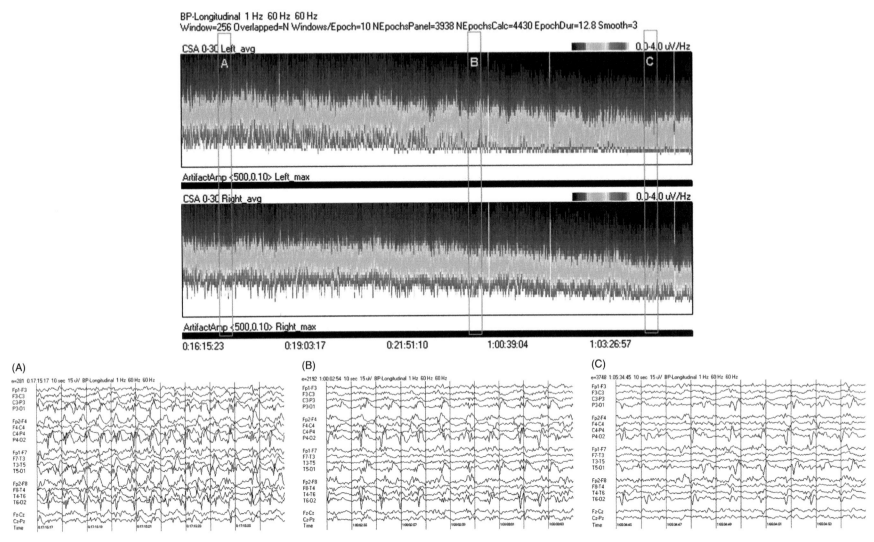

Figure 9.10. Spectrogram basics, long-term trends: gradual resolution of ESE, IIC and BIPDs

Figure 9.10main Twelve-hour spectrogram in a 3-year-old s/p cardiac surgery showing gradual resolution of NCSE/ESE. This example also supports the concept of an ictal-interictal continuum as this patient has smooth, gradual transition from probably ictal to interictal, with no clear cutoff point. (A) EEG at A: posterior-predominant, ~1.5 Hz high amplitude (note sensitivity is at 15 μV/mm) periodic discharges, mostly but not always bisynchronous, often polyspike-and-wave morphology. This pattern is on the ictal-interictal continuum, arguably ictal at this point. (B) EEG at B: similar pattern, but a bit slower, with brief breaks in the rhythmicity for half a second or so, and with more restricted field and more evidence of a bilateral independent pattern. These are BIPDs+F and still on the ictal-interictal continuum, although clearly improved (much less likely to be ictal) compared to earlier in the record. (C) EEG at C: BIPDs with both populations now at < 1 Hz and with resolution of the plus F. Now clearly not ictal at this point.

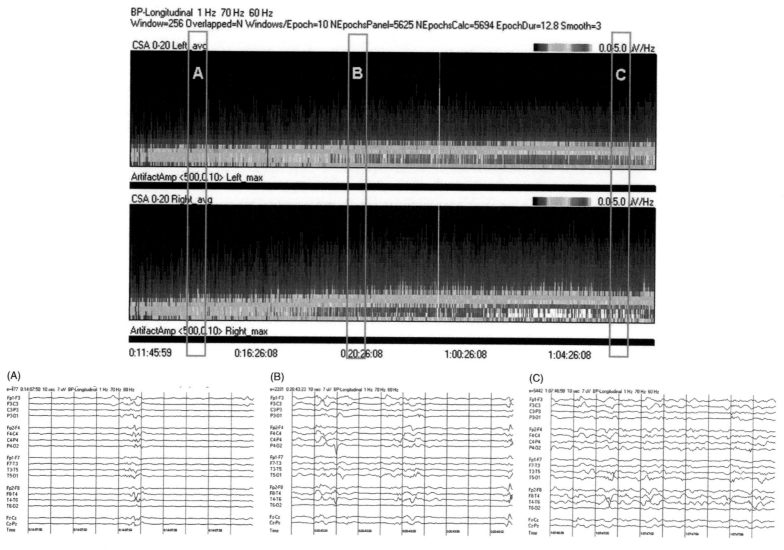

Figure 9.11. Spectrogram basics, long-term trends: wearing off of pentobarbital

Figure 9.11main Spectrogram showing about 20 hours of EEG during pentobarbital-induced coma in a 6-month-old boy with a left frontal hemorrhagic infarct and refractory status epilepticus. By showing this many hours of EEG at once, it is easy to appreciate the long gradual wearing off of the pentobarbital effect. The suppression percent or amplitude-integrated EEG would be additional good QEEG methods for following this (see Figures 9.14 and 9.15). (A) EEG at A: suppression-burst, with just one short burst on this 10 second page. (B) EEG at B: suppression-burst, with more frequent bursts. (C) EEG at C: emergence out of suppression-burst.

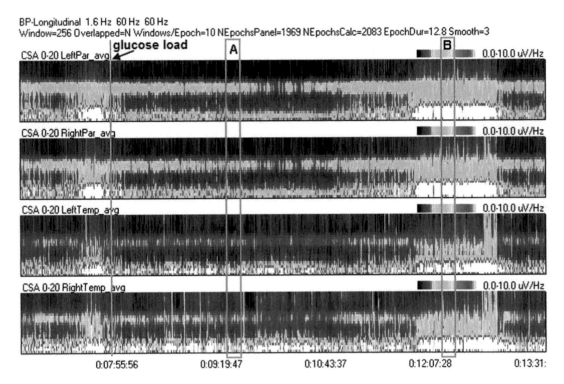

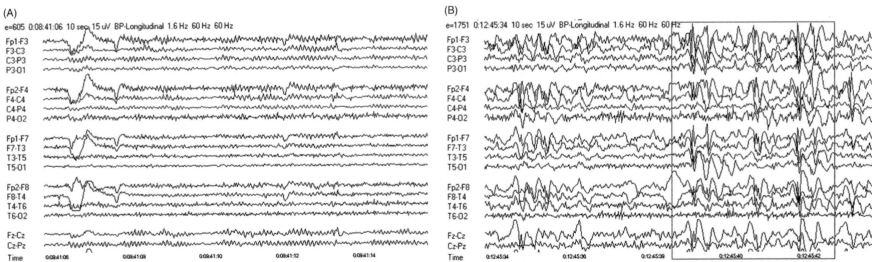

Figure 9.12. Spectrogram basics, long-term trends: glucose load effect in glucose transporter deficiency.

Figure 9.12main Nine hours of QEEG power spectrograms (CSA) in a child with glut-1 deficiency syndrome, a condition with low CSF glucose due to a defect in the glucose transporter glut-1, which transports glucose into the central nervous system across the blood-brain barrier. Many patients with this syndrome have seizures and generalized epileptiform discharges. This example shows periods of high delta power due to frequent generalized spike-wave discharges (before the glucose load, and much later in the record at point B). These resolve with a glucose load (labeled line) and the EEG normalizes (point A). After fasting for 5–6 hours, the generalized epileptiform discharges gradually return (point B). (A) EEG at A: no epileptiform discharges. (B) EEG at B: frequent irregular generalized spike-wave discharges (box), resulting in marked increase in delta power (due to the high voltage delta waves associated with the spikes).

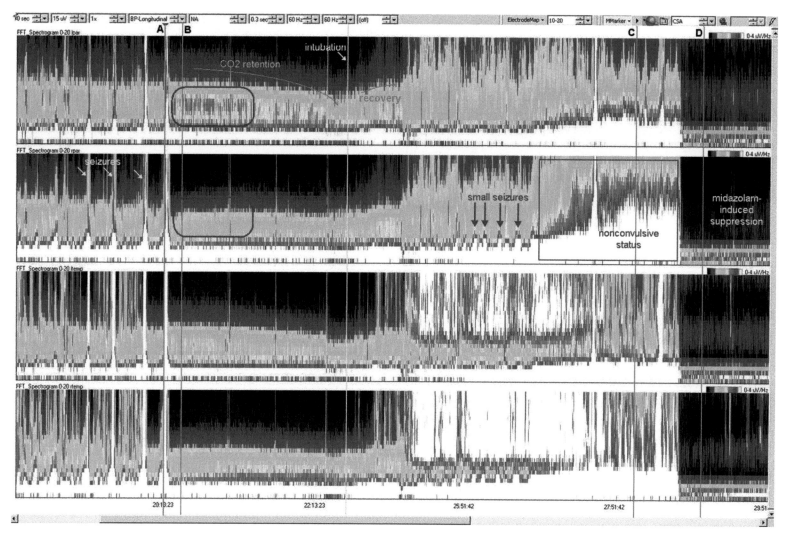

Figure 9.13. Spectrogram basics, long-term trends: CO_2 retention, acidosis and resolution of nonconvulsive seizures

Figure 9.13main: 12 hours of QEEG power spectrogram (CSA) from a man in his 60s with a right-sided subdural hematoma and refractory nonconvulsive seizures. At the beginning of the record, he was still having 2–3 electrographic seizures per hour (labeled arrows, with example at point A; classic 'flame' shape of seizures on CSA). Intubation was being avoided if possible. The seizures resolved without specific intervention, but the patient then became sleepier. When not having seizures, the power spectrograms showed an asymmetry, with attenuation of theta/alpha in the right parasagittal region (purple ellipses starting at point B), likely due to the extra-axial collection on the right. After the

seizures resolved, the background EEG on the healthier side (the left) began to attenuate gradually (orange curved arrow labeled CO_2 retention); arterial blood gas revealed CO_2 retention and acidosis, with a pH of 7.1. He was then intubated (yellow line), and background began to recover (curved arrow labeled recovery) as his CO_2 and pH normalized. However, smaller seizures then appeared (labeled 'small seizures'), followed by NCSE (sample shown at point C) that eventually had a clinical component (ECSE). Midazolam infusion was then started, seizures stopped, and background was attenuated (point D). The respiratory acidosis is probably what stopped the seizures, and when this was corrected, seizures returned.

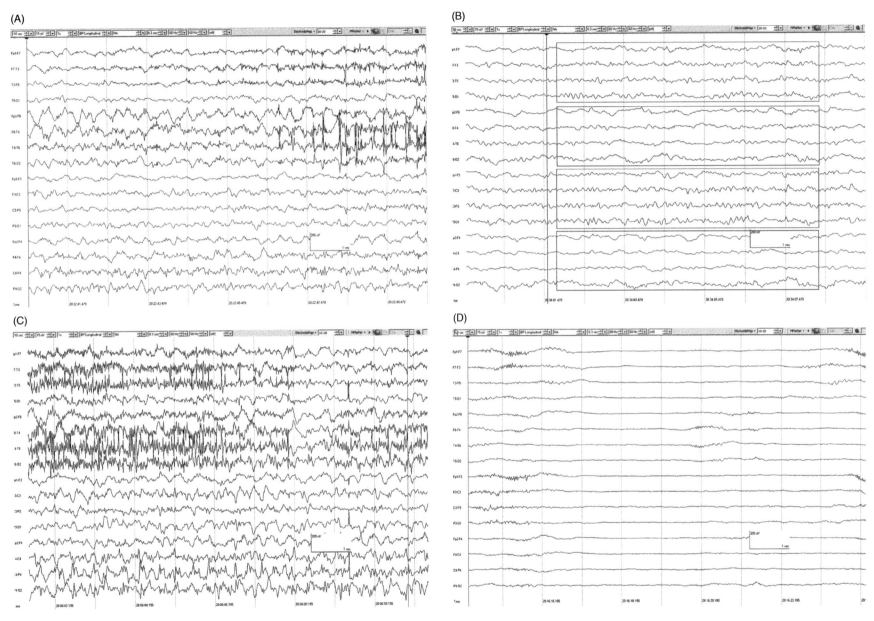

Figure 9.13. (*Continued*) (A) EEG at A: right hemisphere seizure. (B) EEG at B: attenuation of faster frequencies on the right (blue boxes [right] compared to green boxes [left]). (C) EEG at C: status epilepticus, maximal in the right parasagittal region (bottom of the page in this bipolar longitudinal temporal over parasagittal montage). (D) EEG at D: suppressed with low-amplitude beta activity due to midazolam infusion.

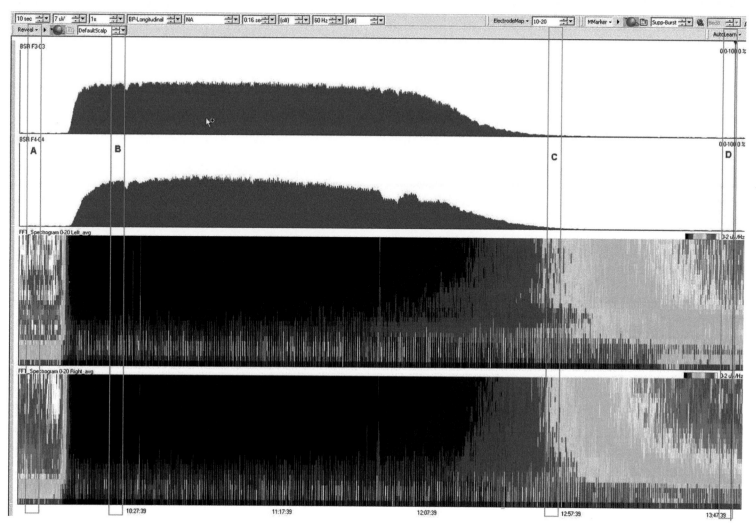

Figure 9.14. QEEG basics, suppression percent: wearing off of neuromuscular blockade and return of shivering artifact.

Figure 9.14main: 4 hours of QEEG in a 75-year-old woman s/p cardiac arrest being treated with hypothermia. The initial EEG (A) is obscured by continuous muscle artifact, likely due to shivering related to hypothermia (often 'micro-shivering' that is difficult to notice clinically). The bottom two rows are the CSAs for the left and right hemisphere. At point A there is a large amount of power filling from the top of the rows (EMG artifact), but little at the very bottom (delta range). A paralytic was administered between A and B, removing all muscle artifact.

The underlying EEG shows marked suppression with low-amplitude bursts(B). The top 2 rows represent the suppression percentages for the left and right hemispheres (labeled 'BSR' in this example [standing for burst-suppression ratio, though it is actually a percentage of suppression, not a ratio]). Suppression percentages (confusingly often called a burst-suppression ratio) refer to the proportion of a record that is suppressed at any given time; 0% indicates continuous cerebral activity (including artifact if not using artifact reduction, such as at point A), and 100% indicates complete suppression. Neuromuscular blockade was administered, and the muscle artifact rapidly ends. The suppression percentages rapidly rise to the accurate amount as the EMG activity has been removed from the record, remains high for a couple hours, before gradually declining before C (causing a humpback whale shape). On the spectrogram, muscle artifact can be seen gradually returning (starting at C) and increasing in power until again prominent at D. The same humpback whale shape of suppression can be seen with administration of highly sedating anti-seizure medication, where cerebral activity becomes rapidly suppressed for a period of time and then slowly recovering. The initial pattern on the spectrogram (top down) in this case, however, indicates this is due to muscle artifact (confirmed by the raw EEG).

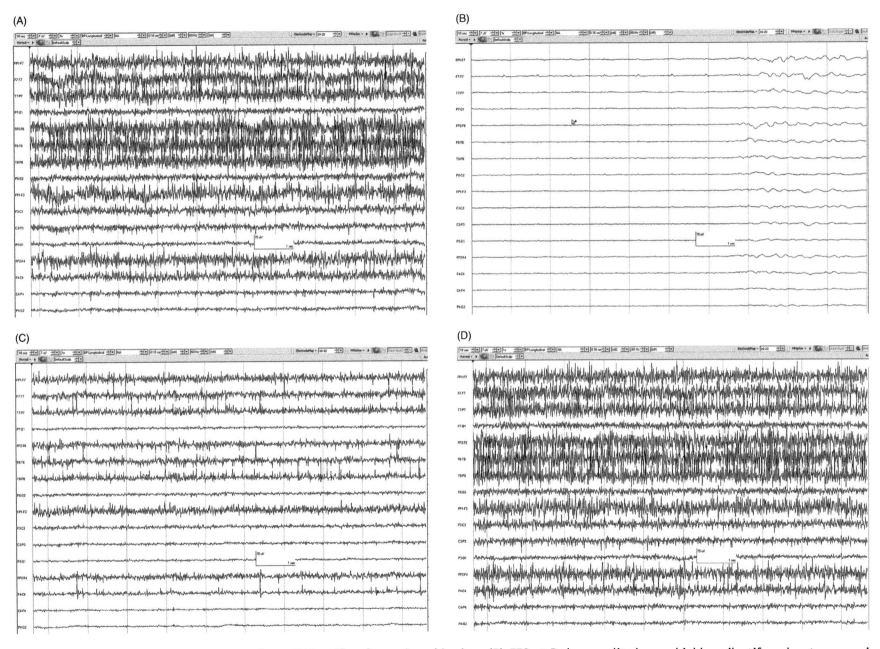

Figure 9.14. (*Continued*) (A) EEG at A: prominent EMG artifact from micro-shivering. (B) EEG at B: low-amplitude non-highly epileptiform burst suppression. (C) EEG at C: slow return of EMG artifact. (D) EEG at D: prominent EMG artifact returns as neuromuscular blockade wears off.

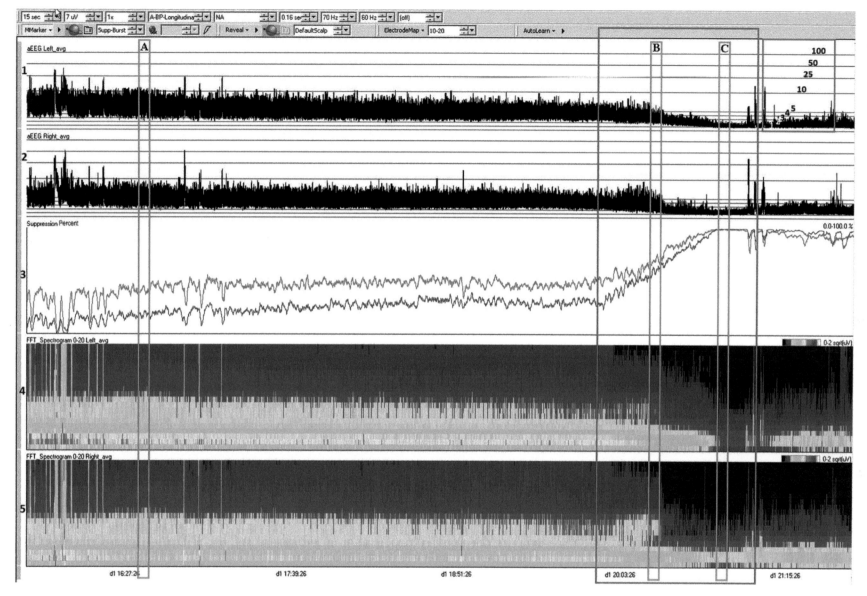

Figure 9.15. QEEG basics, amplitude-integrated EEG and suppression percent: patient death.

Figure 9.15main Six hours of QEEG in a middle-aged woman with cancer, septic encephalopathy and do-not-resuscitate status. The top 2 rows consist of the amplitude-integrated EEG (aEEG) for the left (row 1) and right (row 2) hemispheres. Row 3 is the suppression percent for the left (blue trace) and right (red trace) hemispheres, and rows 4 and 5 are the left and right hemispheric power spectrograms respectively. The aEEG can be thought of as showing both the minimum and maximum amplitudes for each page (short epoch) of EEG.

Thus, the tracing is a band with vertical thickness, or width. The y axis is a semi-logarithmic scale of the amplitudes: the bottom half is a linear scale from 0 to 10 μV (lines shown for 1–5, and for 10 μV), and the upper portion is a logarithmic scale from 10 to 100 μV for higher voltages, with lines shown at 10, 25, 50 and 100 μV. These values have been placed on the right-hand side of row 1 (red box) (units = μV). A very thick band that reaches the bottom of the tracing suggests suppression-burst (parts with very low amplitude and parts with high amplitude in each short epoch or EEG page).

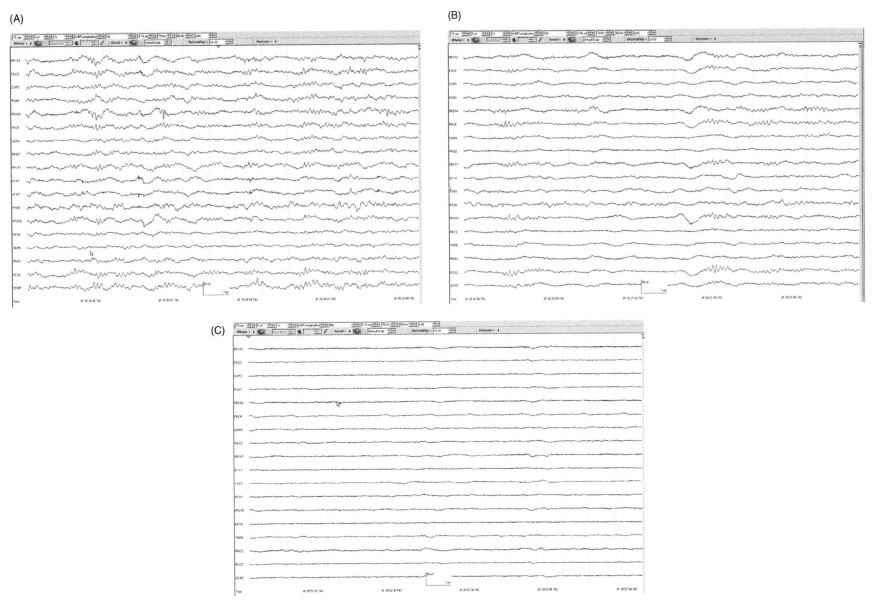

Figure 9.15. (*Continued*) The above description is an oversimplification of aEEG. The raw EEG signal undergoes filtering and mathematical modification prior to amplitude calculations in order to enhance the power of faster frequencies, which are normally lower amplitude than slower frequencies (see Scheuer and Wilson 2004 for technical details of this and many other QEEG techniques). The QEEG panel demonstrates mild asymmetry with more attenuation on the right. This is most evident on the suppression percent (row 3) that is consistently higher on the right (red = right, i.e., it is more suppressed on the right). The asymmetry is appreciable on the aEEG: the left hemisphere (row 1) consistently touches the 10 µV line early in this epoch (for example, see around point A), whereas the right hemisphere (row 2) is consistently below it. The asymmetry can also be seen in the power spectrograms (CSA; bottom 2 rows), with less power through all frequencies on the right (row 5). Near the end of this time period (green box), there is gradual loss of all power on both sides, with suppression rising to 100 percent and amplitudes dropping near zero as cerebral blood flow ceased. (A) EEG at A: mild right-sided attenuation. (B) EEG at B: more attenuation diffusely. (C) EEG at C: suppressed EEG.

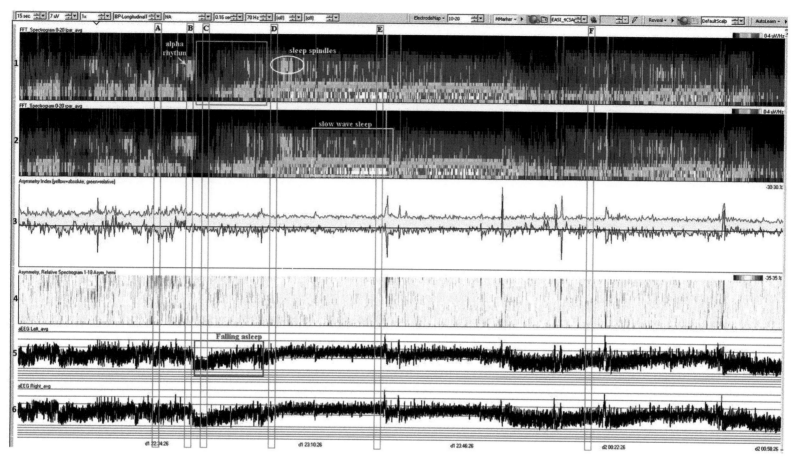

Figure 9.16. QEEG basics, amplitude-integrated EEG and asymmetry measures: normal study with state changes.

Figure 9.16main Three hours of QEEG in a normal middle-aged man. Patient is awake at first (A and B), becomes drowsy (C), then falls asleep (magenta boxes), progressing from stage N2 (D) to stage N3 (slow wave sleep; E and yellow box). In addition to the spectrogram (CSA) (rows 1 and 2), this QEEG panel also includes the absolute EEG asymmetry index (EASI) and overlapped relative EEG asymmetry index (REASI) (row 3), asymmetry spectrogram (row 4), and left and right hemisphere amplitude-integrated EEG (aEEG) (rows 5 and 6). The EASI is shown in yellow and the REASI in green (row 3). The EASI is the absolute difference between the two hemispheres (irrespective of which hemisphere is of greater voltage). This is calculated by comparing asymmetry at each pair of homologous electrodes and summing their absolute values to give a total asymmetry score; this can only be positive and upward on this display. The REASI is supplementary to this because it demonstrates the 'relative' asymmetry, i.e., laterality.

Down-going indicates more power on the left, and upgoing on the right. A way of gathering more information about asymmetry is by using a relative asymmetry spectrogram (row 4). The relative asymmetry spectrogram is similar to the REASI but instead of power as a whole (combining all frequencies), it displays relative power at each frequency from 1–18 Hz averaged over the entire hemisphere. In this example the REASI is mostly downward (power slightly favoring the left), which is confirmed by the asymmetry spectrogram, which is largely blue (favoring the left) across all frequencies. If the power favored the right, the asymmetry spectrogram would be red (red = more power on right, blue = left). The final two rows show the amplitude-integrated EEG (aEEG). aEEG can be applied to a single channel (as is commonly done with neonatal EEG monitoring, sometimes via a bedside device known as a 'cerebral function monitor'), or to a group of channels; in this setup shown, all channels in one hemisphere are averaged into one aEEG trace. aEEG was introduced in Figure 9.15.

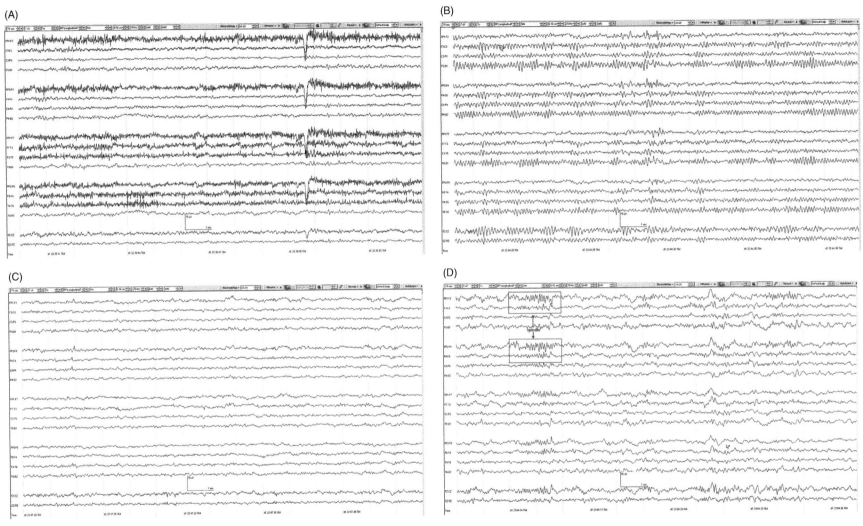

Figure 9.16. (*Continued*) (A) EEG at A: normal awake recording with eyes open. At A power is mostly low, maximal in the theta and alpha range (CSA); the low amplitudes are appreciated in the aEEG as well. (B) EEG at B: eyes closed, with prominent alpha rhythm. Note the band appearing on the spectrogram around 9 Hz due to this activity (labeled 'alpha rhythm' on QEEG). Also note the lack of any delta power at this time to distinguish this pattern on the QEEG from sleep. The amplitude has increased from point A when most rhythms were relatively attenuated by eye opening. (C) EEG at C: typical drowsy EEG. Note that after this, there is gradual increase in power at slower frequencies (mainly delta) seen on the spectrogram as he falls asleep (upper magenta box).

A sudden drop (between B and C), followed by gradual increase in amplitude can also be appreciated on the aEEG. The amplitudes (both minimum and maximum) drop as his alpha rhythm attenuates and drowsiness ensues (C). The amplitudes then gradually increase as the patient falls further asleep (lower magenta box labeled 'falling asleep'). (D) EEG at D: normal N2 sleep with spindles (labeled) and K-complexes. Most of the power sits in the theta and delta range at this point. However, the effect of the presence of spindles can be seen with a broad range of power extending just above the alpha frequency (i.e., the sigma frequency of sleep spindles, 12–15 Hz; white ellipse labeled 'sleep spindles').

(E)
(F)

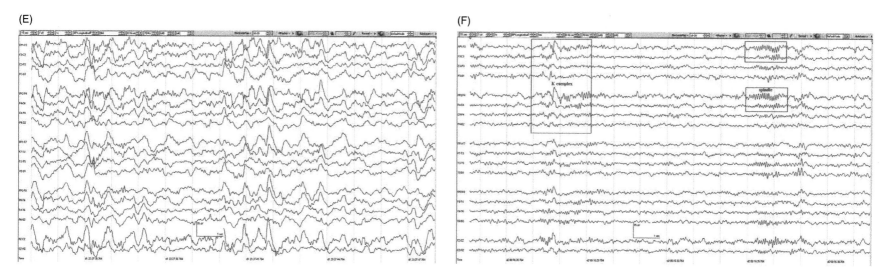

Figure 9.16.   (*Continued*) (E) EEG at E: normal N3 sleep (slow wave sleep), consisting of mostly medium to high voltage delta. (F) EEG at F: back to N2 sleep.

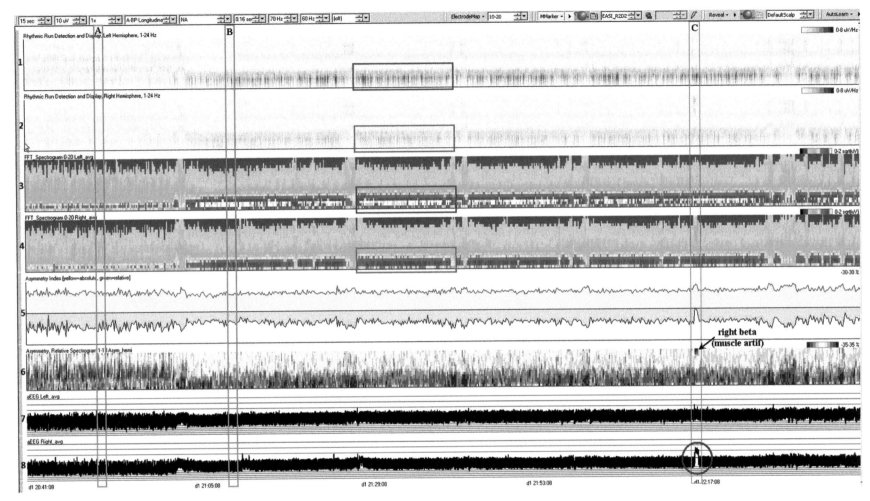

Figure 9.17. QEEG basics, asymmetry measures and rhythmicity spectrogram: subdural hematoma and breach effect, and aEEG 'false positives'

Figure 9.17main Two hours of QEEG in a 70-year-old man with a left hemisphere mass, s/p biopsy and evacuation of a left-sided subdural hematoma. The power spectrograms (rows 3 and 4) show a persistent asymmetry, initially with greater power in all frequencies (A) on the left, later with this difference only notable in the delta frequency (B) with faster frequencies roughly symmetric. This asymmetry is well appreciated with the green REASI (row 5), which is always below zero and down-going (meaning greater power on the left). The asymmetry spectrogram (row 6) adds additional information, again initially showing much greater power on the left (dark blue) in all frequencies (e.g., at A), then only showing dark blue in the lower frequencies with less asymmetry at higher frequencies for most of this page (including at B). Increase in all frequencies on one side is suggestive of a skull defect as in this case: increase in slower frequencies is due to the underlying brain dysfunction (i.e., focal slowing), whereas the increase in faster frequencies is due to the skull defect (breach effect).

The top 2 rows are *rhythmicity detectors*, which in the past were sometimes referred to R2D2 (rhythmic run detection and display), but more appropriately now called rhythmicity spectrograms. Rhythmicity spectrograms are measures of rhythmicity that will become darker when the activity at that frequency becomes more regular (rhythmic or periodic) (i.e., will show a dark band at the frequency of the rhythmic pattern). The pattern with the greatest rhythmicity is a sine wave or very regular periodic pattern such as an EKG. Note that one can have high power (as seen on the CSA) at a given frequency, but low rhythmicity if it is irregular/arrhythmic. Rhythmicity is very useful for the detection of seizures, as will be discussed in Figures 9.21 and 9.22.

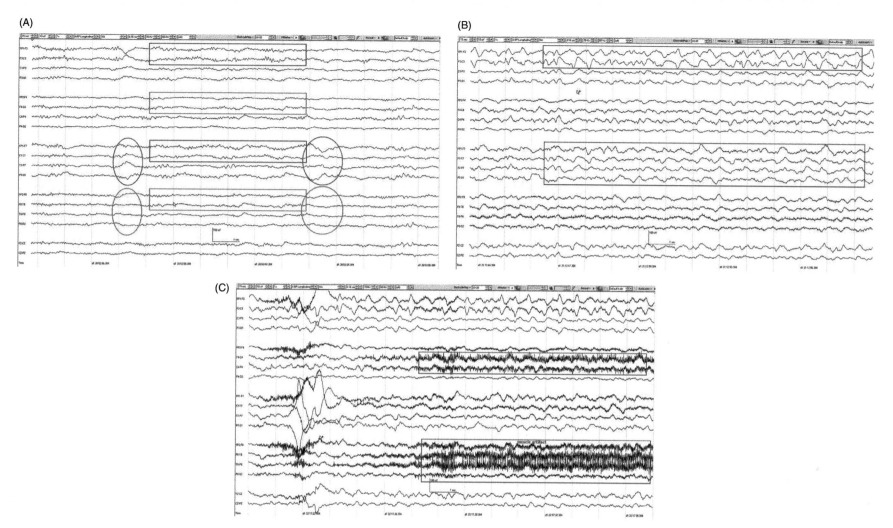

Figure 9.17. (*Continued*) There is an obvious asymmetry in rhythmicity here as well as power, with much higher rhythmicity on the left, especially at lower frequencies (delta; boxes). The left side has fairly rhythmic delta for much of the recording, including at B and C, due to quasi-rhythmic delta on that side. At C, there is a sudden, brief elevation of amplitude seen in the aEEG trace on the right (blue circle), the typical signature of a seizure. However, one can tell that this is likely due to muscle artifact (or accompanied by muscle artifact) via the asymmetry spectrogram, which shows a burst of red (more power on right) at the highest frequencies (arrow labeled 'right beta'). The power spectrogram also shows high-frequency activity on the right at this point, seemingly coming down from the top of the tracing and suggesting artifact. Review of the raw EEG confirms that the change is due to muscle artifact and is a 'false positive' change on aEEG that is not due to seizure. This pattern, which looks identical to a seizure on an aEEG trace, is common, and is one reason it is crucial to never diagnose seizures on an aEEG trace alone (or any single QEEG measure) without reviewing the raw EEG (shown in part c).

(A) EEG at A: there is more delta slowing on the left (blue ellipses= left, compared to green ellipses = right), as well as more prominent faster frequencies on the same side (seen in the ellipses, as well as the rectangles; blue rectangles = left, green rectangles = right). This is due to underlying structural dysfunction (slowing) combined with breach effect (faster frequencies). (B) EEG at B: more delta on the left (blue rectangles), quasi-rhythmic at F3, which results in greater delta power and rhythmicity in the left hemisphere (also becoming more asymmetric in the delta range on asymmetry measures). (C) EEG at C: left frontal quasi-rhythmic delta continues, maximal at F3. Prominent right-sided muscle artifact appears (blue rectangles), leading to the aEEG amplitude change and the burst of fast activity on CSA on the right.

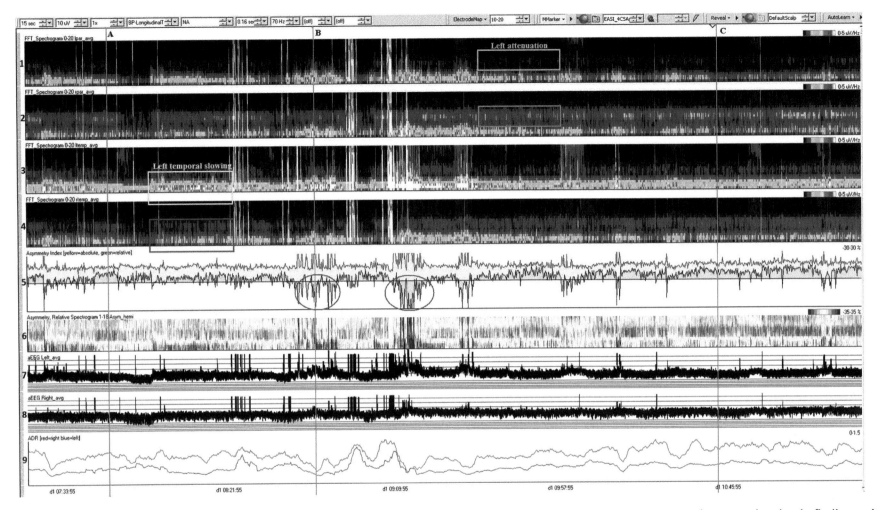

Figure 9.18. QEEG basics, asymmetry measures including alpha/delta ratio: left hemispheric ischemia

Figure 9.18main Four hours of QEEG in a middle-aged man with right hemiparesis after a left carotid endarterectomy. At the time of this study, postoperative CT and MRI had been unremarkable, but hemiparesis and neglect were marked and persistent, and EEG showed findings typical of cortical dysfunction from ischemia. No seizures occurred, clinically or on EEG. Repeat MRI days later showed widespread laminar necrosis through the left hemisphere.

Ischemia on spectrograms: The first four rows show power spectrograms from 0–20 Hz in homologous parasagittal (rows 1–2) and temporal (rows 3–4) regions. Left temporal slowing can be seen as higher delta power (yellow box, compared to pink box in right temporal region). Left hemisphere attenuation (decreased power) of faster frequencies, mainly affecting alpha frequencies, can be seen in the left parasagittal region (green box, compared to orange box on right). These

findings can be seen on the raw EEG at C. These are the classic findings with ischemia: loss of faster frequencies and increased slowing.

Ischemia on asymmetry measures: The EASI/REASI, introduced in Figure 9.16, is show in row 5 and relative asymmetry spectrogram in row 6. The REASI (green tracing) is usually upgoing suggesting more power on the right overall. The asymmetry spectrogram in this case is much more useful than the total asymmetry measures. The asymmetry spectrogram shows that higher frequencies (>~6 Hz) are greater on the right (red) due to attenuation of more physiologic rhythms in the affected hemisphere (left), and slower frequencies (<~4 Hz) are greater on the left (blue) due to focal delta slowing. This is the typical pattern with ischemia, though also seen with other processes that cause both increased slowing and attenuation of faster frequencies on one side. Contrast this with Figure 9.17 where faster frequencies were increased on the side of greater delta slowing, a finding usually suggesting breach effect.

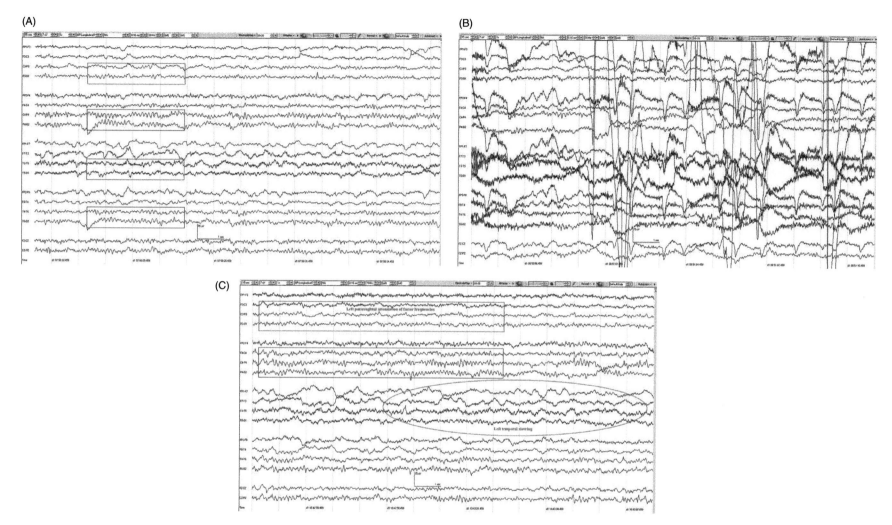

Figure 9.18. *(Continued) Ischemia on alpha/delta ratio:* This figure also shows the alpha/delta ratios (ADRs) for each hemisphere (row 9) (below the aEEG) (red trace = right, blue trace = left). Since alpha frequencies decrease and delta increases with ischemia, the alpha/delta ratio is used to magnify this difference. Note that the ADR is persistently higher on the right, suggesting ischemia on the left. ADRs take all power in the alpha frequency 8–13 Hz and divide this by the total delta power (1–4 Hz). The technique is a sensitive measure of ischemia and often utilized to screen for delayed cerebral ischemia (DCI) after subarachnoid hemorrhage (covered in Chapter 10).

(A) EEG at A: note the attenuation of faster frequencies in the left hemisphere, including the alpha rhythm (8 Hz and fairly well developed on the right, blue boxes; nearly absent on the left, green boxes). There is also continuous left temporal slowing. (B) EEG at B: this is at the point where there appears to be a switch in the direction of overall asymmetry, with the green relative symmetry trace going downward. Review of the raw EEG shows that this is due to movement artifact, most prominent in the left temporal region. (C) EEG at C: the raw EEG at a relatively random point shows the asymmetries already mentioned (labeled).

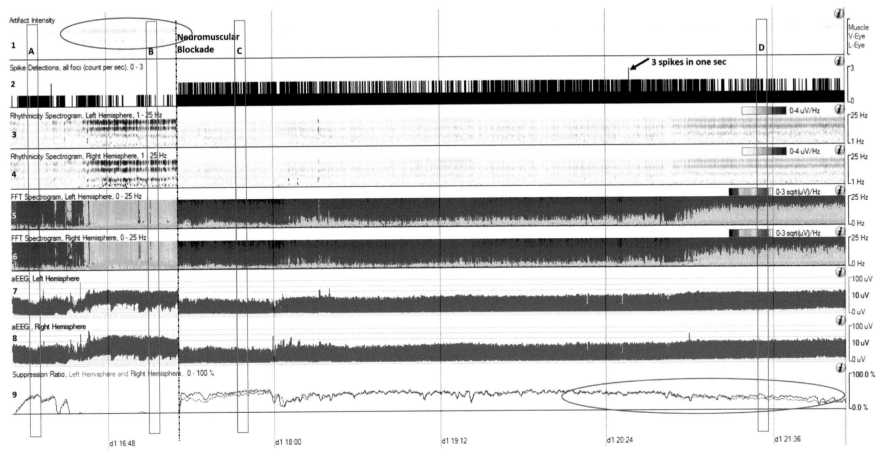

Figure 9.19. QEEG basics, artifact detection, spike detection, and artifact reduction: myoclonic status epilepticus, targeted temperature management and neuromuscular blockade

Figure 9.19main Six hours of QEEG from a 59-year-old man s/p cardiac arrest. At the beginning of the record (A) the EEG is suppressed with occasional sporadic generalized spikes. The spikes can be detected with the spike detector (row 2, 'spike detections'). The y scale of spike detections is 0–3 spikes per second with 1 block indicating 1 spike per second at that time, 2 blocks 2 spikes per second, and 3 blocks 3 blocks per second. At this stage there is little power in any frequency (rows 5 and 6) and the suppression percentages (row 9) are as high as 50%. The patient begins to shiver from targeted temperature management and develops myoclonic status epilepticus (B). The artifact detector (row 1) detects this with a green bar suggesting muscle artifact and intermittent vertical eye movement artifact detected with the blue bars (blue ellipse; horizontal/

lateral eye movements would be in red, as explained on the right end of the first row). In this case the vertical eye movement artifact was from ocular movement with each myoclonic jerk. Prominent muscle artifact at this stage is seen with top-down artifact in the rhythmicity (rows 3 and 4) and power spectrograms and falling of the suppression percentages (row 9) as this artifact gets perceived as brain activity. Neuromuscular blockade is administered at the labeled line. Artifact disappears and a greater number of spikes are detected (previously hidden within artifact, now often 2 per second; 3 is only reached once during this epoch, labeled arrow), the rhythmicity, power and amplitude all plummet and the suppression percentage rapidly increases. As the record continues there is a long-term trend. The suppression percentage slowly reduces over the record (red ellipse) and the rhythmicity and power slowly increase as the discharges become more frequent and of higher voltage (D).

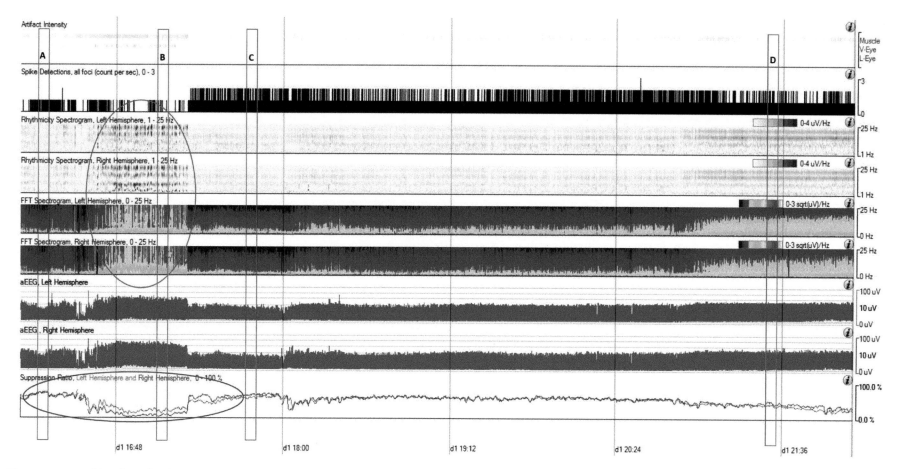

Figure 9.19. (*Continued*) Figure 9.19main2 The same panel of QEEG as Figure 9.19main but with the artifact reduction (AR) turned on. Note the second part of the record is relatively artifact-free (due to neuromuscular blockade) so there is little change to how this has been displayed. The biggest difference was when the patient was shivering and in myoclonic status epilepticus. The AR algorithm has removed a significant amount of rhythmicity and power that was due to muscle artifact (red ellipse). Note it has not removed all of the muscle artifact (a feat that was only achieved by neuromuscular blockade). The result, however, is that for this section there is a more accurate reflection of the EEG, with higher suppression percentages (blue ellipse). The AR software has helped in this instance, but again information has been removed, and no AR algorithm is perfect.

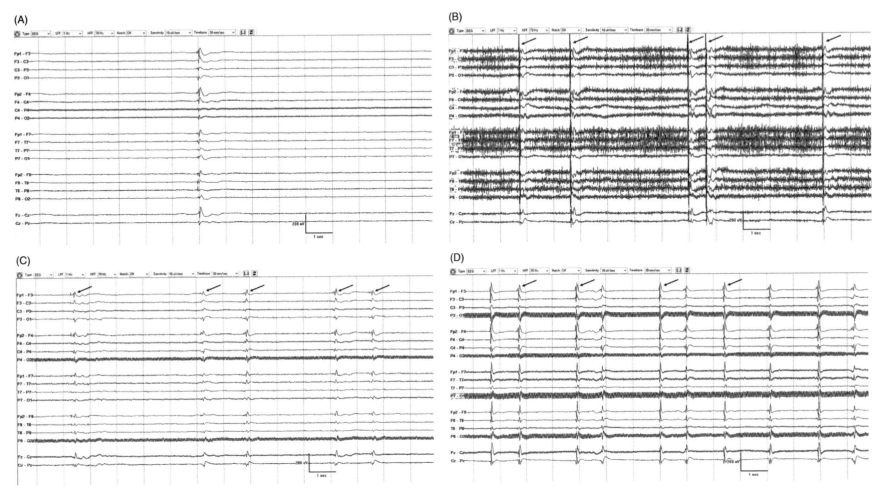

Figure 9.19.   (*Continued*) (A) EEG at A: suppression with occasional sporadic generalized spikes. (B) EEG at B: myoclonic status epilepticus with repeated jerking of eyes and face (arrows showing muscle artifact bifrontally, likely super-imposed on generalized epileptiform discharges) occurring while the patient is shivering (due to targeted temperature management), with a significant amount of muscle artifact. (C) EEG at C: effect of neuromuscular blockade with abrupt cessation of all muscle artifact revealing abundant low voltage generalized spikes (arrows). (D) EEG at D: long-term trend, the generalized spikes gradually (over several hours) became more frequent and of higher voltage (arrows). This trend could be easily detected by the QEEG.

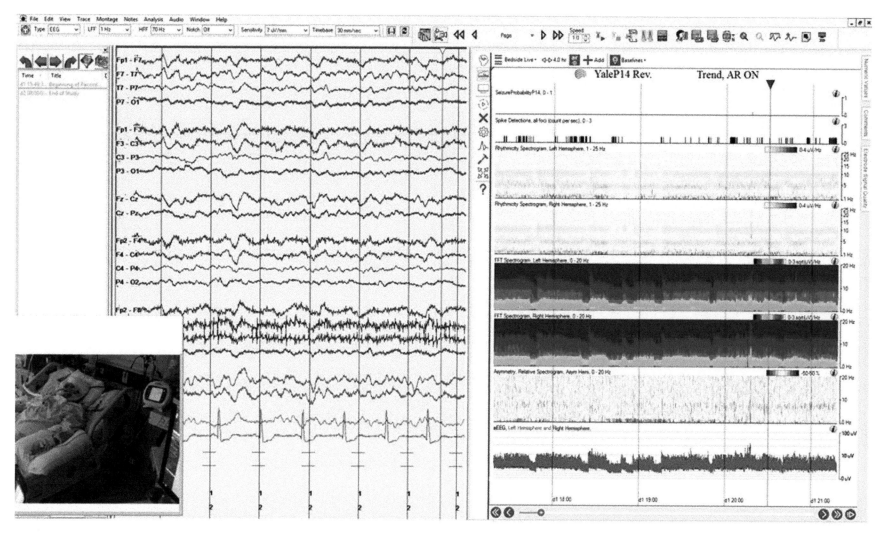

Figure 9.20. QEEG basics, typical bedside display. This demonstrates the typical bedside display while recording EEG in the ICU. As the video (lower left window) and EEG (left half of the screen) are recording the QEEG software is also calculating and displaying the trends (4-hour window shown on the right of the screen). With this configuration it is easy for clinicians at the bedside to see the current page of raw EEG, but also the long-term trends (i.e., improvement, deterioration and response to interventions). The live bedside QEEG trends can also be visualized remotely, such as at a live central review station where EEG technologists can follow several patients at once.

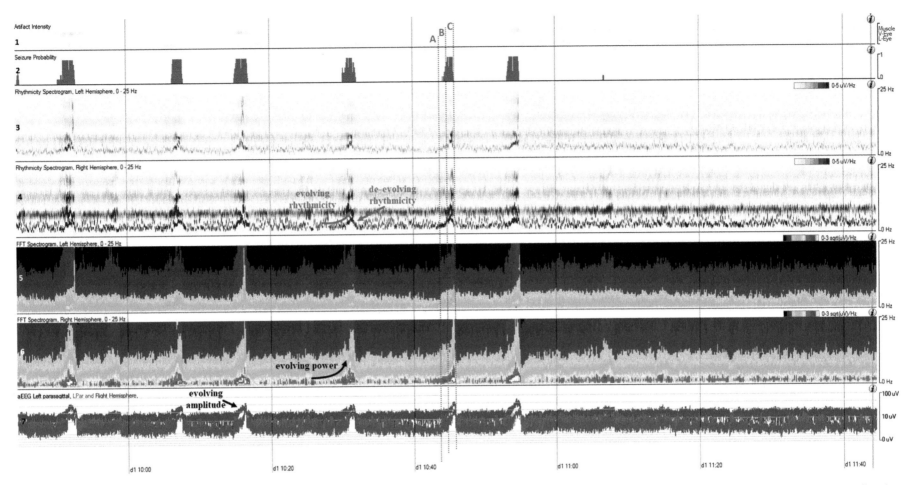

Figure 9.21. QEEG, detection of seizures: evolving nonconvulsive seizures. This 2-hour QEEG is from a 77-year-old man that had a large right hemispheric acute subdural hematoma s/p right hemicraniectomy. There were frequent electrographic seizures arising from the right hemisphere postoperatively. The seizures have a typical pattern of evolving rhythmicity (row 4, labeled red curved arrow, showing gradual change in frequencies that are rhythmic), power (row 6, labeled arrow), and amplitude (row 7, labeled arrow, demonstrating a diagonal increase in amplitude through the right hemisphere [red tracing] that precedes the left [blue trace]. Seizures were treated with anti-seizure medication with no seizures in the final 1/3rd of the page. The seizure probability detector (row 2) also shows the seizures nicely and can be a useful trend that overcomes several pitfalls (see later part of this chapter: Pitfalls and solutions). The seizures build up from an abnormal baseline resulting in a distinctive shape, or 'flame'. The seizure does slow again, this is mostly seen on downward angle on rhythmicity spectrogram (such as that labeled with a straight red arrow).

(A)

(B)

(C)

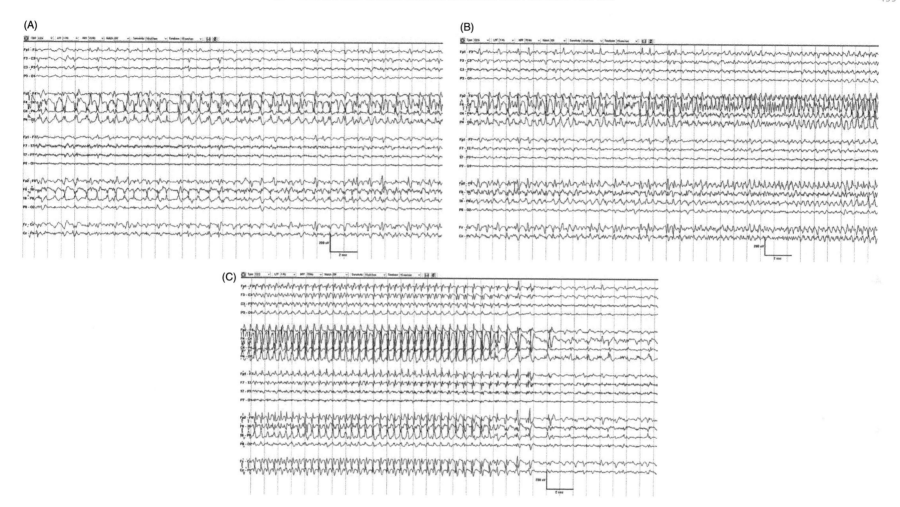

Figure 9.21. (*Continued*) (A) EEG at A: seizure onset, longitudinal bipolar, compressed timescale (15 mm/s): baseline EEG with right hemispheric LPDs at 1–1.5 Hz. These gradually build as the seizure starts towards the end of the page. (B) EEG at B: mid-seizure, compressed timescale (15 mm/s): seizure has begun with epileptiform discharges increasing to 3 Hz at the end of the page (evolution in frequency), involving more of the right temporal region, and also some propagation to the left hemisphere (evolution in location). (C) EEG at C: end of seizure, compressed timescale (15 mm/s): The amplitude significantly increases at C (in both hemispheres; evolution in amplitude), but the frequency has started to slow again (back to 1.5 Hz at the end of the seizure). This 'de-evolution' (still a form of evolution) can also be seen on the rhythmicity spectrogram (labeled arrow).

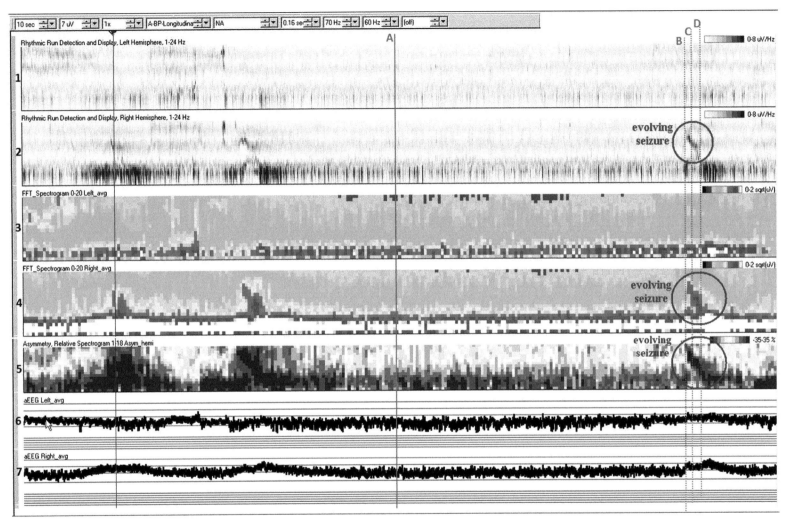

Figure 9.22. QEEG, detection of seizures: 'de-evolving' nonconvulsive seizures.

Figure 9.22main Two hours of QEEG in a 58-year-old man with remote subarachnoid hemorrhage admitted with a generalized convulsion followed by confusion. The power spectrograms (rows 3 and 4) show greater delta on the right throughout, which results in a red lower portion of the asymmetry spectrogram (red = power favoring the right especially in the delta and theta ranges, row 5). A few right-sided seizures are seen with clear evolution visible on the QEEG (e.g., blue circles and B-D). The seizures appear as evolving rhythmicity on the right (row 2), initially above 12 Hz (point B), then gradually decreasing in frequency (points C–D), resulting in a diagonal line (circled), the hallmark of evolution (rhythmicity changing gradually in frequency; in this case, slowing down). Rhythmicity eventually settles into the delta frequency (point D). The same diagonal evolution, in power rather than rhythmicity, can be seen on the power spectrogram (row 4) and the asymmetry spectrogram (in red as the seizures are on the right, row 5). Overall amplitude gradually increases on the right during the seizures, as can be seen on the amplitude-integrated EEG tracing on the bottom panel.

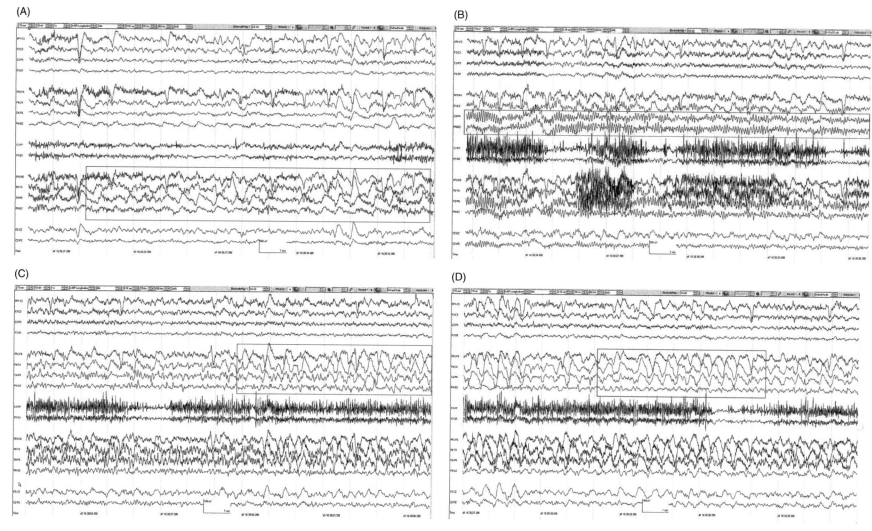

Figure 9.22. (*Continued*) (A) EEG at A: interictal, with delta range slowing in the right temporal region (box). (B) EEG at B: early ictal, with rhythmic 12–13 Hz activity maximal in the right parieto-temporal region (P4-P8) (box). Also seen in Pz at the bottom of the page. (C) EEG at C: mid-ictal, the ictal pattern transitions to slower frequencies, now widespread in the right hemisphere. (D) EEG at D: late ictal, with rhythmic delta in the right hemisphere, mainly ~2 Hz (box).

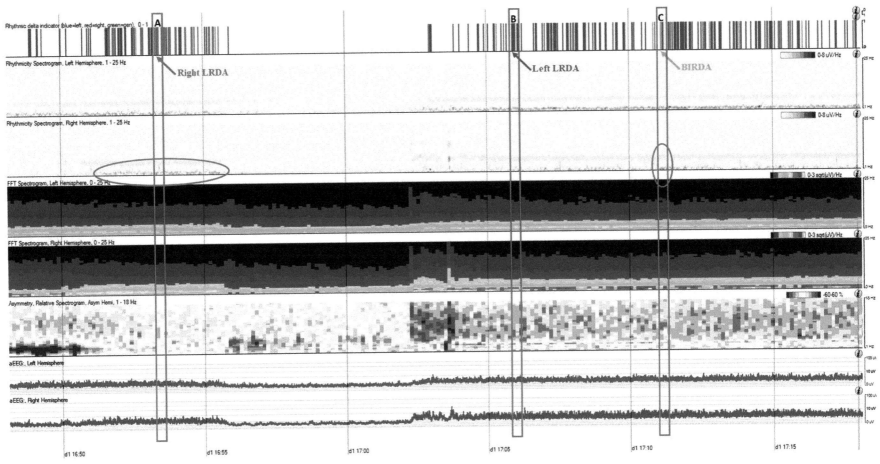

Figure 9.23. QEEG, detection of rhythmic delta activity: bilateral independent rhythmic delta activity (BIRDA).

Figure 9.23main: This 30-minute segment of QEEG is from a 29-year-old woman with a severe traumatic brain injury and BIRDA. A short time frame has been chosen to demonstrate the utility of a rhythmic delta indicator (row 1). At the beginning of the record, the patient transitions from polymorphic right-sided slowing to frequent right temporal LRDA (labeled in row 1; also seen in row 3, in red ellipse as new right-sided rhythmicity in the delta frequency, even though the overall delta power has not increased on the power spectrogram [row 5]). Note the scale of the rhythmicity spectrograms have been set at 0–8 µV/Hz (half as sensitive as conventional), which means that only very rhythmic activity will be detected. At point A, the right LRDA is detected with the RDA detector showing a red bar (red = right). Later in the record, point B, there is left LRDA. Here the RDA detector registers a blue bar (blue = left). When there is BIRDA (i.e., when the two populations of LRDA overlap) this displays as 'generalized' (point C) as it is in both hemispheres (thus a limitation of the RDA detector is that it would not be able to differentiate GRDA from bilateral independent (including multi-focal) RDA). The rhythmicity spectrogram also detects the right-sided rhythmic pattern at point C (second smaller red ellipse).

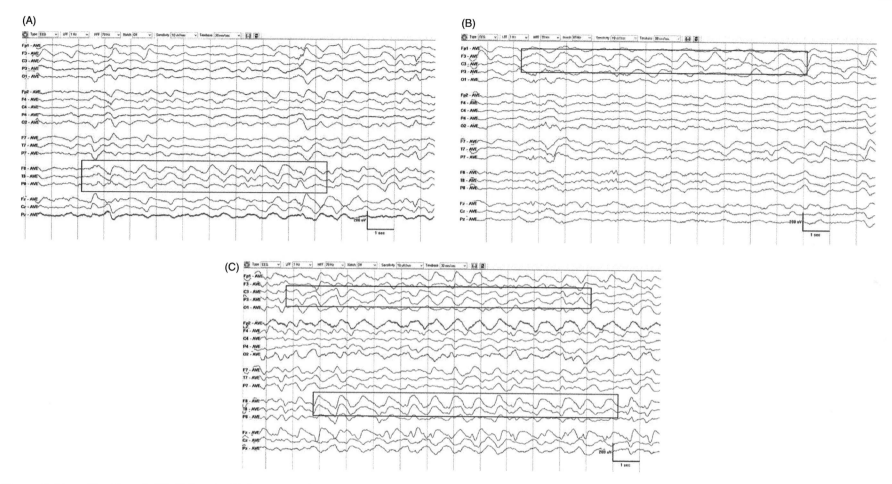

Figure 9.23. (*Continued*) (A) EEG at A. Right temporal 1–1.5-Hz LRDA. (B) EEG at B. Left fronto-central 1-Hz LRDA. (C) EEG at C. BIRDA (left centro-parietal and right temporal RDA, independent of each other [boxes]).

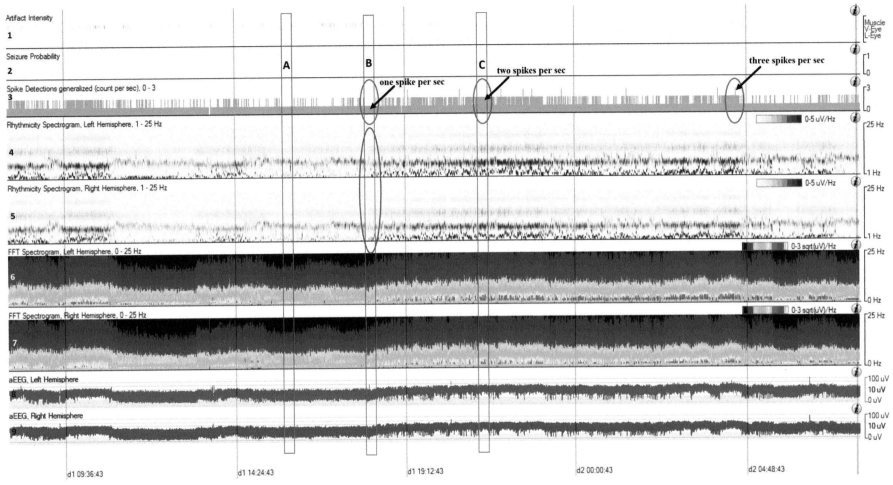

Figure 9.24. QEEG, spike detector to detect typical frequency of GPDs: ictal-interictal continuum (IIC) monitoring.

Figure 9.24main This 16-hour QEEG page is from a 71-year-old woman who had long to very long periods of stimulus-induced generalized sharp waves that became periodic (SI-GPDs) and often qualified for the ictal/interictal continuum (IIC). The QEEG shows how the spike detector can supplement the rhythmicity, FFT and aEEG trends. Looking at the spike detector (row 3, green tracing) it is easily apparent where the spikes are 1 per second (likely interictal, such as at point B, highlighted with red ellipse and labeled), 2 per second (IIC, such as

at point C), and even 3 per second very briefly on occasion (seizure if sustained, as labeled in the ellipse farthest to the right). This can be useful in objectively comparing the burden of IIC and its frequency (from 1 to 2 to 3 Hz) from one record to the next, which can be difficult to compare if using solely rhythmicity or power spectrograms for example. Between A and C, one can see gradual increase spikes (row 3), in rhythmicity (rows 4–5), power (CSAs, rows 6–7) and amplitude (aEEG, bottom 2 rows), all suggesting possible increase in epileptiform activity. These changes were, however, not sufficient to trigger the seizure probability detector (row 2, near top of the page).

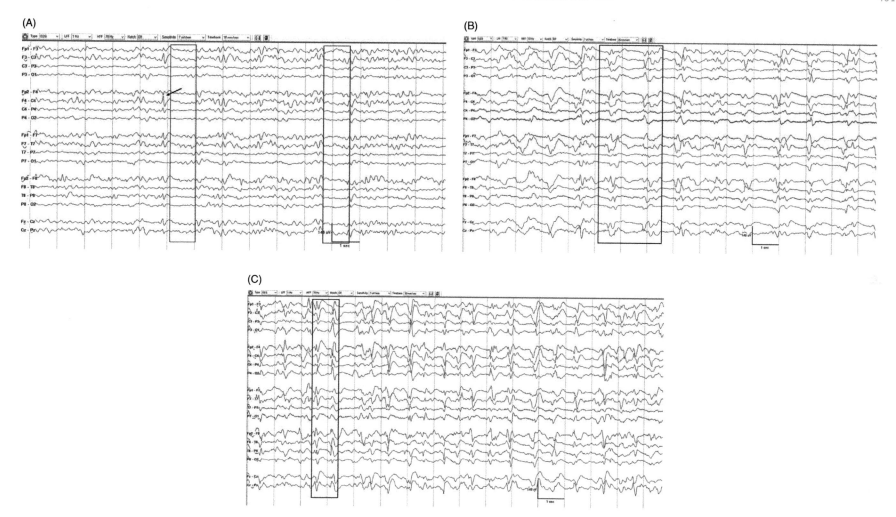

Figure 9.24. (*Continued*) (A) EEG at A. A non-stimulated state. Nearly continuous record (periods of attenuation in boxes) with occasional possible sporadic generalized epileptiform discharges (arrow). (B) EEG at B. This represents the end of a stimulated pattern. There are 1-Hz GPDs (two of them are within the box). This is picked up on the spike detector (arrow within the first red ellipse labeled 'one per sec'). (C) EEG at C. Gradual worsening of the pattern over several hours. GPDs now occurring at approximately 1.5 Hz, occasionally with two occurring within 1 second (box). Note the spike detector now often demonstrates two spikes per second (arrow within second red ellipse, Figure 9.24m).

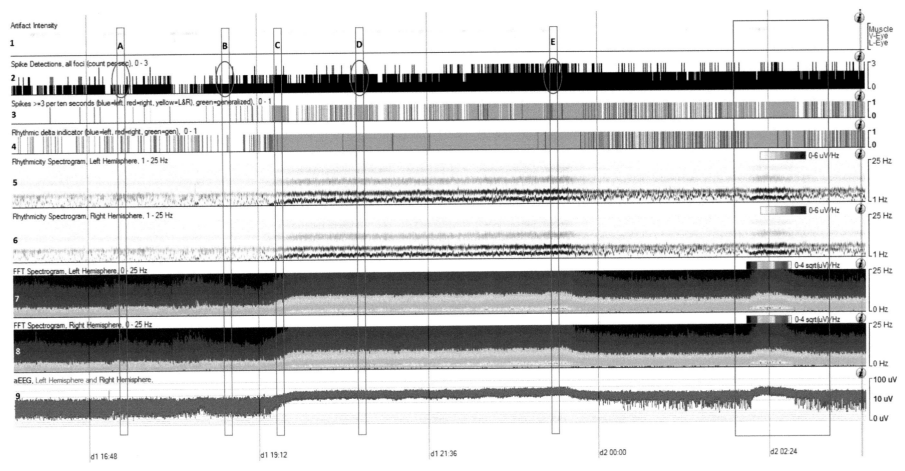

Figure 9.25. QEEG long-term trends, spike detector, rhythmic delta detector: gradual development of nonconvulsive status epilepticus, treatment and recurrence.

Figure 9.25main. This 12-hour QEEG is from a 61-year-old woman status/post cardiac arrest. After 48 hours of therapeutic hypothermia, the patient was rewarmed and had achieved normothermia by the beginning of the record (15:00). The best background (including for the prior 48 hours) was continuous with moderate generalized slowing and abundant sporadic multifocal possible sharp waves (point A), but usually <1/second. The epileptiform discharges slowly increase in frequency (at point B consistently 1 per second [blue ellipse at B]; point C and D, consistently 1–2 per second [blue ellipse at D]; and point E consistently 2–3 per second [blue ellipse at E, i.e., likely to qualify for electrographic status epilepticus, confirmed on raw EEG in this case]). A spike threshold can also be set, in this case ≥3 spikes per 10 seconds (row 3). This is dichotomous, either absent or indicating a line when reached. It can be useful to set a treatment threshold, e.g., if it was desired to minimize the proportion of the record with discharges above 1.5 Hz the spike threshold could be set to ≥15 spikes per ten seconds to easily identify these components. The patient slowly develops ESE over a series of hours with slow evolving power, rhythmicity and amplitude best seen on the FFT (rows 7 and 8; power spectrograms) and aEEG (row 9). The rhythmic delta indicator also registers this change (row 4), as it begins to detect the rhythmicity associated with the discharges (and is green since it is generalized). Anti-seizure medication successfully slowed down and interrupted the continuous electrographic seizure (shortly after point E), but it recurred later in the record (blue box) and was again treated.

(A)

(B)

(C)

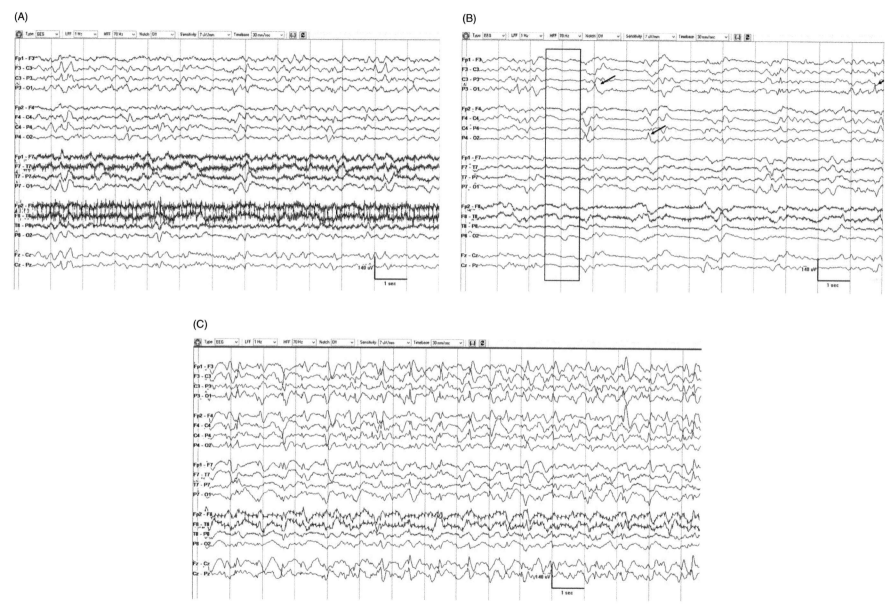

Figure 9.25. (*Continued*) (A) EEG at A. Moderate generalized slowing with scattered multifocal sharply contoured theta waves (possible sharp waves). (B) EEG at B. Episodes of attenuation (box) and the emergence of sharply contoured activity/sporadic sharp waves in several brain regions (arrows), now more frequent and nearly periodic. (C) EEG at C. Spiky GPDs at 1 Hz, clearly ≥3 per 10 seconds as shown on the QEEG (row 3, mostly in green = generalized), and a significant increase in quasi-rhythmic delta activity.

(D)

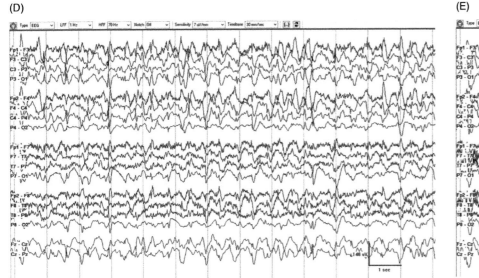

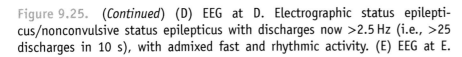

(E)

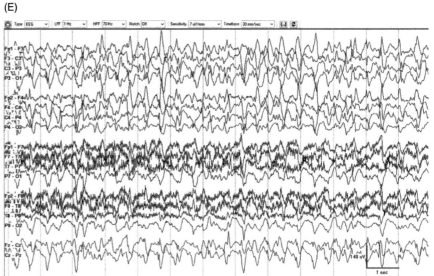

Figure 9.25. (*Continued*) (D) EEG at D. Electrographic status epilepticus/nonconvulsive status epilepticus with discharges now >2.5 Hz (i.e., >25 discharges in 10 s), with admixed fast and rhythmic activity. (E) EEG at E. NCSE/ESE but with even higher voltage and more superimposed faster frequencies. It is difficult to discern the true number of spikes per second in this page, but the spike detector consistently registers 3 per second (QEEG row 2).

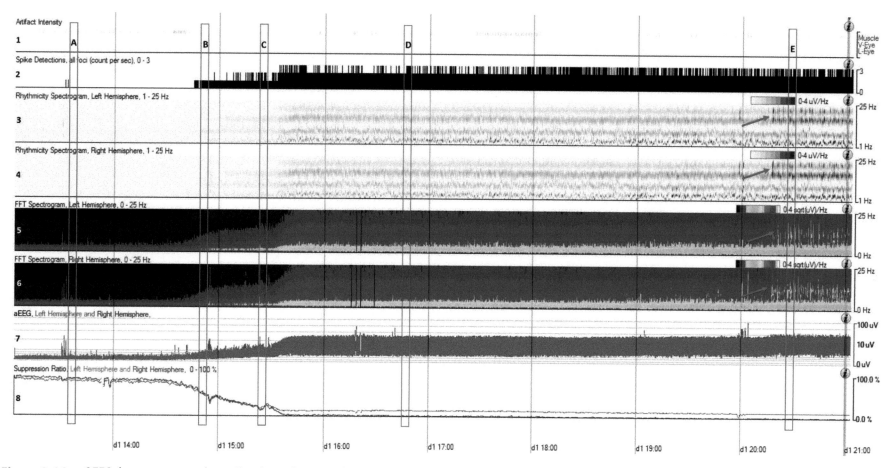

Figure 9.26. QEEG long-term trends, spike detection, amplitude-integrated EEG, and suppression percent: suppression to GPDs to myoclonic status epilepticus.

Figure 9.26main. This 8-hour QEEG is from a 47-year-old woman s/p cardiac arrest. The initial EEG is suppressed with suppression percentages close to 100% (bottom row) (point A). The emergence of very low voltage 0.5–1 Hz GPDs (raw EEG at point B) that are detected on the spike detector (1 per second [row 2]), results in a slight increase in power (rows 5 and 6) and amplitude (row 7), and a reduction in the suppression percentage. As the GPDs become polyspikes and higher voltage, the spike detector starts to show 2 spikes per second, and the suppression percent falls further (point C). Further increase in the frequency of

GPDs then gets detected at 3 spikes per second, and the suppression percent falls to zero as the rhythmicity and power significantly increase (point D). Many of the polyspike discharges are now long enough to qualify as bursts (if part of burst suppression, not yet the case) or BIRDs (if not part of burst suppression). The patient enters myoclonic status epilepticus (point E). The polyspikes are now associated with myoclonic jerking (evidenced by the bi-frontal EMG spikes now superimposed). Note the thick aEEG tracing due to discontinuity, with each page of EEG having low voltage (attenuation) and medium-high voltage (polyspike bursts) activity. In full burst suppression, this is usually even thicker, reaching the bottom of the scale.

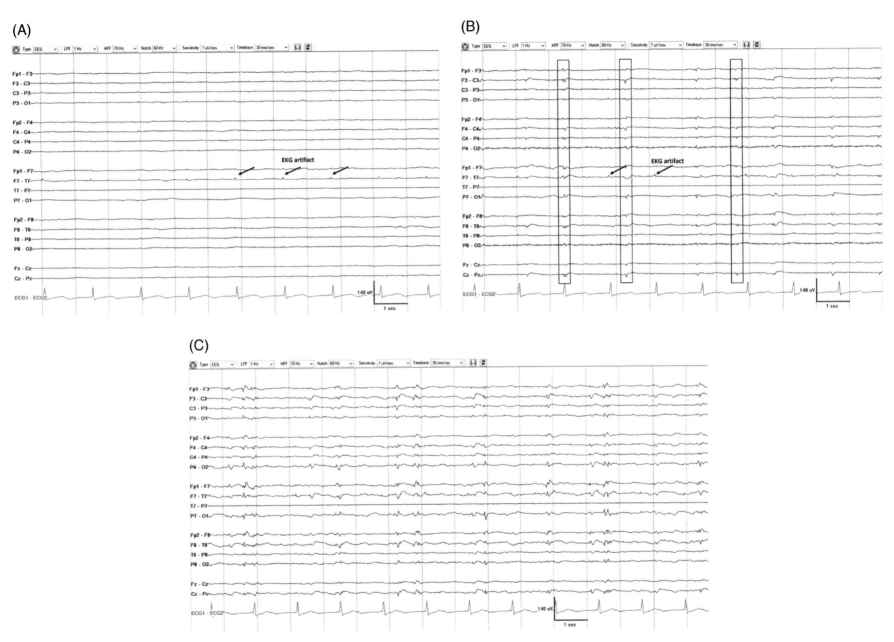

Figure 9.26.   (*Continued*) (A) EEG at A. Background suppression with EKG arti-fact (arrows). (B) EEG at B. Low voltage 0.75 Hz GPDs (boxes) look similar to EKG artifact (arrows). (C) EEG at C. GPDs increase in voltage and frequency, now averaging >1 Hz, and sometimes consisting of polyspikes.

(D)

(E)

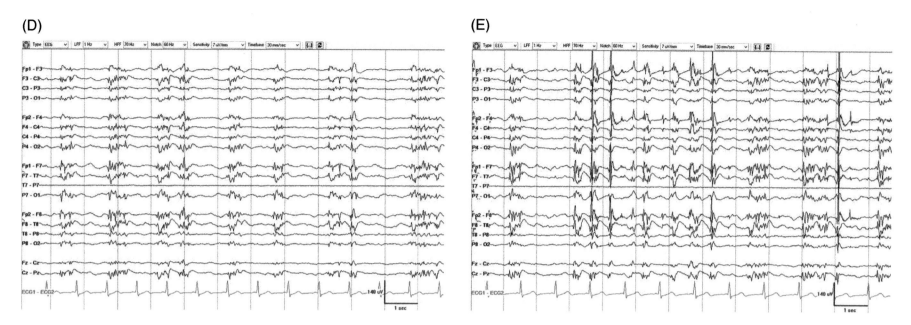

Figure 9.26. (*Continued*) (D) EEG at D. GPDs now become polyspike (sometimes bursts if ≥0.5 seconds). (E) EEG at E. Myoclonic status epilepticus, GPDs now associated with high voltage EMG spikes.

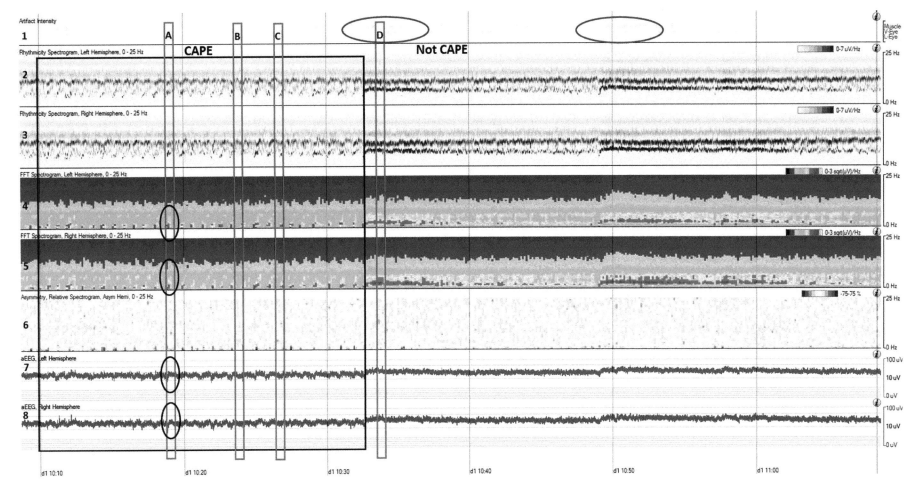

Figure 9.27. QEEG, cyclic patterns: Cyclic Alternating Pattern of Encephalopathy (CAPE)

Figure 9.27main. This 1 hour of QEEG is from a 69-year-old woman s/p right frontal tumor resection. The QEEG demonstrates a cyclic alternating pattern of encephalopathy (CAPE) (black box). CAPE refers to background patterns, each lasting at least 10 s, and spontaneously alternating between the two patterns in a regular manner for at least 6 cycles (but often lasts minutes to hours). In this example the CAPE consists of pattern A: medium to high amplitude delta activity with sharply contoured theta activity that is more prominent in the right parasagittal region due to the breach effect (raw EEG at point A); and pattern B: the less stimulated state that appears more 'normal' with lower voltage, faster activity, predominantly 6–8 Hz) activity (raw EEG at point B). The patterns alternate between each other (i.e., A-B-A-B-A-B), hence the term CAPE. Pattern A is best signified by the significant rise in delta power on the FFT (power spectrogram, rows 4 and 5) and increase in amplitude on aEEG (rows 7 and 8) (black ellipses). Pattern A is the more stimulated pattern despite having a greater amount of delta activity, a very common scenario in patients with encephalopathy. A typical spontaneous transition between states is shown at point C. The patient is stimulated at the end of the black box, with a raw EEG sample at point D: some EMG and eye movement artifacts appear [blue ellipses], the cyclic pattern stops, and the patient then remains in the 'more awake' state with more delta (pattern A).

(A)

(B)

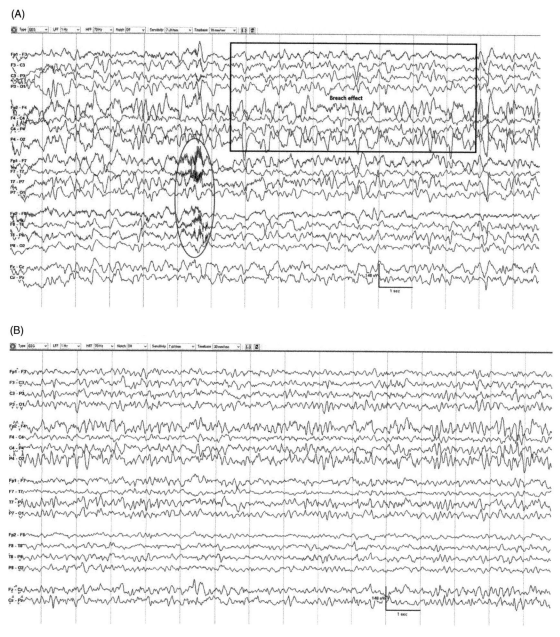

Figure 9.27. (*Continued*) (A) EEG at A: more stimulated (or more 'awake') state, with more slowing and higher amplitudes, and some muscle artifact (blue ellipse). There is breach effect when comparing the parasagittal chains (labeled box). (B) EEG at B: less stimulated (or less awake) state, with lower voltage and faster EEG, with no muscle or movement artifact.

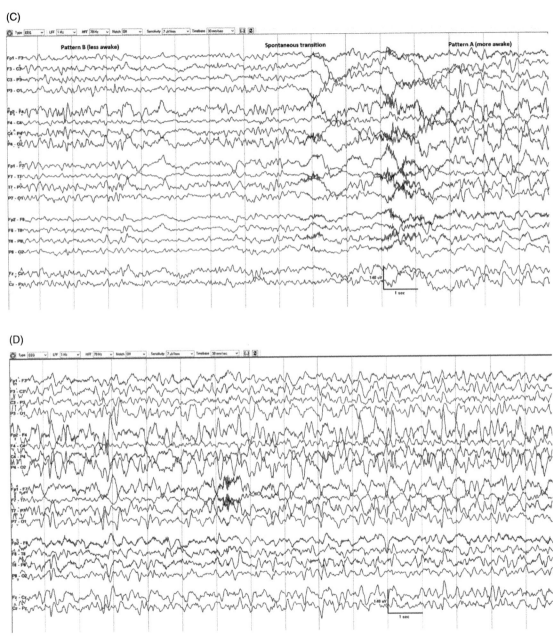

Figure 9.27. (*Continued*) (C) EEG at C: spontaneous transition between the less awake state (pattern B) and more awake state (pattern A). Note the EMG activity as the patient transitions from one state to the other. (D) Post stimulation (for standard patient care; remains in the more awake state for a long time here due to ongoing stimulation).

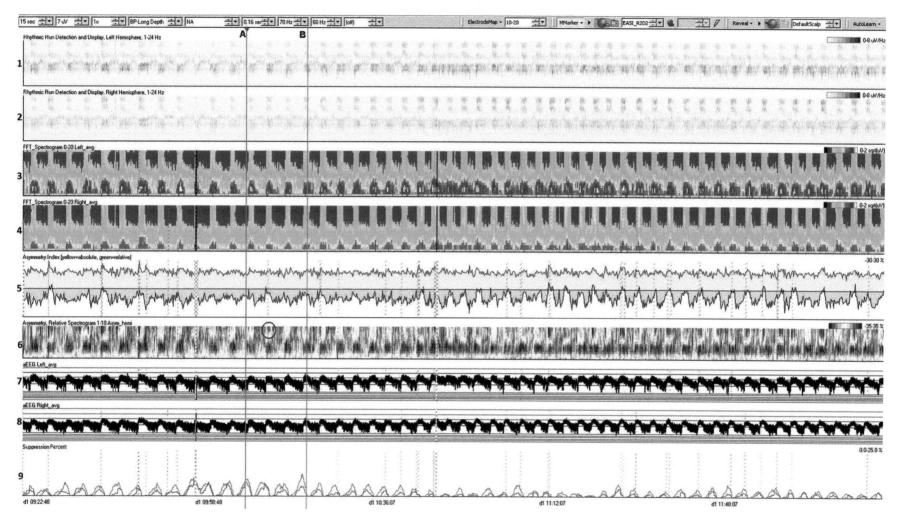

Figure 9.28. QEEG, cyclic patterns: CAPE with cyclic LPDs

Figure 9.28main: 3 hours of QEEG in an elderly man with a large right frontal intracerebral hemorrhage with ventricular extension. A cyclic pattern is evident. In this case, there are left-sided LPDs (from the opposite side of the hemorrhage) coming and going every ~3 minutes. At the same time, muscle artifact appears on the right, best appreciated on the asymmetry spectrogram (row 6, appearing in red at high frequencies; circle). There was no detectable clinical correlate. The cyclic muscle artifact is either due to contralateral 'ictal' muscle tone or cyclic arousal with nonspecific increase in muscle tone when more stimulated, with less muscle activity on the left due to paralysis on that side, and with the LPDs present in the more awake portion of the cycle. Also note the persistent asymmetry, with more power on the left (down-going green relative asymmetry index tracing [REASI, row 5], and blue on the asymmetry spectrogram, maximal in the theta range). Finally, the cyclic pattern can be seen on the suppression percent (bottom row). The asymmetry can also be seen in this tracing, with higher suppression percentages on the right (red) than left (blue).

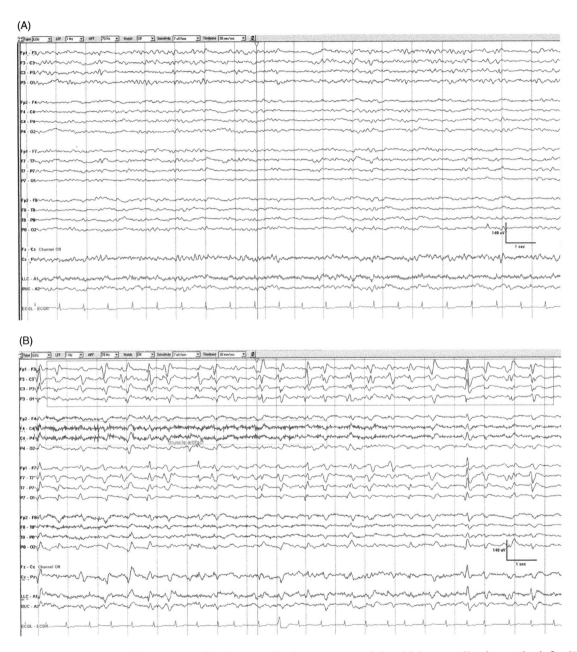

Figure 9.28.   (*Continued*) (A) EEG at A: portion without LPDs, showing mostly theta range activity, higher amplitude on the left. (B) EEG at B: portion with left LPDs (blue box), averaging ~1.5 Hz, with some spread to the right (i.e., sometimes bilateral asymmetric), and right-sided muscle artifact (green box).

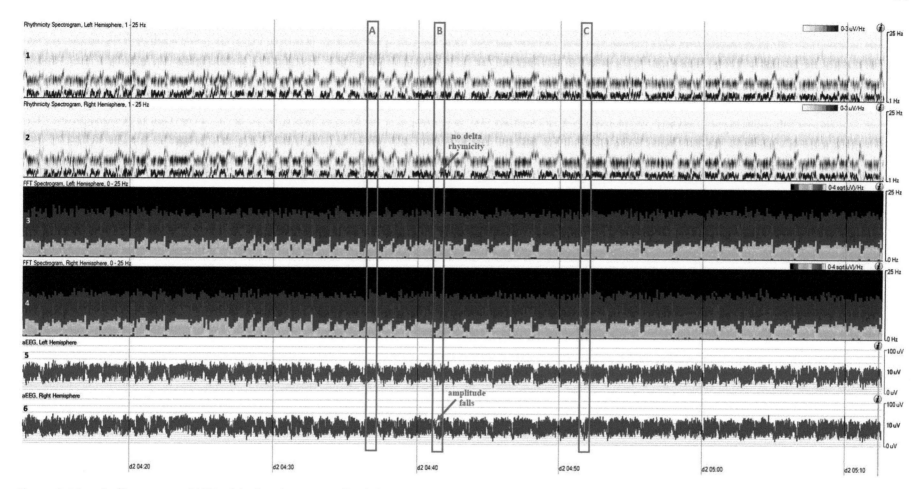

Figure 9.29. Cyclic patterns: CAPE, with abundant generalized sharp waves in the more awake state

Figure 9.29main. This 1-hour segment of QEEG is from a 65-year-old woman with respiratory failure and sepsis. The QEEG demonstrates regular spontaneous cycling between a more stimulated/more awake state (point A, pattern A of CAPE) that consists of abundant, nearly periodic generalized sharp waves, resulting in high theta and delta rhythmicity and power at that point; and a less stimulated/less awake state (point B, pattern B of CAPE) consisting of medium-amplitude theta and spindle-like activity; hence, the QEEG demonstrates little delta power/rhythmicity (labeled red arrow) and the amplitude also falls on aEEG (row 6). The patient regularly transitions from one pattern to the other. Point C (and raw EEG at C) demonstrates the patient spontaneously changing from pattern B to pattern A.

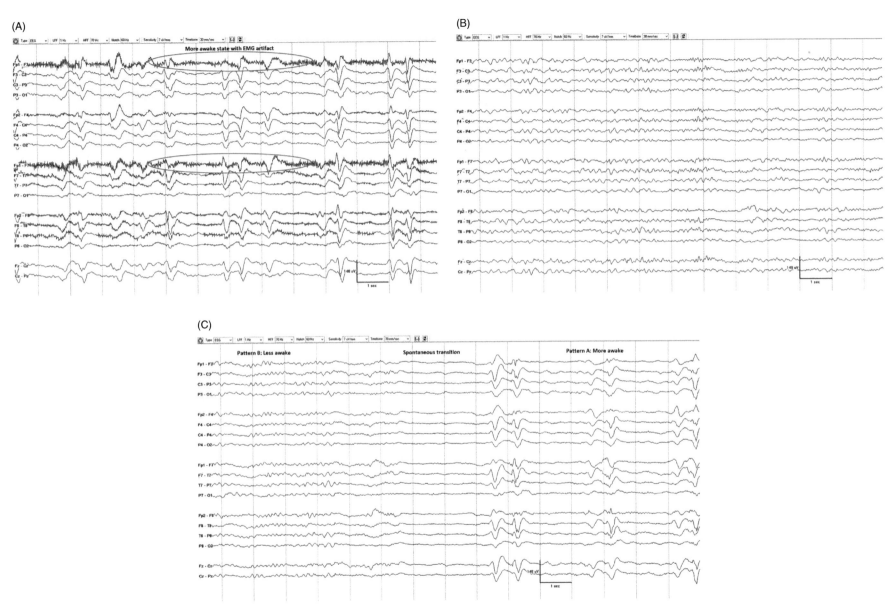

Figure 9.29. (*Continued*) (A) EEG at A: the more awake (more stimulated) pattern A of CAPE, with abundant generalized sharp waves, almost periodic (not quite GPDs on this page as never 6 in a row at regular rate). There is greater EMG in this state (red ellipses) providing evidence for the patient being more awake at this time, compared to when in pattern B. (B) EEG at B: the less awake (less stimulated) pattern B of CAPE, lower voltage and faster EEG without epileptiform discharges. (C) EEG at C: spontaneous transition from pattern B (less awake) to pattern A (more awake).

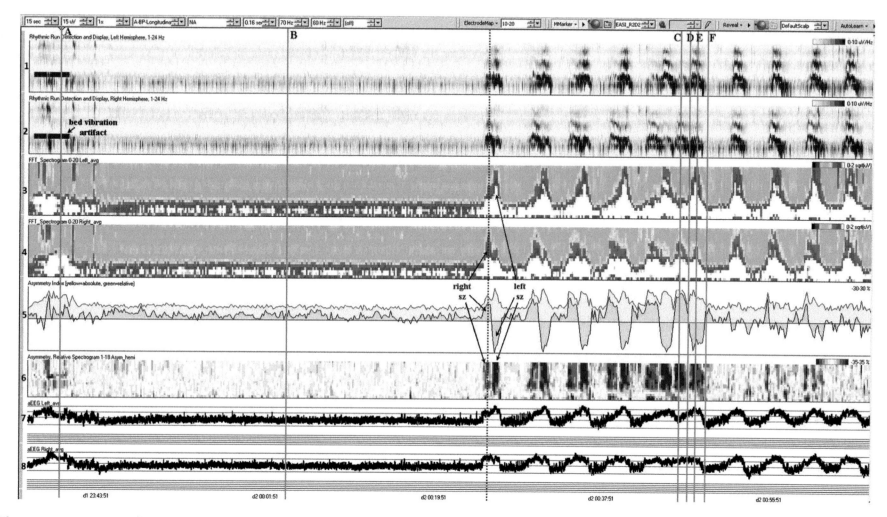

Figure 9.30. QEEG, cyclic patterns: cyclic 'ping-pong' seizures

Figure 9.30main1: 2 hours of QEEG in a 7-year-old boy with refractory nonconvulsive seizures from probable viral encephalitis. Near the beginning, there is classic mechanical artifact (perfect rectangular shape at 5 Hz in the spectrogram at point A) from an oscillating bed. There is then a nondescript period (including point B), followed by the onset of cyclic seizures in the 2nd half of this sample. The QEEG shows that each seizure starts on the right (dotted line labeled 'right sz', with another example at point C) as seen on the power spectrogram (burst on right [row 4] precedes left [row 3]), the green relative asymmetry index (upward first, row 5), the asymmetry spectrogram (burst of red first, row 6), then spreads to the left (labeled 'left sz' with another example at point E) with the green asymmetry index switching to downwards (more power on left) and the asymmetry spectrogram switches to blue.

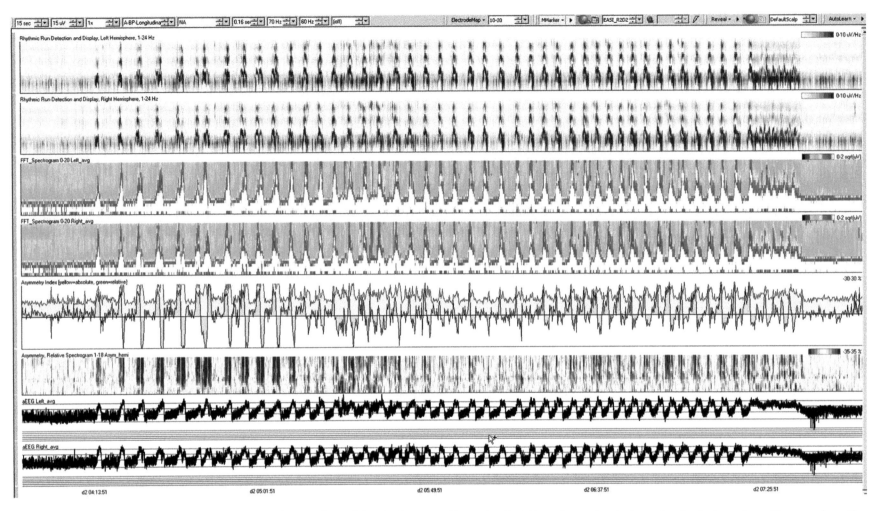

Figure 9.30. (*Continued*) Figure 9.30 main2 Four hours of QEEG beginning 3 hours later. There is a stable pattern of seizures alternating from side to side. This is a form of cyclic seizures that can be referred to as 'ping–pong' seizures. Note also that the seizures begin to cycle at a faster rate as the record continues. This culminates in a continuous bilateral ictal rhythm, just prior to additional anti-seizure medication being administered at the end of the page.

(A)

(B)

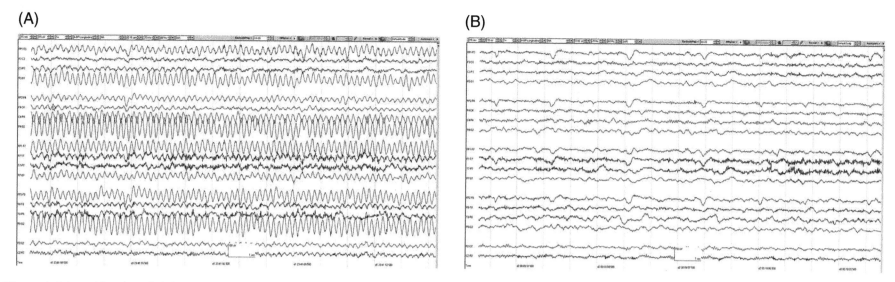

Figure 9.30.   (*Continued*) (A) EEG at A: rhythmic 5 Hz artifact from a vibrating bed. (B) EEG at B: baseline EEG.

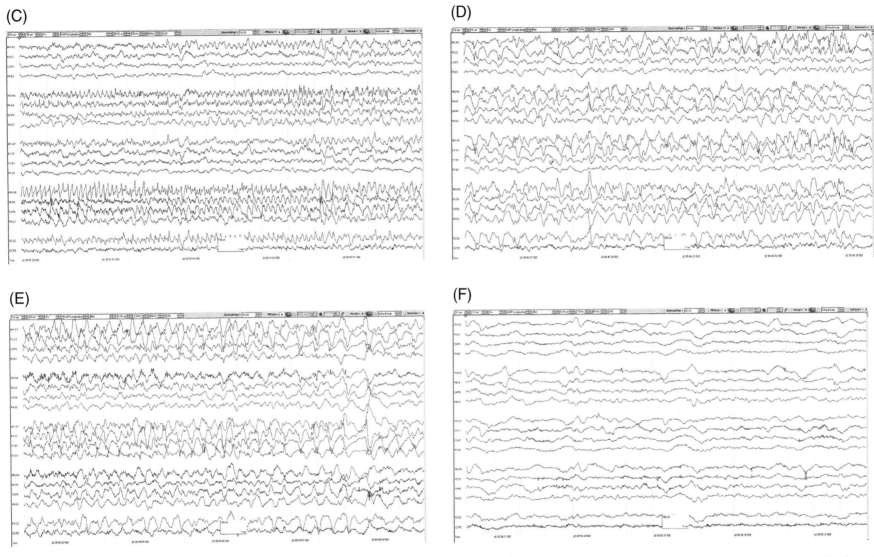

Figure 9.30.   *(Continued)* (C) EEG at C: right-sided seizure. (D) EEG at D: evolving seizure, now bilateral and symmetric; hence the asymmetry measures show no asymmetry at this point. (E) EEG at E: evolving seizure, now maximal on the left. (F) EEG at F: postictal EEG.

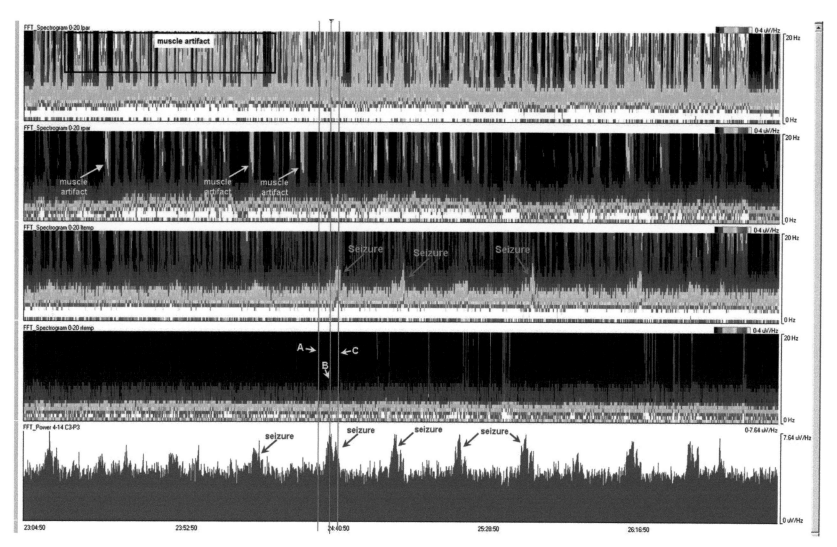

Figure 9.31. QEEG pitfalls and solutions: artifact obscuring highly focal non-convulsive seizures.

Figure 9.31main Four hours of QEEG in a man in his 70s s/p resection of a tumor in the left parietal region. The background shows more power in all frequencies through the left hemisphere. Greater power in both delta and faster frequencies on the same side is typical for a region of dysfunction (causing slowing) and overlying breach effect (resulting in increased faster frequencies) (this was discussed in Figure 9.17). Also note the muscle artifact (coming down from the top of the spectrograms and labeled). This patient was having frequent focal nonconvulsive seizures from P3 (left parietal; B) that remained very focal most of the time and were hard to recognize on the standard spectrogram, mainly because the muscle artifact in the left parasagittal chain obscures the ictal pattern (top row). Thus, an additional row was added to the QEEG panel (bottom) showing total power from 4–14 Hz at C3-P3, the most relevant channel and frequencies (i.e., all the muscle artifact that is >14 Hz has been removed). This tracing showed each seizure rather clearly. Some of the seizures spread to the left temporal lobe and were well visualized on the spectrogram on the temporal row (C, and purple 'seizure' labels). Interictal EEG is shown in A, left parietal seizure in B, and spread to left temporal lobe in C (in the shape of 'flames'). In this case, the limitation of the QEEG to detect seizures was muscle artifact, but with a row specifically removing this and homing in on the channel and pattern of interest, the seizures and effect of anti-seizure medication could be followed easily.

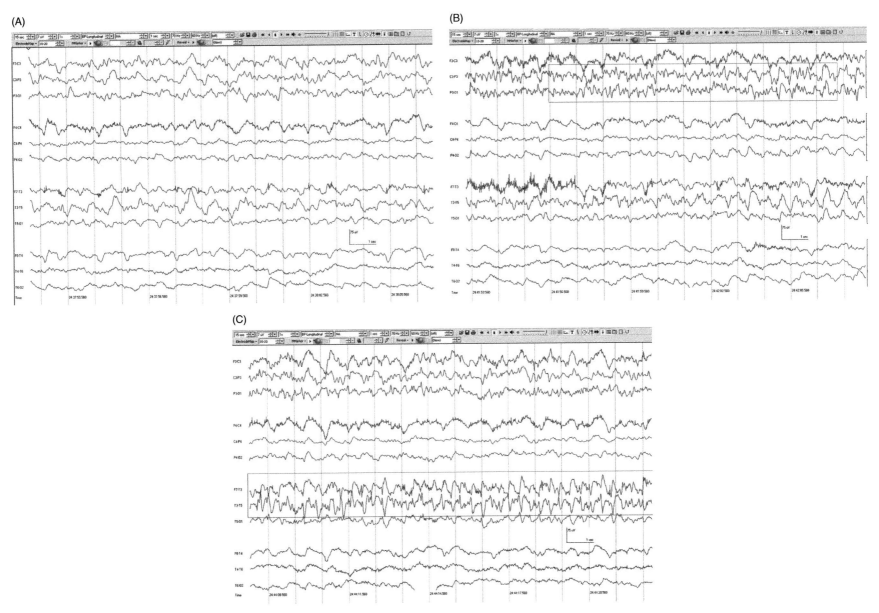

Figure 9.31. (*Continued*) (A) EEG at A: baseline, with prominent slowing and breach effect on the left. (B) EEG at B: evolving ictal pattern predominantly at C3 (box). Note that this portion was readily identifiable on the last row (C3-P3 4–14 Hz total power) but is not visible on the standard spectrograms (due to muscle artifact). (C) EEG at C: ictal pattern has now spread to the left temporal region (box) when it becomes obvious on the left temporal spectrogram as well. Note not all seizures spread and therefore not all seizures are easily detected in the temporal region; for example, the first seizure labeled in the bottom row, around 24:00, is easily detected in the tailored bottom row but hard to see in the regular spectrogram in either the parietal or temporal regions.

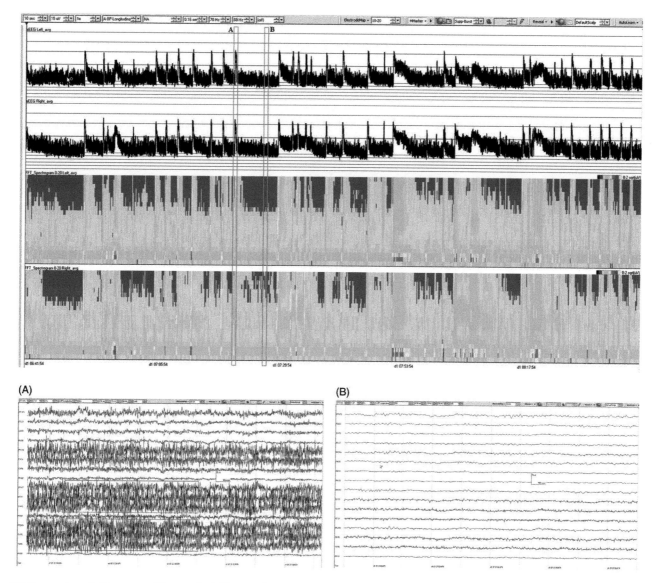

Figure 9.32. QEEG pitfalls and solutions: artifact mimicking seizures on amplitude-integrated EEG (aEEG).

Figure 9.32main Two hours of QEEG in a 44-year-old woman with HIV/AIDS, sepsis, meningitis and prior seizures. Note frequent paroxysmal increases in amplitude (such as A) that look like typical seizures on the aEEG tracing. However, this patient had no seizures, but rather had intermittent muscle artifact. This is a reminder of the dangers of interpreting aEEG traces without expert review of the corresponding raw EEG. It is also valuable to note that the FFT spectrogram is typical of muscle artifact, demonstrating activity suddenly appearing from the top of the trace and lacking the diagonal pattern of evolution that is typical of seizure. This is one of the reasons to view several trends together. Similar to using different montages for raw EEG interpretation, the multiple QEEG trends are complimentary, with information from all trends (and raw EEG) assisting with providing the most accurate interpretation. (A) EEG at A: muscle artifact, which caused the increase in amplitude on aEEG. (B) EEG at B: baseline, with much less muscle artifact.

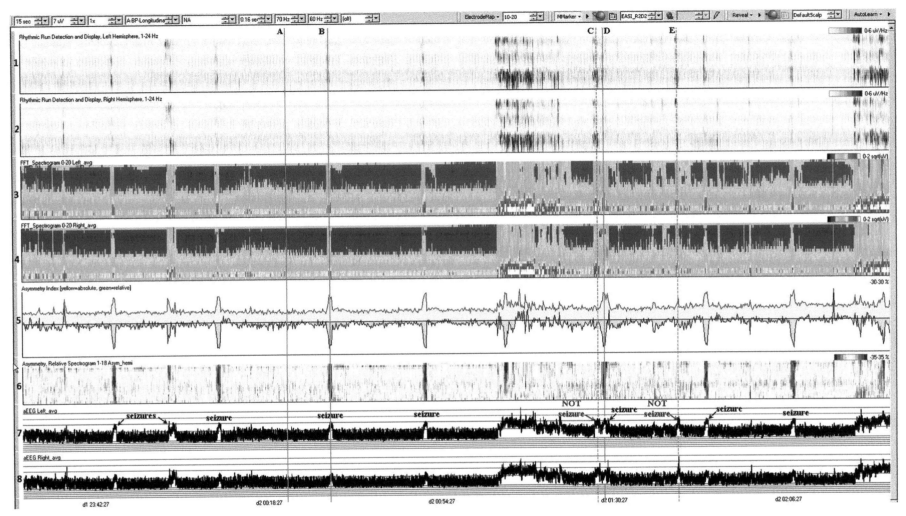

Figure 9.33. QEEG pitfalls and solutions: multiple seizures and identical-appearing false positives on amplitude-integrated EEG (aEEG).

Figure 9.33main 3–4 hours of QEEG from a man in his sixties with a left hemisphere brain tumor, presenting with worsening memory and language. Multiple electrographic seizures were recorded (labeled), maximal on the left as evident on the aEEG (higher amplitudes on left) (bottom two rows), the relative asymmetry index going sharply downward (more power on left) (row 5), and the asymmetry spectrogram turning dark blue with each seizure (row 6). The power spectrogram (rows 3 and 4) and the asymmetry spectrogram both demonstrate involvement of all frequencies, and the rhythmicity spectrogram (rows 1 and 2) shows a burst of rhythmicity with most of them. Note the two episodes labeled 'not seizure' (and with dashed lines). In these instances, the aEEG tracing jumps up in a manner almost identical to the prior and subsequent seizures. However, these are due to muscle artifact. Note that the two asymmetry rows do not show the typical seizure pattern with these artifactual increases in amplitude. This example shows the benefit of using multiple QEEG measures simultaneously, and again stresses the importance of not relying on one measure alone without reviewing the raw EEG.

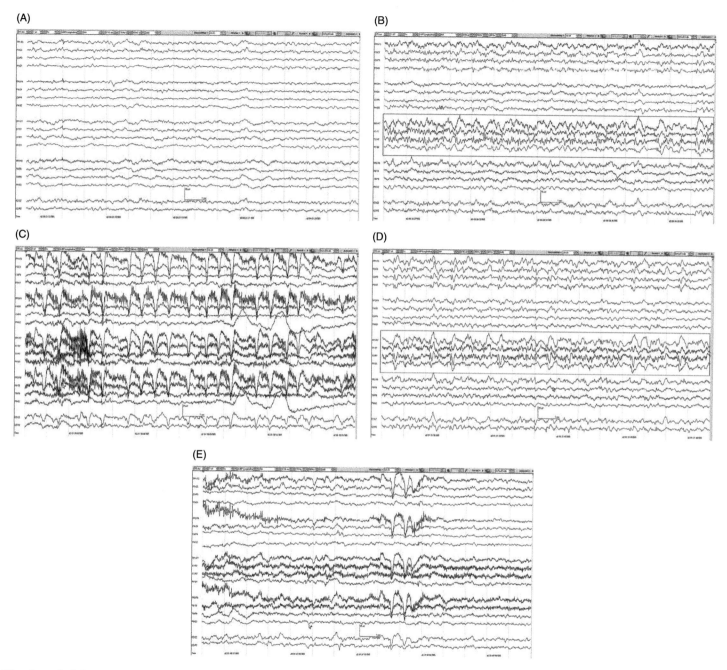

Figure 9.33. (*Continued*) (A) EEG at A: background EEG. (B) EEG at B: left hemisphere seizure, maximal in the temporal chain and composed of mixed frequencies (box). (C) EEG at C: blinking, movement and muscle artifact only. No seizure. (D) EEG at D: another left-sided seizure (box). (E) EEG at E: muscle artifact and a couple of blinks. No seizure.

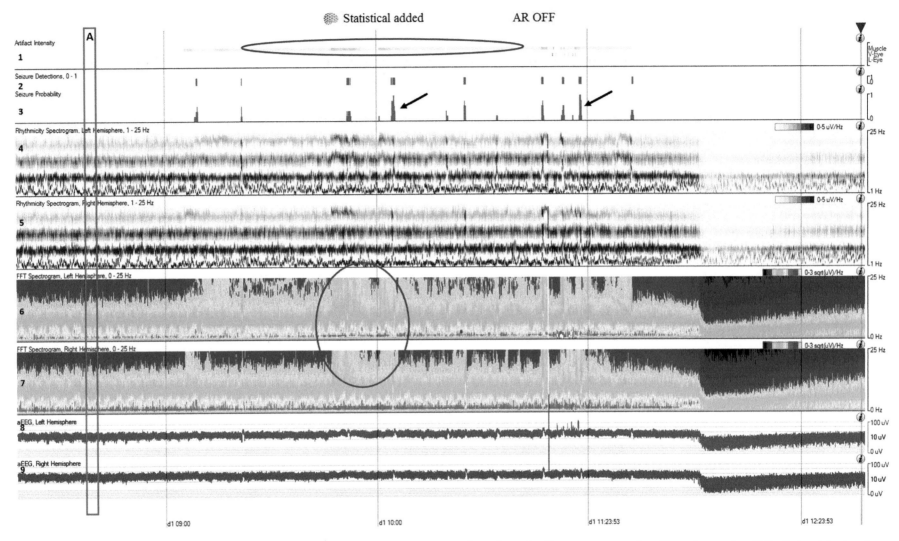

Figure 9.34. QEEG pitfalls and solutions: brief right and left hemispheric seizures in the context of GPDs and muscle artifact.

Figure 9.34main Four hours of QEEG. The baseline EEG in this 32-year-old woman with cryptogenic NORSE (new onset refractory status epilepticus) demonstrates GPDs at 1.5 Hz (raw EEG at point A). An hour into the record there is a significant increase in muscle artifact (blue ellipses around the green artifact detector at the top [row 1], and on the power spectrograms [rows 6 and 7]). In this type of scenario, where the baseline EEG is already significantly abnormal, and/or where there is a significant amount of artifact, it can be difficult to detect seizures (especially if they are brief). A way of screening for this scenario is with automated seizure detectors (row 2) and seizure probability (row 3) algorithms. In this case, these trends suggest the development of brief seizures, but these are difficult to detect with the muscle artifact. Artifact reduction algorithms can be especially useful at reducing muscle artifact and the result of applying this filtering can be seen in the following Figure 9.34main2.

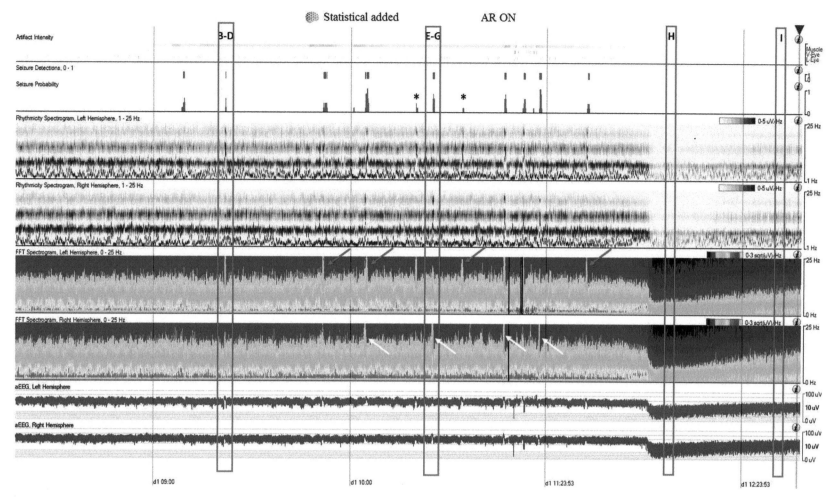

Figure 9.34. (*Continued*) Figure 9.34main2 The same 4 hours of QEEG with the artifact reduction turned on, as indicated at the top of the page with 'AR ON'. It is now clear (especially on the power spectrograms) that there are several seizures starting independently in left (red arrows) and right (white arrows) hemispheres. The seizures are brief, so it could be hard to see the typical diagonal pattern of evolving power, rhythmicity or amplitude. The trend with the best temporal resolution (i.e., calculated and presented the most often or with the smallest time intervals) is the aEEG. For brief seizures the aEEG can often demonstrate the typical pattern of sudden increase in amplitude that may be harder to appreciate on rhythmicity or power spectrograms (as in this case). Points B-D demonstrates a left-sided seizure. Points E-G demonstrates a right-sided seizure. Again, it is valuable to note that no trend is absolute. For example, the seizure probability and seizure detector trends alerted to the presence of seizures, but with refining the QEEG it is evident that there are several seizures (such as those highlighted by the asterisks) that do not register well on the seizure probability or detector trends, but have the same seizure signature on the spectrograms and aEEG tracings. Again, the trends are complimentary. Later in the record (point H), the patient was administered propofol. Rhythmicity and power across all frequencies decrease markedly, and amplitude drops very low as the seizures and GPDs stop. Muscle artifact also stops at this time. The thicker aEEG tracing at H suggests bursting activity, with each page reaching marked suppression (aEEG trace reaching <2 µV) but also having portions close to normal voltage (reaching 10 µV on aEEG trace; see raw EEG at H). GPDs slowly return as propofol wears off (point I). Between H and I, there is a clear gradual trend of increasing amplitudes, power and rhythmicity that suggest that seizures might soon be returning as well. This type of gradual trend is much harder to appreciate on raw EEG then on QEEG traces such as this.

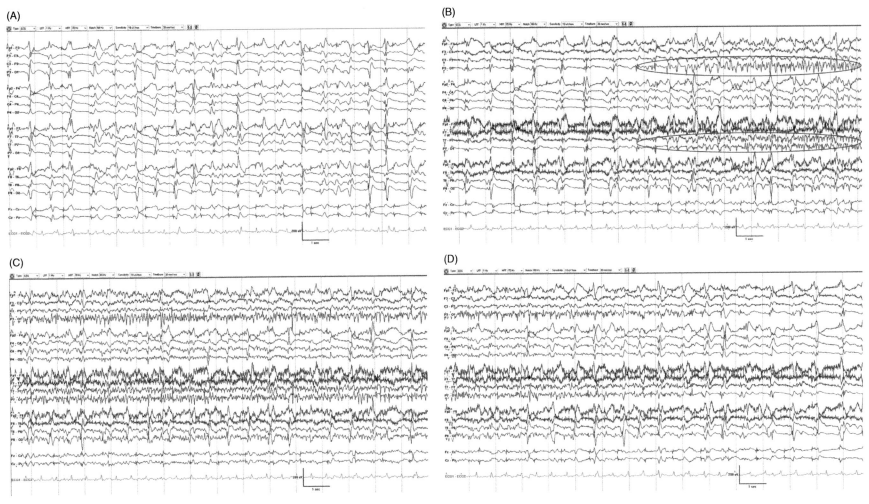

Figure 9.34. (*Continued*) (A) EEG at A: baseline EEG with GPDs at 1.5 Hz. Note the sensitivity has been reduced to 10 μV/mm. (B) EEG at B: ESz beginning in the left posterior quadrant (ellipses), though also seen posteriorly on the right at lower voltage. (C) EEG at C: ESz predominantly in the posterior left hemisphere (still also seen on the right, much lower voltage). (D) EEG at D: end of left hemisphere-maximal ESz.

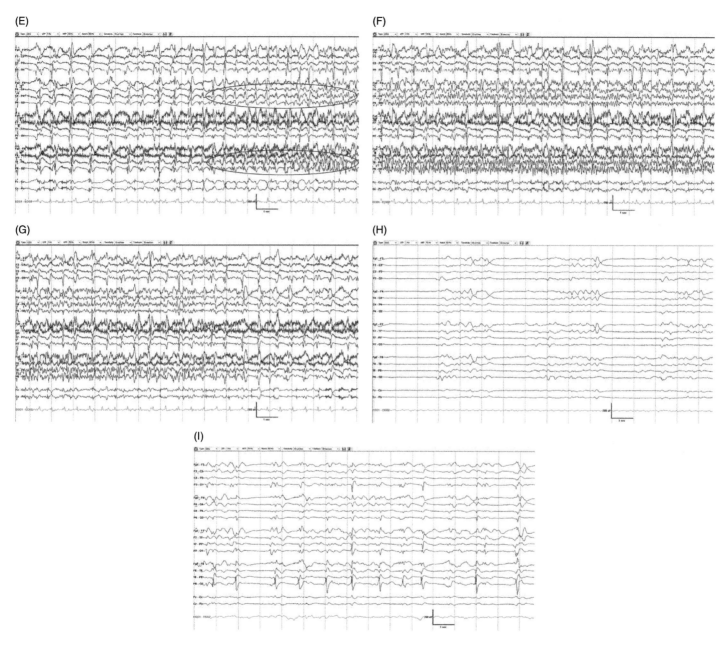

Figure 9.34. (*Continued*) (E) EEG at E: ESz onset, maximal in the right hemisphere (ellipses), though also seen on the left. (F) EEG at F: ESz continues, almost completely in the right hemisphere. (G) EEG at G: end of right hemisphere ESz. (H) EEG at H. After propofol, with resolution of GPDs and a discontinuous (almost burst suppressed) record. (I) EEG at I. Slow return of GPDs (most prominent in the right posterior temporal region in this instance, but as they became more prominent, they again became symmetric and synchronous).

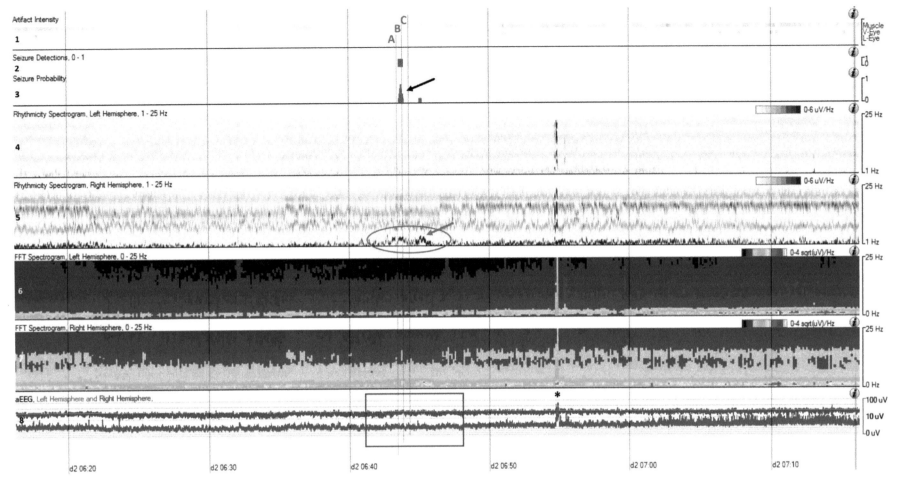

Figure 9.35. QEEG pitfalls and solutions: very focal seizures within breach effect.

Figure 9.35main. 1 hour of QEEG from a 41-year-old woman with TBI and right subdural hematoma s/p right decompressive hemicraniectomy. There is a prominent breach effect and dysfunction of the right hemisphere. The aEEG (row 8) shows the voltage through the right hemisphere is much greater than that on the left; and there is significant rhythmicity (row 5 compared to row 4) and power (row 7 compared to row 6) through all frequencies through the right hemisphere. The patient had very focal electrographic seizures (ESzs; F4 spreading to Fz only) (raw EEGs at A-C). These are very hard if not impossible to see on rhythmicity, power or amplitude trends. The seizure detector (row 2) and seizure probability (row 3) trends do detect the first seizure (black arrow); however, they do not quite detect the second seizure that shortly follows this (red arrow; though the seizure probability does go above zero there, warranting a close look at the raw EEG at that spot). The ictal pattern seen on the raw EEG is predominantly rhythmic activity at a mildly slower and only slightly higher amplitude than the background activity in that hemisphere and limited to two electrodes. Knowledge of this explains why it is difficult to see on the hemispheric QEEG measures, including aEEG (blue box) and power spectrograms; there is a hint of it on the rhythmicity spectrogram with subtle increase in rhythmicity in the delta range (red ellipse). This patient highlights a limitation of the QEEG for very focal, brief seizures, especially in a region of significant abnormality. The sensitivity and specificity can be improved by utilizing a series of trends, tailoring them to the specific patient, channels and ictal pattern once known, and focusing on detailed review of the raw EEG whenever change is detected (including any seizure detection, even if only low probability). This is actually contrasted with a false positive seizure on the aEEG on this QEEG page. (asterisk; similar to example previously demonstrated in Figures 9.32 and 9.33.

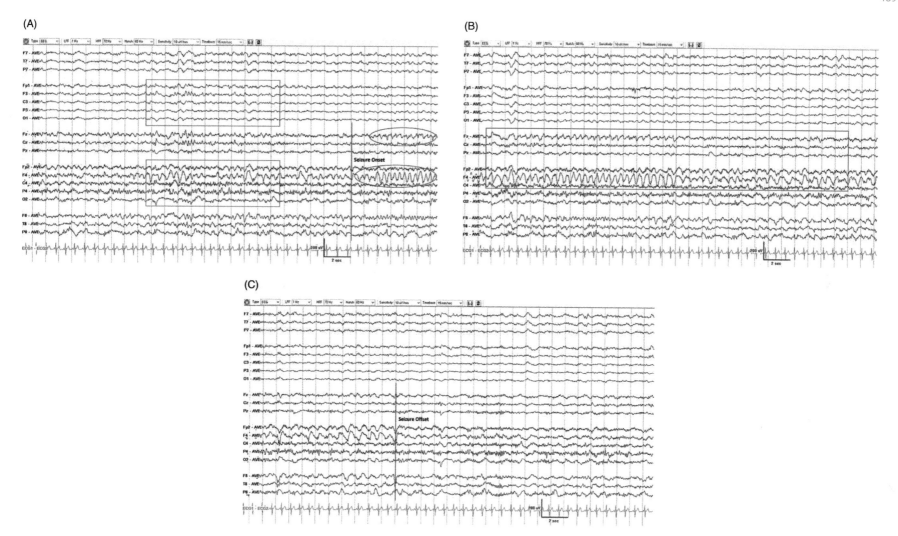

Figure 9.35. (*Continued*) (A) EEG at A: average referential montage (left hemisphere over right hemisphere) at 10 µV/mm and time scale reduced to 15 mm/s (compressed). Asymmetric background with medium-high voltage delta (1.5–2-Hz) in the right parasagittal region (red boxes comparing left and right parasagittal). An ESz begins at the end of the page (labeled line) consisting of evolving rhythmic delta activity at F4 spreading to Fz (blue ellipses). The amplitude and underlying frequencies have not changed much, they just became more rhythmic, and only at F4 and Fz. (B) EEG at B: further evolution of the seizure (again maximal at F4, resolving at Fz in the middle of this page, but now involving Fp2 to some degree) (red box). (C) EEG at C: end of the ESz (labeled line) and return to asymmetric background.

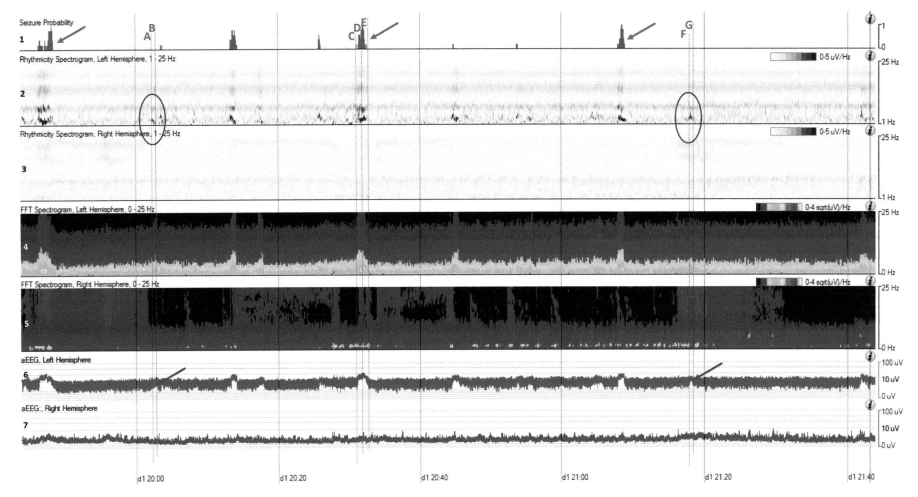

Figure 9.36. QEEG pitfalls and solutions: very focal unilateral independent seizures and regional rhythmicity

Figure 9.36main1. 2 hours of QEEG from a 74-year-old man with severe TBI s/p left hemicraniectomy who had many very focal ESzs (more common with skull defects, esp craniectomies) from three independent foci within the left hemisphere. Although some seizures are easy to detect (red arrows), others are much more subtle (blue ellipses on the rhythmicity spectrogram; also, subtly visible on the left hemisphere aEEG, blue arrows) and are not detected by the seizure detector (row 1 at A-B and at F-G). This is because these highlighted seizures are very focal and therefore do not contribute greatly to the hemispheric trends. This can be overcome by utilizing the regional rhythmicity (rhythmicity spectrograms calculated for each region of the EEG, rather than the hemisphere as a whole), shown in the next figure. It can also be run on individual channels (not shown).

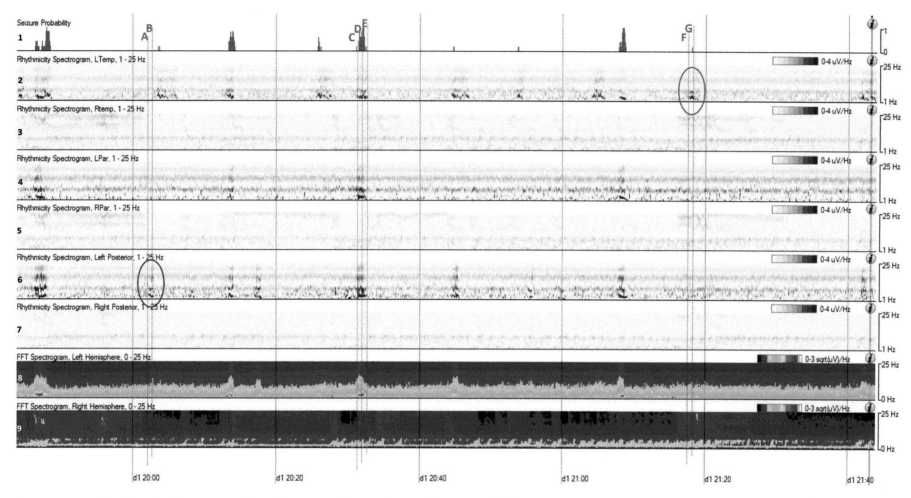

Figure 9.36. (*Continued*) Figure 9.36main2. The same 2 hours of QEEG but rhythmicity spectrograms are now presented by region (row 2, left temporal: 3, right temporal: 4, left parasagittal: 5, right parasagittal: 6, left posterior: 7, right posterior). The hemispheric power spectrograms remain at the bottom. Now at A-B typical burst of unilateral evolving rhythmicity can be detected in the left posterior region (blue ellipse). This is due to a very focal seizure at O1. C-E shows a left hemispheric seizure, which is easily detected on the seizure probability and the hemispheric FFT (row 8). The ESz at F-G only involves the left temporal region (red ellipse). The example highlights how the raw EEG and QEEG are complimentary. Knowledge of the ictal patterns and regions involved on the raw EEG allow for the QEEG trends to be tailored so the most information can be extracted. In this case the independent regions of seizure generation can be easily assessed with regional rhythmicity, and any new regions of excitability would be easily evident.

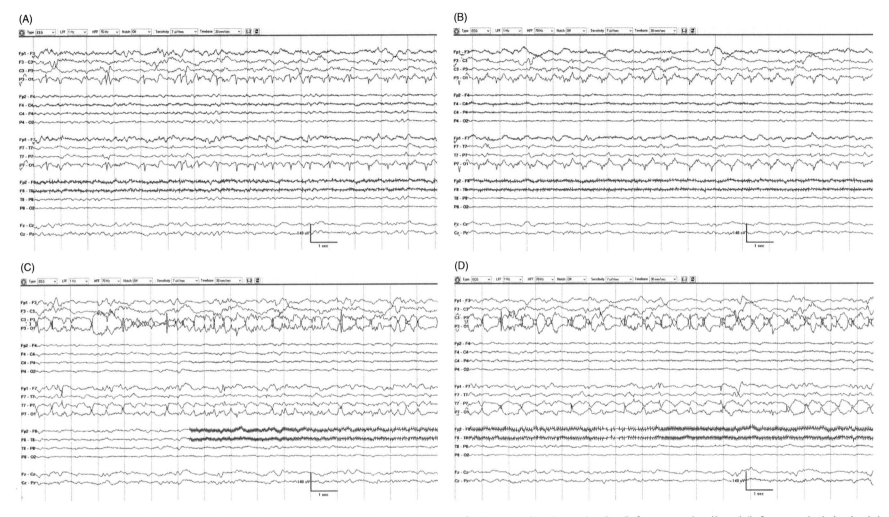

Figure 9.36. (*Continued*) (A) EEG at A: very focal ESz beginning at O1 (seen only in the 'left posterior' rhythmicity trend on the QEEG, likely related to having a craniectomy). (B) EEG at B: further evolution of ESz at O1. (C) EEG at C: start of ESz at P3/O1 (seen in the 'left parasagittal' and 'left posterior' rhythmicity trends). (D) EEG at D: further evolution of ESz at P3/O1 > P7.

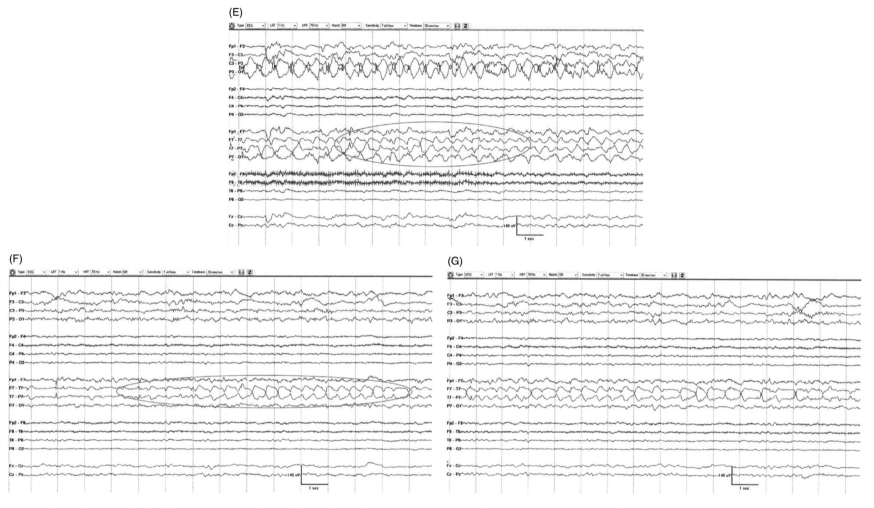

Figure 9.36. (*Continued*) (E) EEG at E: propagation of ESz to T7 (left temporal, red ellipse). (F) EEG at F: very focal ESz emerging at T7 (red ellipse). (G) EEG at G: further evolution and end of ESz at T7. Note there is very little involvement of other electrodes, an unusual seizure, especially with slow frequencies (likely related to severe contusion and hemicraniectomy), but it is clearly an evolving seizure nonetheless, with a pattern similar to the spread pattern in the prior seizure (part E).

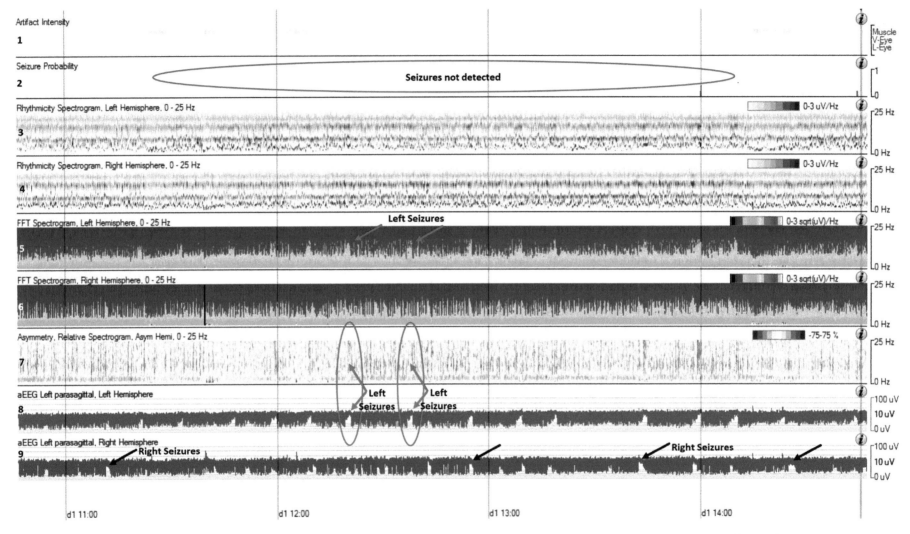

Figure 9.37. QEEG pitfalls and solutions: bilateral independent BIRDs and seizures.

Figure 9.37main1 This 4-hour QEEG is from a 57-year-old woman with multiple brain metastases and altered mental status. The example has been mainly included as it demonstrates a case where the patient is clearly in electrographic status epilepticus, but the seizure probability indicator does not register as such (red ellipse). It again highlights that QEEG trends are complementary and no one trend/algorithm is 100% sensitive/specific. The reason for the seizure probability not registering seizures is likely because the background EEG is so abnormal that seizures are not drastically different from this, discussed in Figure 9.37main2. The frequent left-sided seizures are easier to appreciate. There appears evolving power (labeled red arrows, row 5) and amplitude (red ellipses and labeled with arrows), with reversal of the asymmetry spectrogram to favor the left at the time of seizures (also red ellipse). Right-sided seizures are suggested by sudden increased in amplitude on the aEEG (labeled arrows), but they are hard to appreciate on rhythmicity or power spectrograms. These could be better appreciated by spreading out the QEEG panel; very brief events are often apparent when looking at a smaller time window (see Figure 9.37main2).

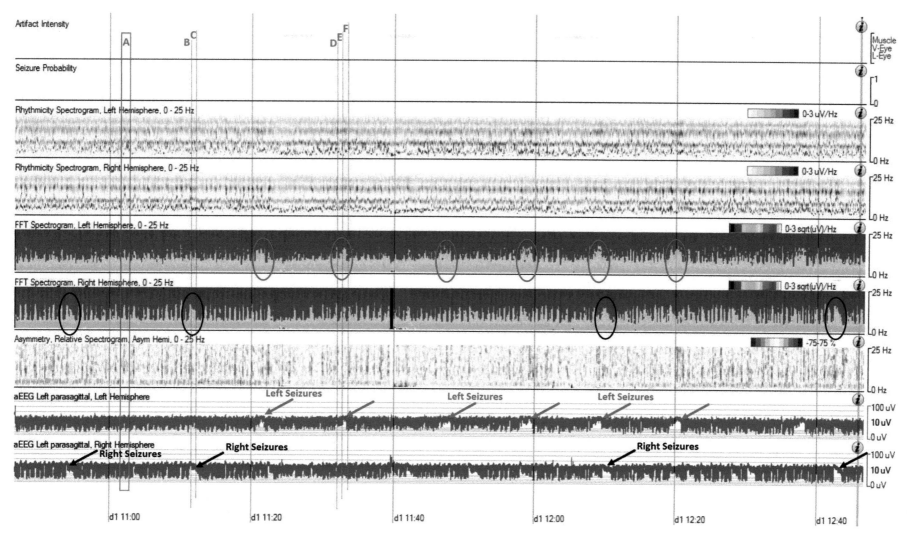

Figure 9.37. *(Continued)* Figure 9.37main2 The QEEG panel has been reduced from 4 hours (Figure 9.37main1) to 2 hours (the first 2 hours of the prior figure). The background EEG (see raw EEG A) is suppressed, with BIPDs+F and bilateral independent BIRDs. The result of these are broad or thick bars on the aEEG. This is similar to burst suppression, i.e., each page of EEG consists of low voltage activity interrupted by high voltage activity. This also forms a 'striped' or 'spiculated' pattern on the power spectrogram. Evolving power of right hemispheric seizures (e.g., points B-C) is now easier to appreciate (several highlighted with ellipses, although evolution is again best detected on aEEG [right seizures labeled with arrows]). This example again highlights that the aEEG has a better temporal resolution than rhythmicity and power spectrograms, and it is much easier to identify the seizures despite a background of abundant BIRDs with aEEG in this case. Left-sided seizures are also highlighted in red ellipses on power spectrogram and labeled with red arrows on aEEG.

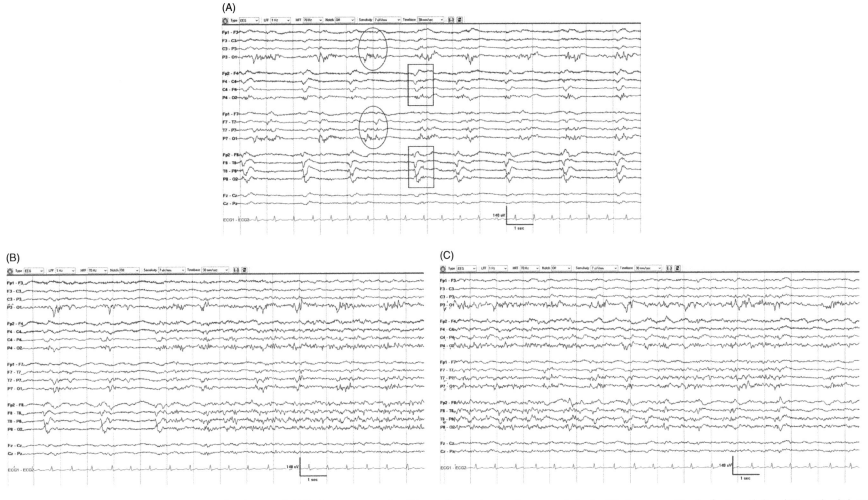

Figure 9.37.   (*Continued*) (A) EEG at A: background EEG is suppressed with BIPDs+F at times qualifying as bilateral independent BIRDs (when >0.5 seconds in duration). The left posterior periodic complexes (ellipses) mostly consist of fast activity that lasts for ≥0.5 seconds (BIRDs). The right hemispheric PDs (boxes) are also associated with low-amplitude fast activity (PDs+F). (B) EEG at B: onset of a right hemispheric ESz. (C) EEG at C: right hemispheric maximal ESz continues and ends.

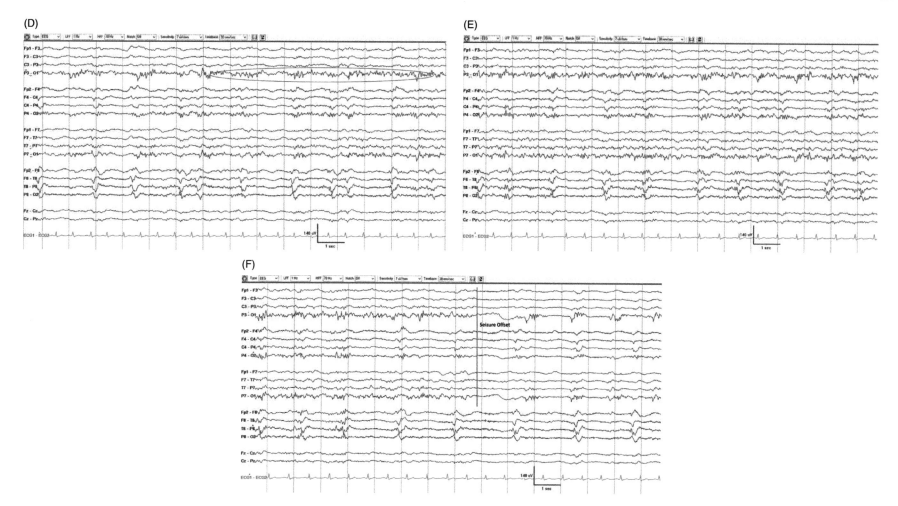

Figure 9.37. (*Continued*) (D) EEG at D: onset of a left hemispheric ESz, O1 maximal (also seen at O2). The seizure begins with the periodic BIRDs in the left posterior quadrant coalescing and evolving (blue ellipse). (E) EEG at E: left occipital-maximal ESz continues. Note the PDs+F continue in the right temporal region. (F) EEG at F: left hemispheric ESz ends (labeled line). EEG returns to baseline pattern of BIPDs+F (sometimes BIRDs as discussed above).

10 Quantitative EEG: special applications and multimodal monitoring

10.1 Delayed ischemia detection

As cerebral blood flow decreases, the EEG changes in the following manner: First, there is subtle loss of faster frequencies (beta and alpha, sometimes including sleep spindles). Then, as flow drops further, slowing appears – first excess theta, then excess delta. All of this occurs while ischemia is at a reversible stage and standard anatomical imaging, including MRI with diffusion weighted imaging, remains normal. As flow continues to decline, there is suppression of all frequencies, which corresponds with irreversible neuronal death (infarction) (these changes are summarized in Figure 10.1). Thus, EEG can detect ischemia when standard imaging cannot, although perfusion imaging can also detect this. This ability of EEG to detect ischemia early with a procedure that can be done continuously is the basis for continuous EEG monitoring in patients at high risk for ischemia such as those with subarachnoid hemorrhage. Several quantitative measures can be used, which all rely on the same principle: with the development of ischemia there is loss of the more physiologic faster frequencies (activity > ~6 Hz), and a greater degree of slowing (mostly activity <6 Hz).

10.2 Quantitative thresholds and alarms

Having multiple objective quantified trends to follow allows for the setting of thresholds and alarms to those thresholds. Alarms can alert clinicians to the earliest undesirable change so that reactive changes in therapy can be made as earliest as possible. For example, if a patient was in refractory status epilepticus and the goal was to maintain a certain level of sedation, then an alarm could be set if the power increased above a certain threshold (absolute value or relative to a defined baseline), or if the suppression percent dropped below a certain value. Seizure alarms can also be set. These often have a significant false positive rate; however, if a patient has a reliably detectable seizure pattern with little other activity, then an alarm can alert the clinician to the earliest seizure recurrence. Alarms can also be used to detect changes in cerebral function, such as delayed ischemia after subarachnoid hemorrhage (SAH). For example, an alarm can be set if the alpha/delta ratio falls below a certain value, prompting clinician review of the patient and EEG. Many variants of the fast:slow ratio can be used, and these are sensitive and fairly specific measures of ischemia. Other changes that suggest ischemia are decreases in EEG

Hirsch and Brenner's Atlas of EEG in Critical Care, Second Edition. Lawrence J. Hirsch, Michael W.K. Fong, and Richard P. Brenner.
© 2023 John Wiley & Sons Ltd. Published 2023 by John Wiley & Sons Ltd.

variability, including in the variability of relative alpha (alpha power/total power), and increase in epileptiform activity.

10.3 Multimodal monitoring, including intracranial EEG

With further advances in technology, multimodal monitoring has become more widely available and even a standard of care in many neurological/neurosurgical ICUs. Multimodal systems allow the integrated recording of invasive and non-invasive physiological parameters. Non-invasive measures such as heart rate, oxygen saturation, blood pressure and surface EEG can be recorded synchronously with arterial pressure, intracranial pressure, CSF measurements including lactate and neuron specific enolase, and intracranial EEG strip or depth electrode recordings. Transcranial Dopplers and near-infrared spectroscopy can be included as well. Other invasive monitoring techniques include use of intracerebral microdialysis (sample of the interstitial fluid to measure lactate, pyruvate, glucose, glutamate, glycerol, etc.), brain tissue oxygen levels, focal cerebral blood flow, brain temperature, pH and more. Such multimodal monitoring has allowed advances in our understanding of epileptiform patterns, and most importantly how these epileptiform patterns affect brain and systemic physiology.

Intracranial EEG recordings in the ICU can be obtained via subdural strips (usually placed in the operating room if neurosurgery is being performed) or intraparenchymal 'depth' electrodes, which can be placed bedside (or in the operating room); both types can be removed bedside and have been reported to add little if any morbidity to patients already getting other invasive brain monitoring. These electrodes can detect seizure activity that is otherwise not visible on the scalp, can provide artifact-free recordings for real-time monitoring and setting highly specific alarms, can help clarify equivocal patterns seen on the scalp EEG, and can detect peri-injury depolarization (PIDs). PIDs are related to cortical spreading depression and seem to be very common in acute brain injury, including ischemia, trauma and hemorrhages. Similar to seizures, they seem to contribute to secondary neuronal injury and are potentially treatable or preventable.

Figure list

Ischemia detection and setting of alarms

Figure 10.1 Cerebral ischemia.

Figure 10.2 Ischemia detection: multimodality monitoring for delayed cerebral ischemia after subarachnoid hemorrhage (SAH); alpha-delta ratio.

Figure 10.3 Ischemia detection: multimodality monitoring for delayed cerebral ischemia after SAH; ADR, and alpha variability.

Figure 10.4 Ischemia detection: multimodality monitoring for delayed cerebral ischemia after SAH, using depth electrode and alarms.

Figure 10.5 Setting of alarms: multimodality monitoring; pentobarbital coma, suppression-burst, depth electrode and QEEG alarms.

Figure 10.6 Setting of alarms: hydrocephalus and multiple QEEG alarms.

Figure 10.7. Setting of alarms: envelope (amplitude) trend analysis for neonatal seizure recognition.

Figure 10.8 Setting of alarms: envelope (amplitude) trend analysis for multiple seizures in an adult.

Figure 10.9. Ischemia detection: Brain Symmetry Index during carotid clamping.

Figure 10.10 Ischemia detection and setting of alarms: Brain Symmetry Index (BSI), seizures and alarm sent to a mobile device.

Multimodality monitoring

Figure 10.11. Multimodality monitoring: electrocorticogram (ECoG) of peri-injury depolarizations and cortical spreading depression (CSD).

Figure 10.12 Multimodality monitoring: electrocorticogram (ECoG) of peri-injury depolarizations (PIDs).

Figure 10.13 Multimodality monitoring of hemorrhagic transformation of a large infarct, including with ICP, brain tissue oxygen tension, cerebral microdialysis and depth electrode.

Figure 10.14 Multimodality monitoring of seizures on intracranial EEG after meperidine bolus, including ICP, cerebral microdialysis and depth electrode.

Figure 10.15 Multimodality monitoring of traumatic brain injury (TBI), including ICP, brain tissue oxygen tension, cerebral microdialysis and depth electrode.

Figure 10.16. Multimodal monitoring of traumatic brain injury (TBI), including ICP, brain tissue oxygen tension, cerebral microdialysis and depth electrode.

Figure 10.17 Multimodality monitoring: ictal-appearing SIRPIDs on intracranial EEG only.

Figure 10.18. Multimodality monitoring: Cyclic seizures on intracranial EEG only.

Figure 10.19 Multimodality monitoring: TBI, seizures and periodic discharges on intracranial EEG only, QEEG applied to intracranial EEG.

EEGs throughout this atlas have been shown with the following standard recording filters unless otherwise specified: LFF 1 Hz, HFF 70 Hz, notch filter off.

Suggested reading

Baang HY, Chen HY, Herman AL, et al. The utility of quantitative EEG in detecting delayed cerebral ischemia after aneurysmal subarachnoid hemorrhage. *J Clin Neurophysiol.* 2021.

Claassen J, Hirsch LJ, Frontera JA, Fernandez A, Schmidt M, Kapinos G, Wittman J, Connolly ES, Emerson RG, Mayer SA. Prognostic significance of continuous EEG monitoring in patients with poor grade subarachnoid hemorrhage. *Neurocrit Care* 2006;**4**(2):103–112.

Claassen J, Hirsch LJ, Kreiter KT, et al. Quantitative continuous EEG for detecting delayed cerebral ischemia in patients with poor-grade subarachnoid hemorrhage. *Clin Neurophysiol.* 2004;**115**(12):2699–2710.

Claassen J, Hirsch LJ, Kreiter K, Du YE, Connolly ES, Emerson RG, Mayer SA. Quantitative continuous EEG for detecting delayed cerebral ischemia in subarachnoid hemorrhage. *Clin Neurophysiol* 2004;**115**:2699–2710.

Claassen J, Perotte A, Albers D, et al. Nonconvulsive seizures after subarachnoid hemorrhage: multimodal detection and outcomes. *Ann Neurol.* 2013;**74**(1):53–64.

de Vos CC, van Maarseveen SM, Brouwers PJ, van Putten MJ. Continuous EEG monitoring during thrombolysis in acute hemispheric stroke patients using the brain symmetry index. *J Clin Neurophysiol.* 2008 Apr;**25**(2):77–82.

Dohmen C, Sakowitz OW, Fabricius M, Bosche B, Reithmeier T, Ernestus RI, Brinker G, Dreier JP, Woitzik J, Strong AJ, Graf R; Co-Operative Study of Brain Injury Depolarisations (COSBID). Spreading depolarizations occur in human ischemic stroke with high incidence. *Ann Neurol.* 2008 Jun;**63**(6):720–728.

Dreier JP, Woitzik J, Fabricius M, Bhatia R, Major S, Drenckhahn C, Lehmann TN, Sarrafzadeh A, Willumsen L, Hartings JA, Sakowitz OW, Seemann JH, Thieme A, Lauritzen M, Strong AJ. Delayed ischaemic neurological deficits after subarachnoid haemorrhage are associated with clusters of spreading depolarizations. *Brain.* 2006 Dec;**129**(Pt 12):3224–3237.

Fabricius M, Fuhr S, Bhatia R, Boutelle M, Hashemi P, Strong AJ, Lauritzen M. Cortical spreading depression and peri-infarct depolarization in acutely injured human cerebral cortex. *Brain.* 2006 Mar;**129**(Pt 3):778–790.

Fabricius M, Fuhr S, Willumsen L, Dreier JP, Bhatia R, Boutelle MG, Hartings JA, Bullock R, Strong AJ, Lauritzen M. Association of seizures with cortical spreading depression and peri-infarct depolarisations in the acutely injured human brain. *Clin Neurophysiol.* 2008 Sep;**119**(9):1973–1984.

Foreman B, Claassen J. Quantitative EEG for the detection of brain ischemia. *Crit Care.* 2012;**16**(2):216

Foreman B, Albers D, Schmidt JM, et al. Intracortical electrophysiological correlates of blood flow after severe SAH: A multimodality monitoring study. *J Cereb Blood Flow Metab.* 2018;**38**(3):506–517.

Hartings JA, Andaluz N, Bullock MR, et al. Prognostic value of spreading depolarizations in patients with severe traumatic brain injury. *JAMA Neurol.* 2020;**77**(4):489–499.

Kim JA, Zheng WL, Elmer J, et al. High epileptiform discharge burden predicts delayed cerebral ischemia after subarachnoid hemorrhage. *Clin Neurophysiol.* 2021.

Kramer AH, Kromm J. Quantitative continuous EEG: Bridging the gap between the ICU bedside and the EEG interpreter. *Neurocrit Care.* 2019;**30**(3):499–504.

Leão AAP. Spreading depression of activity in the cerebral cortex. *Journal of Neurophysiology.* 1944;**7**(6):359–390.

Mikell CB, Dyster TG, Claassen J. Invasive seizure monitoring in the critically-ill brain injury patient: current practices and a review of the literature. *Seizure.* 2016;**41**:201–205.

Ponten SC, Ronner HE, Strijers RLM, et al. Feasibility of online seizure detection with continuous EEG monitoring in the intensive care unit. *Seizure.* 2010;**19**(9):580–586.

Rathakrishnan R, Gotman J, Dubeau F, Angle M. Using continuous electroencephalography in the management of delayed cerebral ischemia following subarachnoid hemorrhage. *Neurocrit Care.* 2011;**14**(2):152–161.

Rosenthal ES, Biswal S, Zafar SF, et al. Continuous electroencephalography predicts delayed cerebral ischemia after subarachnoid hemorrhage: A prospective study of diagnostic accuracy. *Ann Neurol.* 2018;**83**(5):958–969.

Rots ML, van Putten MJ, Hoedemaekers CW, Horn J. Continuous EEG monitoring for early detection of delayed cerebral ischemia in subarachnoid hemorrhage: a pilot study. *Neurocrit Care.* 2016;**24**(2):207–216.

Sheikh ZB, Maciel CB, Dhakar MB, Hirsch LJ, Gilmore EJ. Nonepileptic electroencephalographic correlates of episodic increases in intracranial pressure. *J Clin Neurophysiol.* 2020.

Strong AJ, Anderson PJ, Watts HR, Virley DJ, Lloyd A, Irving EA, Nagafuji T, Ninomiya M, Nakamura H, Dunn AK, Graf R. Peri-infarct depolarizations lead to loss of perfusion in ischaemic gyrencephalic cerebral cortex. *Brain.* 2007 Apr;**130**(Pt 4):995–1008.

Tu B, Assassi NJ, Bazil CW, Hamberger MJ, Hirsch LJ. Quantitative EEG is an objective, sensitive, and reliable indicator of transient anesthetic effects during Wada tests. *J Clin Neurophysiol.* 2015;**32**(2):152–158.

van Putten MJ. The revised brain symmetry index. *Clin Neurophysiol.* 2007 Nov;**118**(11):2362–2367. Epub 2007 Sep 20.

van Putten MJ. Extended BSI for continuous EEG monitoring in carotid endarterectomy. *Clin Neurophysiol.* 2006 Dec;**117**(12):2661–2666.

van Putten MJ, Tavy DL. Continuous quantitative EEG monitoring in hemispheric stroke patients using the brain symmetry index. *Stroke.* 2004 Nov;**35**(11):2489–2492.

Vespa P, Tubi M, Claassen J, et al. Metabolic crisis occurs with seizures and periodic discharges after brain trauma. *Ann Neurol.* 2016;**79**(4):579–590.

Vespa PM, Nuwer MR, Juhász C, Alexander M, Nenov V, Martin N, Becker DP. Early detection of vasospasm after acute subarachnoid hemorrhage using continuous EEG ICU monitoring. *Electroencephalogr Clin Neurophysiol.* 1997 Dec;**103**(6):607–615.

Vespa PM, Nuwer MR, Nenov V, et al: Increased incidence and impact of nonconvulsive and convulsive seizures after traumatic brain injury as detected by continuous electroencephalographic monitoring. *J Neurosurg.* 1999;**91**(5):750–760.

Waziri A, Claassen J, Stuart RM, et al. Intracortical electroencephalography in acute brain injury. *Ann Neurol.* 2009;**66**(3):366–377.

Witsch J, Frey HP, Schmidt JM, et al. Electroencephalographic periodic discharges and frequency-dependent brain tissue hypoxia in acute brain injury. *JAMA Neurol.* 2017;**74**(3):301–309.

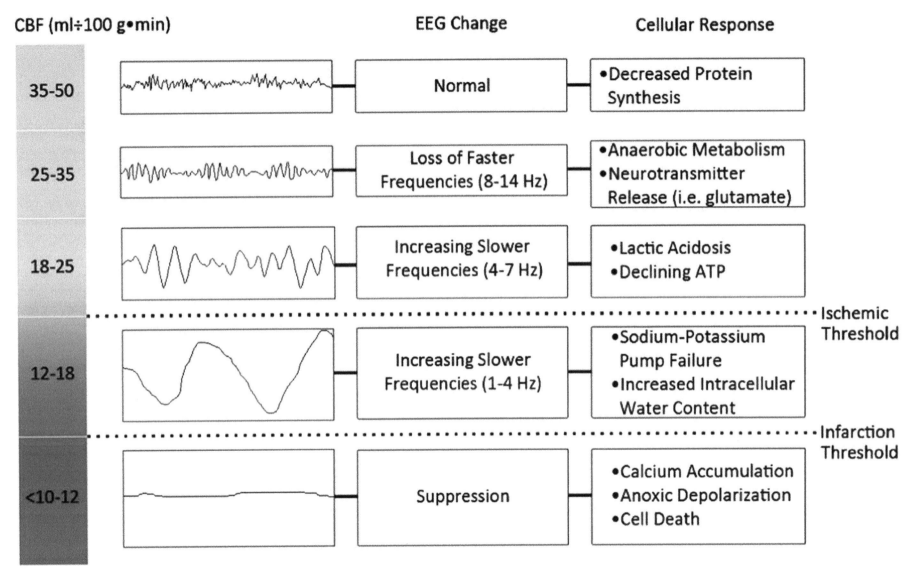

Figure 10.1. Cerebral ischemia. The table outlines the cerebral blood flow (CBF) and the respective estimates of the cellular and molecular changes, and EEG changes (middle column). With falling CBF the brain switches to anaerobic metabolism that results in falling cerebral glucose and increasing lactate. These changes can be detected with regular intracerebral sampling (as seen in Figures 10.13–10.16). The EEG changes are well described, with progressive loss of more 'physiologic' rhythms (alpha and beta), with gradual increase in theta and delta activity. These changes occur while there is still 'reversibility', and therefore the goal of ischemia detection is to use these changes to prompt an intervention to prevent non-reversible ischemia/infarction. ATP, adenosine triphosphate.

Reproduced from Foreman B, Claassen J. Quantitative EEG for the detection of brain ischemia. Crit Care. 2012;16(2):216, with permission.

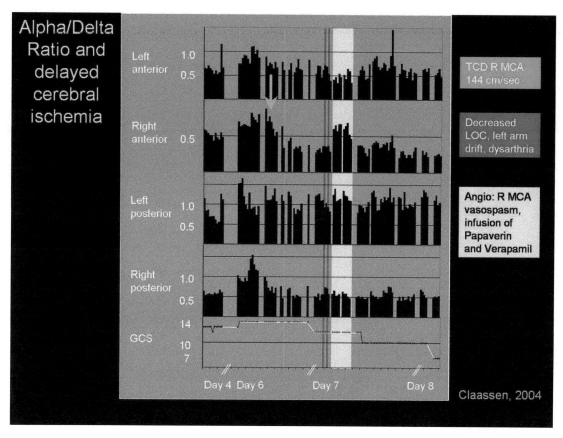

Figure 10.2. Ischemia detection: multimodal monitoring for delayed cerebral ischemia after subarachnoid hemorrhage (SAH); alpha-delta ratio.

Figure 10.2main: This 57-year-old woman was admitted for an acute subarachnoid hemorrhage (admission Hunt and Hess grade 4) from a right posterior communicating aneurysm. The aneurysm was clipped on SAH day 2. No infarcts were seen on postoperative CT, day 2 (shown, Figure 10.2A). Postoperatively she had a Glasgow Coma Score (GCS) of 14. CEEG monitoring was performed from SAH days 3 to 8 to monitor for seizures and delayed cerebral ischemia. The figure shows the Alpha/delta ratio (ADR) calculated every 15 minutes and the Glasgow Coma Score (GCS), shown for days 6–8 of continuous EEG (cEEG) monitoring. The alpha/delta ratio progressively decreased after day 6, particularly in the right anterior region (green arrow), to settle into a steady trough level later that night, reflecting loss of fast frequencies and increased slowing over the right hemisphere in the raw EEG (also shown, Figure 10.2B). On SAH day 6, right middle cerebral artery (MCA) blood flow velocity (measured using transcranial doppler) was marginally elevated (144 cm/s), but the patient remained clinically stable with hypertensive-hypervolemic therapy (systolic blood pressure >180 mmHg). On day 7, the GCS dropped from 14 to 12 and a CT scan showed a right internal capsule and hypothalamic infarction (see day 7 CT). Angiography demonstrated severe distal right MCA and left vertebral artery spasm; however, due to the marked tortuosity of the parent vessels and the location of vasospasm, a decision was made not to perform angioplasty, but to infuse verapamil and papaverine. This resulted in a marked, but transient increase of the right anterior and posterior alpha/delta ratios (yellow shaded area). Later that day the patient further deteriorated clinically to a GCS of 7, with a new onset left hemiparesis, and ultimately died on SAH day 9 from widespread infarction due to vasospasm (see day 8 CT).

Reproduced from Claassen J, Hirsch LJ, Kreiter K, Du YE, Connolly ES, Emerson RG, Mayer SA. Quantitative continuous EEG for detecting delayed cerebral ischemia in subarachnoid hemorrhage. Clin Neurophysiol 2004;115:2699–2710, with permission.

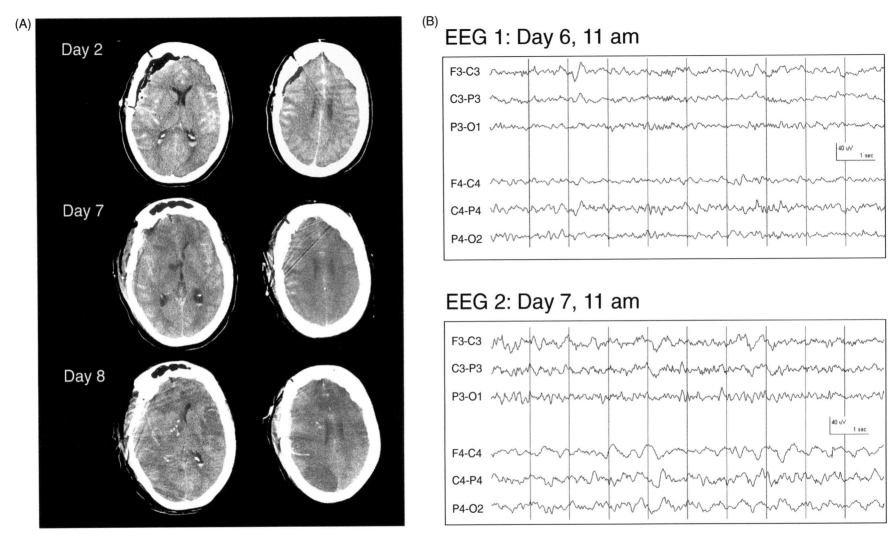

Figure 10.2. (*Continued*) (A) CT scans. CT scans obtained on SAH days 2, 7 and 8. (B) EEG samples. Sample of raw EEG prior (SAH day 6) and during (SAH day 7) change in the alpha/delta ratio. There is an increase in delta and decrease in faster activity, more pronounced on the right (bottom 3 channels) in EEG 2 compared to EEG 1.

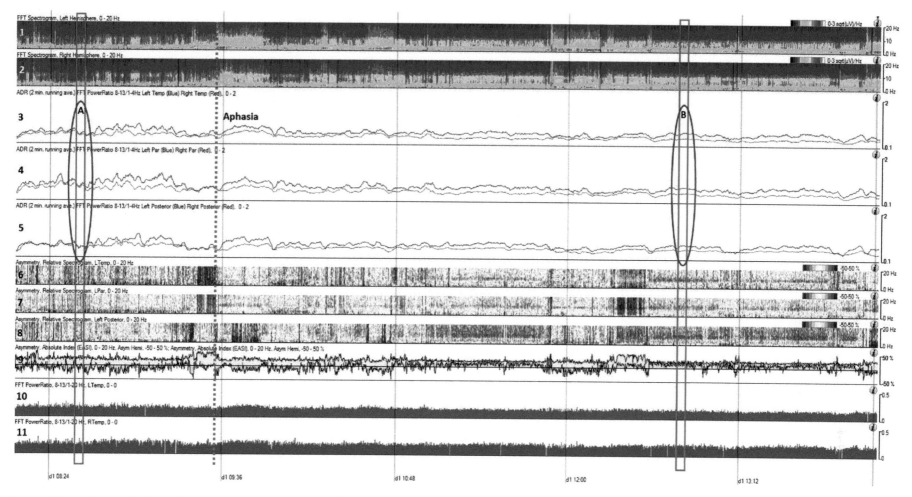

Figure 10.3. Ischemia detection: multimodal monitoring for delayed cerebral ischemia after SAH; ADR, and alpha variability.

Figure 10.3main1 This 6 hours of QEEG is from a 48-year-old woman s/p SAH (Hunt and Hess grade II), due to a left distal ICA/proximal MCA aneurysm. Day 0 angiogram (Figure 10.3C) confirmed the aneurysm and mild left ICA vasospasm (purple ellipse on angiogram, Figure 10.3C). The aneurysm was coiled, and the vasospasm successfully treated with 10mg of intra-arterial verapamil. The patient had no deficit after coiling. CEEG was commenced for monitoring of seizures and repeated vasospasm/DCI. The EEG at the beginning of the record is near normal (Figure 10.3A). At point A the activity between the hemispheres is relatively similar. The ADRs are symmetric in all vascular territories (temporal/

MCA [row 3], parasagittal/ACA [row 4], posterior/PCA [row 5]) (blue ellipse at A). The asymmetry spectrogram suggests slightly greater power on the left; however, the REASI (row 9) is only marginally down-going (i.e., the degree to which activity favors the left is small). In the first hour, there is also reasonable variability in both the ADR tracing and in relative alpha (RAV) (relative alpha tracing for the temporal regions shown in the bottom 2 rows). RAV can be another measure of ischemia. The total alpha (8–13 Hz) is placed as a fraction over the total amount of activity (1–20 Hz). The alpha variability of a normal record is said to represent a bustling city skyline. Loss of this variability to a flat plateau is suggestive of ischemia.

(A)

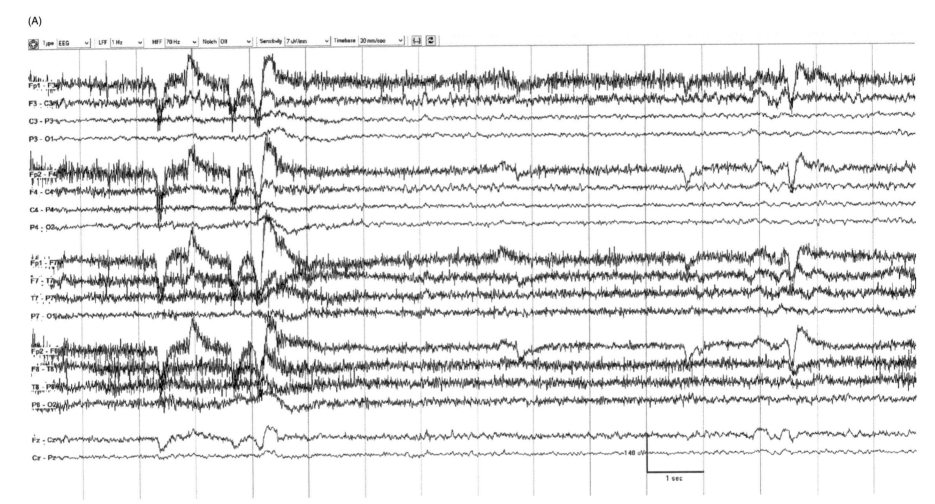

Figure 10.3. (*Continued*) Shortly after A, there develops consistent separation of the ADR tracings, higher on the right throughout, a sign of significant asymmetry, worrisome for ischemia on the left. Variability was maintained until about 09:30, just before clinical symptoms were noted. The patient then developed aphasia (dotted red line labeled 'aphasia'). ADRs in this software package are calculated with a 2-minute rolling average. Vasopressor medications were attempted to increase perfusion, but this did not improve the ADRs. At point B the ADRs are still asymmetric, the asymmetry spectrograms have all turned red in higher frequencies (i.e., activity in theta and above ranges has been lost on the left [greater on the right]), and this is confirmed with the REASI that is now upgoing (favoring right hemisphere). Variability remained poor. The asymmetry spectrograms also show increased slowing (delta, blue) in the left MCA and ACA territories for the final >1 h of this page. This switch of color around 5–6 Hz is classic for ischemia (attenuation of frequencies faster than that, but more slowing on the ischemic side). The patient was taken back to angiogram, which confirmed a recurrence of vasospasm (Figure 10.3D).

(A) EEG at A: appearing almost normal in the awake state.

(B)

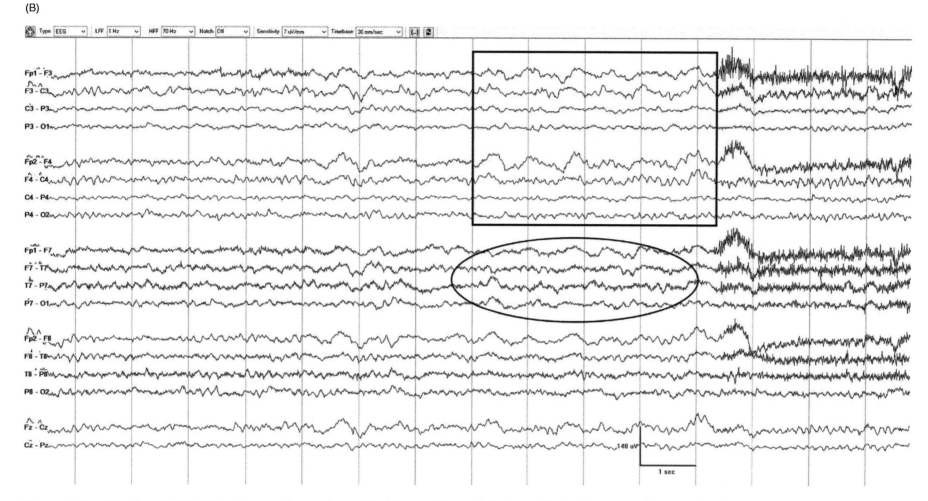

Figure 10.3. (*Continued*) (B) EEG at B: more drowsy, but still with reactivity to eye opening in the last few seconds of the page. There is greater delta activity in the left temporal region (ellipse), and the bifrontal slowing favors the left (especially F3-C3 compared to F4-C4) with loss of the more physiologic 7 Hz activity on the left (box).

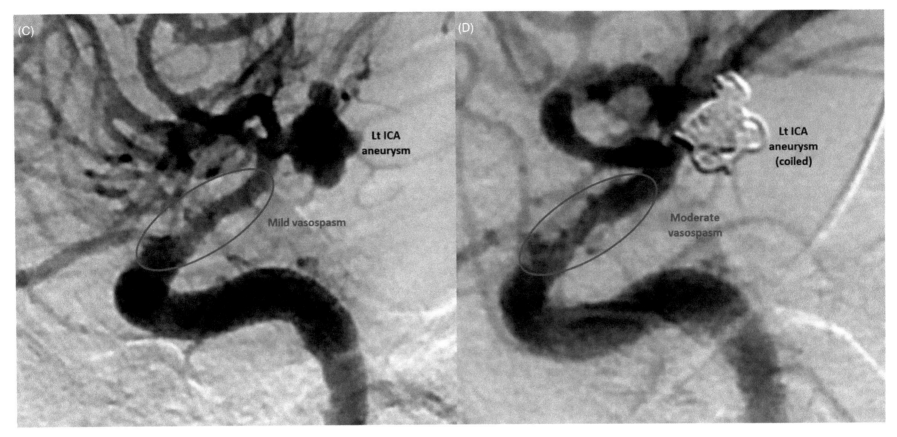

Figure 10.3. (*Continued*) (C) Angiogram on presentation with a left terminal ICA aneurysm and mild vasospasm (blue ellipse). (D) Angiogram at time of developing aphasia with persistent reduction in left hemispheric ADRs. The left ICA aneurysm has been coiled in the interim, and there is worsening of left ICA vasospasm. This was treated with angioplasty and 20mg total of intra-arterial verapamil. Aphasia gradually resolved and the ADRs normalized.

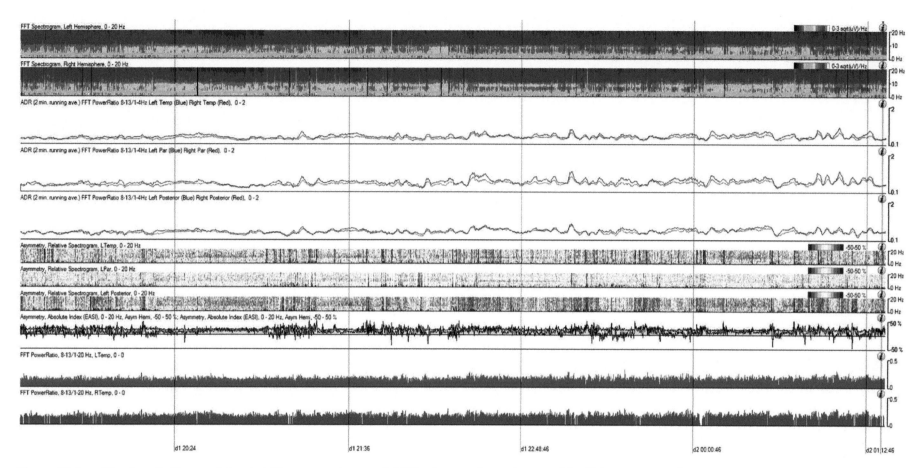

Figure 10.3. (*Continued*) Figure 10.3main2 The next 6 hours of QEEG after the second angiogram (i.e., after angioplasty and additional 20mg total of intra-arterial verapamil). The next 6 hours show the QEEG is stable and actually improves by the end of the window. Compared to the beginning (where the patient would still have some sedative medication in effect) the ADRs are greater at the end of the page (and remain largely symmetric/overlapping for the entire parge), and there is even greater variability of both the ADR tracings and the relative alpha tracings at the bottom.

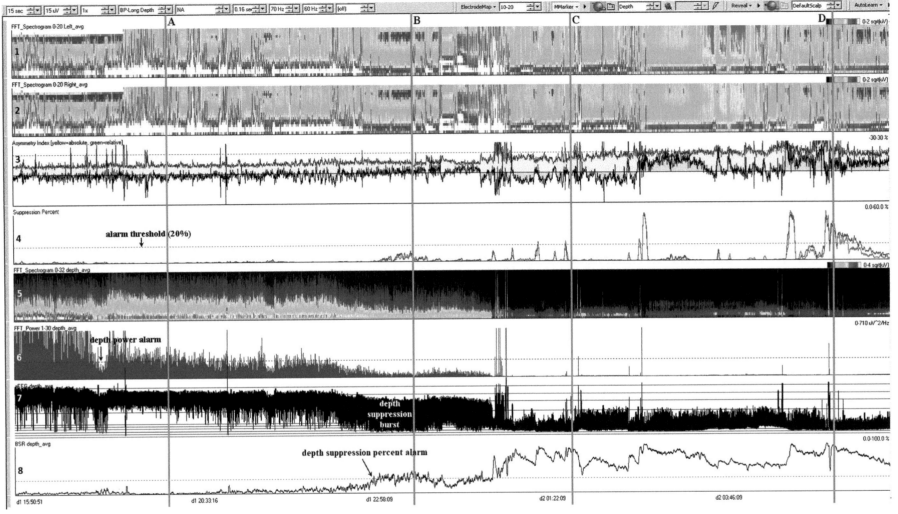

Figure 10.4. Ischemia detection: multimodal monitoring for delayed cerebral ischemia after SAH, using depth electrode and alarms.

Figure 10.4main Sixteen hours of QEEG in a 70-year-old woman s/p Hunt and Hess grade 3–4 subarachnoid hemorrhage. The patient developed sepsis, bilateral vasospasm and bilateral infarcts during this time period. The top 4 rows (rows 1–4) are based on the standard scalp EEG, whereas the bottom four (rows 5–8) are based on intracranial EEG recorded from a miniature, 8 contact, cortical mini-depth electrode placed in the right frontal lobe (see scout X-rays, parts E and F); this is also referred to as intracortical EEG, or ICE. Alarm thresholds can be seen as dotted red lines, set on the scalp asymmetry index (row 3), the scalp suppression percent (row 4), depth total power (1–30 Hz) (row 6), depth average amplitude using the aEEG tracing (red line not shown) (row 7), and depth suppression percent (row 8). On the scalp QEEG tracings, it is difficult to appreciate major changes until the 2nd half of this time period, when asymmetry increases and the suppression percent eventually rises, at least intermittently. On the depth QEEG tracings, the changes can be seen much earlier and more clearly, and a long gradual dramatic trend can be seen in the first third of this sample. The bottom 3 rows all triggered alarms, beginning with a drop in total power in the depth (labeled 'depth power alarm'), then a drop in average amplitude (not shown), then a rise in the suppression percent (labeled 'depth suppression percent alarm'). Also note the thick band that developed in the depth amplitude-integrated EEG row (labeled in 2nd row from bottom) corresponding to intracranial suppression-burst (both high and low amplitudes in every page or epoch). By the 2nd half of this time period, the depth EEG pattern appears to be nearly flat, with low power in all frequencies, low amplitudes and high suppression percents. The patient went on to develop bilateral anterior cerebral artery and left middle cerebral artery infarcts with rising intracranial pressure by the end of this time period. She died 2–3 days later.

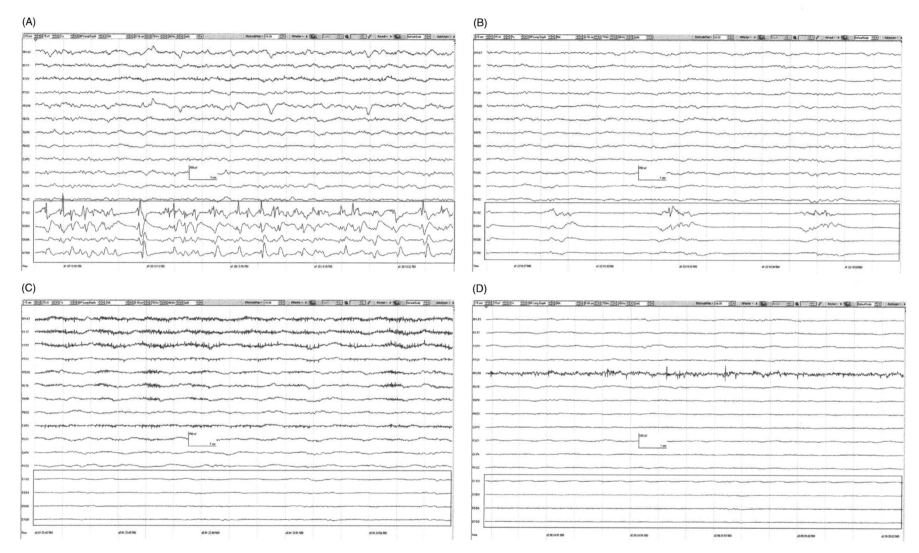

Figure 10.4. *(Continued)* (A) EEG at A: diffuse slowing on the scalp EEG, but continuous highly epileptiform activity in the depth EEG (bottom 4 channels, in box). This is not an unusual occurrence, with seizure-like activity on the depth recording only. (B) EEG at B: diffuse slowing and attenuation on the scalp, and suppression-burst in the depth EEG (bottom 4 channels, in box). (C) EEG at C: depth EEG recording (box) is now flat, with the scalp EEG showing some muscle artifact and diffuse attenuation. The scalp recording is not quite low enough to qualify as suppressed in the scalp suppression percent calculation, possibly due to the muscle artifact. (D) EEG at D: scalp and depth recordings are now flat. The suppression percent on the scalp (as well as the depth) is now above 50%.

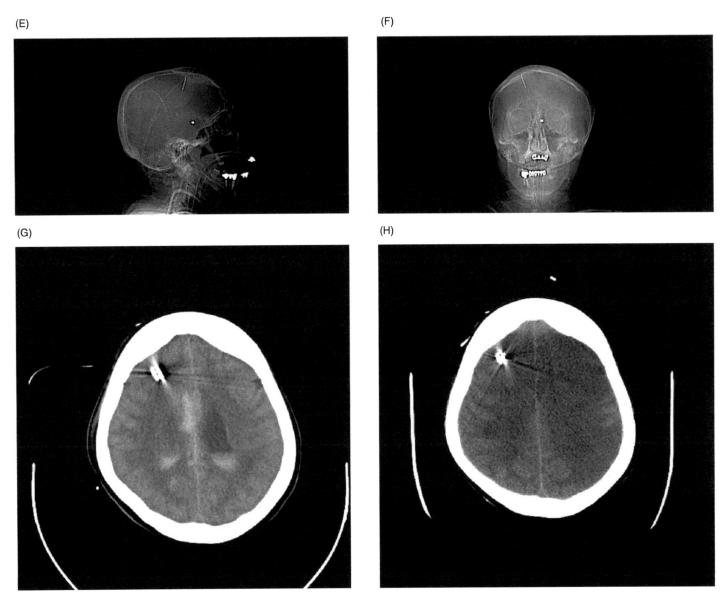

Figure 10.4. (*Continued*) (E) and (F) Skull X-ray (scout views during the CT scan), showing the 8-contact mini-depth electrode in the right frontal lobe; there is a ventricular catheter right next to it (placed via same burrhole). (G) CT scan before the vasospasm and infarcts. The artifact in the right frontal lobe is from the ventricular catheter and the depth electrode combined. Bilateral intraventricular blood can be seen. (H) CT scan after the vasospasm and infarcts, showing bilateral infarcts, worse on the left.

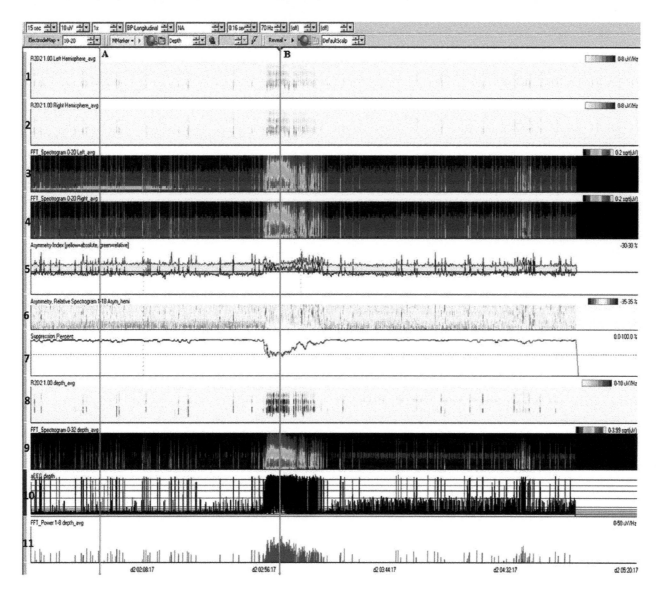

Figure 10.5. Setting of alarms. Multimodal monitoring; pentobarbital coma, suppression-burst, depth electrode and QEEG alarms

Figure 10.5main Four hours of QEEG in a 27-year-old woman with encephalitis. The patient was being treated with pentobarbital for refractory status epilepticus, with a goal of near-complete suppression because frequent seizures continued to arise from any lower degree of suppression. Note the suppression percent (the percent of the record that is 'flat', or below 5 μV in this setup; 7th row) was around 100 percent for most of the record. It then dropped down to just under 50 percent (B), crossing the alarm threshold set at the bedside (dotted red line on the suppression percent row) and resulting in an increase in pentobarbital. Alarms can be set on almost any QEEG parameter, and can result in bedside alarming and/or multiple forms of remote notification. The bottom 4 rows in this case show QEEG calculations on a single miniature 8 contact depth electrode traversing the cortex that is placed at the time of placement of other invasive monitoring devices. EEG from these intracranial electrodes has much improved signal to noise ratio, allowing much more reliable setting of QEEG alarms for detection of brain events, including seizures and ischemia. Note the very thick aEEG tracing on the depth electrode at point B (2nd to last row), signifying burst suppression with high amplitude bursts.

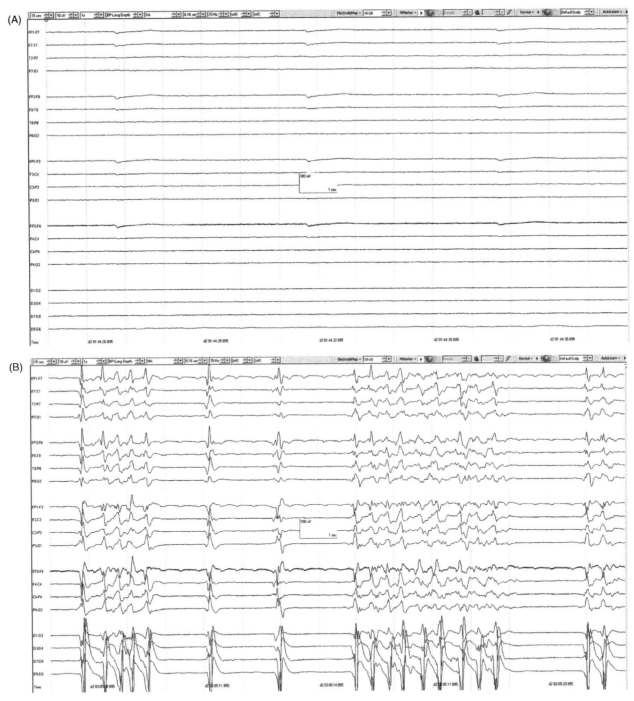

Figure 10.5. (*Continued*) (A) EEG at A: complete suppression, including on the depth electrode (bottom 4 channels). (B) EEG at B: suppression-burst, with about 40% of the record suppressed, and the rest containing medium to high amplitude epileptiform discharges. This is the pattern that led to alarming of the suppression percent (became too low), though it could also have been due to increased total power, mean amplitude or rhythmicity on the depth channels (bottom 4 channels). Alarms on any of these could have been sensitive and specific for this change.

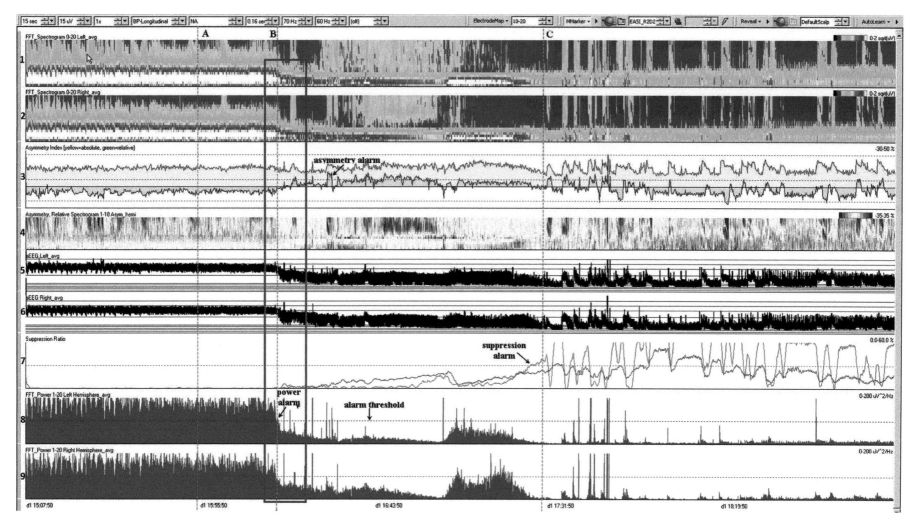

Figure 10.6. Setting of alarms. Hydrocephalus and multiple QEEG alarms.
Figure 10.6main1 Four hours of EEG in a 61-year-old woman with hepatic encephalopathy, cryptococcal meningitis, and a lumbar drain to help manage raised intracranial pressure (ICP). The drain stopped functioning and ICP went up (purple box). Total power (bottom 2 rows) rapidly dropped, and dropped below the alarm threshold (dashed red line) resulting in an alert (labeled 'power alarm'). Shortly after, the asymmetry alarm threshold is crossed (labeled 'asymmetry alarm'), followed by the suppression alarm about an hour later (suppression percent above 25% in this example). The case demonstrates that alarms can be set for a number of trends, and the threshold for each alarm (dashed red lines in each respective trend) can be tailored for a given patient. Alarms can also be set on the aEEG tracing using the average amplitude (not shown). In this case, the EEG change was rapidly noted, and led to discovery of the non-functioning lumbar drain.

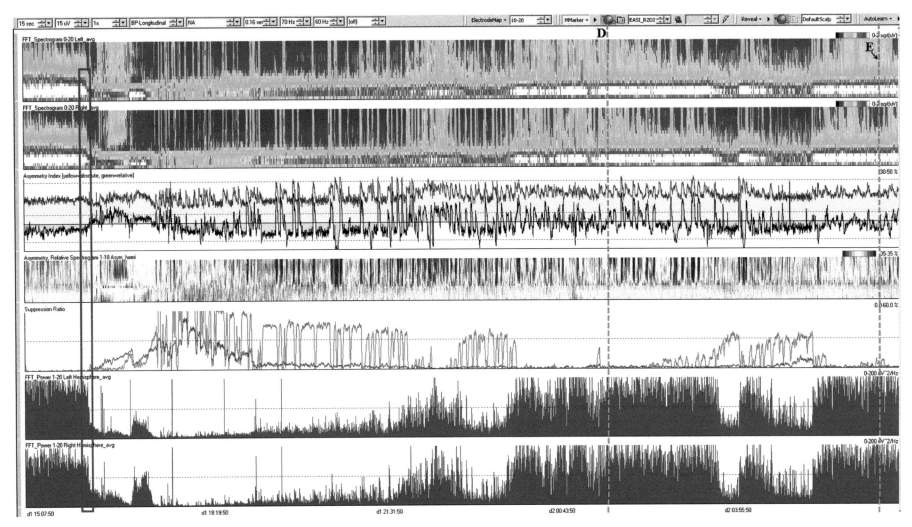

Figure 10.6.   (*Continued*) Figure 10.6main2. Sixteen-hour view in the same patient starting at the same time. The acute changes can be seen in the first few hours. By the second half of this 16-hour period, EEG has begun to recover after the lumbar drain was fixed and ICP came back down.

(A)

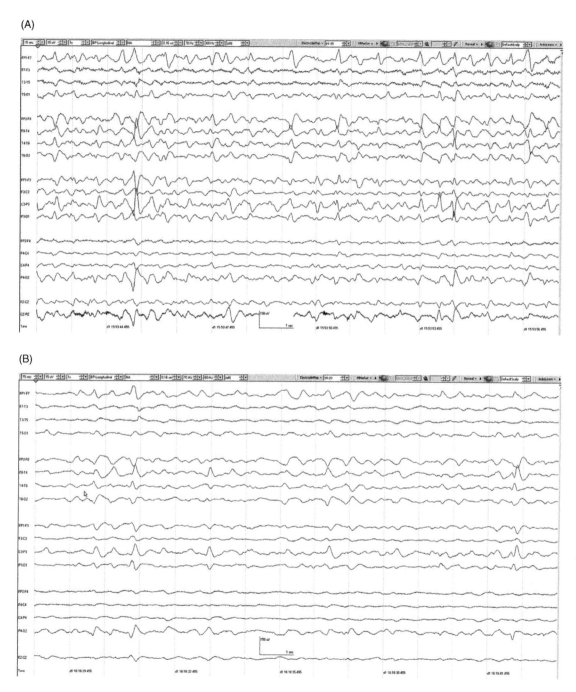

(B)

Figure 10.6. (*Continued*) (A) EEG at A: baseline abnormal EEG. (B) EEG at B: diffuse attenuation compared to baseline as ICP rises.

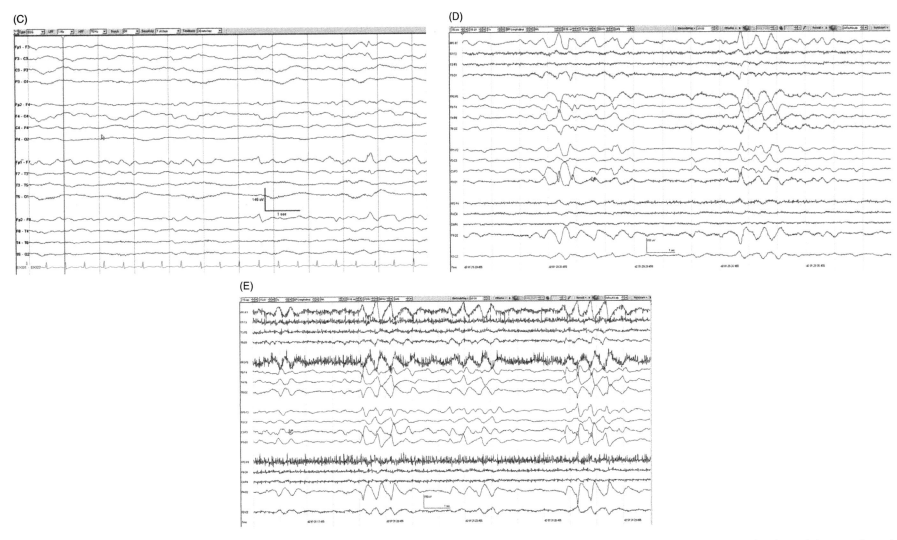

Figure 10.6. (*Continued*) (C) EEG at C: more attenuated (and now unreactive, not shown). (D) EEG at D: early recovery of EEG; now reactive (reactivity not shown). (E) EEG at E: further recovery of EEG (almost back to baseline).

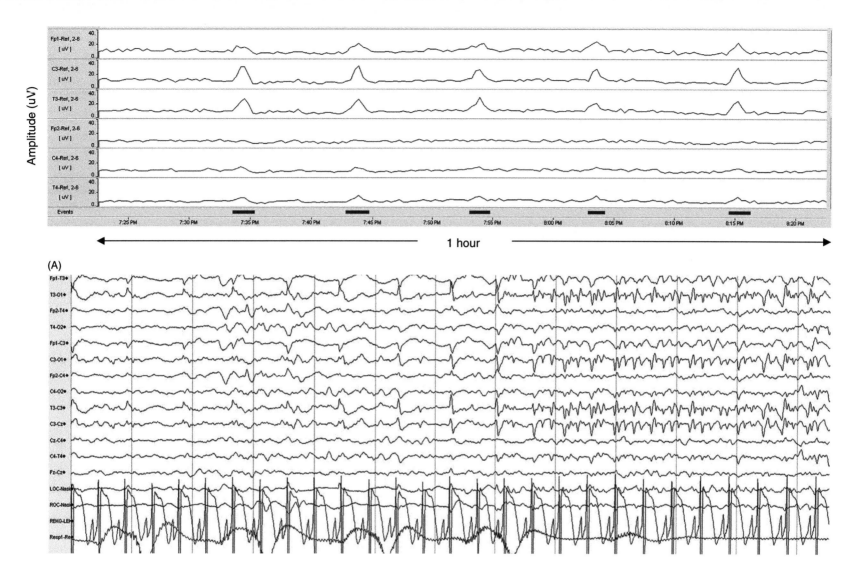

Figure 10.7. Setting of alarms. Envelope (amplitude) trend analysis for neonatal seizure recognition.

Figure 10.7main One-hour envelope trend tracing in a term neonate with discrete recurrent seizures secondary to hypoxic ischemic encephalopathy. Envelope trending selects waveforms within a specified frequency range (e.g. 2–6 Hz as in this example) and plots the median amplitude of waveforms within this frequency range over a specified period of time (usually 10–20 s). The vertical axis is in microvolts, and the horizontal axis is time. Display of 2–4 hours per screen is usually optimal for seizure detection with envelope trend. In neonates with acute encephalopathy, the background is often slow or discontinuous and suppressed. Seizures contain a rhythmic series of waves, often in the 2–6 Hz range, and thus result in an increase in the median amplitude within that range, which is displayed as an upward deflection. Plotting the median amplitude rather than the mean amplitude reduces false detections from brief artifacts such as movement or electrode artifact, making it more suitable for alarms. In this example, the flatter periods contain delta activity that is excessively discontinuous. The large upward deflections in the left hemisphere (C3, T3) are seizures, as confirmed on the corresponding raw EEG (which is always necessary). Seizures identified by standard EEG interpretation are marked by the black bars below the envelope trend. (A) EEG showing onset of the first marked seizure using a standard neonatal montage.

Images courtesy of Nicholas Abend, MD and Susan T. Herman, MD, U.S.A.

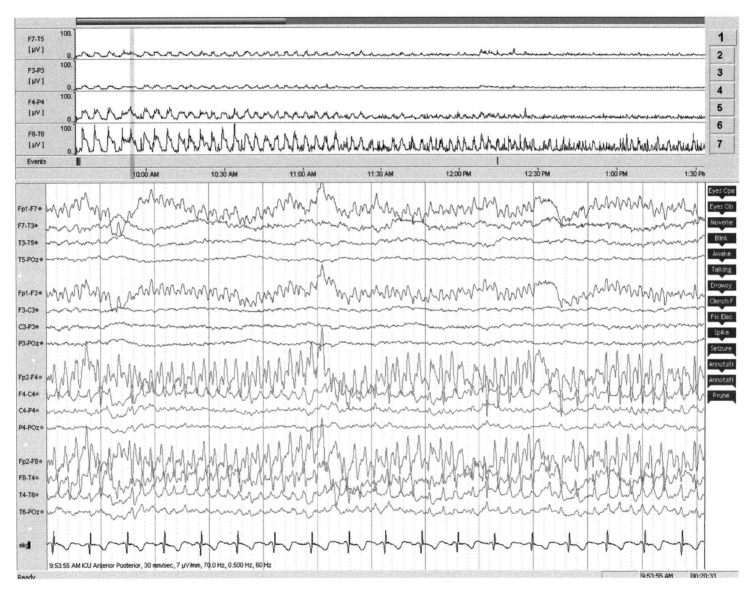

Figure 10.8. Setting of alarms. Envelope (amplitude) trend analysis for multiple seizures in an adult.

Figure 10.8main1: This QEEG is from a 61-year-old woman s/p right frontal meningioma resection and prolonged confusion postoperatively. Envelope (amplitude) trend reveals frequent, periodic amplitude peaks on the right, each

corresponding to an electrographic seizure (raw EEG example corresponding to the gray bar is shown below).

Images courtesy of Suzette Laroche, MD, U.S.A.

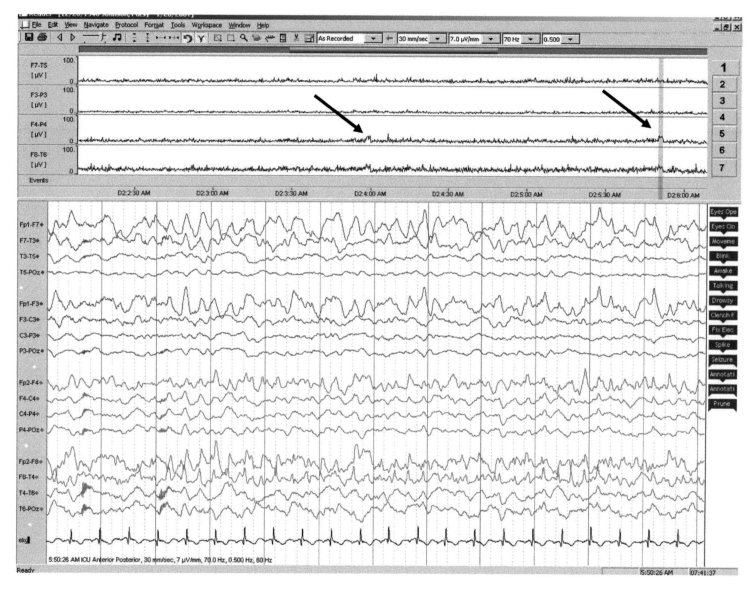

Figure 10.8. (*Continued*) Figure 10.8main2: Same patient 2 days later, after treatment for focal nonconvulsive status epilepticus. Envelope trend reveals two small peaks in amplitude corresponding to more subtle, isolated electrographic seizures, maximal at F8 (example at the gray bar shown). Again, envelope trending (plotting median amplitude) is less prone to false positive detections, compared to aEEG. Prior examples of false positive aEEG detections have been shown in Figures 9.17 and 9.33. Therefore, envelope trending carries a greater specificity, which is a feature that is valuable when setting QEEG alarms, especially if they are alarming at the bedside.

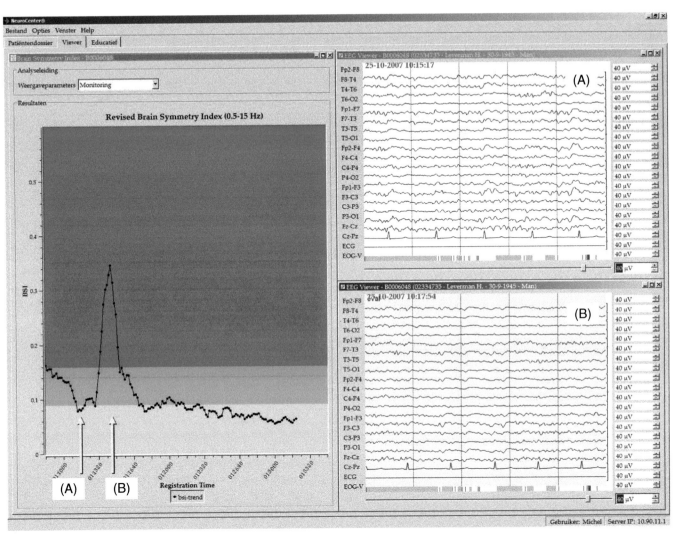

Figure 10.9. Ischemia detection: Brain Symmetry Index during carotid clamping.

The Brain Symmetry Index, or BSI, is a single numerical measure of total asymmetry, essentially summing the absolute values of the differences at each homologous electrode pair for all frequencies (similar to the yellow total absolute asymmetry index in prior images; see Figures 9.16 and 9.17 for initial description). This example shows the rise in asymmetry after clamping of the carotid artery during an endarterectomy. Note the right side attenuation after clamping on the raw EEG (B). The BSI correlates with clinical stroke scales and has been used to follow the evolution of stroke and the effects of tPA administration (see van Putten 2004, 2007; de Vos 2008).

Image courtesy of Michel JAM van Putten, MD, PhD, The Netherlands.

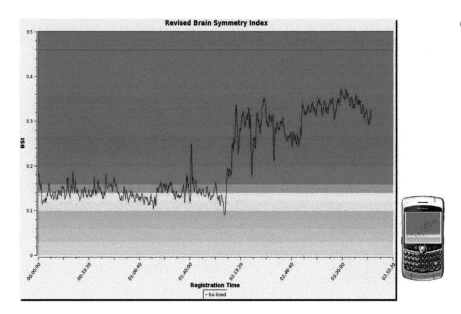

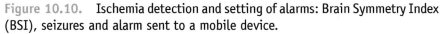

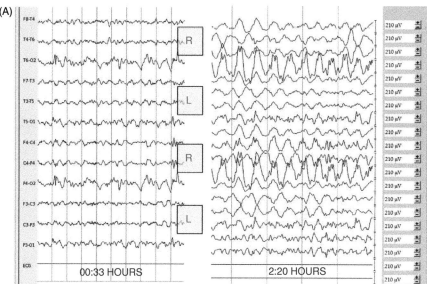

Figure 10.10. Ischemia detection and setting of alarms: Brain Symmetry Index (BSI), seizures and alarm sent to a mobile device.

Figure 10.10main A 4-hour tracing of the BSI in a 3-year-old with right hemisphere seizures. The prominent and sustained rise in BSI (increasing asymmetry) was due to seizure activity on the right. The inset shows the ability to have screenshots sent remotely to a handheld device. (A) EEG before and after the rise in BSI. The 2nd EEG shows ictal activity maximal in the posterior right hemisphere.

Images courtesy of Michel JAM van Putten, MD, PhD, The Netherlands.

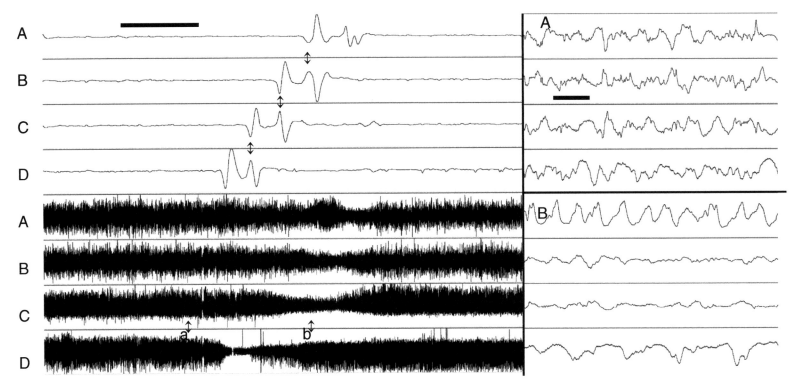

Figure 10.11. Multimodal monitoring: electrocorticogram (ECoG) of peri-injury depolarizations and cortical spreading depression (CSD).

Intracranial recordings have demonstrated that cortical spreading depression and peri-injury depolarizations are very common in patients with acute brain injuries, including trauma, infarct and subarachnoid hemorrhage. Furthermore, there is extensive evidence that they contribute to secondary injury. This example is from a 65-year-old woman, who four days previously suffered a subarachnoid hemorrhage and an intracerebral hematoma due to a ruptured aneurysm of the left middle cerebral artery. After clipping of the aneurysm on the second day, a subdural strip was placed over the left frontal cortex. Four channels of electrocorticography (ECoG) were recorded from five platinum electrodes, 1 cm apart, and connected in a bipolar chain (A–D). The initial 40 hours of recording showed irregular delta activity and intermittent trains of spikes. Over the subsequent 70 hours, 16 episodes of CSD were recorded. The patient died 10 days post ictus due to respiratory failure.

Left panel: 60 min recording, bar: 10 minutes. *Upper four traces:* 0.05 Hz low pass filtered (thus only infraslow activity recorded), full scale 4 mV. *Lower four traces:*

same recording as upper traces, but now 0.5 Hz high pass filtered (closer to standard EEG filtering), full scale 1 mV. *Right panels:* (A) and (B): high resolution samples from points a and b labeled in the lower left panel, bar: 1 s, same amplification and filtering as lower left. (A) shows background activity a few minutes before onset of CSD commencing in channel D and subsequently spreading to channel C, B and A. (B) indicates the time when activity is depressed in channel B and C, but not yet in channel A, while channel D is recovering after CSD. CSD is caused by a severe, long lasting depolarization of the cortical tissue as evidenced by the huge change of the DC-potential recorded in the same channels and visualized in the upper four, low pass filtered, curves. A slow potential change (SPC) commences in channel D and spreads from electrode to electrode as evidenced by the phase shift of the SPC between channel D-C, C-B and B-A (double arrows). CSD spreads at 3 mm/min in accordance with Leão's observations in the rabbit.

Image courtesy of Martin Fabricius, MD, Denmark.

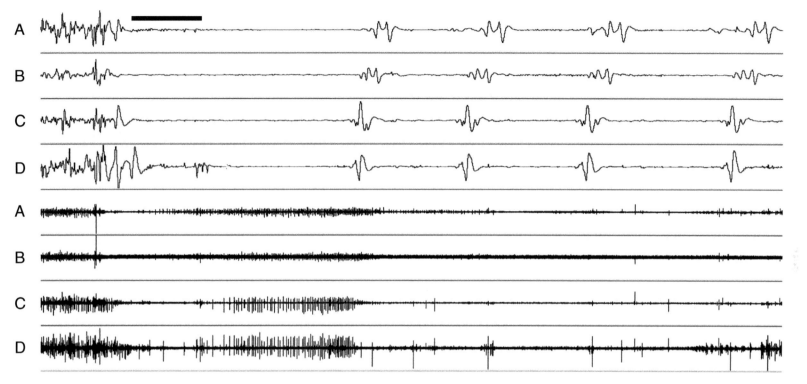

Figure 10.12. Multimodal monitoring: electrocorticogram (ECoG) of peri-injury depolarizations (PIDs)

67-year-old man had a fall and was admitted with a right frontal lobe contusion and acute subdural hematoma. After evacuation of the hematoma, a subdural strip was placed over the right middle frontal gyrus. Baseline ECoG activity showed burst-suppression pattern with long periods of suppression. The patient remained comatose and died 2 days later. *Upper four traces:* 0.05 Hz low pass, full scale 4 mV. *Lower four traces:* same recording as upper traces, but now 0.5 Hz high pass, full scale 2 mv. Bar: 20 minutes. 200 minutes of the recording is shown commencing 18 hours after ictus. Two episodes of cortical spreading depression (CSD) accompanied by stereotyped slow potential changes (SPCs) are seen at the far left (channel A to D) and in the middle (D to A), one hour apart. Recovery of ECoG background activity after the first CSD was delayed and incomplete, but after the second CSD the ECoG activity remained depressed in all channels. Then another three episodes of very stereotyped SPCs are seen spreading from channel D to A at a velocity of 2–3 mm/min and occurring at approximately 30 min intervals. Arterial oxygen saturation remained >90% and no extra sedative was administered to the patient in this period to explain the lack of cortical activity. The ECoG remained depressed indicating compromised metabolism. The event was therefore classified as a PID, i.e. a depolarization wave spreading slowly through an area of the cortex where perfusion is too low to maintain nerve cell signaling, but where the cells are still viable. Animal experiments suggest that repeated PIDs expand the final volume of injured cortex by energy depletion and vasospasm.

Images courtesy of Martin Fabricius, Denmark, and Anthony J. Strong, United Kingdom.

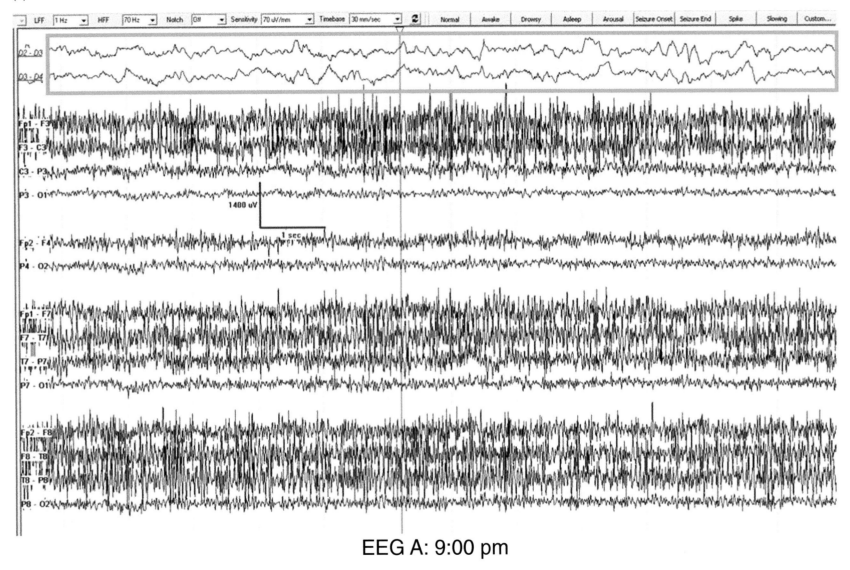

EEG A: 9:00 pm

Figure 10.13. Multimodal monitoring of hemorrhagic transformation of a large infarct, including with ICP, brain tissue oxygen tension, cerebral microdialysis and depth electrode.

Figure 10.13(A)–(E) 73-year-old man with a large right hemisphere infarct (see CT scan, part G) undergoing invasive monitoring for raised intracranial pressure (ICP), and being treated with hypothermia. An 8-contact miniature depth electrode was placed in the right frontal lobe in the ischemic penumbra, along with the ICP monitor, a brain tissue oxygen tension monitor, and a cerebral microdialysis catheter.

Baseline EEG at 9:00 pm is shown in A, including continuous mixed frequency in the depth electrode recordings (top 2 channels, and in green box); scalp recording is obscured by muscle artifact, likely from micro-shivering (see Figure 9.19). The scale legend y axis represents 1400 μV for the depth channels, and 140 μV for the scalp channels for all EEGs in this case.

Reproduced from Waziri A, Claassen J, Stuart RM, et al. Intracortical electroencephalography in acute brain injury. Ann Neurol. 2009;66(3):366–377, with permission.

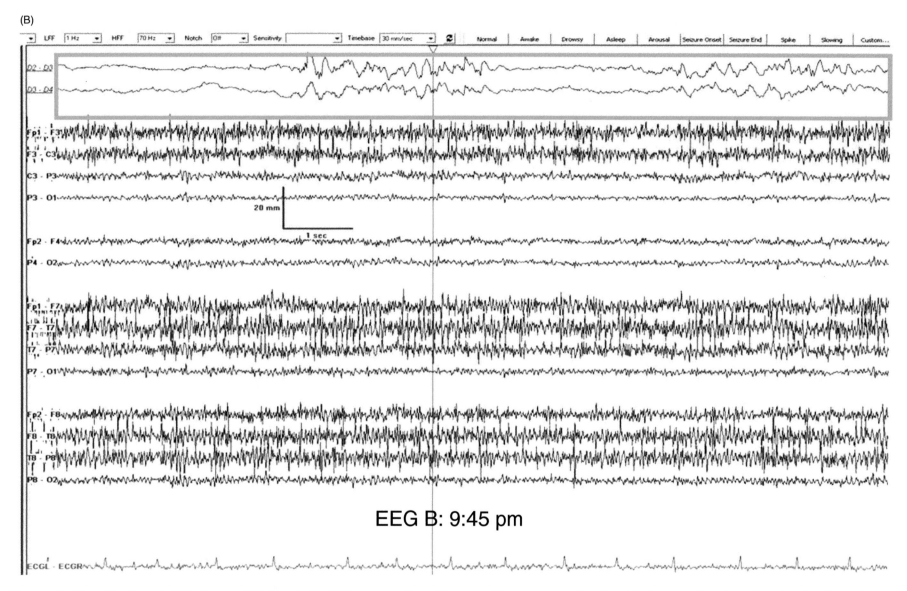

Figure 10.13. (*Continued*) At 9:45 p.m. (B), the depth EEG becomes discontinuous, with suppression-burst suddenly appearing, later found to be due to hemorrhagic transformation of the infarct; the scalp shows no significant change.

(C)

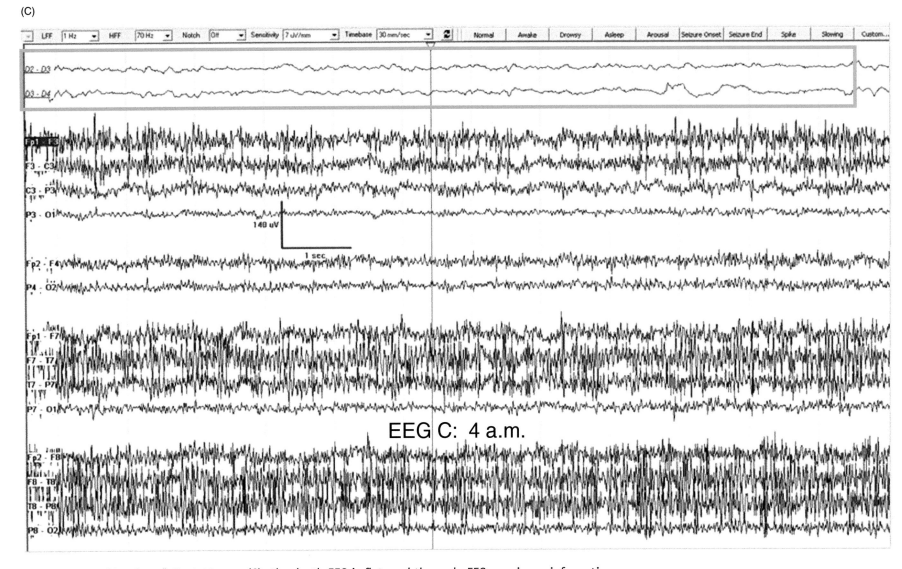

Figure 10.13.   (*Continued*) By 4:00 a.m. (C), the depth EEG is flat, and the scalp EEG remains uninformative.

(D)

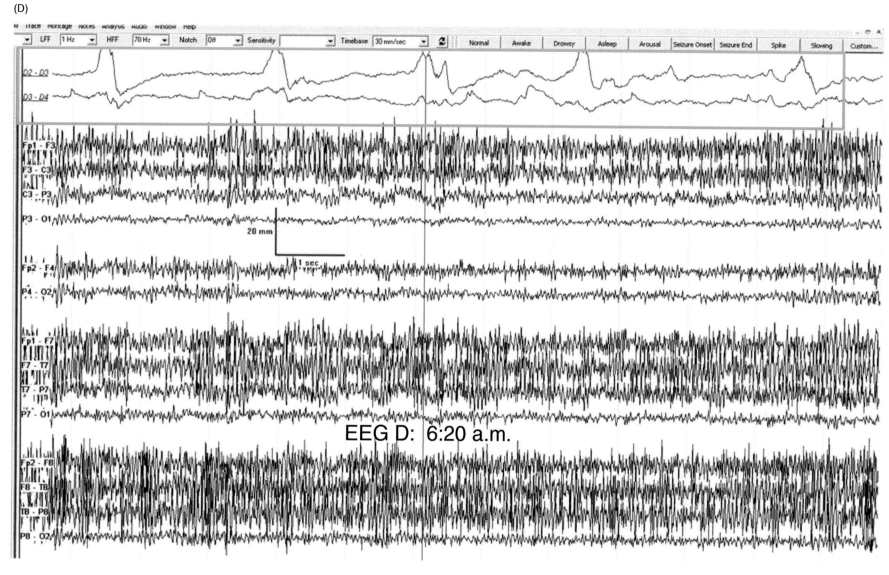

Figure 10.13. (*Continued*) The intracranial EEG begins to recover, with periodic delta waves by 6:20 a.m. (D), and resumption of a continuous pattern by 7:25 a.m. (E).

(E)

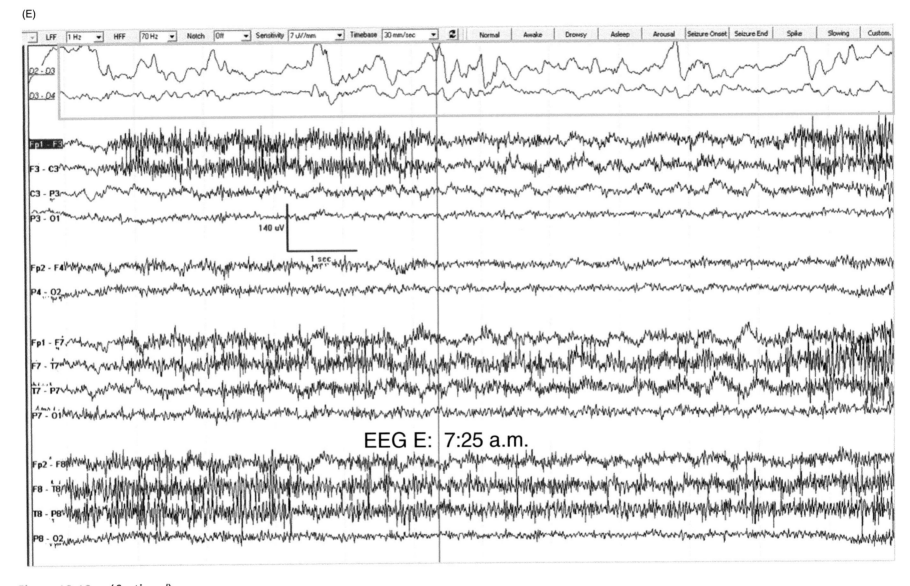

Figure 10.13.   (*Continued*)

(F)

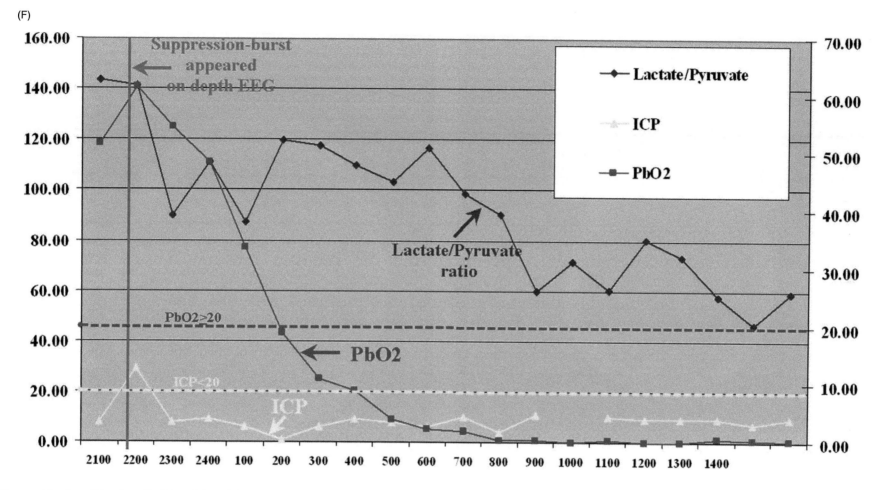

Figure 10.13. (*Continued*) (F) Multimodal graph: the prominent EEG change (green line) occurred a few hours before brain tissue oxygen tension dropped significantly. ICP bumped slightly above normal at the probable time of the hemorrhagic transformation, but rapidly returned to normal. The parenchymal microdialysate lactate/pyruvate ratio (a standard measure of neuronal stress, with normal <30) was markedly elevated throughout and thus was not helpful (it was actually improving during this time). No clinical change was noted until the next day. Thus, intracranial EEG seemed to be the earliest and best indicator of an acute event in this case. It also allowed monitoring of the EEG without paralyzing the patient, which would have been necessary to monitor using the scalp EEG.

(G)

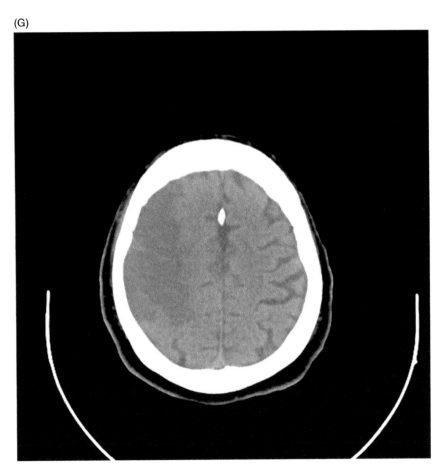

(H)

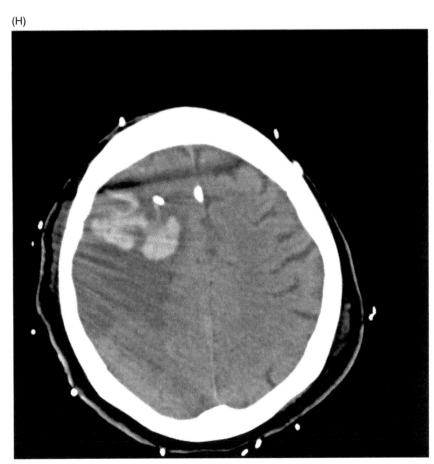

Figure 10.13. (*Continued*) (G) Head CT scan prior to placement of invasive monitors, showing the large right hemisphere infarction. Falx calcification can also be seen. (H) Head CT scan after hemorrhagic transformation. A ventricular catheter can be seen as well; the miniature depth electrode was more superior (and more superficial, as it barely reaches the white matter).

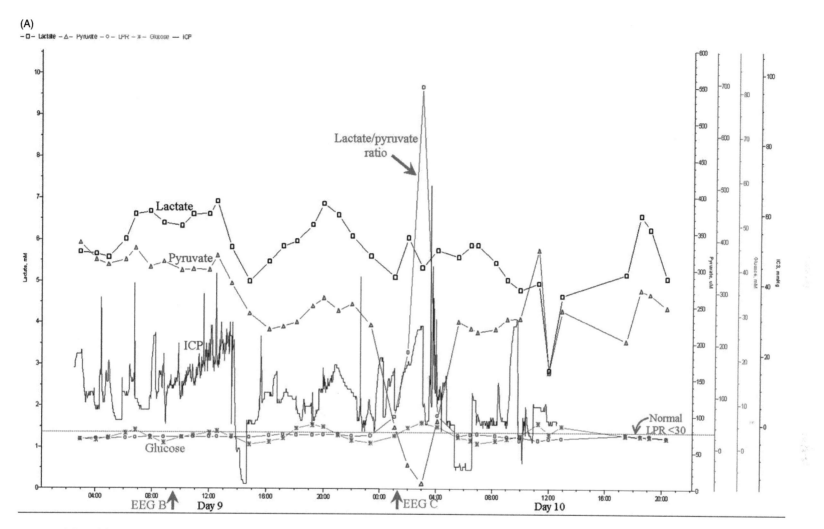

Figure 10.14. Multimodal monitoring of seizures on intracranial EEG after meperidine bolus, including ICP, cerebral microdialysis and depth electrode Figure 10.14A-C: 61-year-old woman with a Hunt and Hess grade V subarachnoid hemorrhage, s/p placement of a left frontal 8-contact mini-depth electrode and cerebral microdialysis catheter, and a right frontal ventricular drain. Almost 48 hours of multimodal data shown in the graph (A). There was a dramatic rise in the lactate/pyruvate ratio (red tracing) from 1–4 a.m., which occurred shortly after administration of meperidine. The increase in this ratio was not due to a rise in lactate as is seen with ischemia, but rather to a drop in pyruvate, as can be seen with increased substrate utilization, such as with seizures. Intracranial pressure (ICP) went up as well, but had been quite variable prior to this.

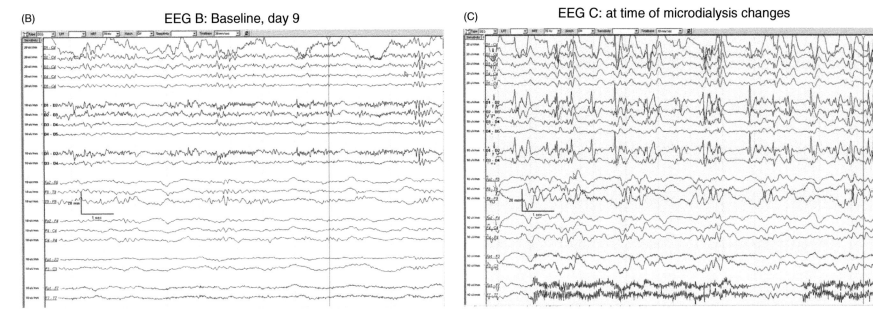

(B) **EEG B: Baseline, day 9**

(C) **EEG C: at time of microdialysis changes**

Figure 10.14. (*Continued*) EEG at baseline (B) showed no epileptiform discharges. At the time of the dramatic rise in lactate/pyruvate ratio (C), the depth electrode (top 11 channels, with labels starting with 'd') showed nearly continuous epileptiform discharges, especially with any alerting stimuli (SIRPIDs, or stimulus-induced rhythmic, periodic or ictal discharges). The scalp EEG (bottom 10 channels) did not show any definite epileptiform discharges.

This example presumably shows the adverse physiological effects (markedly elevated lactate/pyruvate ratio [LPR] with decreasing pyruvate) of these epileptiform discharges. When an epileptiform EEG pattern is associated with this type of physiological effect in a given patient, we are more likely to treat it aggressively than if these changes are not seen. In this case, it resolved after a few hours, and meperidine was avoided to prevent recurrence. Without the intracranial recording, we would not have known that seizure activity was the explanation for the rising LPR, though this physiological pattern (rising LPR with dropping pyruvate) raises that possibility even if depth EEG is not being recorded.

(A)

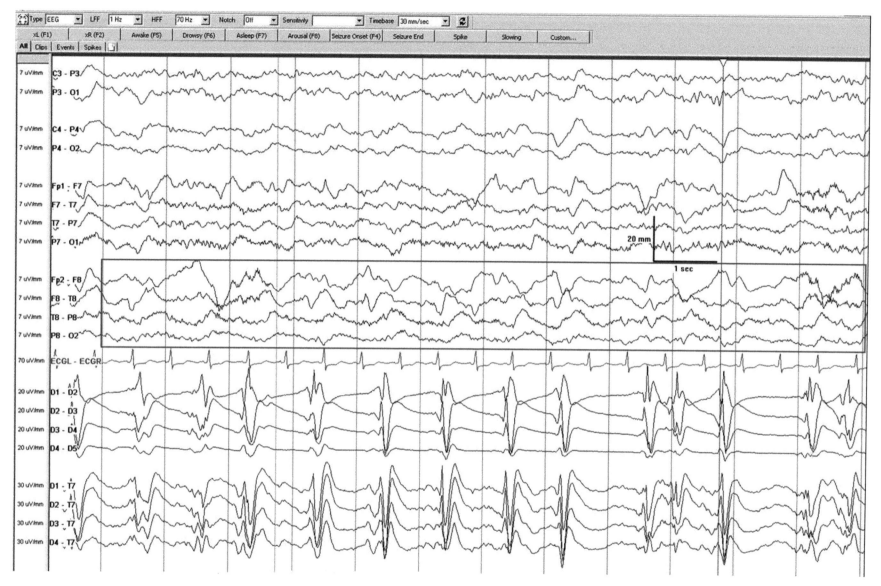

Figure 10.15. Multimodal monitoring: Seizures and periodic discharges on intracranial EEG only.

Figure 10.15(A)–(B): 2 samples of EEG from an older woman with a poor-grade subarachnoid hemorrhage, ventricular extension and right frontal intraparenchymal hemorrhage. The bottom 8 channels are from an 8-contact, mini-depth electrode placed in the superficial cortex of the right frontal lobe near the hemorrhage, but in normal-appearing brain. The remaining channels are from standard scalp electrodes. For much of the record there were prominent periodic epileptiform discharges (EEG at A) on the depth channels; this was sometimes accompanied by quasi-rhythmic delta (almost LRDA, but not rhythmic enough) (blue box). There were frequent episodes where the periodic discharges were replaced by an ictal-appearing rhythm on intracranial EEG (EEG at B) but no hint of a correlate on the scalp. When the seizure began the, the scalp EEG appeared to normalize (quasi-rhythmic delta resolved; 'pseudo-normalization').

(B)

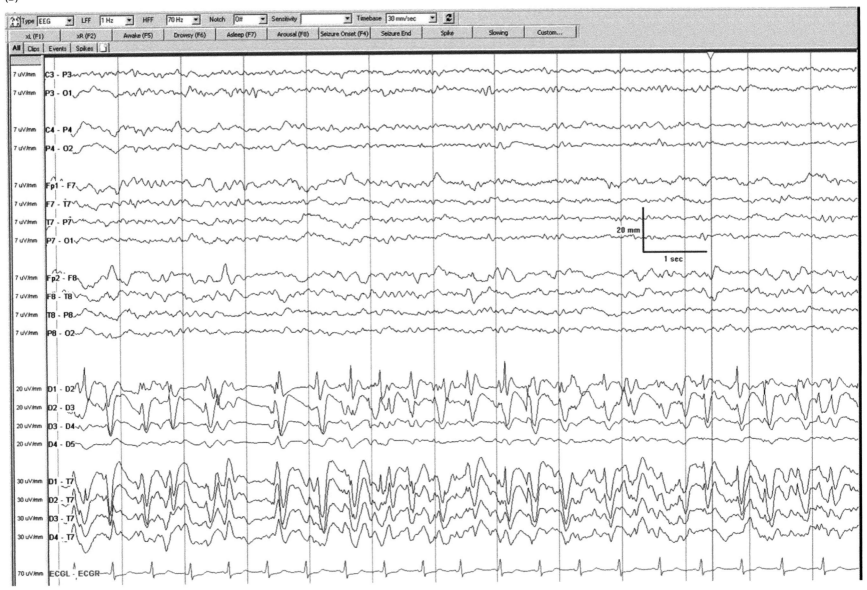

Figure 10.15. (*Continued*)

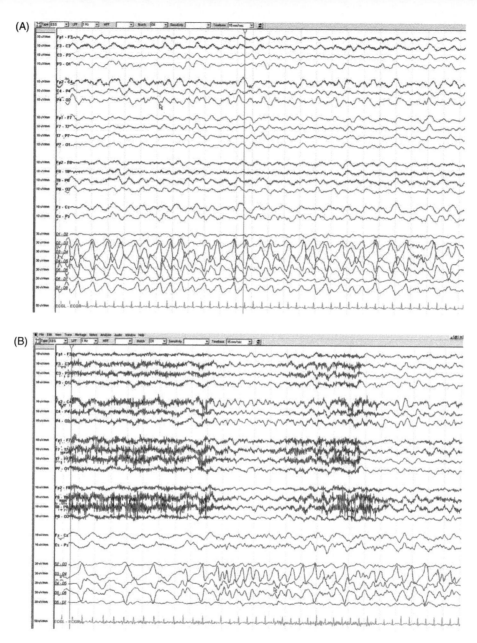

Figure 10.16. Multimodal monitoring of traumatic brain injury (TBI), including ICP, brain tissue oxygen tension, cerebral microdialysis and depth electrode. (A) 20-year-old pedestrian hit by a car, sustaining a small right frontal contusion with subarachnoid hemorrhage, intraventricular hemorrhage and basilar skull fracture. She was rousable to painful stimuli only. No clinical seizures were noted. Invasive monitors were placed in the right frontal lobe, including an 8-contact mini-depth electrode, brain tissue oxygen tension monitor, intracranial pressure (ICP) monitor, and cerebral microdialysis catheter. Scalp EEG (A and B, all but the bottom 5 channels) showed only moderate diffuse slowing, but depth (intracranial) EEG (bottom 5 channels on A and B, labeled as 'D#') showed new appearance of rhythmic, high amplitude, sharply contoured delta, sometimes evolving. This pattern waxed and waned but became more prominent and persistent over 1–2 days.

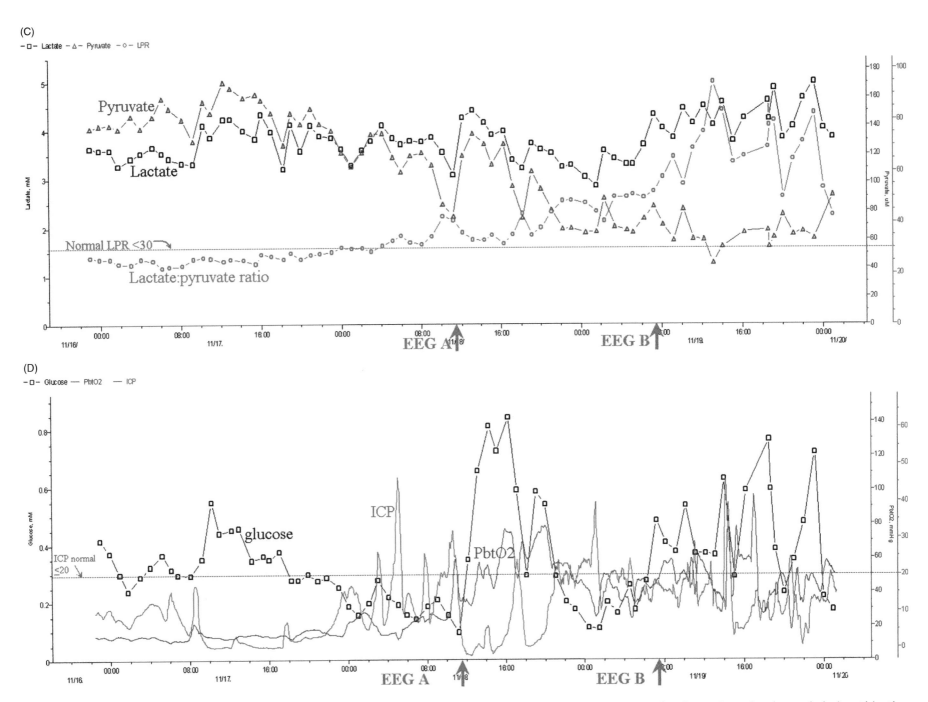

Figure 10.16. (*Continued*) Figure 10.16C + D: Multimodal graphs (3–4 days shown) reveal that the lactate/pyruvate ratio was gradually rising on the days of the above findings. This was due to declining pyruvate, not rising lactate, suggesting excessive substrate utilization such as that seen with seizure activity, rather than ischemia. ICP was also intermittently elevated during this time period. Thus, due to this evidence of neuronal stress with potentially permanent secondary neuronal injury, this pattern was treated more aggressively.

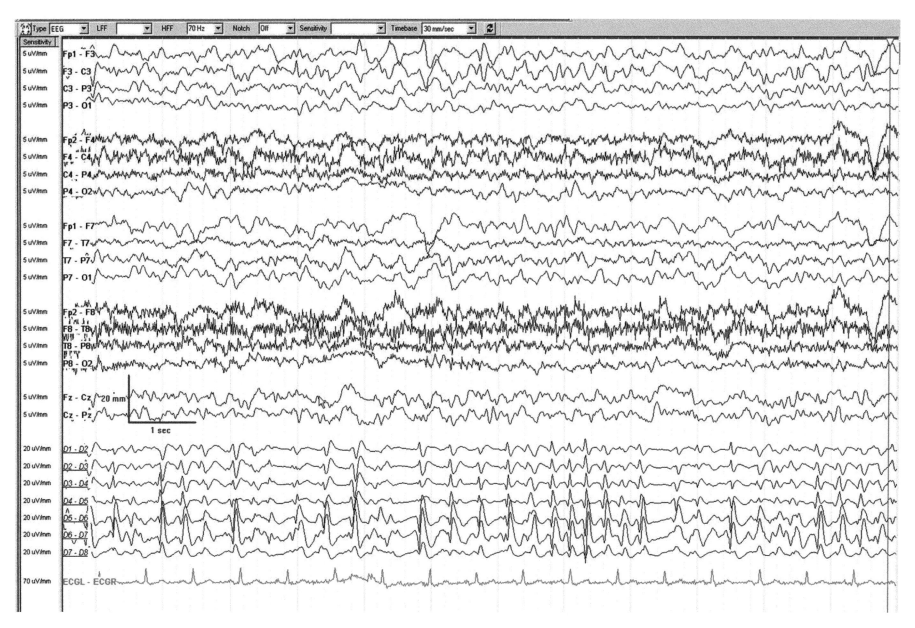

Figure 10.17. Multimodal monitoring: Ictal-appearing SIRPIDs on intracranial EEG only.

Figure 10.17: EEG sample from another older woman with a subarachnoid hemorrhage and a left frontal 8-contact mini-depth electrode. When stimulated (suctioning, examination, loud noise, pain, etc.), she had ictal-appearing runs in the depth EEG only, as shown here. The bottom 7 EEG channels are from the depth. There was left hemisphere slowing, but no hint of seizures or epileptiform patterns on the scalp recording. Thus, these were ictal-appearing SIRPIDs (stimulus-induced rhythmic, periodic or ictal discharges) that were visible on the intracranial EEG but not the scalp.

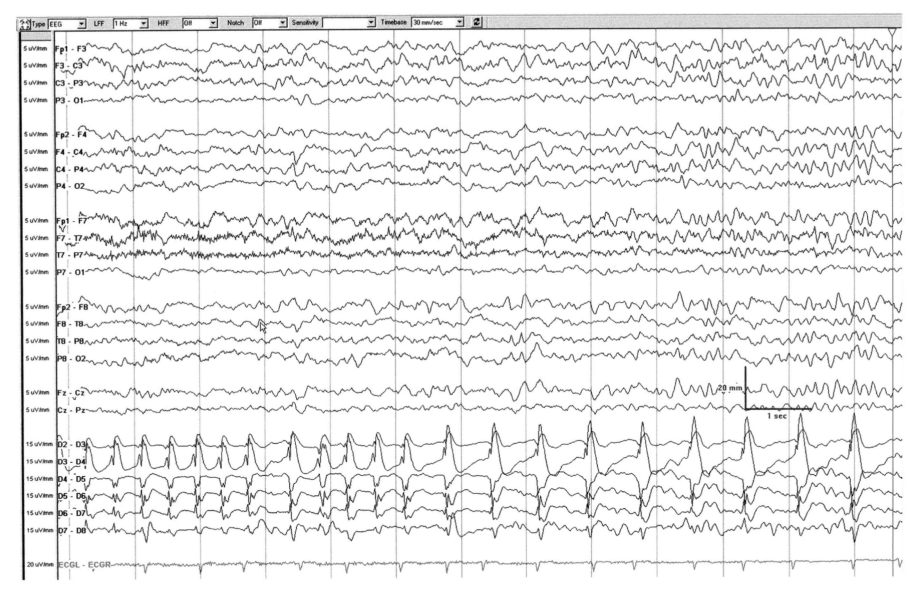

Figure 10.18. Multimodal monitoring: cyclic seizures on intracranial EEG only. Figure 10.18: EEG sample from an older woman with a Hunt and Hess grade III subarachnoid hemorrhage and a left frontal mini-depth electrode. She had no seizures for some time, then had a 5-hour period with cyclic seizures in the depth electrode only, each lasting about one minute and recurring every few minutes. A typical seizure is shown here. The bottom six channels show a clearly evolving seizure, with no hint of it seen on the scalp channels despite a high-quality recording with no missing electrodes.

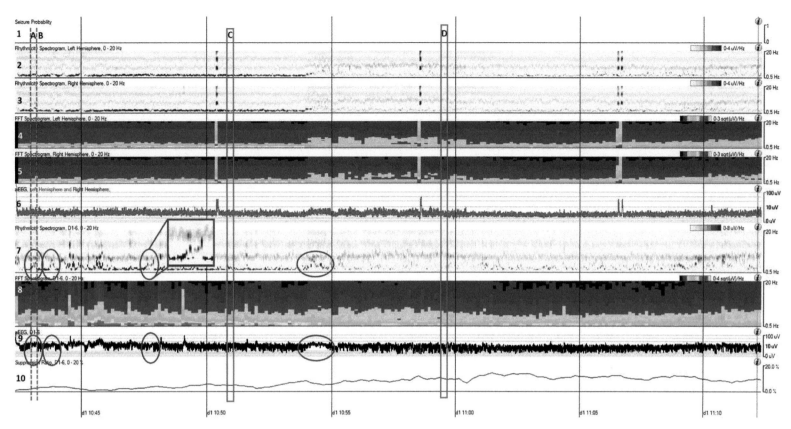

Figure 10.19. Multimodal monitoring of TBI, seizures and periodic discharges on intracranial EEG only, with QEEG applied to intracranial EEG.

Figure 10.19main This 30 minutes of QEEG is from a 54-year-old man s/p TBI. A 6-contact mini-depth electrode was placed via a multi-lumen bolt. The baseline EEG is shown at point C. There is high voltage generalized but frontally predominant quasi-rhythmic delta activity (Figure 10.19C). The depth electrode (presented in referential [D1-D6-ref] and bipolar [bottom 5 channels] formats) demonstrates very high voltage periodic discharges at this point. On the scalp QEEG there is prominent delta power and rhythmicity (at 1 Hz), whereas the QEEG applied to the depth electrode has greater rhythmicity in higher frequencies (from the sharp-wave discharges) (row 7). Note the QEEG applied to the scalp electrodes does not even suggest in the slightest that this person is having seizures (rows 1–6). There is no probability of seizure detected in row 1 (seizure detector), and no patterns of evolving rhythmicity (rows 2–3), power (rows 4–5), or amplitude (row 6). Contrast this with the same QEEG trends applied to the intracranial EEG (D1-D6) (rhythmicity spectrogram [row 7], power spectrogram/CSA [row 8], aEEG [row 9], suppression percent [bottom row]). From the beginning of the record there are several seizures (blue ellipses, showing evolving rhythmicity and amplitude, appearing as diagonals, especially on the rhythmicity spectrogram [expanded in the 3rd seizure]). When reviewing the raw EEG (points A and B), the periodic discharges are clearly interrupted by an evolving electrographic seizure (on intracranial EEG only) before the periodic pattern resumes. Interestingly the scalp EEG 'normalizes' at the time of seizures, as seen in this example where the seizure leads to the spontaneous cessation of the generalized delta activity and only shows low voltage (non-evolving) beta activity. The delta activity returns when the intracranial seizure stops. Additional anti-seizure medication was administered following a more prolonged intracranial seizure (last pair of blue ellipses). Following this the scalp EEG improved to only mild generalized slowing (theta range) and attenuation, and the intracranial EEG became burst suppressed (point D). This can be appreciated with loss of rhythmicity and power, and rising suppression percentage when applied to the intracranial EEG. The case is a valuable reminder that the scalp EEG is a summation of series of cortical dipoles from wide regions of the brain. The activity of a single discrete brain region (such as the region of traumatic contusion where the bolt was placed) may not be reflected well, or at all (as in this case), on the scalp EEG.

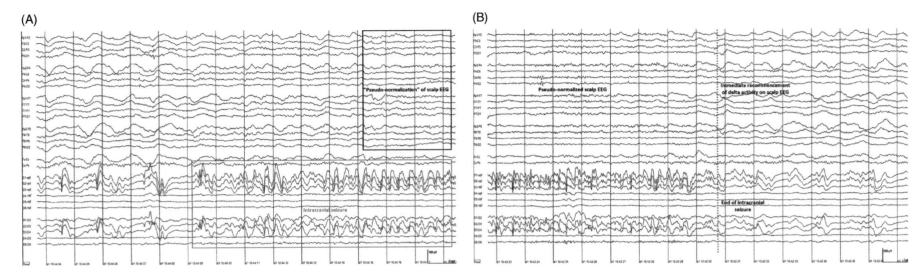

Figure 10.19. (*Continued*) (A) Standard 10-20 bipolar montage top part of the page (conventional settings, gain 7 µV/mm, LFF 1 Hz, HFF 70 Hz, no notch filter). Intracranial EEG (6-contact depth electrode) presented in both referential (D1-ref to D6-ref) (gain 10 µV, LFF 1.6 Hz, HFF 70 Hz, no notch filter) and bipolar montages (gain 7 µV, LFF 1.6 Hz, HFF 70 Hz, no notch filter). An intracranial seizure evolves over the second half of the page (red box). This leads to 'pseudo-normalization' of the scalp EEG (black box). (B) End of intracranial seizure (labeled dotted red line). The low voltage beta activity (pseudonormalized EEG) ends, and the bifrontal delta activity recommences. In this case the 'ictal' scalp rhythm was attenuation of delta activity with new appearance of low voltage (non-evolving) fast activities, appearing to be an improvement. Looking at the scalp EEG alone, it would be impossible to recognize this as an electrographic seizure (or any epileptiform pattern).

(C)

(D)

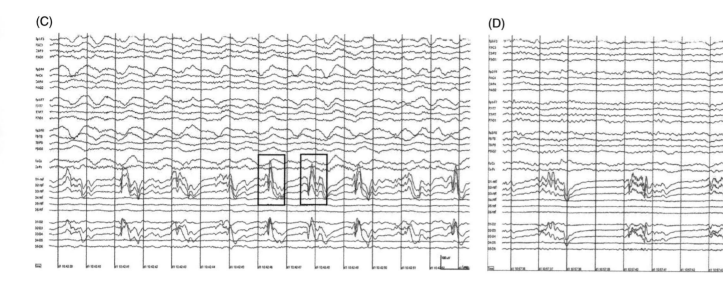

Figure 10.19. (*Continued*) (C) Baseline EEG with quasi-rhythmic delta activity on the scalp EEG, and high voltage periodic discharges on intracranial EEG (two highlighted on the referential montage with boxes). (D) Following treatment of intracranial seizures. Additional ASM resulted in burst suppression recorded on the intracranial EEG. Note following resolution of intracranial seizures the scalp EEG is completely different. The scalp EEG now just demonstrates normal voltage theta range activities. It does not demonstrate the higher voltage delta activity (that correlated with intracranial PDs), and this is clearly different than the scalp EEG pattern of low voltage fast activity (at the time of intracranial seizures). However, without the intracranial EEG it would be impossible to realize that those prior scalp EEG patterns were associated with intracranial seizures or a highly epileptic focus.

A ACNS standardized critical care EEG terminology 2021 (condensed version)

A. Background EEG

1. **Symmetry:**
   a. Symmetric
   b. Mild asymmetry (consistent asymmetry in amplitude on referential recording of <50%, or consistent asymmetry in frequency of 0.5–1 Hz)
   c. Marked asymmetry (>50% in amplitude or >1 Hz in frequency)

2. **Predominant background frequency:** Beta (>13Hz), Alpha, Theta, Delta. If 2 or 3 frequency bands are equally prominent, record each one.

3. **Posterior dominant "alpha" rhythm:** Specify frequency (to the nearest 0.5 Hz) or absent.
   NOTE: When the background is asymmetric, describe the predominant frequency and posterior dominant rhythm separately for each hemisphere.

4. **Continuity:**
   a. Continuous.
   b. Nearly Continuous: continuous, but with occasional (1–9% of the record) periods of *attenuation (periods of lower voltage ≥10 μV but <50% of higher voltage background)* or *suppression (periods of lower voltage <10 μV).*
   c. Discontinuous: 10–49% of the record consisting of attenuation or suppression.
   d. Burst-suppression/Burst-attenuation: 50–99% of the record consisting of attenuation or suppression, with bursts alternating with attenuation or suppression; also specify the following:
      i. Localization of the bursts (G/ L/ BI/ UI/ Mf)
      ii. Typical duration of bursts and interburst intervals
      iii. Sharpest component of a typical burst
      iv. Highly Epileptiform Bursts (present or absent): Present if 2 or more epileptiform discharges (spikes or sharp waves) occur within the majority (>50%) of bursts and occur at an average of 1 Hz or faster within a single burst; OR a rhythmic, potentially ictal-appearing pattern occurs within the majority (>50%) of bursts.
      v. Identical Bursts (Present or absent): Present if the first 0.5 s or longer of each burst (or of each stereotyped cluster of 2 or more bursts) appears visually similar in all channels in the vast majority (>90%) of bursts.

Hirsch and Brenner's Atlas of EEG in Critical Care, Second Edition. Lawrence J. Hirsch, Michael W.K. Fong, and Richard P. Brenner.
© 2023 John Wiley & Sons Ltd. Published 2023 by John Wiley & Sons Ltd.

e. Suppression: >99% of the record suppressed (<10 uV, as defined above).

NOTE: Bursts must average ≥0.5 s and have at least 4 phases (polyphasic); if shorter or fewer phases, then they are single discharges. Bursts within burst-suppression or burst-attenuation can last up to 30 s.

5. **Reactivity:** Change in cerebral EEG activity to stimulation: Reactive, Unreactive, *SIRPID*s only, Unclear, Unknown. Reactivity may include change in amplitude (including attenuation) or frequency. Note strength and/or nature of stimulation. Appearance of muscle activity or eye blink artifacts does not qualify as reactive.

6. **State changes**
   a. Present with normal stage N2 sleep transients (K-complexes and spindles)
   b. Present but with abnormal stage N2 sleep transients
   c. Present but without stage N2 sleep transients
   d. Absent

7. **Cyclic Alternating Pattern of Encephalopathy (CAPE):** Present, Absent, or Unknown/unclear. Present if changes in background patterns, each lasting at least 10 s, and spontaneously alternating between the two patterns in a regular manner for at least 6 cycles (but often lasts minutes to hours). *If present, then describe whether seen in the patient's more awake/stimulated state or less awake state, the characteristics of each pattern, and the typical duration of each pattern.*

8. **Voltage:**
   a. High (most or all activity ≥150 μV in longitudinal bipolar with standard 10-20 electrodes, [measured from peak to trough])
   b. Normal
   c. Low (most or all activity <20 μV in longitudinal bipolar with standard 10-20 electrodes, [measured from peak to trough])
   d. Suppressed (all activity <10 μV). If nearly continuous or discontinuous, then this refers to the higher amplitude portion

9. **Anterior-posterior (AP) gradient:** Present, absent or reverse. An AP gradient is present if at any point in the epoch, there is a clear and persistent (at least 1 continuous minute) anterior to posterior gradient of voltages and frequencies such that lower amplitude, faster frequencies occur in anterior derivations, and higher amplitude, slower frequencies occur in posterior derivations. A reverse AP gradient is defined identically but with a posterior to anterior gradient of voltages and frequencies.

10. **Breach effect:** Present, absent, or unclear. *If present record location or hemisphere.*

B. Sporadic Epileptiform Discharges

Quantify spikes and sharp waves as:

a.	Abundant:	≥1 per 10 s, but not periodic
b.	Frequent:	≥1/min but less than 1 per 10 s
c.	Occasional:	≥1/h but less than 1/min
d.	Rare:	<1/h

C. Rhythmic or Periodic Patterns (RPPs)

All patterns recorded must consist of main term #1 followed by #2, with modifiers added as appropriate.

Main Terms

1. **Generalized (G) OR Lateralized (L) OR Bilateral Independent (BI) OR Unilateral Independent (UI) OR Multifocal (Mf)**
   Additional localizing information:
   For **G**: Specify frontally, occipitally, or midline predominant, or "generalized, not otherwise specified"
   For **L or UI**: Specify unilateral, bilateral asymmetric, or bilateral asynchronous; and lobe(s) most involved or hemispheric

NOTE: For UI specify for each pattern separately

For **BI** or **Mf**: Specify symmetric or asymmetric; and lobe(s) most involved or hemispheric in both hemisphere

2. **Periodic Discharges (PDs)** OR **Rhythmic Delta Activity (RDA)** OR **Spike-Wave (SW**; includes sharp-wave and polyspike-wave)

NOTE: A pattern can qualify as rhythmic or periodic as long as it continues for at least 6 cycles (e.g. 1/s for 6 s, or 3/s for 2 s).

NOTE: If a pattern qualifies as both PDs and RDA simultaneously, it should be coded as PDs+R rather than RDA+S

Major Modifiers

a. **Prevalence:** Specify % of record or epoch that includes the pattern. This should be based on the percent of seconds that include or are within the pattern. If ≥ 2 patterns are equally or almost equally prominent, record presence and persistence of each.

i.	Continuous	$\geq 90\%$ of record or epoch
ii.	Abundant	50–89% of record or epoch
iii.	Frequent	10–49% of record or epoch
iv.	Occasional	1–9% of record or epoch
v.	Rare	<1% of record or epoch

b. **Duration**: Specify typical duration of pattern if not continuous.

i.	Very long	≥ 1 hour
ii.	Long	10–59 minutes
iii.	Intermediate duration	1–9.9 minutes
iv.	Brief	10–59 seconds
v.	Very brief	<10 seconds

c. **Frequency** = Rate (cycles per second): Specify typical rate and range (minimum-maximum) for all patterns.

Categorize as <0.5/s, 0.5/s, 1/s, 1.5/s, 2/s, 2.5/s, 3/s, 3.5/s and 4/s.

NOTE: if >4/s would either be classified as a BIRD if <10 s (section E) or a seizure if ≥ 10 s (section D).

d. **Phases** = Number of baseline crossings of the typical discharge (in longitudinal bipolar and in the channel in which it is the most readily appreciated). Applies to PDs and the entire spike-and-wave or sharp-and-wave complex of SW (includes the slow wave) but not to RDA. Categorize as 1, 2, 3 or >3.

e. **Sharpness**: Specify for both the predominant phase (phase with greatest amplitude) and the sharpest phase if different. Applies only to PDs and SW, not RDA. If SW, specify for the spike/sharp wave only. For both phases, describe the *typical* discharge.

   i. Spiky (duration of that component [measured at the EEG baseline] is <70 ms)

   ii. Sharp (duration of that component is 70–200 ms)

   iii. Sharply contoured (>200ms but with sharp morphology)

   iv. Blunt (>200ms)

f. **Voltage** [of PDs, SW or RDA; not background EEG]:

   i. *Absolute*: Typical amplitude measured in standard longitudinal bipolar 10-20 recording in the channel in which the pattern is most readily appreciated. For PDs, this refers to the highest amplitude component. For SW, this refers to the spike/sharp wave. Amplitude should be measured from peak to trough (not peak to baseline). Specify for RDA as well. Categorize amplitude as:

a)	Very low	$<20\,\mu V$
b)	Low	$20\text{--}49\,\mu V$
c)	Medium	$50\text{--}149\,\mu V$
d)	High	$\geq 150\,\mu V$

   ii. *Relative:* For PDs *only* (PDs require two amplitudes, absolute and relative). Typical ratio of amplitude of the highest amplitude component to the amplitude of the background between discharges measured in the same channel and montage as absolute amplitude. Categorize as ≤ 2 or >2.

g. **Stimulus-Induced (SI) or Stimulus-Terminated (ST)** = Repetitively and reproducibly brought about by (Stimulus-Induced [SI]) or reproducibly terminated by (Stimulus-Terminated [ST]) an alerting stimulus, with or without clinical alerting, when the patient is in their less stimulated state; may also occur spontaneously. If never clearly induced by stimulation, then categorize as *spontaneous*. If unknown, unclear or untested, then categorize as "**unknown**". Specify type of stimulus (*auditory*; *light tactile*; patient care and other *non-noxious* stimulations; or *noxious*: suction, sternal rub, nostril tickle or other).

h. **Evolving** OR **Fluctuating** OR **Static**: Terms refer to changes in *either frequency, location or morphology.* If neither evolving nor fluctuating applies, then categorize as **static**.

  i. **Evolving**: an unequivocal sequential change in frequency or location lasting for at least 3 cycles each or an unequivocal sequential change in morphology with each morphology or each morphology plus its transitional forms lasting for at least 3 cycles; The criteria for evolution must be reached without the pattern remaining unchanged in frequency, morphology and location for 5 or more minutes.

    a) Evolution in *frequency:* a change in the same direction for 2 consecutive time periods by at least 0.5/s

    b) Evolution in *morphology*: at least 2 consecutive changes to a novel morphology

    c) Evolution in *location*: sequential spread into or sequentially out of at least two standard 10-20 electrode locations

  ii. **Fluctuating:** ≥ 3 changes, not more than one minute apart, in frequency (by at least 0.5/s), ≥ 3 changes in morphology, or ≥ 3 changes in location (by at least 1 standard inter-electrode distance), but *not qualifying as evolving*. Change in amplitude or sharpness alone would not qualify as evolving or fluctuating.

i. **Plus (+)** = additional feature(s) rendering a pattern more ictal-appearing than the usual term without the plus. Applies to PDs and RDA only. Categorize as follows:

  i. "**+F**": superimposed *fast* activity. Can be used with PDs or RDA.
  Extreme Delta Brush (EDB): A specific subtype of +F:
  Definite EDB: Consists of either abundant or continuous:

A. RDA+F, in which the fast activity has a stereotyped relationship to the delta wave (e.g., always maximal on the upstroke, crest, or downstroke of the wave); OR

B. PD+F, in which each PD contains a single blunt delta wave with superimposed fast activity, and in which the fast activity has a stereotyped relationship to the delta wave (i.e., periodic delta brushes)

Possible EDB:
Satisfying criterion A) or B) above EXCEPT either:

  a) only occasional or frequent (rather than abundant or continuous) OR

  b) the superimposed fast activity lacks a stereotyped relationship to the delta wave; continuous, invariant fast activity during RDA would fall into this category.

  ii. "**+R**": superimposed *rhythmic* or *quasi-rhythmic* activity. Applies to PDs only.
  iii. "**+S**": superimposed *sharp* waves or *spikes, or sharply contoured*. Applies to RDA only.
  iv. "**+FR**": superimposed *fast* activity and *rhythmic* or *quasi-rhythmic* activity. Applies to PDs only.
  v. "**+FS**": superimposed *fast* activity and *sharp* waves or *spikes, or sharply contoured*. Applies to RDA only.
  vi. "No +"

NOTE: Bilateral "+" vs. unilateral: If a pattern is bilateral and qualifies as plus on one side, but not on the other, the overall main term should include the plus (even though one side does not warrant a plus).

NOTE: "+F": If a pattern qualifying as RDA or PDs has superimposed continuous fast frequencies, this can and should be coded as +F if the fast activity is not present in the background activity when the RDA or PDs is not present. In other words, if the superimposed fast activity is part of the RDA or PD pattern and not simply part of the background activity.

D. Electrographic and Electroclinical Seizures

1. **_Electrographic seizure_ (ESz)** (largely based on the Salzburg criteria) is defined as either:
   a) Epileptiform discharges averaging >2.5 Hz for ≥10 s (>25 discharges in 10 s), OR
   b) Any pattern with definite evolution as defined above and lasting ≥10 s.

2. **Electrographic status epilepticus (ESE)** is defined as an electrographic seizure for ≥10 continuous minutes or for a total duration of ≥20% of any 60-minute period of recording.

3. **_Electroclinical seizure_ (ECSz)** is defined as:
   Any EEG pattern with either:
   a) Definite clinical correlate time-locked to the pattern (of any duration), OR
   b) EEG **_AND_** clinical improvement with a parenteral (typically IV) anti-seizure medication.

4. **Electroclinical _status epilepticus_ (ECSE)** is defined as an electroclinical seizure for _≥10 continuous minutes or for a total duration of ≥20% of any 60-minute period_ of recording. An ongoing seizure with bilateral tonic-clonic (BTC) motor activity only needs to be present for ≥5 continuous minutes to qualify as ECSE. In any other clinical situation, the minimum duration to qualify as SE is ≥10 mins.

4b. **_Possible_ ECSE** is a RPP that qualifies for the IIC that is present for ≥10 continuous minutes or for a total duration of ≥20% of any 60-minute period of recording, which shows EEG improvement with a parenteral anti-seizure medication **_BUT_** without clinical improvement.

E. Brief Potentially Ictal Rhythmic Discharges (BIRDs)

Focal (including L, BI, UI or Mf) or generalized rhythmic activity >4 Hz (at least 6 waves at a regular rate) lasting ≥0.5 to <10 s, not consistent with a known normal pattern or benign variant, not part of burst-suppression or burst-attenuation, without definite clinical correlate, and that has at least one of the following features:

   a. Evolution ("evolving BIRDs", a form of definite BIRDs)

   b. Similar morphology and location as interictal epileptiform discharges or seizures in the same patient (definite BIRDs)

   c. Sharply contoured but without (a) or (b) (possible BIRDs)

F. Ictal-Interictal Continuum (IIC)

A pattern on the IIC is a pattern that does not qualify as definite seizure, but there is a reasonable chance that it may be contributing to impaired alertness, causing other clinical symptoms, and/or contributing to neuronal injury. Such patterns include:

1. Any PD or SW pattern that averages >1.0 Hz and ≤2.5 Hz over 10 s (>10 and ≤ 25 discharges in 10 sec); or

2. Any PD or SW pattern that averages ≥0.5 Hz and ≤1 Hz over 10 s (≥5 and ≤10 discharges in 10 sec), and has a plus modifier or fluctuation; or

3. Any lateralized RDA averaging >1 Hz for at least 10 s (at least 10 waves in 10 s) with a plus modifier or fluctuation

AND

4. Does not qualify as an ESz or ESE.

Index

Hirsch and Brenner's Atlas of EEG in Critical Care, Second Edition. Lawrence J. Hirsch, Michael W.K. Fong, and Richard P. Brenner.
© 2023 John Wiley & Sons Ltd. Published 2023 by John Wiley & Sons Ltd.